EDITION
11

# Introduction to Clinical Pharmacology

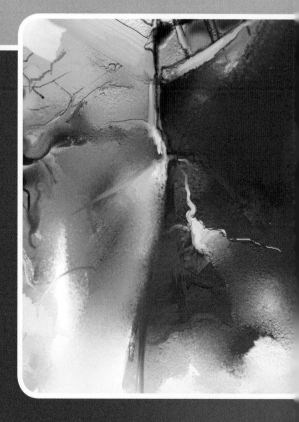

**Constance G. Visovsky,** PhD, RN, ACNP, FAAN
Professor and Lewis & Leona Hughes Endowed Chair
    in Nursing Science
College of Nursing
University of South Florida
Tampa, Florida

**Cheryl H. Zambroski,** PhD, RN
Associate Professor
College of Nursing
University of South Florida
Tampa, Florida

**Shirley Meier Hosler,** RN, BSN, MSN
Adjunct Faculty
Santa Fe Community College
Santa Fe, New Mexico

ELSEVIER

Elsevier
3251 Riverport Lane
St. Louis, Missouri 63043

INTRODUCTION TO CLINICAL PHARMACOLOGY, 11TH EDITION                    ISBN: 978-0-443-11336-9

Previous editions copyrighted 2016, 2019, and 2022.

**International Standard Book Number: 978-0-443-11336-9**

*Senior Content Strategist:* Brandi Graham
*Content Development Specialist:* Andrew Schubert
*Publishing Services Manager:* Deepthi Unni
*Project Manager:* Nayagi Anandan
*Design Direction:* Renee Duenow

Printed in India

Last digit is the print number: 9 8 7 6 5 4 3 2 1

Working together
to grow libraries in
developing countries

www.elsevier.com • www.bookaid.org

# Contributor

**M. Linda Workman, PhD, RN, FAAN**
Visiting Professor
Case Western Reserve University
Cleveland, Ohio

# Reviewers

**Larissa Brown, MSN, RN**
Educator
Three Rivers College
Poplar Bluff, Missouri

**Tammy R. Dean, BSN, RN**
Director
Prince William County School of Practical Nursing
Manassas, Virginia

**Diane Duffy, RN, BSN, MEd**
Practical Nursing Director
Chisholm Trail Technology Center
Omega, Oklahoma

**James Graves, PharmD, MBA**
University of Missouri Health Care
Columbia, Missouri

**James D. Holland, PhD, RN, CNL, RRT, RCP**
Associate Dean of Nursing and Allied Health
North Florida College
Madison, Florida

**Denise King, MSN, RN**
Practical Nursing Program Lead Instructor
Beaufort County Community College
Washington, North Carolina

**Jill Kirk, RN, BSN**
Director of Nursing
Tennessee College of Applied Technology
Paris, Tennessee

**Leslie Merritts, RN, BSN**
Director of Practical Nursing
Treasure Coast Technical College
Vero Beach, Florida

**Tina Spagnola, MSN, RN, NPD-BC, NE-BC**
Program Chair & Nursing Instructor
Pinellas Technical College
Clearwater, Florida

# Preface

This 11th edition of *Introduction to Clinical Pharmacology* offers updated drug information from a team of committed authors who have years of experience in clinical care, in nursing education, and in teaching pharmacology content. Understanding and retaining knowledge of pharmacology are critical components of nursing care and patient safety. The author team strived to make the pharmacology learning experience one that combines updated information with drug safety cues and memory joggers to initiate information recall. In addition, features such as Lifespan Considerations link the information to care of the patient across all ages as appropriate. Each chapter contains a brief review of the body system and potential health problems. This format promotes high levels of content retention and also incorporates the newest NCLEX® testing blueprint format.

This textbook is written using the second person throughout to engage students and help them understand the nursing responsibilities required for use in the clinical setting. The textbook's new organization and style are intended to engage students and help them develop an in-depth understanding of the "need to know" content that is critical for safely administering medications in all environments in which licensed practical nurses/vocational nurses (LPNs/VNs) are employed. The components of the nursing process aligning with the LPN/LVN role are emphasized. All chapters, test questions, case studies, and illustrations have been greatly expanded to explain drug actions and techniques for administration. In addition, the 11th edition has an added chapter focused on drugs for anesthesia and analgesia and cancer therapeutics.

The textbook uses current terminology for education and healthcare practice. For example, more settings include nurse practitioners and physician assistants as legal prescribers in addition to the physician. To reflect this change, the term healthcare provider is used throughout. When discussing individuals receiving nursing care, the authors prefer the use of the term *patient* as opposed to the term *client*.

Learning Outcomes now replace Chapter Objectives. These outcomes concisely and clearly let the student know which content represents the *highest priority* for safe medication administration. All drugs and drug categories no longer in common usage, or those that do not apply to the LPN/VN role, have been eliminated. The textbook also helps students learn to make use of prevailing technology in drug delivery. Internet resources and references have been identified and highlighted within the Bookmark This feature.

Newly created drug tables are divided by drug category and organized to provide students with concise access to mechanisms, common adult drug dosages, and essential nursing implications for administration and patient teaching. Key terms critical for pharmacology are listed at the beginning of each chapter and include phonetic pronunciations, definitions, and page numbers where each term is first used. This textbook takes advantage of the use of medical and nonpharmacologic terminology, with short definitions placed alongside the terms and in the Glossary to aid student reading and retention.

Throughout this textbook, ensuring patient safety remains a major theme. The safety features are the Top Tip for Safety boxes that highlight very specific precautions, unusual drug dosages, or critical nursing interventions. This author team deeply believes that it is critical to provide patient safety information to reduce drug errors. In addition, patients and families who understand the why of directions are more likely to adhere to them. Toward this purpose, nursing actions are accompanied by the appropriate rationale. In the discussion of each drug category, the sections on patient and family teaching provide direct examples of exactly what to teach patients and families, as well as the rationales for why these actions or precautions are necessary. Specific content on Lifespan Considerations for drug administration related to older adults and pediatric patients and for pregnancy and lactation are appropriately placed for maximum retention.

Other user-friendly learning techniques provided in this streamlined and updated edition include features such as Memory Jogger and mnemonics. End-of-chapter review questions have been changed to reflect the latest NCLEX® format for developing clinical judgment, including multiple-choice, "select all that apply," and Next-Generation NCLEX–style questions. These formats help the student to think through responses rather than focus on rote memorization. All clinical chapters have newly developed case studies designed to help students learn to apply specific content.

The Student Study Guide has been revised. The instructor's TEACH resource is completely updated based on the revised Learning Outcomes for each chapter. The test bank has also been revised with newly formatted Next-Generation NCLEX® questions that require the student to apply knowledge and prepare for the NCLEX® examination.

## ORGANIZATION AND FEATURES

This textbook has been updated to include updated drugs, to remove drugs and terms that are no longer used in practice, and to add tables for each drug classification that list common drugs for each class and normal adult dosage ranges. Throughout this text, medications are referred to as drugs, and the drug prescriber is called the healthcare provider because this can be a physician, advanced practice nurse, certified registered nurse anesthetist, or physician's assistant. The text has been reorganized into three units totaling 23 chapters to streamline access to specific content areas. Chapter-ending Get Ready for Next-Generation NCLEX® Examination questions have been updated and revised throughout the text and use mostly application questions and Next-Generation NCLEX-style questions to provide students with practice in answering these types of examination questions.

### UNIT I

The first unit provides an overview of general principles of pharmacology, including the nursing process as it relates to drug administration, and safe practices in drug administration that set the knowledge base for understanding specific drug categories. For example, this edition includes information on unique aspects of the contemporary LPN/LVN practice environment, including working in teams with medication assistants, the registered nurse, the healthcare provider, and other healthcare professionals.

Safe practice is accentuated throughout Chapter 1, with a guide to planning and giving drugs to patients. The updated *9 Rights of Drug Administration* is presented in detail and includes the right of the patient to refuse a drug. Although giving drugs properly is important, equally important are evaluating the expected drug response, understanding common side effects, and knowing how to handle adverse events from drugs.

In Chapter 2, the legal, regulatory, and ethical content related to giving drugs in the LPN/LVN role has been updated to include a thorough discussion of schedule drugs, drug diversion, and a distinction between addiction, drug abuse and misuse, and physical dependence. Technology-associated patient identification, drug orders, and the giving and recording of drugs in either a standard Kardex or electronic health record are covered. In Chapter 3, the student is acquainted with the Principles of Pharmacology, including drug absorption, distribution, metabolism and elimination to provide a basis for the drug knowledge in the following chapters.

### UNIT II

Unit II is dedicated to the principles and calculations related to drug administration. The beginning of the unit focuses on drug calculation methods, such as fractions, ratio, and proportion, and dimensional analyses to give an in-depth review of drug calculation approaches used in different educational settings. Unit II is concerned with drug calculation, preparation, and administration. LPN/LVNs work in a variety of settings, including acute care, but are often employed in assisted nursing centers, nursing homes, and care centers in which high-tech drug administration systems may not be used. Thus they need to be able to give medications safely and accurately, relying on their own ability to calculate the drug dosages accurately. Chapter 4 includes the "need to know" content related to drug calculation and includes basic fractions, ratio and proportion, and dimensional analysis, a mathematical technique that is being adopted by many nursing programs for drug calculation. Intravenous drugs, oral drugs, parenteral drugs, and intravenous infusion calculation are presented in an organized, step-by-step manner. The application of topical, transdermal, mucous membrane, and eye and ear drugs is also presented with accompanying illustrations to help the student visualize the process while reading the material.

### UNIT III

Drug classification groups provide essential information for student retention on select drug categories. Unit III focuses on content that has application to treatment purpose (i.e., anti-infective drugs), and chapters are associated with body systems, such as renal, urinary, and cardiovascular systems. By grouping drugs using the drug classification system, students quickly learn about individual drugs by understanding their drug class. The narrative content in the text focuses on major drug groups, and coverage of specific drugs appears in reference tables. A brand-new chapter covering drugs for cancer treatment has been added. In addition, special attention has been placed on drugs for reproductive health, the treatment of thyroid and adrenal problems and osteoporosis. All chapters have been updated in this edition to represent the latest clinical drug treatment information. Each drug class is presented in a consistent format with a separate Patient and Family Teaching section. Even though additional drug references can be used by students, the author team believes it is critical that students have a base knowledge of the potential dosage ranges for adult drugs to promote safe, effective practice. Thus drug dosage ranges are included in tables with each chapter in Unit III.

Chapter-ending NCLEX® Examination questions and Case Studies require the student to apply information gained from each chapter to address patient scenarios. Suggested answers to the questions and Case Studies are provided online in the TEACH Instructor Resources on Evolve at http://evolve.elsevier.com/Visovsky/LPNpharmacology.

## TEACHING AND LEARNING PACKAGE FOR THE INSTRUCTOR

### TEACH INSTRUCTOR RESOURCES

TEACH Instructor Resources on Evolve, available at http://evolve.elsevier.com/Visovsky/LPNpharmacology, provide a wealth of material to help you make your pharmacology instruction a success.

In addition to all of the Student Resources, the following are provided for faculty:

- The Exam View Test Bank has been completely updated with approximately 480 questions that feature Next-Generation NCLEX–style questions. Each question is coded for the correct answer, rationale, page reference, and cognitive level.
- TEACH Lesson Plans, based on textbook chapter Learning Objectives, serve as ready-made, modifiable lesson plans and a complete roadmap to link all parts of the educational package. These concise and straightforward lesson plans can be modified or combined to meet your particular scheduling and teaching needs.
- PowerPoint Presentations provide approximately 450 text slides for classroom or online presentations.
- Open-Book Quizzes for each chapter in the textbook help to ensure that your students are reading and comprehending their textbook reading assignments.
- An Image Collection includes all the illustrations and photos from the textbook.
- Suggestions for Working with Students Who Speak English as a Second Language help you promote the success of ESL learners.
- Answer Keys to the Critical Thinking Questions, Case Studies, and Study Guide activities and exercises are available for your own use or for distribution to your students.

## FOR THE STUDENT

Evolve Student Resources, available at http://evolve.elsevier.com/Visovsky/LPNpharmacology, include more than 400 interactive Review Questions for the NCLEX-PN® Examination, Video Clips, an Audio Glossary with pronunciations for more than 150 Key Terms, 12 Interactive Drug Dosage Calculators, newly proposed FDA Guidelines on Pregnancy and Lactation, and links to updated information on the Top 200 Prescription Drugs, a Bibliography, and a detailed Glossary.

A comprehensive Study Guide, available separately, includes Worksheets and Review Sheets with an enhanced focus on critical thinking, prioritizing, care of older adults, and cultural considerations. The exercises focus on promoting medication safety and prevention of drug errors.

In working with patients, the nursing student will quickly learn that giving medications is one of the most challenging parts of the nursing role. A nurse who develops the knowledge and skills needed to correctly give medications will be noticed and recognized with respect by both patients and colleagues in the healthcare system. Both the responsibilities and the personal rewards are great.

**Constance G. Visovsky, PhD, RN, ACNP, FAAN**
**Cheryl H. Zambroski, PhD, RN**
**Shirley Meier Hosler, RN, BSN, MSN**

# Acknowledgments

The eleventh edition of *Introduction to Clinical Pharmacology* represents a collaboration among three experienced nurse educators and clinicians who have taught pharmacology to all levels of nursing students. The 11th edition brings these authors back together with updated information, new drugs, and what the LPN/LVN needs to know to administer medications safely and monitor the patient for both expected and adverse effects. I remain grateful to my colleagues, Dr. Zambroski and Ms. Hosler, for their excellence and dedication to this work and for providing a textbook and test bank that will prove to be critical resources for the LPN/LVN student and faculty.

The author team remains extremely grateful to Dr. M. Linda Workman, our dear friend and mentor, who continues to provide her support and guidance to this author team. Lifetime mentors are few and far between, so we acknowledge her commitment and support.

The author team is grateful for the Elsevier editorial, production, marketing, and design staff. Special thanks to Brandi Graham, Senior Content Strategist, for her guidance to this author team; and to Andrew Schubert, Content Development Specialist, for his editorial guidance and support to keep the text production on track.

On behalf of the author team, I would like to express our eternal gratitude to our families and friends, who supported our endeavors on this project and were our cheerleaders throughout the process. I would like to acknowledge the love and support of my husband, Bob Visovsky, who sustained me during this project. Thank you to my students, who inspire me every day to be a better teacher. Last, I would like to thank my God for presenting this opportunity to me and for providing the fortitude to take this textbook to completion.

**Constance (Connie) G. Visovsky,
PhD, RN, ACNP, FAAN**

Thank you to my terrific colleagues, Dr. Visovsky, Ms. Hosler, and Dr. Passmore, as well as to our students, who challenge and cheer us as we continue to learn each day. A special thank you to my husband, James, for his ongoing love and support during this project.

**Cheryl H. Zambroski, PhD, RN**

Thanks to every student who has shared a path with me along the way: I could never have achieved the process of learning how to write if you hadn't first taught me how to teach. To my colleagues, Connie, Cheryl, and Denise, you are the best of the best!

**Shirley Meier Hosler, RN, BSN, MSN**

# About the Authors

## CONSTANCE G. VISOVSKY, PHD, RN, ACNP, FAAN

**Constance (Connie) G. Visovsky** received her BS and MS degrees in nursing from the University of Rochester, Rochester, New York, and her PhD from Case Western Reserve University, Cleveland, Ohio. She is an acute care nurse practitioner, specializing in the treatment of patients with cancer. She is considered an expert in the area of chemotherapy-induced peripheral neuropathy and has grants and publications on this topic to her credit. Dr. Visovsky is an experienced nurse educator and scientist. She is currently Professor and the Lewis & Leona Hughes Endowed Chair in Nursing Science at the University of South Florida, College of Nursing.

## CHERYL H. ZAMBROSKI, PHD, RN

**Cheryl H. Zambroski** received her diploma in nursing from Rockford Memorial Hospital School of Nursing, her BS and MS in Nursing from the University of Illinois, and her PhD in Nursing from the University of Kentucky. Her clinical experiences focused on adult health in areas that include emergency nursing, critical care, and medical-surgical nursing. She also worked as a clinical nurse specialist in cardiovascular and thoracic nursing. Her teaching career began at Jefferson Community College in Louisville, Kentucky. She later taught a variety of courses in the undergraduate program and the clinical nurse specialist track at the University of Louisville. Currently, Dr. Zambroski teaches pharmacology, public health, and mental health nursing at the University of South Florida College of Nursing.

## SHIRLEY MEIER HOSLER, RN, BSN, MSN

**Shirley Meier Hosler** received her AAS from Maria College in Albany, New York, later receiving her BSN from the University of New Mexico and MSN from the University of Illinois, Chicago. Shirley has more than 40 years of clinical, administrative, educational, and academic experience, having worked as a staff nurse, held numerous administrative nursing positions, and served on the faculty of colleges and universities. Her educational accomplishments include the development of online and classroom programs for nursing, emergency medical personnel, and paramedic professionals. Shirley has a broad base of expertise with specific concentration in the areas of prehospital medicine, adult medicine, and critical care. She has received numerous awards for her unique and innovative educational accomplishments.

# To the Student

## READING AND REVIEW TOOLS

- **Learning Outcomes** introduce the chapter topics.
- **Key Terms** are listed with page number references, and difficult medical, nursing, or scientific terms are accompanied by simple phonetic pronunciations. Key terms are considered essential to understanding the professional language and chapter content. Key terms are defined within the chapter, are in color the first time they appear in the narrative, and are briefly defined in the text, with complete definitions in the Glossary.
- Each chapter ends with a **Get Ready for the Next-Generation NCLEX® Examination!** section that might include (1) **Key Points** that reiterate the chapter outcomes and serve as a useful review of concepts, (2) an extensive set of **Review Questions for the NCLEX® Examination** with answers located on the Evolve site, (3) **Case Studies** with answers located on the Evolve site, and (4) **Drug Calculation Review Questions** with answers located on the Evolve site.
- A complete **Bibliography** section in the back of the text cites evidence-based information and provides resources for enhancing knowledge.

## CHAPTER FEATURES

**Procedures related to giving drugs** are presented in a logical format with a defined purpose and relevant illustrations and are clearly defined and presented in a logical set of steps.

**Memory Jogger** boxes restate key points from anatomy, physiology, or pharmacology that are important for students to remember and serve as foundational information for giving and monitoring drug therapy. Basic principles of drug calculation are presented in easy-to-follow steps to reinforce learning.

**Top Tip for Safety** boxes identify the important knowledge that will aid students in giving particular drugs and will provide critical information and warnings of adverse effects of drugs that are important to patient safety.

**Lifespan Considerations** boxes draw attention to information that is especially important to remember when giving a specific drug to older adults, children, or pregnant/lactating women.

**Safety Alerts** indicate a particularly important factor to remember about a specific drug or drug class.

**Canadian Drugs** indicated within the tables point out brands available only in Canada.

**Video Clips** located in the margins of the text indicate available relevant videos located on the Evolve site.

**Bookmark This** boxes list useful websites that provide important resources for all nurses.

# Contents

# Pharmacology and the Nursing Process in LPN Practice

**1**

http://evolve.elsevier.com/Visovsky/LPNpharmacology

## Learning Outcomes

1. Explain how licensed practical or vocational nurses (LPNs/VNs) use the clinical problem-solving process (nursing process) in practicing safe drug administration.
2. Discuss the differences between subjective and objective data related to drug administration.
3. Describe the specific actions involved in using the nursing process to safely give drugs.
4. List specific nursing activities related to assessing, planning, implementing, and evaluating the patient's response to drugs.
5. Compare the steps of the nursing process to the skills needed in applying the clinical judgment model.
6. Describe each of the *9 Rights of Drug Administration* as essential components of safe drug administration.

## Key Terms

**9 Rights of Drug Administration** A series of nursing actions to protect the patient from drug error.

**adverse effect** A drug effect that is more severe than expected and has the potential to damage tissue or cause serious health problems. It may also be called *adverse effect, toxic effect*, or *toxicity* and usually requires an intervention by the prescriber.

**assessment** The first step of the nursing process; involves gathering information about the patient that will be used in planning care.

**clinical judgment** The observed outcome of critical thinking and decision making; an iterative process that uses nursing knowledge to observe and assess presenting situations, identify a prioritized client concern, and generate the best possible evidence-based solutions in order to deliver safe client care (National Council of State Boards of Nursing [NCSBN], 2019).

**clinical problem-solving process (nursing process)** A system to guide the nurse's work in a logical way; consists of five major steps: (1) assessment, (2) diagnosis, (3) planning, (4) implementation, and (5) evaluation.

**contraindication** Health-related reason for not giving a specific drug to a patient or a group of patients.

**diagnosis** A name (or label) for the patient's disease or condition.

**evaluation** The process of determining the right response by looking at what happens to the patient when the

nursing care plan is put into action. It is an appraisal of the treatment effectiveness.

**expected side effects** Unintended but not unusual effects of a drug that occur in many people taking the drug; the effects are usually mild and do not require the drug to be stopped.

**healthcare setting** Any setting in which the LPN/VN practices nursing.

**identifiers** Information used to reliably prove that an individual is the person for whom the drug treatment is intended; may include the person's full name, medical record identification number, birthdate, or telephone number.

**implementation** The act of carrying out the planned interventions.

**objective data** Information that can be seen, heard, felt, or measured by someone other than the patient.

**planning** Using information about the patient gathered in the nursing assessment to set short-term and long-term goals.

**precaution** Health-related reason that a drug may be given that requires more monitoring to avoid adverse events (precautions).

**subjective data** Reports of what the patient says he or she is feeling or thinking.

**therapeutic effect** The intended action of the drug, also known as a drug's beneficial outcome.

## THE LPN/VN'S ROLE AND THE NURSING PROCESS

Licensed practical or vocational nurses (LPNs/VNs) play a vitally important role in providing nursing care for patients and families across the lifespan. In fact, in December 2022 there were nearly 1,000,000 LPNs in the United States. The need for a well-educated LPN/

VN workforce is predicted to grow about 6% between 2021 and 2031, with projections of nearly 59,000 job openings annually over the decade. The factors that increase the demand for LPNs/VNs include an aging nursing workforce reaching retirement age, an aging population in general, and an increased number of people who are living with chronic and complex illnesses.

LPN/VN practice has shifted dramatically over the past decades, from the time when most graduates practiced in acute care settings (hospital-based care) until today, when graduates practice in a wide variety of long-term and community-based settings. LPNs/VNs practice in nursing homes, assisted living facilities, outpatient clinics, home health agencies, psychiatric/behavioral health facilities, hospices, rehabilitation centers, and other settings. No matter the setting, as an LPN/VN, you will share a responsibility with registered nurses (RNs) and other members of the healthcare team to provide safe, quality, and cost-effective care.

Wherever you choose to practice, it is likely that drug administration will be a significant part of your role. A survey of new LPNs/VNs revealed that over half of their work hours were involved in providing care related to giving drugs and to monitoring patients receiving drugs, including parenteral therapies. These new nurses rated knowledge of "client safety" and "medication" as the most important for safe and effective professional practice regardless of the setting.

Before we begin discussing specific drugs, we review the client clinical problem-solving process as it relates to drug administration. Although you may be familiar with the nursing process, we focus on how you will use it as you safely give drugs to patients in a variety of settings. To review, the client problem-solving process (nursing process) is a system that guides the nurse's work in a logical way (Fig. 1.1). The nursing process consists of five major steps: (1) assessment, (2) diagnosis, (3) planning, (4) implementation, and (5) evaluation.

## ASSESSMENT

Assessment is the first step in the nursing process, and it involves collecting important information (also called *data*) about the patient that will be used in planning care. Depending on the clinical setting, an RN is assigned as the staff member who must perform the initial full assessment for each patient. However, as an LPN/VN, you will often make vital contributions to this assessment and may even be asked to provide full nursing assessment via protocols. This step of the nursing process is important because it provides initial information as you begin to make a record for developing the plan of care.

The first part of assessment related to drug administration involves gathering information about the patient and the patient's health condition before you give the drugs. When the patient is admitted to the healthcare setting (any setting in which LPNs/VNs practice nursing), you can obtain that information by talking to the patient (or to his or her caregiver if necessary), checking the patient closely for signs and symptoms of illness, viewing past medical records, and reviewing

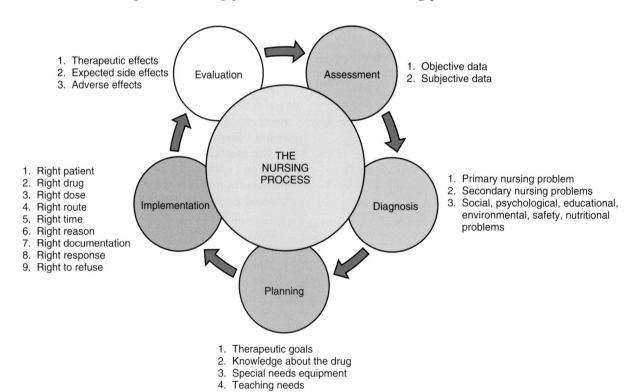

FIG. 1.1 The nursing process and examples of considerations associated with each step.

information the patient may have brought to the setting. Ask carefully about current health problems, a history of illnesses or surgeries, and drugs taken now and in the past (including over-the-counter [OTC] drugs and herbal or dietary supplements). This information is important for all team members and helps everyone to plan the patient's care. Information in the patient's history often directs the nurse and the physician to look for certain physical signs of illness that may be present.

Information you gather through assessment falls into two groups: subjective data and objective data. Subjective data are what the patient reports feeling and thinking. For example, if a patient reports feeling nauseated after taking a drug, you must accept the patient's word. You cannot see, hear, or feel the patient's nausea—that is why the data are subjective. A patient may report trouble breathing. Although you may observe rapid breathing, the degree of difficulty the patient feels cannot be measured. Information is subjective if you have to rely on the patient's words or if the symptoms cannot be felt by anyone other than the patient. In such cases you would report, "The patient states that. . . ." Other examples of subjective data that you may learn about from a patient interview include:

- The chief problem according to the patient (in the patient's own words)
- The patient's belief about what caused the problem
- The patient's description about what relieves the problem
- The patient's report of the severity of the problem

Objective data are data that can be seen, heard, felt, or measured by someone other than the patient. They include information obtained when the healthcare provider performs a physical examination or orders laboratory tests, x-rays, or other diagnostic tests. The RN or physician typically conducts a comprehensive physical assessment. As an LPN/VN, it is important for you to assess vital signs (respiratory rate, pulse, blood pressure, weight, height, temperature), physical findings based on careful observation, auscultation (listening with the stethoscope), and light palpation as appropriate for your clinical setting and your state's Nurse Practice Act. Other examples of objective data include:

- Presence of edema
- Quality of a cough
- Percentage of foods eaten at a meal
- Measures of intake and output

It is especially important to gather subjective and objective assessment data when the patient is first seen or on admission to the healthcare setting. This initial information can be used as a baseline for comparison as care progresses. In addition to the physical examination, it is important to gather a thorough patient history. Asking questions and listening carefully to the patient may be just as important as the physical examination or the results of laboratory tests. The LPN/VN is often with the patient, so he or she plays a very important role in continuing to listen to what the patient says and reporting new information to the other healthcare team members.

The nurse may not always be the one gathering the subjective and objective data; however, the nurse and everyone else on the healthcare team should learn whatever information they can from the chart, the physician, the family, and other team members and use that information to plan the patient's care. Understanding the difference between subjective and objective information can help you in reporting, or charting, the information. Based on our previous example and because you do not objectively *see* nausea, if the patient reports nausea (subjective information), your charting should specify "The patient reports nausea" rather than "The patient is nauseated." However, if the patient vomits (objective information), you will record the time, color, and amount.

Much of your role in assessment may be reporting data you collect to the RN or to other members of the healthcare team. The primary role you play in assessing the patient is defined by your state's Nurse Practice Act, which lists what actions LPNs/VNs may and may not perform. Your role also may vary according to your healthcare setting's policies and procedures.

**Factors to Consider in Assessing the Patient**
Certain information is very helpful in planning the care of the patient who is receiving drug therapy. The baseline nursing assessment is conducted at the time of the patient's admission to the healthcare setting. An important part of the assessment is the patient's drug history. The patient is typically the best source; however, you may also include reports from caregivers (e.g., spouse, close relatives, friends) and past medical records (often in the electronic medical record [EMR]).

When asking about the patient's drug history, you will want to collect data in the following areas:
1. Symptoms, signs, or diseases that explain the patient's need for a drug (such as high blood glucose levels, high blood pressure, or pain)
2. The names and, when possible, dosages of all the drugs the patient is taking, including:
   - Prescription drugs (in this category, patients often forget to mention birth control pills and implanted birth control measures)
   - OTC drugs such as aspirin, vitamins, laxatives, cold and sinus preparations, and antacids
   - Alcohol or street drugs used for recreational purposes (e.g., marijuana, cocaine)
   - Alternative therapies such as herbal agents or nutritional supplements
3. Any problems that the patient has had with drug therapy, for example:
   - Allergies (include the name of the drug and the symptoms the patient experienced)
   - Diseases that may prohibit or limit use of some drugs (e.g., sickle cell disease, glucose-6-phosphate dehydrogenase deficiency, drug addiction, immune deficiencies)

Data collection in all of these areas is important because this information can help prevent drug interactions or complications of drug therapy. You will also use this information as you monitor the patient's response and any changes in patient condition or status that may influence drug therapy during the time the patient is in the healthcare setting. This will help you determine whether the drug is helping the patient.

 **Memory Jogger**

Nursing assessment is the use of your observational, questioning, and listening skills to learn information about the patient that can be used to ensure that you are giving drugs safely.

## DIAGNOSIS

After all data have been collected, the nurse and other healthcare team members must identify the patient problems. This is determined through data **diagnosis**. The RN interprets the assessment data to identify the patient problem. The physician uses select data to make the medical diagnoses. As an LPN/VN, your knowledge about the patient allows you to make a significant contribution to the overall plan of care, including the plan of care around drug administration. The following are examples of follow-up questions you will need to ask related to giving drugs:

* What are the major health-related problems of this patient?
* What drugs is the patient likely to require?
* What special knowledge or equipment is required in giving these drugs?
* What special concerns or cultural beliefs does the patient have?
* How much does this patient understand about the prescribed treatment and drugs?
* What factors affect the patient's ability for self-care?

Answers to these questions (1) help you contribute to the goals of nursing care, (2) affect strategies you will use to care for the patient, and (3) tell you what type of patient teaching will be needed. Answering these questions may be more challenging with children, older adults, or people whose language or culture is different from yours. However, just as a physician must have the correct diagnosis to prescribe the right treatment, finding the correct answers to these questions helps you to plan the best care for the patient.

## PLANNING

Based on the data you help collect, the medical and nursing diagnoses are made, goals are set, and nursing care plans are written. As a member of the healthcare team, the LPN/VN will be able to assist with the **planning** step. The nursing care plan involves collaboration with nurses and patients or caregivers to determine the expected patient outcomes. Using the information gathered in the assessment about the patient's history, medical and social problems, risk factors, and how ill the patient may

be, goals are set on a short-term or a long-term basis. For example, the following short-term goal may be written: "The patient will describe pain at a level of 3 or below, on a scale of 0 to 10, 30 minutes after receiving a drug for pain." An example of a long-term goal is "The patient will demonstrate how to rotate injection sites for using his insulin pen by the time of discharge."

 **Memory Jogger**

When collecting the drug history, be sure to include the patient's use of OTC drugs, such as herbal and dietary supplements, because they may interfere with prescription drugs.

## Drug Orders and the Nursing Care Plan

Physicians, nurse practitioners, nurse midwives, nurse anesthetists, clinical nurse specialists, and physician assistants may write drug orders according to individual state laws. Large hospitals may have a staff *hospitalist*—a physician or nurse practitioner who practices in the hospital to oversee care for all patients. Teaching hospitals may employ resident doctors who are still in educational programs.

After a drug is ordered, the nurse must verify that the order is accurate. This is usually done by checking the drug administration record or EMR against the original order. You will need to learn and follow the procedures of the agency where you work when checking drugs and drug orders. In all care environments, you must carefully check each time you give a drug. This is essential to maintaining patient safety and minimizing the risk for errors or adverse effects.

The nurse must also apply knowledge about the drug to the specific drug order to determine whether the drug and the dose ordered seem to be correct. No part of the order or the reason for giving the drug should be unclear. (Chapter 2 presents the information required for a clear and legal drug order.) Any questions about whether a drug is appropriate or safe for that patient must be answered before the drug is given. The EMR may alert the nurse if there is a problem with the order. However, good clinical judgment in carrying out the drug order is very important. If you determine that (1) any part of the order is incorrect or unclear, (2) the patient's condition would be made worse by the drug, (3) the person ordering the drug may not have had all the information needed about the patient when drug therapy was planned, or (4) there has been a change in the patient's condition and a question has arisen about whether the drug should be given, the drug should be *withheld* (i.e., not given) until the healthcare provider has been called and the question has been answered. If you think there is a problem with the drug order and the provider cannot be contacted or does not change the order under question, notify the charge nurse and the nursing supervisor as soon as possible. Most hospitals have clear policies about whom to contact, how to report this problem, and what to do next.

After you have the drug order and have decided to give the drug, include in your plan any patient problems that may increase the risk of issues related to the drug's side effects. For example, a patient who has poor vision may have a risk of falling in an unfamiliar hospital or nursing home setting. This is important if you are giving a diuretic and the patient needs to go to the bathroom frequently. You must plan ahead so that the patient can safely get to the bathroom. The importance of these problems may change over time as the patient's condition changes. Ongoing communication between nurses and the healthcare team is important to maintain safe, quality, and cost-effective patient care.

### Factors to Consider in Planning to Give a Drug

Planning to give a drug involves four important steps:
1. Know the reason you are giving the patient the drug. In other words, what is this drug supposed to do for the patient?
2. Learn specific information about the drug, including:
   - The major action of the drug
   - Negative side effects that may develop
   - The usual dosage, route, and frequency
   - Situations in which the drug should not be given (**contraindications**)
   - Health-related reasons in which the drug should be given with greater consideration to avoid adverse events (**precautions**)
   - Main drug interactions (i.e., the possible influence of another drug given at the same time)
3. Plan for special storage requirements, procedures, techniques, or equipment needs, including:
   - Does the solution need to be shaken before it is given?
   - Should the drug be refrigerated?
   - Do you need a specific syringe (such as an insulin syringe)?
   - What special techniques are necessary for giving the drug, such as using an inhaler or not applying pressure to the site after giving certain injectable drugs?
4. Develop a teaching plan for the patient, including:
   - What the patient needs to know about the drug's action and side effects
   - What the patient needs to know to take the drug correctly
   - What the patient needs to report to the nurse or physician if there are any problems

As you develop your plan, be sure to use the data you gathered in the assessment and your knowledge about the drug. You will use this information as you prepare to implement your plan. Whether or not to give the drug will depend on your assessment, your knowledge, and your professional judgment.

Regarding drug orders, make certain that you understand each part of the drug order. Do not give the drug if you have a question about any part of the order.

 **Top Tip for Safety**

**CHECK THE EXPIRATION DATES INCLUDED ON THE DRUG LABELS: OUT WITH THE OLD!**
Expired medications can be less effective and may adversely affect the patient's health.

The planning step of the nursing process is also the time to:
- Ensure that you have a place to gather the drugs that is quiet and free of interruption.
- Gather any special equipment you will need to give the drug (such as intravenous [IV] infusion pumps, alcohol wipes, or nebulizers).
- Review special procedures you will need to give the drug (such as the Z-track injection technique), to properly administer eye or ear drops, or to deliver a rectal suppository.

All of this information is documented in the nursing care plan in the paper chart or EMR so that other team members can see the plan.

### IMPLEMENTATION

**Implementation** involves carrying out your plan of care as you safely give drugs to the patient. In planning the patient's care, you learned why each drug was ordered, the drug's actions, and how to safely give the drug. You will apply this knowledge during implementation of the plan. For example, if you are giving an angiotensin-converting enzyme inhibitor (see Chapter 9) to a patient with high blood pressure, you will need to check the patient's blood pressure before giving the drug. If you are planning to give the ordered penicillin antibiotic (see Chapter 5) and you notice that the patient has a red rash on his or her chest and arms, you would withhold the next dose of the drug until you have reported the rash to the healthcare provider, because it may indicate an allergic reaction. After you have carried out the plan, you will record in the patient's chart or EMR that you have given the drug.

### The 9 *Rights of Drug Administration*

A major strategy for giving drugs to patients is the **9 Rights of Drug Administration**. The nurse must always keep in mind these nine commonly recognized rights of drug administration (Box 1.1). Chapter 4 provides specific details about preparing and giving drugs.

You may have heard nurses in the clinical setting discuss the importance of the *five rights, six rights*, or *eight rights*. Over time, nursing has continued to emphasize those essential components of safe drug administration, and more rights have been added.

For our purposes, the nine rights ensure that you identify the *right patient* and give the *right drug* with the *right dose* using the *right route* at the *right time* for the *right reason*. Then you use the *right documentation* to record that the dose has been given. You then monitor the patient to assess the *right response*. The final right is that patients have the *right to refuse* the drug. You might

**Box 1.1    The *9 Rights of Drug Administration***

- The right patient—Use at least two identifiers.
- The right drug—Check the drug label at least three times.
- The right dose—Make sure that you use the right amount of the drug; double-check the dose.
- The right route—Never change the route of administration without an order.
- The right time—Make sure that the drug has not been given recently or should be given at a different time of day.
- The right reason—Does this make sense for this patient? Know your patient and the drug.
- The right documentation—Document after you have given the drug, never before.
- The right response—How is the patient responding to the drug? Does it work?
- The right to refuse—Patients have the right to refuse; ask the patient to clarify his or her reason, provide good patient teaching, and document.

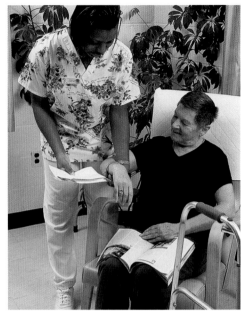

FIG. 1.2 Nurse checking the patient's wristband for identification. (From Hoffmann Wold, G. (2012). *Basic geriatric nursing* (5th ed.). Mosby.)

wonder how you can remember nine things. A runner who really enjoyed racing in 15K races (9.3 miles) said that he liked them the best because he could divide them into three 5Ks (3.1 miles each) so it seemed easier. You can do the same with the nine rights.

This section reviews each right and explains the reason each is essential for safe, quality, and cost-effective care.

 **Memory Jogger**

**THE *9 RIGHTS OF DRUG ADMINISTRATION* (THREE AT A TIME)**
- Right patient, right drug, right dose
- Right route, right time, right reason
- Right documentation, right response, right to refuse

***The Right Patient.*** Before you give any drug, make sure that you identify the right patient. The National Patient Safety Goals claim that the purpose of this approach is (1) to reliably identify the individual as the person for whom the treatment is intended and (2) to match the treatment to the person. To properly identify the patient, you use at least two identifiers. **Identifiers** are information that is used to reliably prove that an individual is the person for whom the drug treatment is intended. Identifiers may be the person's full name, medical record identification number, birthdate, or telephone number. These may be compared with the patient's identification bracelet (wristband) in appropriate situations. Healthcare agencies may specify the main identifiers to be used in the setting and/or use a barcode system to scan the drug to the wristband.

For patients who are alert and oriented, asking them their full name and birthdate and comparing the information with the medical record is a straightforward process. However, for those who are hard of hearing, confused, very young or very old, or critically ill, be sure to compare the name, birthdate, or medical record number against the patient's wristband (Fig. 1.2). Best practice is to directly instruct the patient: "Tell me your full name." This is much safer than asking "Are you Joe Jones?" A patient who is confused may not understand the question and may say yes or no regardless of whether that is the correct name.

In the hospital setting, never give a drug to a patient who is not wearing a wristband. Some long-term care settings use photographs of patients to assist the nurse in identifying patients who might be confused. Never identify the patient solely by the room or bed number.

◆ ***The Right Drug.*** Each drug that is prescribed for the patient has a particular intended action. You will need to make sure that you give the right drug. Carefully compare the drug order with the drug label. Do not assume that the correct drug has been sent by the pharmacy.

Make sure that the drug is in the form prescribed because some drugs can come in multiple forms (e.g., tablets, capsules, syrup). Many drugs have names that look or sound almost the same as the names of other drugs; these are sometimes called *look-alike, sound-alike drugs.* The Institute for Safe Medication Practices (ISMP) has published a list of easily confused drug names (Table 1.1). The US Food and Drug Administration and ISMP also recommend the Tall Man lettering system to reduce confusion for look-alike drug names (Table 1.2). In this system, for example, Lamisil (brand name for an antifungal drug) is written as LamISIL. This helps highlight the "ISIL" part of the name so that the nurse does not confuse it with Lamictal (an antiseizure drug), written as LaMICtal. The Tall Man lettering system has been embraced by healthcare agencies as one more strategy to reduce drug errors.

Drugs may come individually wrapped in a unit-dose system package or as a prescription filled for one person; in rare cases, they may be taken from a unit's stock drugs. Sometimes the drug label includes a bar-code that is scanned by a computer. However it is packaged, you must read the drug label at least three times.

### Top Tip for Safety

Read the drug label three times!
1. Before taking the drug from the unit-dose cart or storage area
2. Before preparing or measuring the prescribed dose of drug
3. At the bedside before you give it to the patient

◆ **The Right Dose.** As an LPN/VN, you will want to make sure you are giving the right dose. The amount of drug to be given is typically ordered by the healthcare provider as a dose for the "average" patient. A patient who is older, who has experienced severe weight loss as a result of illness, or who is small or very obese may require changes in the usual dosages. Pediatric patients often have doses ordered based on how much they weigh. Geriatric or older adult patients may be very sensitive to many drugs and may require a change in dosage. If the patient has poor liver or kidney function, changes in dosage may be necessary for the desired effect. The healthcare provider may order a specific dosage of the drug when treatment begins and may adjust the dose later based on changes in the patient's condition.

Giving the correct dose of a drug also requires that you use the proper equipment (e.g., insulin must be measured in an insulin syringe), the proper drug form (e.g., oral or rectal, water or oil based, scored tablets or coated capsules), and the proper concentration (e.g., 0.25% versus 0.5% solution for eye drops), and you must accurately calculate the right drug dose. For high-alert drugs (see Chapter 2), many healthcare settings have policies that require two nurses to check any drug dose that must be calculated—particularly for drugs such as narcotics, heparin, insulin, and IV drugs—to reduce the risk for error.

◆ **The Right Route.** Each drug must be given by the right route. The drug order must state how the drug is to be given (route of drug administration). The nurse must never change routes without obtaining a new order. Although many drugs may be given by different routes, the dose is often different for each route.

The oral route is the preferred route if the patient is oriented (i.e., awake and able to understand) and can swallow without choking. In some cases, faster delivery or a higher blood level of a drug is needed, and the drug may be given parenterally (e.g., subcutaneously or intravenously; see Chapter 4). Special precautions may be needed for drugs given through these routes (such as how fast they can be given or in what dosage). Review your drug references to ensure that you are giving the drug correctly.

For patients with breathing problems such as asthma, drugs that previously were given orally can now be given by an inhaler. This decreases the number of side effects by getting the drug directly to where it is needed: in the lungs. You will need to teach the patient techniques to achieve the greatest benefit from the inhaler. Other routes that you will see in practice are drugs given as eye drops, ear drops, topical agents,

**Table 1.1  Examples from Institute for Safe Medication Practices Commonly Confused Drug Names**

| DRUG NAME[a] | CONFUSED DRUG NAME | DRUG NAME | CONFUSED DRUG NAME |
|---|---|---|---|
| Aciphex | Accupril | Diprivan | Ditropan |
| Adderall | Inderal | Flonase | Flovent |
| Allegra | Viagra | Lantus | Lente |
| Benadryl | benazepril | Lexapro | Loxitane |
| Bextra | Zetia | Microzide | Micronase |
| Captopril | carvedilol | Paxil | Plavix |
| Cozaar | Zocor | Pyridium | pyridoxine |

[a]Brand name drugs always start with a capital letter. Generic drug names always start with a lowercase letter.

**Table 1.2  Examples from Institute for Safe Medication Practices List of Drug Names with Tall Man Letters**

| DRUG NAME WITH TALL MAN LETTERS[a] | CONFUSED DRUG NAME | DRUG NAME WITH TALL MAN LETTERS | CONFUSED DRUG NAME |
|---|---|---|---|
| busPIRone | buPROPion | SOLU-Medrol | Solu-CORTEF |
| chlorproMAZINE | chlorproPAMIDE | SandIMMUNE | SandoSTATIN |
| Glipizide | glyBURIDE | SEROquel | SINEquan |
| NIFEdipine | niCARdipine | ZyPREXA | ZyrTEC |
| cefTRIAXone | ceFAZolin | FLUoxetine | PARoxetine |
| KlonoPIN | cloNIDine | HumaLOG | HumuLIN |
| PriLOSEC | PROzac | hydroOXYzine | hydrALAZINE |

[a]Brand name drugs always start with a capital letter. Generic drugs typically start with lowercase letters. NOTE: Some generic drug names incorporate Tall Man letters. Generic drugs that start with Tall Man letters are identified with an asterisk.

or part of shampoos. The most important thing is that you give the right form of the drug for the right route.

◆ *The Right Time.* The drug order should say when and how often the drug is to be given. In many situations you will work with the RN (and/or pharmacist) to determine the right time. Most healthcare agencies have guidelines that specify what time drugs will be given when they are ordered (e.g., drugs given once a day are given at 9:00 a.m.). You must be familiar with your agency guidelines for general times of administration. Nevertheless, it will be important for you to report if the information suggests timing that conflicts with the usual guideline. For example, some statin drugs (given once a day) should be given before bedtime for best effect rather than in the morning. If you have any questions, make sure to notify the RN or the healthcare provider. It is always better to ask the question than to risk a mistake.

To be effective, many drugs must be given exactly on schedule, day and night, to keep the level of drug constant in the body. For example, if a patient is taking warfarin (an anticoagulant) to decrease the risk for blood clots, the drug must be given at the same time every day. Patients with infections should follow a very regular schedule to maintain a consistent level of antibiotics and decrease the risk for antibiotic resistance.

You may need to plan around other patient activities when you give drugs. A patient with a newly diagnosed infection may need to have a blood culture drawn *before* starting antibiotic therapy. If the patient is scheduled for an ultrasound, you may want to *hold* giving a diuretic in the early morning (i.e., wait until later) so that the patient does not experience urinary urgency while having the procedure. As you go through each chapter on drugs, you will learn more on this topic.

Drugs are usually given when there is the best chance for the body to absorb them and the least risk of side effects. Some drugs should be given when the patient's stomach is empty, and others should be given with food to prevent gastrointestinal side effects. Some drugs require that the patient not eat certain foods. Others do not mix well with alcohol. Antacids interfere with the absorption of a number of drugs and therefore need to be given 2 hours before or 2 hours after taking those drugs. When a patient is taking several drugs, check to ensure that the drugs do not interfere or interact with each other. (For example, some antibiotics can interfere with the action of birth control pills, and a sexually active woman taking both could become pregnant if she does not use another form of contraception.) Whenever you are giving a new drug or one you have never seen before, use your drug references to ensure that the timing is correct.

It is especially important to confirm the timing of one-time-only, as needed, and emergency drugs. *The nurse must be certain that no one else has already given the drug and that it is the appropriate time to give the drug.* Narcotics (opioids) are often ordered as "stat" (to be

| Box **1.2** | **Factors to Consider in Giving a Drug at the Right Time** |

- Always confirm the last time the drug was given to avoid giving too much in too short a time period.
- Understand and follow the rules of your hospital regarding the times to give scheduled drugs.
- Check drug references for the best times to achieve the best drug absorption and to limit risks for interactions with other drugs.
- Give drugs at times ordered to help keep blood levels of the drug constant.
- Plan drug therapy while keeping in mind other diagnostic and laboratory testing that your patient may be experiencing.

given within a few minutes of the order) or "PRN" (as needed). Note on the patient's record as soon as possible that you have given a narcotic so that it is clear the patient has been given the drug. (For more information, see Chapter 2.) Box 1.2 lists the main factors to remember in giving a drug at the right time.

Even though it may be tempting if you are on a busy unit, never leave a drug at the bedside for the patient to take later. If the patient cannot take the drug when you bring it, you should return later with the drug. As a nurse, you must document the time the patient actually takes the drug. If you are not present when the patient takes the drug, you cannot document it.

### ⬦ Top Tip for Safety

**MAKE CERTAIN THE PATIENT TAKES THE DRUG**
Never leave a drug at the bedside for the patient to take later.

*The Right Reason.* All medications are prescribed for a clear purpose. As a LPN, you should have a good understanding of your patient's health problems. The prescribed drugs should make sense to you, even if you may not fully understand the specific disease pathophysiology. As you learn pharmacology, you will learn the basic uses of the specific drugs and this will help you apply what you have learned to your patients. For example, you may have a patient with a diagnosis of high blood pressure, you would expect the patient to have an antihypertensive drug in their plan of care. If you have a patient with decreased mobility, you would understand that a stool softener would be helpful in decreasing the risk of constipation. On the other hand, if you have a patient with a viral infection, and the patient is prescribed an antibiotic typically prescribed for a bacterial infection (for example ampicillin or doxycycline), you would double check with the charge nurse or other healthcare provider for the reason the patient is receiving this drug. If you have a patient who is having severe diarrhea, you would question why the patient is scheduled to receive a laxative (and you would hold the medication until you have talked to the healthcare provider). Never be afraid to ask the charge nurse or healthcare provider to better understand why the patient is receiving the drug.

*The Right Documentation.* Increasingly, electronic health record and charting systems are being used in healthcare settings. Whether the nurse records giving the drug in a paper chart or uses an electronic chart, the basics are the same: You need to make the right documentation. Record the time, route, and site of administration (if parenteral) after you have given the drug. It is very important to record this right away; do not delay or wait until later. As a tool of communication, failure to record means that you did not give the drug. In an emergency or when a drug is used only once or twice, such a failure is very important.

The documentation must always list the drug given, the dose, and the time it was actually given, not the time it was supposed to be given. In some offices or clinics where immunizations are given, the policy may require that the lot number listed on the bottle be recorded in the patient's chart. Most charting systems include a place to record the patient's response to the drug. Any patient reports of problems or adverse effects must be noted in the chart and reported immediately to the head nurse and the physician.

It is vitally important that you *never record drugs that were not given or record them before they are given*. If a patient does not receive the drug for any reason, notify the nurse in charge or the healthcare provider according to the policies of your healthcare setting.

Following the rules of your healthcare setting and carefully following the rights of drug administration can reduce the risk for drug error. If an error is made, talking about it honestly and taking quick action to correct any damage are vitally important to protect the patient from harm. Acknowledging error is an essential, and ethical, part of nursing practice.

*The Right Response.* As every drug is prescribed for a right reason, you will want to determine if the patient is having the expected response. Your evaluation of the response, whether expected or unexpected, guides your next actions. For example, if a patient is prescribed an antihypertensive for a patient with high blood pressure, you will monitor the blood pressure to determine if the drugs have achieved the desired result. If, on the other hand, the patient experiences severe side effects from the drug, you will report to healthcare provider. Knowing the basic actions of the drug and the overall plan of care will help you to determine your actions.

*The Right to Refuse.* Patients do have the right to refuse drugs based on the principle of autonomy (right to self-determination). Although we recognize that patients can refuse (with rare exception; see the following paragraph), it is important to talk with patients regarding their reasons for refusal. In many cases, refusals are based on a lack of understanding about the purposes

of the drug, and talking about it gives you the opportunity to teach or clarify information about the drug. Another example is a patient who refuses a laxative because he or she has diarrhea—clearly a good reason! Whatever the reason, if the patient refuses after you have answered all of his or her questions, make sure to document the refusal in the medical record.

In some clinical areas (e.g., psychiatric units), patients may be a danger to themselves or to others. In those situations, know your state laws that allow emergency treatment orders. If there is any question, make sure to check with the RN or the healthcare provider.

## EVALUATION

**Evaluation** is the process of determining the right response and looking at what happens to the patient when the nursing care plan is put into action. It is the appraisal of the treatment's effectiveness. Evaluation requires the nurse to watch for the patient's response to a drug, noting both expected and unexpected findings. For example, when antipyretics (i.e., drugs that reduce fever) are given, you will take the patient's temperature to determine whether the drug lowered the fever. When drugs are given to reduce blood pressure, you will do regular blood pressure checks. For drugs used to reduce pain, you will evaluate whether the drug reduced the patient's pain according to your agency's pain scale.

Evaluation of what happens when you give a drug helps the healthcare team decide whether to continue the same drug or make a change. Gathering such information is also a part of the continuing assessment of a patient during care that the nurse will record in the patient's chart. The nursing process may be seen as a circle (see Fig. 1.1). For example, the patient's temperature can be part of the evaluation step of the nursing process, but it may also be part of the assessment step when you notice that the patient's temperature remains elevated, indicating that the patient needs a different dose of the drug, a different drug altogether, or some additional treatment measures.

 **Top Tip for Safety**

**EVALUATE RESPONSE TO DRUG**
It is important to watch the patient and look for any signs of improvement as well as any side effects, adverse effects, or allergic responses.

### Factors to Consider in Evaluating Response to Drug

The nurse checks for three types of responses to drug therapy: therapeutic effects, expected side effects, and adverse effects.

**Therapeutic effects** are seen when the drug does what it was supposed to do. If you understand why the drug is being given (i.e., the therapeutic goal of the drug), you will be able to decide whether that goal is being met. For example, if the patient's blood glucose level is high and regular insulin is given, you should see a lower blood glucose level when it is next checked. If the patient is constipated and takes a laxative, the patient should have a bowel movement.

**Expected side effects** are unintended but not unusual effects that occur in many people taking the drug; they are usually mild and do not require the drug to be stopped. One example of an expected side effect is the sleepiness that most patients feel when taking an opioid (narcotic) for pain. All drugs have side effects, but not all patients have every side effect listed for a single drug. Always document side effects. Side effects such as nausea or vomiting sometimes can be stopped by decreasing the dosage or by giving the drug with food. Telling the healthcare provider about the side effects helps him or her decide whether the patient should keep taking the drug or it should be stopped.

**Adverse effects** are seen when patients do not respond to their drugs in the way they should or develop new signs or symptoms. For example, a patient with pneumonia may be given penicillin. Although this antibiotic may be working to control the infection, the patient may develop shortness of breath, which could be an allergic reaction to the drug; in that case, the penicillin must be stopped. A patient taking an anticoagulant to prevent blood clots must be closely watched for signs of bleeding or bruising that would indicate the patient has taken too large a dose or has had a larger-than-expected response to the drug. *If you suspect a patient is having an adverse effect, report it to the RN or the healthcare provider immediately.* When serious adverse effects occur in response to a drug, the healthcare provider usually discontinues (stops) the drug.

The nurse is the healthcare worker who is most often with the patient and is therefore in an important position to notice the patient's response to drug therapy. Carefully and repeatedly evaluating the patient and documenting your findings in the patient's medical record is vitally important in the delivery of safe, quality, and cost-effective care.

 **Top Tip for Safety**

Use the *9 Rights of Drug Administration* each and every time you give a drug to a patient!

## USING THE CLINICAL JUDGMENT MODEL

In 2023, the National Council of State Boards of Nursing (NCSBN) altered the format of the National Council Licensure Exam (NCLEX®) to include questions evaluating the new LPN/VN's ability in clinical decision making, also called **clinical judgment**. This requires you to be able to translate your nursing knowledge into clinical practice. The NCSBN definition of *clinical judgment* is "the observed outcome of critical thinking and decision making. This iterative process uses nursing knowledge to observe and assess presenting situations, identify a prioritized client concern, and

generate the best possible evidence-based solutions to deliver safe client care" (NCSBN, 2019, p. 1). This definition builds on and expands the nursing process and indicates that clinical judgment skills are not linear steps that are followed in a particular sequence.

After developing the definition of clinical judgment, the NCSBN developed a Clinical Judgment Measurement and Action Model. Six cognitive (thinking) skills—called *cognitive processes*—were identified as essential for nurses to make appropriate clinical judgment. These skills help nurses identify changes in a patient's clinical condition and know what actions to take and why. The six essential cognitive skills of clinical judgment are Recognize Cues, Analyze Cues, Prioritize Hypotheses, Generate Solutions, Take Action, and Evaluate Outcomes (NCSBN, 2019):

- **Recognize Cues**

  Cues are elements of assessment data that provide important information for the nurse as a basis for making client decisions. In a clinical situation, the nurse determines which data are *relevant* (directly related to client outcomes or the priority of care) and of immediate concern to the nurse, or *irrelevant* (unrelated to client outcomes or priority of care). *For example, you recognize the specific lab values that are critical to whether or not you administer a certain medication. Of the patient's available lab work, you determine which values are relevant to the medication you are giving.*

- **Analyze Cues**

  When using this skill, the nurse considers the context of the client's history and situation and interprets how the identified relevant cues relate to the client's condition. Data that support or contradict a particular cue in the client situation are determined, and potential complications are identified. *For example, once you are aware that a patient has a potassium level of 3.5 mEq/L, consider the effect of giving or withholding a furosemide diuretic for this patient.*

- **Prioritize Hypotheses**

  For this skill, the nurse needs to examine all possibilities about what is occurring in the client situation. The urgency and risk for the client are considered for each possible health condition. The nurse determines which client conditions are the *most likely* and *most serious*, and why. *For your patient with the potassium level of 3.5 mEq/L, there is a risk of heart rhythm disturbances if the furosemide diuretic is given and the potassium drops too low. Although the patient may need diuretics for the heart failure, it is a priority to make sure that it can be given safely.*

- **Generate Solutions**

  To generate solutions, the nurse first identifies expected client outcomes. Using the prioritized hypotheses, the nurse then plans specific actions that may achieve the desirable outcomes. Actual or potential evidence-based actions that should be *avoided* or are *contraindicated* are also considered because some actions could be harmful for the client in the given situation. *For the considered patient, holding the furosemide until plans are made to supplement oral potassium can prevent hypokalemia and allow administration of the diuretic.*

- **Take Action**

Using this skill, the nurse decides which nursing actions will address the highest priorities of care and determines in what priority these actions will be implemented. Actions can include, but are not limited to, additional assessment, health teaching, documentation, requested primary healthcare provider orders, performance of nursing skills, and consultation with healthcare team members. *Recognizing the problem, you contact the healthcare provider with the information and receive an order for 20 mEq KCl orally to be given with the furosemide.*

- **Evaluate Outcomes**

After implementing the best evidence-based nursing action, the nurse evaluates the actual client outcomes in the situation and compares them to expected outcomes. The nurse then decides if the selected nursing actions were effective, ineffective, or made no difference in how the client is progressing. *The patient avoids irregular heart rate, lung sounds are clear, and the patient has no peripheral edema.*

As mentioned, the six clinical judgment skills build on and expand the nursing process. The following table shows a comparison of the steps of the nursing process and the essential cognitive skills needed for sound clinical judgment.

| STEPS OF THE NURSING PROCESS | COGNITIVE SKILLS FOR CLINICAL JUDGMENT |
|---|---|
| Assessment | Recognize Cues |
| Diagnosis | Analyze Cues |
| Diagnosis | Prioritize Hypotheses |
| Planning | Generate Solutions |
| Implementation | Take Action |
| Evaluation | Evaluate Outcomes |

# Get Ready for the Next-Generation NCLEX® Examination!

## Key Points

- Use the *9 Rights* each and every time you give a drug to a patient.
- Nursing assessment is using your observational, questioning, and listening skills to learn information about the patient that can be used to ensure that you are safely giving drugs.
- When assessing a patient, always ask carefully about current health problems, history of illnesses, history of surgeries, and drugs taken (including OTC and herbal drugs), both now and in the past.
- Always know why you are giving the patient the drug.
- Check the label of each drug you are giving three times to ensure that it is the right drug.
- Do not give a drug that was made for one route by any other route.
- When giving a one-time-only drug, take extra precautions to make certain that it has not already been given by someone else.
- Never record drugs that were not given or record them before they are given.
- Always use two unique patient identifiers when giving a patient a drug.
- If a patient refuses to take a drug, clarify the patient's reason and make sure to document the refusal.
- All drugs have side effects, but not all patients have every side effect listed for any single drug.
- Any questions about whether a drug is appropriate or safe for that patient *must* be answered before the drug is given.
- If you suspect a patient is having an adverse effect, report it immediately to the RN or the healthcare provider.
- Never leave a drug at the bedside for the patient to take later.
- In the hospital, never give a drug to a patient who is not wearing an identification band.

## Clinical Judgment and Next-Generation NCLEX® Examination-Style Questions

1. **Which of the following is considered a therapeutic effect?**

   1. Tachypnea
   2. Decreased nausea
   3. Edema of left foot
   4. Irregular heart rate

2. **Which of the following examples would be considered objective data? Select all or any that apply.**

   1. "I have pain in my chest."
   2. Blood pressure is 140/70.
   3. Skin is warm and dry.
   4. "I had an appointment last week with my doctor."
   5. Child's mother states, "His temperature was 102 degrees before we came to the hospital."
   6. Weight gain of 3 pounds in 4 days.
   7. Patient states she has trouble breathing or "catching" her breath.

3. **Which of the following would be considered examples of the *9 Rights*? Select all or any that apply.**

   1. Right patient
   2. Right time
   3. Right room number
   4. Right to refuse
   5. Right documentation
   6. Right reason

4. **Which of the following examples would be considered a contraindication?**

   1. Giving a drug for pain to a patient who has a fractured left ankle
   2. Giving a drug that causes birth defects to a patient who is 8 weeks pregnant
   3. Giving a drug that may cause dizziness to a patient with high blood pressure
   4. Giving a drug that may cause an increase in heart rate to a patient who has asthma

5. **The LPN/VN is giving a patient her morning drugs due at 9:00 a.m. After you have already prepared the drug, the patient states, "No, I don't want that pill today." What is your best first action?**

   1. Tell the patient she has to take the drug because it was ordered by the doctor.
   2. Ask the patient to tell you her reason for not taking the drug.
   3. Teach the patient why she needs it and give the drug.
   4. Ask the patient if she has any questions about the drug.

6. **A patient recently began taking an antibiotic for a wound infection and presents for a follow-up appointment. The office nurse reviews the patient's temperature and checks for wound drainage. Which stage of the nursing process corresponds to this review?**

   1. Assessment
   2. Diagnosis
   3. Planning
   4. Intervention
   5. Evaluation

7. **For which patient should the LPN/VN contact the healthcare provider to obtain a new order for an alternative route of drug administration?**

   1. The patient who is a newly diagnosed diabetic
   2. The patient who must take the drug with food
   3. The patient who is experiencing nausea and vomiting
   4. The patient who is receiving a drug for pain after surgery

8. **Based on the following data, the risk for a drug error to be made is highest in which patient?**

   1. An 87-year-old patient who is drowsy after receiving pain medication
   2. A 14-year-old patient who is in traction after experiencing a broken leg
   3. A 65-year-old patient who has just undergone a knee replacement
   4. A 24-year-old pregnant patient who speaks both Spanish and English fluently

9. **What is the best way to check that you are giving the drug to the right patient?**

   1. Ask the patient's name.
   2. Compare the patient with the room number.
   3. Check the patient's wristband.
   4. Check two unique patient identifiers.

10. The LPN is caring for a patient transferred from the acute care setting to a skilled nursing facility for rehabilitation following diagnosis of post-COVID syndrome. The patient describes generalized weakness, fatigue, difficulty sleeping, anxiety, and shortness of breath with minor activity. While in the hospital, the patient had intermittent episodes of confusion but was oriented to person, place, and time at admission. Admission vital signs were BP 160/70, HR 78, RR 18. The patient is to receive an oral blood pressure tablet.

    **For each potential step to give the drug, place an X in the box to indicate whether the action would be *Essential* (appropriate or necessary), *Non-Essential* (makes no difference or not necessary), or *Contraindicated* (could be harmful).**

| NURSING ACTIONS FOR DRUG ADMINISTRATION | ESSENTIAL | NON-ESSENTIAL | CONTRA-INDICATED |
|---|---|---|---|
| Assess the patient's mental status. | | | |
| Use two patient identifiers before giving the drug. | | | |
| Check the patient's blood sugar. | | | |
| Lay the patient flat in bed. | | | |
| Check the patient's blood pressure before administration of the drug. | | | |
| Document that the drug has been given following administration. | | | |
| Teach the patient that drugs for blood pressure may cause dizziness. | | | |
| Get the patient up in the chair before giving her the medication. | | | |

# Legal, Regulatory, and Ethical Aspects of Drug Administration

## 2

## Learning Outcomes

1. Describe the legal, regulatory, and ethical responsibilities of a nurse for drug administration.
2. Explain the meaning of controlled substances (scheduled drugs) and why drugs are placed in this category.
3. Describe the legal responsibilities for managing controlled substances.
4. List the information required for a legal drug order or prescription.
5. Describe the four different types of drug orders.
6. List what you need to do if you make a drug error.

## Key Terms

**as needed or PRN drug order** An order for a drug to be given as needed based on a nurse's judgment about safety and patient need.

**black box warning** A special designation from the FDA indicating that the drug has a higher-than-normal risk for causing serious or life-threatening problems in addition to its positive benefits for some people.

**controlled substances** Drugs that are highly regulated because they are commonly abused; also known as *scheduled drugs*.

**emergency or stat drug order** A one-time drug order to be given immediately.

**high-alert drugs** Drugs that have the potential to cause significant harm to patients.

**legal responsibility** The nurse's authority as defined by the Nurse Practice Act in each state. It involves the nurse's judgment and actions while performing professional duties. All nurses must know what is legal in regard to drugs in the state in which they practice.

**Nurse Practice Act** The state law that licenses LPNs/VNs, registered nurses, nurse anesthetists, nurse practitioners, and nurse midwives. It describes the minimal educational preparation and professional requirements needed to perform specific functions, including drug administration, to protect the public safety.

**over-the-counter (OTC) drugs** Category of drugs identified by federal legislation that pose a low risk to patients; they may be purchased without a prescription, have a low risk for abuse, and are safe when directions are followed.

**physical dependence** The physical symptoms that occur with drug withdrawal (e.g., shaking, increased heart rate, pain, confusion, seizures).

**prescription drugs** Category of drugs regulated by federal legislation because they are dangerous, and their use must be controlled; they may be purchased only when prescribed. Examples are antibiotics and oral birth control pills.

**prescriptive authority** The authority designated by an individual state that determines who is legally permitted to write an order or prescription for drugs.

**professional responsibility** The obligation of nurses to act appropriately, ethically, and to the best of their ability as healthcare providers.

**psychological dependence** Feeling of anxiety, stress, or tension when a patient does not have access to a medication.

**single drug order** A one-time order to be given at a specified time.

**standing drug order** A drug order that indicates the drug is to be given until discontinued or for a certain number of doses.

## INTRODUCTION

As a nurse you must understand the legal, ethical, and professional responsibilities associated with drug administration, as your decisions can result in consequences for the patient. The nurse's responsibilities include a thorough understanding of the drugs to be given, drug delivery systems, the accurate interpretation of drug orders, safe medication administration practices, and the nursing process as it relates to drug therapy. Failure of the nurse to carry out these responsibilities can result in serious drug errors and patient harm. There are also ethical issues that may occur while giving drugs to patients. For example, in assisted living or nursing home facilities, it is a common practice to mix drugs with food or drink, mainly to help patients swallow their prescribed drugs more easily. Before you decide to give drugs mixed in food or drink, you should consider several things: You have an ethical responsibility to inform the patient's care provider, the patient, and the family that you will be giving the drugs in this manner. Failure to inform the provider, patient, or family of this practice is considered *covert drug administration*, which, although not illegal, is not considered a best practice in drug administration. The mixing of drugs with food or drink must be documented in the patient's care plan and on the drug administration chart to address the legal aspects of this practice. Additionally, certain foods or drinks, such as grapefruit juice, should not be taken with certain drugs because this practice may influence the effect of that drug. It is important to check your drug handbook before mixing drugs with food or drink.

It also is important to know which types of drugs cannot be crushed or have the capsule opened. For example, a 325-mg, enteric-coated aspirin pill may be difficult for some patients to swallow, but crushing the drug affects the speed at which it is absorbed and increases the chance that the patient will develop a stomach ulcer. Some drugs have a coating that slows the release of the drug. Crushing capsules and tablets releases all of the drug at once, instead of slowly over time, and can result in accidental overdose. The Institute for Safe Medication Practices (ISMP) has published a "do not crush" list that can be used for reference: http://www.ismp.org/tools/donotcrush.pdf.

Another important legal and ethical issue facing nurses is known as *drug diversion*. Drug diversion is defined as the illegal transfer of regulated drugs (e.g., narcotics) from the patient for whom they were prescribed to another person (e.g., a nurse), for use by themselves or others. When a nurse diverts a prescribed drug, it can result in significant threats to patient safety and is a liability for the healthcare organization that employs the nurse. The American Nurses Association (ANA) has defined an *impaired nurse* as one who cannot meet the professional code of ethics because of excessive use of alcohol or drugs. When drug diversion is suspected, the organization is required to launch a full-scale investigation. The nurse involved will most likely face disciplinary charges that will include treatment resources for the nurse with drug or alcohol addiction and may include suspension or permanent loss of the nurse's license.

Nurse leaders have a legal and ethical obligation to protect patients and the profession from impaired nurses. Some behaviors that may signal a drug or alcohol dependency problem in a nurse include increased absences, lateness to work, unexplained disappearance from the assigned unit, and decreased alertness. Drug diversion should also be suspected if patients continually report pain despite appropriate drug treatment and if inaccurate counts are noted.

## REGULATION OF DRUG ADMINISTRATION

Nurses who give drugs are required to follow three levels of rules:
1. Federal laws, which describe rules that control how certain drugs may be given
2. State laws and regulations, or rules, which specify who may prescribe, dispense (give a supply), or give drugs and the process to be used
3. Individual hospital or agency rules, which may specify other guidelines or policies regarding how and when drugs are given and the records that must be kept recording drug treatment

### FEDERAL LAWS

Congress is responsible for passing laws that make drugs as safe as possible for patients to take and to create measures that ensure that drugs do what they claim to do (effectiveness). Congress created the US Food and Drug Administration (FDA) to monitor or watch over the testing, approval, and marketing of new drugs. These regulations are very strict, and US drugs are some of the purest and most protected drugs in the world. Many laws have been passed to control drugs that might easily be abused and are dangerous. These laws define the three drug categories in the United States:
1. **Controlled substances**, which include opioids (narcotics) and some sedatives or tranquilizers
2. **Prescription drugs** such as antibiotics and oral contraceptives
3. **Over-the-counter (OTC) drugs** that are available without a prescription

### Substance Abuse and Misuse
It is important for nurses to understand and be able to distinguish the differences between substance (drug) abuse and misuse. Substance abuse or *drug abuse* is *defined* as harmful or hazardous use of psychoactive substances, including alcohol and illicit drugs. The danger of psychoactive substances is that they pose a significant risk for addiction. However, *drug misuse* is defined as the use of illegal drugs and the inappropriate use of legal substances, such as alcohol and tobacco. It is important to note that *drug misuse* also applies to prescription medications and over-the-counter medications. In essence, drug misuse means the patient is using the drug in a way other than what was intended. Substance use disorders occur when the chronic use of alcohol and/or drugs causes significant health problems, disability, and failure to meet major responsibilities at work, school, or home.

### Controlled Substances
Regulations are written for controlled substances because they are most often abused by patients and the general public. The Controlled Substances Act of 1970 classified such drugs into five schedules, and they became known as *scheduled drugs*. Each schedule rates

the likelihood that the drugs in that category will be abused, causing dependency or addiction.

For example, Schedule I drugs, such as heroin, have no medical use and are considered highly addictive. At the other end of the schedules are Schedule V drugs, such as cough medicine with low-dose codeine, which have a low potential for abuse. The degree of control, the recordkeeping required, the order forms, and other regulations are different for each of these five classes. Table 2.1 describes the five drug schedules, with examples of drugs in each category. Drugs are sometimes moved from one class to another if it becomes clear they are being abused by the public. Many states have approved the medical use of marijuana for the treatment of certain conditions, mostly in cases of terminal illness.

> ### Memory Jogger
>
> - **Physical dependence** refers to the *physical symptoms* occurring during drug withdrawal. Symptoms such as shaking, increased heart rate, pain, confusion, seizures, and other troubling symptoms can occur.
> - **Psychological dependence**, or addiction, is a *mental desire* associated with taking certain substances, such as cocaine or alcohol. Symptoms of mental dependence such as anxiety, anger, or depression can occur with psychological dependence.

Federal and state laws make it a crime for anyone to have controlled substances without a prescription. Each state has a practice act that lists which healthcare providers may dispense or write prescriptions for controlled substances. Almost all states have programs for prescription monitoring of controlled substances received by patients from several different providers to prevent prescription drug abuse. Physicians, dentists, nurse practitioners, physician assistants, and sometimes nurse midwives may write prescriptions for controlled substances. Pharmacists dispense the drugs according to the provider's orders. Licensed practical nurses (LPNs) or licensed vocational nurses (LVNs) may give controlled substances to a patient only if the state board of nursing permits it in its scope of practice, and they must be under the direction of a healthcare provider who is licensed to prescribe these drugs.

### Legal Responsibilities in Drug Administration

LPNs/VNs work in many different settings. Some settings may have high levels of technology for securing controlled substances, and others may use a double-lock system. Each state and healthcare agency has laws and policies that cover ordering, receiving, storing, and recordkeeping of controlled substances.

### Table 2.1   Classification of Controlled Substances in the United States

| SCHEDULE | DESCRIPTION | EXAMPLES |
|---|---|---|
| I | High potential for abuse<br>No accepted medical use in treatment<br>Lack of accepted safety for use of the drug or other substance under medical supervision | More than 80 drugs or substances, of which the following are best known: alpha-acetylmethadol, gamma-hydroxybutyric acid (GHB), heroin, lysergic acid diethylamide (LSD), marijuana, mescaline, peyote, methaqualone (Quaalude) |
| II | High potential for abuse<br>Currently accepted use for treatment<br>Abuse may lead to severe psychological dependence or physical dependence | More than 30 drugs or substances, of which the following are best known: amphetamines, cocaine, codeine, fentanyl, hydromorphone (Dilaudid), meperidine (Demerol), methadone, methylphenidate (Ritalin), morphine, oxycodone (Percodan), pentobarbital, secobarbital |
| III | Potential for abuse less than the drugs or substances in Schedules I and II<br>Currently accepted medical use for treatment<br>Abuse may lead to moderate or low physical dependence or high psychological dependence | Most drugs are compounds containing some small amounts of the drugs from Schedule II along with acetaminophen or aspirin, such as acetaminophen with codeine (Tylenol #3 or #4) and aspirin/butalbital/caffeine (Fiorinal)<br>Other drugs include anabolic steroids such as testosterone preparations and sodium oxybate (Xyrem), a drug that contains GHB for use with the sleep disorder narcolepsy |
| IV | Low potential for abuse relative to the drugs or substances in Schedule III<br>Currently accepted medical use for treatment<br>Abuse may lead to limited physical dependence or psychological dependence relative to the drugs or substances in Schedule III | Includes diet drugs containing propionic acid<br>Other well-known drugs include benzodiazepines such as lorazepam (Ativan), flurazepam (Dalmane), diazepam (Valium), midazolam (Versed), and alprazolam (Xanax) and the following: chloral hydrate, paraldehyde, pentazocine (Talwin), phenobarbital |
| V | Low potential for abuse relative to the drugs or substances in Schedule IV<br>Currently accepted medical use<br>Abuse may lead to limited physical dependence or psychological dependence relative to the drugs or substances in Schedule IV | Includes cough preparations containing small amounts of codeine and drugs for diarrhea that also contain small amounts of opioids, such as diphenoxylate with atropine (Lomotil) |

From U.S. Drug Enforcement Administration (DEA), Title 21 U.S.C. Section 812.

Opioids (narcotics) are scheduled drugs, and all of them must be counted during every shift. Records must be kept for every dose given. Agency policy determines which nurses will be held responsible for handing over the control of controlled substances from one shift to the next and for counting and securing controlled substances. All controlled substances that are ordered for a patient but not used during the hospital stay are sent back to the pharmacy when the patient is discharged.

Nurses may never borrow a drug ordered for one patient to use for another patient, and they may never use these drugs for themselves. In a time when drug abuse is so common, the nurse who has responsibility for the controlled substances must remain alert. With about 8% to 15% of healthcare professionals having a history of substance abuse, there is a risk for drug diversion. Some potential clues for identifying drug diversion include a pattern of drugs frequently being "dropped" or "spilled" or unrelieved pain in patients who received large or more frequent doses of drugs. As a nurse, you must know the federal, state, and agency rules about giving any type of drug, including controlled substances. The rules that govern controlled substances are very clear and very strict. If you violate the controlled substance laws, you may be punished by a fine, a prison sentence, or both. Nurses with drug abuse problems can temporarily or permanently lose their license to practice. Nurses have an ethical and a legal responsibility to report suspected drug diversion. In most states, the state board of nursing has a program to help nurses with substance abuse that affects their ability to carry out their nursing duties.

*Distribution of Controlled Substances and Drugs.* Federal and state laws and institutional policies are clear about how controlled substances are handled in hospitals and other agencies. The goal of all regulations and policies is to verify and account for all controlled substances. In some cases, a paper-based system may be used. When controlled substances, particularly opioids (narcotics), are ordered from the pharmacy, they come in single-dose units or prefilled syringes and are attached to a special inventory count sheet. The nurse receiving the order from the pharmacy must inspect the drug and return to the pharmacy a signed record stating that all of the drug ordered was received and correct as verified by two nurses. As each drug is used, it must be accounted for on the inventory sheet by the nurse giving the drug. The use of opioids (narcotics) is carefully monitored on the unit. Controlled substances are stored in a special double-locked cabinet. The keys to this cabinet are kept in a locked box with code access or carried by the charge nurse or a nurse responsible for accounting for opioids (narcotics) on the unit. The nurses who are responsible for the narcotics key has the legal responsibility for overseeing the use and recording of

all opioids during a shift, regardless of whether he or she personally gives the drugs to the patients.

There are also automated drug dispensing systems such as the Pyxis. These systems may include dispensing of opioids, routinely stocked drugs, and drugs specifically prescribed for individual patients. Nurses withdraw drugs by giving a password or fingerprint instead of using a key to open a locked cabinet. One issue to note is that drug orders can be overridden in the Pyxis under specific circumstances, such as when an emergency verbal order is received from the provider. A record is kept of what is ordered and used for patients in these circumstances, but overriding drug orders can result in critical drug errors if not done carefully.

When controlled substances are ordered for a patient, the nurse who will give the drug first checks the order, dosage, and last time the drug was given before obtaining the controlled substance. All nurses giving controlled substances must officially sign out all the controlled drugs given during the shift. The agency's inventory report is completed before the drug is removed from the cabinet or Pyxis. This report may be in the form of a written document, or a patient's barcode may be used instead. The report form should include the patient's name, date, drug, dosage, and signature of the nurse giving the drug. A follow-up note about the patient's response to the drug may also be required. If a dose is ordered that is smaller than that provided (so that some of the drug must be discarded) or the drug is accidentally dropped, contaminated, spilled, or otherwise made unusable and unreturnable, *two nurses* must sign the inventory report and describe the situation. Institutional policy may require additional actions.

If a key or keys are used to access controlled substances in a cabinet, at the end of each shift the responsibility for the keys is transferred to another authorized nurse from the new shift. Keys or electronic access to controlled substances are never given to physicians or any other unauthorized healthcare worker. The contents of the locked cabinet are counted together by one nurse from each shift. The numbers of each ampule, tablet, and prefilled syringe in the cabinet must match the numbers listed on the inventory report form. Sealed packages are kept sealed. Opened drug packages must each be inspected and counted. Prefilled syringes must be examined to make sure they all have the same color, the same fluid levels, and the same amounts of air within them. Both nurses must sign the inventory report, officially stating that the records and inventory are accurate at that time.

Occasionally, the inventory and the written report do not agree. Any disagreement between the number of remaining doses and the number listed in the inventory report must be explained. All nurses who have access to the cabinet keys or the locked Pyxis must be asked about the controlled substances they have given.

Steps must be retraced to see if someone forgot to record any drug. Patient charts can also be checked to see if a controlled substance was given that was not signed for on the inventory report. If errors in the report cannot be found, both the pharmacy and the nursing service office must be notified, and an investigation is opened to determine if drug diversion has occurred. Depending on the type and magnitude of the issue, the institution or agency administrator and security police also may be contacted.

### Top Tip for Safety

**CONTROLLED SUBSTANCES**

Verify all orders for controlled substances. Only authorized nurses can be responsible for access to and delivery of controlled substances, and for the LPN/LVN, this authority may differ between states and provinces. Follow all regulatory policies and procedures for safety and security of controlled substances. Report any suspicious findings that may point to possible drug diversion.

## Prescription Drugs

In the United States, the safety and effectiveness of prescription drugs are regulated by the Federal Prescription Drug Marketing Act (1987), and it is the responsibility of the Food and Drug Administration (FDA) to decide which drugs will require a prescription to be obtained. This regulation is in place to prevent prescription drug misuse and abuse. The ability to write prescriptions is provided to only a few healthcare professionals (e.g., physicians, dentists, nurse practitioners, physician assistants).

Misuse or abuse of prescription drugs can lead to adverse drug events, including those caused by dangerous drug interactions. The most commonly abused prescription drugs include narcotics (opioids) and drugs given for sleep or anxiety disorders.

The Omnibus Budget Reconciliation Acts of 1989, 1990, and 1991 placed further controls on drugs for Medicare or older adult patients. According to one study, as many as 15% of older adults are at risk for potentially major drug–drug interactions. Older patients are at high risk for problems with prescription drugs. They may not take the drug properly because of poor eyesight, memory, or coordination; they may take many drugs that interact with each other; or they may have chronic diseases that interfere with how the drug works.

Medicare Plan D provides coverage of some types of drugs for those who pay for this insurance option. More and more, insurance and government groups that pay for drugs limit the types and numbers of drugs that may be ordered to those on a "preferred" drug list. The preferred drug list may require the use of cheaper generic drugs to control costs because new or brand-name drugs usually are more expensive. Many drugs are not FDA approved as safe and effective for children or pregnant women. Prescription drugs make up most of the drugs given to patients in assisted living centers, nursing homes, or hospitals. Prescription drugs are carefully tested for safety and effectiveness before they are put on the market. However, even though much may be known about a particular drug, each patient can have different reactions to it. You must know the expected and adverse effects of drugs given to your patients and watch for signs that the drug is working the way it should. Any adverse reactions that may develop must be reported to the ordering provider. Patients often take several drugs at the same time, and the interaction among the drugs may make it hard to tell how each drug affects the patient, making your nursing knowledge of these drugs a critical part of safe nursing practice.

### Over-the-Counter Drugs

The FDA has also found that many drugs are safe enough not to need a prescription. These drugs are known as over-the-counter (OTC) drugs. OTC drugs are used to treat many common minor problems, such as colds, allergies, headaches, minor burns, constipation, or upset stomach. These drugs may be purchased easily at a drugstore or pharmacy. They are often the first thing patients try before they go to the doctor. Although OTC drugs are widely available, they are not without some risk. Like all drugs, some OTC drugs may produce adverse effects in some patients. There is also the possibility of adverse drug or food interactions or harm caused by excessive doses. Patients should be taught to read the drug facts label that is included with all OTC products and to consult with their pharmacist or other healthcare provider if they have additional questions concerning OTC drug use.

Accidental overdoses of common cold drugs in children have occurred because of confusion by parents about the correct dosage to give, and these drugs are no longer recommended for use in pediatric patients. Studies have shown that 40% of parents give their children incorrect dosages of liquid drugs. Cold and allergy products that contain pseudoephedrine and can be used to make illegal drugs are now stored behind the pharmacy counter and are sold in limited quantities. OTC drugs that are given in assisted living centers, nursing homes, and hospitals require a legal prescriber's order before they are given. Without an order in these settings, patients cannot take even the OTC drugs they brought with them.

### CANADIAN DRUG LEGISLATION

The Health Products and Food Branch of Canada's Department of National Health and Welfare is like the FDA of the US Department of Health and Human Services. This branch is responsible for the administration and enforcement of federal laws such as the Food and Drugs Act, the Proprietary or Patent Medicine

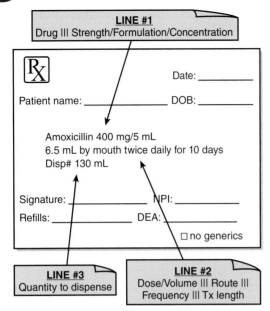

**LINE #1**
Drug III Strength/Formulation/Concentration

Rx

Date: _____

Patient name: _____ DOB: _____

Amoxicillin 400 mg/5 mL
6.5 mL by mouth twice daily for 10 days
Disp# 130 mL

Signature: _____ NPI: _____

Refills: _____ DEA: _____

☐ no generics

**LINE #3**
Quantity to dispense

**LINE #2**
Dose/Volume III Route III
Frequency III Tx length

Fig. 2.1 Example of a valid prescription.

Act, and the Controlled Drugs and Substances Act. These acts, together with provincial acts and regulations that cover the sale of drugs and those that cover the healthcare professions, are designed to protect the Canadian consumer from health hazards; misleading ads about drugs, cosmetics, and devices; and impure food and drugs. The Canadian Food and Drugs Act divides drugs into various categories. Regulations covering the various categories or schedules of drugs differ from those in the United States. There are three major classes of drugs under the Food and Drugs Act: nonprescription drugs, prescription drugs, and restricted drugs.

The Proprietary or Patent Medicine Act provides for a class of products that may be sold to the general public by anyone. The drug formula is proprietary (a trade secret); it is not found in the official drug manuals or printed on the label. The formulas for all such proprietary nonpharmacologic drugs must be registered, and a license must be issued under the Proprietary or Patent Medicine Act. The nurse needs to be aware of patients taking such drugs in the case of possible drug interactions.

The Canadian Controlled Drugs and Substances Act covers the possession, sale, manufacture, production, and distribution of opioids (narcotics) in Canada. Only authorized people may have opioids in their possession. All people authorized to be in possession of an opioid must keep a record of the names and quantities of all opioids dispensed, and they must ensure their safekeeping. Nurses are in violation of this act if they are guilty of illegal possession of opioids.

OTC drugs are regulated in Canada by the Canadian Food and Drugs Act. These drugs can be purchased without a prescription, but there are rules about packaging, labeling, and dispensing of the drugs. Nurses

must be aware of the risks these drugs have and watch for possible adverse effects and interactions with other drugs. OTC drugs available in Canada differ from those available in the United States.

## THE DRUG ORDER

### LEGAL PRESCRIPTIONS

Both state law and agency policy require that all drugs given in hospitals and long-term care facilities must be ordered by licensed healthcare providers acting within their scope of practice. This generally restricts prescriptive authority (the authority to write an order or prescription for drugs) to licensed physicians, dentists, nurse practitioners, nurse midwives, nurse anesthetists, and physician assistants. Providers who write the prescriptions are also called *prescribers*. Prescriptions for a hospitalized patient are written in the specified area of a patient's chart or recorded in the electronic record, and the pharmacy is notified. In some agencies, the order must be transcribed or rewritten by an authorized individual onto a special pharmacy order form, which is then sent to the pharmacy. Assisted living facilities and long-term care facilities may have providers who evaluate the patients and order or issue recurring orders for patient drugs. Every time a patient has a prescription filled, the pharmacy is required to give information about the drug and how it is to be given.

A legal prescription order must contain:
- Patient's full name
- Date
- Name of drug
- Route of administration
- Dose
- Frequency
- Duration
- Signature of prescriber

Additional details about how to give the drug may also be written—for example, "Take with meals," "Avoid milk products with this drug," "(number of) refills available," "May cause drowsiness," or "Please label." Pharmacies also require the patient's age and address on the prescription. This information may help the pharmacist ensure the right drug dosage for the patient (e.g., child, older adult) and verify the patient's identity (Fig. 2.1).

In emergencies or if the provider is not available on site, a *verbal order*, usually over the telephone, may be given. All agencies that employ nurses have policies about verbal orders. The agency decides who is authorized to take, transcribe, and implement verbal orders. The nurse taking the order is responsible for writing the order on the order form in the medical record, including the name of the nurse and the name of the prescriber. Many institutions also require that a note be written to indicate that the order was read back to the prescriber for validation. The prescriber must then cosign the order, usually within 24 hours, for it to be valid. The receiving and transcribing of verbal telephone orders may be the responsibility of the registered nurse (RN). *It is your responsibility as an LPN/ VN to be very familiar with the verbal order policy of the institution where you are practicing.*

## TYPES OF DRUG ORDERS

Drug orders are classified into one of four types: the standing order, the emergency or stat order, the single order, and the as needed or PRN order.

A **standing drug order** indicates that the drug is to be given until discontinued or for a certain number of doses. Hospital or institutional policy usually dictates that most standing orders expire after a certain number of days. A renewal order, such as the following, must then be written by the prescriber before the drug may be continued:
- amoxicillin 500 mg orally every 8 hours for 10 days
- ibuprofen 600 mg orally every 6 hours prn

An **emergency or stat drug order** is a one-time order to be given immediately, such as the following:
- diphenhydramine 50 mg IV stat

A **single drug order** is a one-time order, such as the following, to be given at a specified time:
- cefazolin 1 g IV at 10:00 a.m. before surgery

An **as needed or PRN drug order** is an order for a drug to be given as needed based on a nurse's judgment of safety and patient need, such as the following:
- docusate 100 mg orally at bedtime as needed for constipation

## STATE LAW AND HEALTHCARE AGENCY POLICIES

Although many regulations about giving drugs come from federal laws, details about who may prescribe and who may give drugs are set by each individual state. This authority is spelled out for nurses in the **Nurse Practice Act** of each state and can be found at the National Council of State Boards of Nursing Web site.

| Bookmark This! |

National Council of State Boards of Nursing:
https://www.ncsbn.org/npa.htm

Differences in practice from state to state make it essential that nurses learn what is legal regarding drug administration and that they make sure they abide by the rules and regulations. Because nurses may move from state to state, they must know exactly what is in the Nurse Practice Act of each state where they are licensed to work. Nurses often move between jobs, and some states recognize the nursing license of another state through an agreement called the *Nurse Licensure Compact*. There is a growing list of states that participate in the compact (available at https://www.ncsbn .org).

State rules about nursing practice often list the basic or minimum standards of practice. Agency or institutional policies and guidelines may be more specific or more restrictive than state Nurse Practice Acts. Agencies that employ nurses must provide written policy statements about the educational preparation for nurses permitted to give drugs and an orientation to particular policies, procedures, and recordkeeping rules of the agency. When you accept a nursing job, it is implied that you are willing to obey the policies or procedures of that institution. It may be an agency's policy to require employment for a certain period, completion of special orientation and training sessions, and passage of a probation period before a nurse is permitted to give drugs. Even when you have the legal authority to give drugs, a valid drug order signed by an authorized prescriber is needed.

Giving drugs is a responsibility reserved for nurses who are named by law to give drugs and who can document the appropriate educational preparation to do so. Nurses who give drugs to patients accept **professional responsibility** for giving drugs correctly, ethically, and legally. This means nurses must accept *ethical and legal* responsibility for good judgment and actions in drug administration and monitoring the effects of drugs given. Agencies expect nurses to carry out the steps of the nursing process, and you are responsible for good assessment, planning, implementation, and evaluation of the patient when drugs are given. You will be held responsible for failure to perform any of these steps well.

### Medication Technician or Aides

More than half the states have recognized the role of medication technician or aide in the giving of drugs to patients under the supervision of a licensed nurse. Medication technicians or aides are unlicensed assistive personnel who may obtain certification by taking the Medication Aide Certification Exam. As unlicensed assistive personnel, the medication technician or aide must hold the Certified Nurse Assistant/Aide (CNA) credential, complete a state-approved Medication Assistant program, and meet all other state requirements to become registered, which includes a written competency examination and may, in some instances, include a clinical competency evaluation. The responsibilities of a medication technician or aide include the preparation, distribution, and monitoring of the effects of a patient's prescribed drugs. A national survey of 3,455 medication aides (Budden, 2012) found that medication technicians or aides were asked to perform duties for which they were not trained, such as calling physicians to change medication orders, giving controlled drugs, and making decisions about giving or not giving insulin. These activities are all beyond the scope of an aide because they require assessment skills and nursing judgment. As an LPN/LVN, you are responsible for the supervision of medication technicians or aides as they carry out their duties regarding administering drugs to patients under your care.

### The *9 Rights of Drug Administration*

The nursing process is a helpful system to be used when giving drugs. There is a professional requirement and an implied ethical and legal requirement that nurses use this process. You must learn information about the patient's medical diagnosis, medical history, current symptoms, allergies, and current drugs taken. You are responsible for learning about all your patients' prescribed drugs, including the dosage, route of administration, expected response, adverse reactions, and the monitoring needed to ensure that the drug is working as it should and to observe for drug interactions. You are also responsible for following all laws and agency policies that are related to giving drugs, including the *9 Rights of Drug Administration* (Table 2.2). You also are responsible for teaching the patient and the family what they need to know for continued and safe administration of this drug.

## DRUG ADMINISTRATION SYSTEMS

One critical nursing responsibility is to check that the drug orders for your patient are correct. You may need to confirm the order you have (using a drug Kardex or other paper drug system or using the electronic medical record [EMR] in a computerized system) against the original order by the provider. Every agency has its own drug order, distribution, and recording system for the patient's health record. Agency policy will tell you what information is to be placed in each section. After you give the drug or drugs ordered, you must record all required drug administration information.

An EMR system is a software platform that allows the electronic entry, storage, and maintenance of digital medical data. Integrated within an EMR, many facilities now use a barcoded drug administration system to allow drug orders to be sent to the pharmacy when they are written; the drugs are sent to the patient's room or floor, and the drug is then taken to the patient's bedside. The patient's barcoded wristband and the barcode on each drug are scanned by the nurse using a handheld device (Fig. 2.2). This ensures that the right patient is getting the right drug as noted in the drug order. As the patient is observed taking the drug, the nurse notes that the drug has been given and the chart is electronically updated with this information.

An EMR and an integrated barcoded drug system have several advantages. The use of a computer to create the record prevents illegible clinician handwriting, a common cause of drug errors. These systems also avoid having orders transcribed several times as they are sent to the pharmacy, given to the nurse, and so on; this results in fewer errors. Many systems are designed to indicate whether the dose ordered by the clinician is out of the acceptable dosage range or would interact

| **Table 2.2** | **The *9 Rights of Drug Administration*** |
|---|---|
| **RIGHT PATIENT** | **CHECK THE PATIENT'S NAME USING TWO METHODS TO IDENTIFY THE PATIENT.** |
| Right drug | Check drug order. Check drug label. |
| Right dose | Check drug order. Confirm drug dose is appropriate. |
| Right route | Confirm the drug can be given by the route ordered. Confirm the patient can take or receive the drug by the route ordered. |
| Right time | Confirm the times the drug is ordered are correct. Check for correct time before giving the drug. Check the last time the drug was given. |
| Right reason | Confirm the reason or need for the drug. |
| Right documentation | Document drug administration after the drug is given. Chart the time, route, and any other specific information as necessary. |
| Right response | Confirm the drug has had the desired effect. Document any monitoring needed or adverse effects as needed. |
| Right to refuse | The patient has a right to refuse any prescribed drug. |

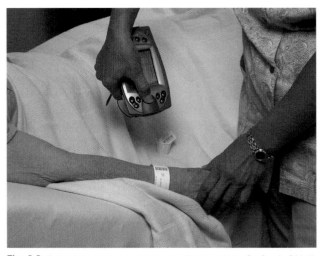

Fig. 2.2 Electronic scan of wristband. (From deWit, S. C., & ONeill, P. (2014). *Fundamental concepts and skills for nursing* (4th ed.). Saunders.)

with another ordered drug, whether there are other dosing errors, or if the patient has a recorded allergy to a prescribed drug.

### KARDEX AND ELECTRONIC DRUG SYSTEMS

The Kardex is a pen-and-paper, flip-file card system that has been used for many years. It contains

**MEDICATION KARDEX**

PRN MEDICATIONS

| Order date initials | Expir. date | Medication dose/frequency/route | Doses given | | |
|---|---|---|---|---|---|
| | | | Date | | |
| | | | Time | | |
| | | | Initials | | |
| | | | Date | | |
| | | | Time | | |
| | | | Initials | | |
| | | | Date | | |
| | | | Time | | |
| | | | Initials | | |
| | | | Date | | |
| | | | Time | | |
| | | | Initials | | |
| | | | Date | | |
| | | | Time | | |
| | | | Initials | | |
| | | | Date | | |
| | | | Time | | |
| | | | Initials | | |
| | | | Date | | |
| | | | Time | | |
| | | | Initials | | |
| | | | Date | | |
| | | | Time | | |
| | | | Initials | | |
| | | | Date | | |
| | | | Time | | |
| | | | Initials | | |
| | | | Date | | |
| | | | Time | | |
| | | | Initials | | |

**IM Injection Site Code**
1. Rt. posterior gluteal
2. Lt. posterior gluteal
3. Rt. anterior gluteal
4. Lt. anterior gluteal
5. Rt. anterolateral thigh
6. Lt. anterolateral thigh
7. Rt. deltoid
8. Lt. deltoid

Indicate the number of the site used with each IM dose given.

Record site with time.

Signatures/Initials

_____
_____
_____
_____
_____
_____
_____
_____
_____
_____
_____
_____

ALLERGIES _____        DIAGNOSIS _____

ROOM NO. _____   NAME _____   DOCTOR _____   AGE _____

Fig. 2.3 An example of a Kardex drug card.

important patient information and the physician's orders. It is regularly updated and changed to reflect current orders. This format keeps important information about the patient easily available for all team members. When a unit-dose system is used, all drugs are listed in the Kardex or drug profile sheet (Fig. 2.3).

 **Memory Jogger**

In every organization, the patient has either a paper or an electronic chart or record. The chart or record's content and format depend on the type of healthcare organization. You are required to document all drug administration according to the agency policy. You are also required to record the patient's response to the drugs given and any adverse effects.

Pyxis (BD Pyxis MedStation) is another type of drug delivery system. The Pyxis is an automated drug dispensing system that provides computer-controlled storage, dispensing, and tracking of prescribed drugs. These automated systems are thought to improve efficiency in giving drugs while ensuring patient safety (Fig. 2.4)

## DRUG ERRORS

The National Coordinating Council for Medication Error Reporting and Prevention (NCC MERP) defines a medication or drug error as any preventable event that may cause or lead to inappropriate medication use or patient harm while the medication is in the control of a healthcare provider, patient, or consumer. Drug or medication errors are costly to patients who as a result suffer adverse effects or even death. Organizations pay a financial price for drug errors that occur. Every drug error that is prevented saves the agency approximately $7,000. Drug errors can occur at any of three points in the drug administration process: (1) preparing the drug, (2) bringing the drug to the patient, and (3) giving the drug to the patient. Studies have pointed to the fast pace of current clinical practice, lower staffing levels, multitasking, and interruptions during the process of preparing and giving drugs as potential causes of drug errors. Efforts to minimize interruptions during all three points of drug administration can reduce errors.

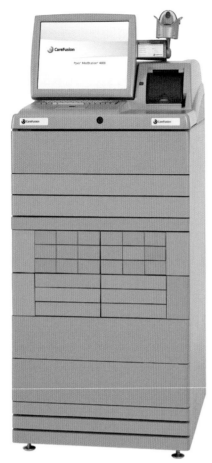

Fig. 2.4 An example of a Pyxis MedStation. (Courtesy and © Becton, Dickinson and Company.)

**? Did You Know?**

These are the three most common points where drug errors are made:
- Preparing the drug
- Bringing the drug to the patient
- Giving the drug to the patient

Each agency has policies and procedures that cover what to do when a drug error is made. Treating drug errors with blame and fear may lead to fewer nurses reporting errors when they occur. Nurses have an ethical responsibility to report drug errors because of possible harm to the patient. Regardless of whether the nurse thinks the error may result in harm to the patient, all errors must be reported. If you suspect an error was made, immediately check the patient, notify the healthcare provider promptly, and follow any orders the provider gives to reduce the effect of the drug error. It is critical to watch the patient's condition by measuring vital signs, drawing blood for tests, or using any other method ordered by the provider. Also notify the nursing supervisor and fill out all agency-required reports.

After the reports are made, an investigation into how and why the error occurred will be conducted. The investigation will include how similar errors might be avoided in the future and will consider any training of the nursing staff that may be needed. Consequences of drug errors vary and are often related to how severe the error was and whether the patient was harmed. If the nurse was careless or negligent, she or he may be held professionally and/or legally liable. Although almost every nurse has made one drug error, repeated errors will not be ignored. Research in each institution helps determine whether the mistakes made in that institution are most commonly caused by a "system error," a unique mistake, failure to follow the *9 Rights of Drug Administration*, or deliberate wrongdoing.

In 2000, the Institute of Medicine (IOM) published a very important report, entitled *To Err Is Human* (IOM, 2000), about the number of errors made in medical care. Estimates suggest that adverse events, which include medical errors, occur in 3% to 4% of patients. The IOM report and other studies have calculated that the costs of medical errors in the United States, including lost income, disability, and the need for additional healthcare, may be between $17 billion and $136.8 billion or more annually. These costs come from a variety of drug-related problems, including patient compliance issues and medical or drug errors. Unfortunately, estimates suggest that more than half of the adverse medical events each year are caused by medical errors that could be prevented. In response to this report, most agencies have tightened ways to report and follow up on drug errors, and some improvement has been confirmed in the most recent studies.

In response to this landmark report, the development and use of healthcare technology have contributed to reducing drug errors. In addition to barcode administration systems, computerized order entry systems work to prevent drug errors by guiding the prescriber to the preferred drug dosages, route, and frequency of administration. Clinical decision support systems are integrated into the EMR and provide the prescriber with notifications, clinical guidelines to guide treatments, and disease-specific drug orders (Alotaibi & Federico, 2017). Nurses must make every effort to follow agency policies and work to minimize interruptions to prevent drug errors.

An independent, not-for-profit organization, The Joint Commission (TJC), accredits and certifies almost 21,000 healthcare organizations and programs in the United States. TJC accreditation and certification are recognized nationwide as symbols of quality that reflect an organization's commitment to meeting certain performance standards. To cut down on drug errors, TJC has discouraged healthcare workers from using any abbreviations that might lead to confusion. Certain abbreviations that were used in the past—such as "hs" for nighttime, "cc" for cubic centimeter, "QD" for daily, and "QOD" for every other day—are no longer used in hospitals that wish to maintain their accreditation. Table 2.3 lists TJCs official "Do Not Use" abbreviations.

| Table **2.3**    The Joint Commission's Official "Do Not Use" List[a] | | |
| --- | --- | --- |
| **DO NOT USE** | **POTENTIAL PROBLEM** | **USE INSTEAD** |
| U, u (unit) | Mistaken for "0" (zero), the number "4" (four), or "cc" | Write "unit" |
| IU (International Unit) | Mistaken for IV (intravenous) or the number 10 (ten) | Write "International Unit" |
| Q.D., QD, q.d., qd (daily) <br> Q.O.D., QOD, q.o.d., qod (every other day) | Mistaken for each other <br> Period after the Q mistaken for "I" and the "O" mistaken for "I" | Write "daily" <br> Write "every other day" |
| Trailing zero (X.0 mg)>* <br> Lack of leading zero (.X mg) | Decimal point is missed | Write X mg <br> Write 0.X mg |
| MS <br> $MSO_4$ and $MgSO_4$ | Can mean morphine sulfate or magnesium sulfate <br> Confused for one another | Write "morphine sulfate" <br> Write "magnesium sulfate" |

*Exception: A "trailing zero" may be used only where required to demonstrate the level of precision of the value being reported, such as for laboratory results, imaging studies that report size of lesions, or catheter/tube sizes. It may not be used in medication orders or other medication-related documentation.
Adapted from The Joint Commission. (2019). *Facts about the Official "Do Not Use" List of Abbreviations.* https://www.jointcommission.org/resources/news-and-multimedia/fact-sheets/facts-about-do-not-use-list/

 **Bookmark This!**

**INSTITUTE FOR SAFE MEDICAL PRACTICES LIST OF ABBREVIATIONS, SYMBOLS, AND DOSE DESIGNATIONS**
https://www.ismp.org/tools/errorproneabbreviations.pdf
   Another list of dangerous abbreviations can be found at http://www.nccmerp.org/dangerous-abbreviations.

## HIGH-ALERT DRUGS

A small category of drugs has a high risk of harm when associated with a drug error. They are called **high-alert drugs** because the consequences of the errors are very serious. A high-alert drug can cause harm to the patient who receives it in error (was not prescribed to receive it) and to those who receive too high a dose, receive too low a dose, or do not actually receive a prescribed dose. High-alert drugs are often packaged, stored, and given differently than others. Some agencies may require extra steps in the drug procedures before high-alert drugs are given.

Categories of common high-alert drugs can be remembered using the acronym PINCH. **P** is for potassium, **I** is for insulin, **N** is for narcotics (opioids), **C** is for cancer chemotherapy drugs, and **H** is for heparin or any drug type that interferes with blood clotting. Information about high-alert drugs in hospital, community, and long-term care settings can be found online (https://www.ismp.org/recommendations).

 **Memory Jogger**

High-alert drug groups are *p*otassium, *i*nsulin, *n*arcotics, *c*ancer chemotherapy agents, *h*eparin, and all other drugs that have interference with blood clotting as their main effect.

## BLACK BOX DESIGNATION

An additional way that some drugs are categorized is by their ability to harm the person taking them. Some drugs are assigned a **black box warning** by the FDA. This means that the drug has a higher-than-normal risk for causing serious and even life-threatening problems in addition to its positive benefits for some people. A black-bordered box is found on the drug insert sheet and may be included on the patient instruction sheet provided by some pharmacies. Fig. 2.5 shows an example of a black box warning. Prescribers must take extra care in deciding whether to prescribe a drug that has a black box warning. The patient should be made aware of the potential problems the drug can cause. When you give a drug that carries a black box warning, you will need to monitor the patient even more closely than usual for possible problems.

## MEDICATION RECONCILIATION

Medication (drug) reconciliation is the practice of comparing the patient's drug orders to all of the drugs that the patient has been taking. By doing so, you can avoid drug errors caused by wrong dosages, duplication of drugs, and leaving out a drug. Medication or drug reconciliation becomes most important during *transitional care*, leaving one healthcare setting for another. For example, the patient is transferred from long-term care to the hospital or is discharged to home. Reports suggest that effective transitional care can reduce the risk of readmission within 30 days of discharge by up to 50% (Polinski et al., 2016). Most medication errors come from lack of communication between healthcare providers during transitions of care.

The role of the nurse in medication reconciliation includes a review of all medications, identifying and reporting any discrepancies in the list of patient drugs, and providing medication education and support to patient and family. When the nurse compares the list of current drugs to the list of prescribed drugs, this list should include all OTC drugs, herbal supplements and vitamins, and prescription drugs the patient takes on a daily basis. Nurses should teach patients to carry their

```
WARNING: RISK OF THYROID C-CELL TUMORS
See full prescribing information for complete boxed warning.
• Liraglutide causes thyroid C-cell tumors at clinically relevant
  exposures in rodents. It is unknown whether Victoza causes
  thyroid C-cell tumors, including medullary thyroid carcinoma
  (MTC), in humans, as human relevance could not be
  determined by clinical or nonclinical studies (5.1).
• Victoza is contraindicated in patients with a personal or family
  history of MTC or in patients with Multiple Endocrine Neoplasia
  syndrome type 2 (MEN 2) (5.1).
```

Fig. 2.5 An example of a black box warning. This warning was included in the Victoza package insert. (From Novo Nordisk. (2010). *A black box warning*. https://www.accessdata.fda.gov/drugsatfda_docs/label/2010/022341lbl.pdf.)

most recent drug list with them to all healthcare provider appointments and to update this list as changes are made.

## PROTECTION OF HEALTHCARE WORKERS

Safe work practices are needed to prevent the exposure of nurses and other healthcare workers to potential infection or injury. This issue became very apparent during the recent COVID-19 pandemic when personal protective equipment (PPE) became less available, potentially exposing healthcare workers to respiratory infection with COVID-19 before vaccines became available. The World Health Organization (WHO) called for the development and implementation of national programs for occupational health for healthcare workers in line with national occupational health and safety policies. The appropriate PPE should be provided as determined by the risk for infection as it relates to drug administration, including masks, gowns, gloves, and eye shielding.

In addition, unsafe clinical practices, such as recapping of syringe needles, can result in needlestick injuries and exposure to bloodborne pathogens. Needlestick injuries expose nurses to serious infectious diseases such as hepatitis B, hepatitis C, and human immunodeficiency virus (HIV) infection. Regulations require hospitals to have a written plan for reducing the risk for needlestick injuries among healthcare workers. Employers are required to provide the safest equipment available, regardless of cost. Such equipment includes needleless products and equipment with engineering controls that have built-in safety features to reduce risk. Sharps disposal units must be available in areas where needed. If a needlestick injury does occur, it must be carefully recorded in the agency's needlestick injury documentation system. The exposure control plan, selection of safety products, and needlestick injury documentation system must be reviewed at least once every year.

> **⚠ Safety Alert!**
>
> Safe disposal of drugs is a primary concern for the health and safety of the population. The following tips are used for the safe disposal of prescription drugs:
> • Follow the disposal directions on the drug packaging or insert.
> • Unless directed, do not flush drugs down the toilet because they can pollute the environment.
> • Bring unused or expired drugs to a local drug take-back program.
> • Consult with a pharmacist about drug disposal guidelines.

## Get Ready for the Next-Generation NCLEX® Examination!

### Key Points

• You are legally required to exercise judgment and responsibility in carrying out drug administration.
• Follow the agency's policy and the state's Nurse Practice Act as it pertains to supervision of medication technicians or aides.
• Know the scope of your practice for drug administration as defined by your state's Nurse Practice Act.
• Always verify orders for all drugs to be given.
• Always account for all controlled substances prescribed for and given to patients.

• Be aware of using unapproved abbreviations in transcribing drug orders for administration.
• Document all drugs given to a patient according to agency policy.
• Assess for and document the patient's responses to drugs you have given.
• Use extreme caution in preparing and giving high-alert drugs.
• Follow all clinical guidelines and agency policies to reduce drug errors and prevent injury to healthcare personnel.
• Use approved methods for disposing or returning unused drugs.

## Clinical Judgment and Next-Generation NCLEX® Examination-Style Questions

1. The nurse who is responsible for the narcotics count is reviewing the institution policy with a new employee regarding the nursing responsibilities for controlled substances.

   **Instructions: Complete the following sentences by choosing the option for the missing information that best corresponds with the numbered list of options provided below.**

   Controlled substances are stored in _____**1**_____. The nurse responsible for controlled substances has the legal responsibility for _____**2**_____. All nurses giving controlled substances must _____**3**_____.

   | OPTION 1 | OPTION 2 | OPTION 3 |
   |----------|----------|----------|
   | The pharmacy<br>A double-locked cabinet<br>Each patient's medication drawer | Overseeing the use and recording of all opioids<br>Giving all needed opioids during the shift<br>Counting all of the opioids used at the end of the shift | Ask the charge nurse to sign out the narcotics given<br>Never discard unused controlled substances<br>Sign out all the controlled drugs given during the shift |

2. Which of the following scenarios may be a sign of possible drug diversion on a unit? **Select all or any that apply.**

   1. A patient is dissatisfied with the drug administration schedule.
   2. A patient receiving oral antibiotics has an excess number of pills.
   3. A patient is unaware that the nurse mixed a drug in applesauce.
   4. A patient receiving opioids reports increased pain.
   5. A nurse reports that the narcotic count is inaccurate.
   6. A patient brings his pain medication from home to the hospital.

3. Which of the following is an example of a standing drug order?

   1. Ketorolac 30 mg IV before surgery
   2. Amoxicillin/clavulanate 825/125 mg by mouth every 12 hours for 10 days
   3. Benadryl 50 mg by mouth stat
   4. Ibuprofen 800 mg by mouth every 8 hours as needed

4. Which drug is classified as a Schedule II controlled substance?

   1. Mescaline
   2. Morphine
   3. Pentazocine
   4. Tylenol #3

5. Which action is most likely to ensure that you are giving the right drug to the right patient?

   1. Checking the patient's bed number
   2. Asking the patient if he is Mr. Jones
   3. Asking the patient if he has taken this drug before
   4. Checking the name on the patient's wristband

6. Which information is required for a prescription to be legal? **Select all or any that apply.**

   1. Patient's name
   2. The instruction "Take with meals"
   3. Prescriber's signature
   4. How often the drug is to be taken
   5. When to notify the prescriber
   6. Drug dose
   7. Name of the pharmacist
   8. Route of administration
   9. How long to take the drug

7. What is the most important action to perform after giving a patient a drug that has a black box designation?

   1. Report the event as a drug error.
   2. Observe the patient closely for an adverse reaction.
   3. Be sure to sign out the drug according to agency policy.
   4. Remind the patient to stay in bed for 2 hours after receiving the drug.

A nurse is caring for the client in the emergency department and reviews the client's history and physical, nurse's notes, flowsheet, orders, and imaging studies.

### History and Physical
### 1500

A 38-year-old female client presents to the emergency department after a motor vehicle accident. The client has a right upper arm air cast in place.
Physical Exam:
General: uncomfortable, tearful
Respiratory: breath sounds clear bilaterally
Cardiovascular: tachycardic, regular rhythm
Musculoskeletal: right arm immobilized, deformity noted; crepitus with palpation with soft tissue damage and an external wound noted to the right upper arm; capillary refill < 3 seconds
Skin: approximately 1 inch (2.5 cm) external wound noted to the right upper arm
Home Medications: None
Allergies: NKDA

### 1540

Provider at the bedside evaluating the client. Orders received.

### Nurse's Notes
### 1540

Provider at the bedside evaluating the client. Orders received.

### Flow Sheet
### 1500

Blood Pressure: 108/68 mm Hg
Heart Rate: 104/min
Respiratory Rate: 20/min
Temperature: 98.6°F (37°C)
Pain score: 7/10

### 1530

Blood Pressure: 98/64 mm Hg
Heart Rate: 108/min
Respiratory Rate: 20/min
Temperature: 98.6°F (37°C)
Pain score: 10/10

### Orders
### 1545

Cefazolin 1 g IV BID x 3 days
Morphine 4 mg IV every 4 hours PRN pain
Normal saline 0.9% 1000 mL IV bolus STAT
Tetanus immunization IM today at 1800

### Imaging Studies
### 1520

Right arm x-ray: transverse humerus fracture with significant localized edema and hematoma formation with soft tissue damage

Choose the most likely options for the information missing from the statement(s) by selecting from the lists of options provided.

The nurse should first _____1_____ and then _____2_____.

| OPTIONS FOR 1 | OPTIONS FOR 2 |
| --- | --- |
| Administer the client's immunization | Administer the client's pain medication |
| Assess the client's allergies | Report the suspected drug diversion |
| Administer the normal saline | Initiate a peripheral IV |
| Administer the client's antibiotics | Use the override process in the Pyxis MedStation to obtain the client's pain medication |

See answer on Evolve at http://evolve.elsevier.com/Visovsky/LPNpharmacology/.

# Principles of Pharmacology

## Learning Outcomes

1. Define the keywords used in pharmacology and drug administration.
2. Explain the differences between the chemical, generic, and brand names of drugs.
3. Compare the drug actions of agonists, partial agonists, and antagonists.
4. Describe the four basic physiologic processes that affect drug actions in the body.
5. Explain the differences between side effects and adverse effects.
6. Discuss personal factors that influence drug therapy.
7. Describe how drugs affect persons at different lifespan stages.

## Key Terms

**absorption** Drugs enter the body and pass into the circulation to reach the parts of the body they need to affect through the processes of diffusion, osmosis, and filtration.

**additive effect** Occurs when giving two drugs together either makes one of the drugs stronger or makes the action of the two drugs more powerful.

**adverse reaction** Severe symptoms or problems that can cause great harm.

**agonist** A drug that works by activating or unlocking cell receptors, causing the same actions as the body's own chemicals.

**allergy** An antigen–antibody response that can cause hives, rashes, itching, or swelling.

**anaphylactic reaction** A severe, life-threatening form of an allergic reaction.

**antagonist** A drug that attaches at a drug receptor site but does not activate or unlock the receptor.

**bioequivalent** Drug products that are chemically the same or identical.

**biotransformation** The transformation or altering of a drug into either active or inactive chemicals after it has been absorbed.

**brand name** The proprietary name that a manufacturer gives to a specific drug. Also known as a *trade name*.

**buccal** (route) Drug placement against the inner cheek.

**chemical names** The names of the chemicals that actually form the drug.

**desired action** The drug does what it is supposed to do.

**distribution** Movement of a drug in the body to reach its site of action by way of the blood and lymph systems.

**drug interaction** When one drug changes the action of another drug.

**enteral** (route) Giving a drug by way of the gastrointestinal system oral, feeding tube, sublingual, or rectal.

**excretion** The process by which waste products are eliminated from the body.

**first-pass (effect)** After they are consumed, drugs are inactivated in the liver before being distributed to other parts of the body.

**generic name** The most common drug name, used by the manufacturer in all countries; also known as the *nonproprietary name*.

**half-life** The time it takes the body to remove 50% of the drug from the body.

**hepatotoxic** Adverse drug effects that can result in liver damage.

**hypersensitivity** An exaggerated response to a drug. An allergy is an example of a hypersensitive response.

**idiosyncratic response** A response to a drug that is peculiar and unpredicted.

**intramuscular (IM)** (route) Giving a drug by way of an injection deep into the muscle.

**intravenous (IV)** (route) Giving a drug by way of an injection into a vein or into tubing that is connected to a catheter that is inserted into a vein.

**metabolism** Physical and chemical reactions that happen inside the body and either build up or break down compounds.

**nephrotoxic** Adverse drug effects that can result in kidney damage.

**paradoxical effect** An effect that is opposite to the effect that would normally be expected.

**parenteral** Giving a drug by way of an injection or infusion underneath the skin.

**partial agonist** A drug that attaches to the receptor site but produces only a partial effect rather than a full (agonist) effect.

**percutaneous** (route) Giving a drug by way of absorption through the skin. Topical creams, patches, and devices under the skin are common examples. Also known as *nonparenteral*.

**pharmacodynamics** The effects of a drug on body functions (what a drug does to the body).

**pharmacokinetics** The metabolism of a drug within the body (what the body does to a drug).

**pharmacotherapeutics** The use of drugs in the treatment of disease.

**prodrug** A drug that must be metabolized before it is active.

**receptor site** Small, locklike areas of cell membranes that control what substances either enter the cell or change its activity.

**side effect** Mild but annoying responses to a drug. Nausea and headache are common and usual side effects to many drugs.

**solubility** The ability of a drug to dissolve in body fluids.

**subcutaneous** (route) Drug placement into fatty tissue.

**sublingual** (route) Drug placement under the tongue.

**synergistic effect** The effect of two drugs taken at the same time is greater than the sum of the effects of each drug given alone.

**topical** (route) Application of a drug directly to the area of the skin that requires treatment; the most common forms are creams, lotions, and ointments.

**trade name (TRĀD)** The proprietary name that a manufacturer gives to a specific drug. Also known as a brand name.

## INTRODUCTION

This chapter provides an overview of very basic information from chemistry, physics, anatomy, and physiology that explains the action of drugs in the body (**pharmacokinetics**, or what the body does to a drug). This involves the processes of absorption, distribution, metabolism/biotransformation, and excretion. It also covers basic information on the effects of drugs on body functions (**pharmacodynamics**, or what the drug does to the body). This information is vital in understanding **pharmacotherapeutics**, or the use of drugs in the treatment of disease.

## DRUG NAMES

Drugs have several different names that may be confusing when you first learn to work with drugs. It is very important to know the different names of a drug so that the wrong drug is not given to a patient. Sometimes a drug is ordered by one name and the pharmacist labels it with another name for the same drug. For example, Valium (trade name) is also known as diazepam, its generic name. It is also common that one trade name drug is substituted for another trade name in the pharmacy. For example, Atarax and Vistaril are two different trade names (brand names) of hydroxyzine (generic name) made by two different manufacturers. When one drug name is ordered and a drug with another name is supplied, it is important for you to know whether the drug is the same or a different drug.

The most common drug name used is the generic name. This is the name the drug manufacturer uses for the drug, and it is the same in all countries. The generic name is also called the *nonproprietary name*—it is the name given to a drug before there is any specific trade name or when the drug has been available for many years and more than one company makes the drug. Examples are ibuprofen and acetaminophen. The American Pharmaceutical Association, the American Medical Association, and the US Adopted Names Council assign generic names. Generic names are not capitalized when written. It is becoming common in hospitals, extended care facilities, and other settings for drugs to be ordered by their generic names.

The trade name, or brand name, is the proprietary name or the name for the drug manufactured by one company. This name is often followed by the symbol ®, which indicates that the name is registered to a specific drug maker or owner and no one else can use that name for a drug. This is the drug name used in advertisements. It is often descriptive, easy to spell, or catchy sounding so that prescribers will remember it easily and be more likely to use it. The first letter of a trade name is capitalized. Examples of trade names are Motrin, Tylenol, and Mylanta.

Chemical names are often difficult to remember because they include all of the chemicals that make up the drug. These names are usually long and hyphenated, and they describe the atomic or molecular structure of the drug. An example is ethyl 1-methyl-4-phenylisonipecotate hydrochloride, the chemical name for meperidine (Demerol). The chemical name is rarely, if ever, used by nurses or physicians and does not need to be remembered for safe drug administration.

## DRUG ATTACHMENT

Drugs take part in chemical reactions that change the way the body acts. They do this most commonly when the drug forms a chemical bond at specific sites on body cells. **Receptor sites** are small, locklike areas of cell membranes that control what substances either enter the cell or change its activity (Fig. 3.1). The chemical reactions between a drug and a receptor site are possible only when the receptor site and the drug can fit together like pieces of a jigsaw puzzle or a key fitting into a lock. Drugs that activate or unlock receptors and have the same actions as the body's own chemicals are known as receptor **agonists**. Here is an example: The drug morphine (key) activates the opiate receptors (lock) and produces analgesia (pain relief). In the body, deep breathing (key) triggers the same opiate receptors (lock) to release the body's own endorphins to decrease pain. (You can teach patients to use this technique to decrease pain.)

Some drugs attach to the receptor site but produce only a partial effect. Thus these drugs are called **partial agonists**. An example of a partial agonist is buspirone (BuSpar). When the drug is given, it partially locks into the serotonin receptors and helps relieve anxiety and depression. Although buspirone can be used alone, it is frequently used to boost the effects of other drugs for depression (such as Prozac) that are full serotonin agonists.

When a drug attaches at a drug receptor site but does not activate or unlock it, there is no increase in cell activity, and the drug is called an **antagonist**. An important feature of an antagonist is that as long as the antagonist is attached to a receptor site, agonists cannot bind there. This antagonist effect blocks the action of agonists. An example of an antagonist is naloxone (Narcan). In an opiate overdose, naloxone is given to completely reverse the effects of the opiate that otherwise would bind to the opiate receptor sites.

The Memory Jogger box summarizes the various types of receptor site activity, and this is key information to memorize and understand.

 **Memory Jogger**

*Agonist:* Drug attaches at the receptor site and activates the receptor; the drug has an action similar to that of the body's own chemicals.

*Antagonist:* Drug attaches at the receptor site, but no chemical drug response is produced, and the drug prevents activation of the receptor.

*Partial agonist:* Drug attaches at the receptor site, but only a slight chemical action is produced.

## BASIC DRUG PROCESSES

Drugs must be changed chemically in the body to become usable. Four basic processes are involved in drug utilization in the body: absorption, distribution, metabolism, and excretion. Drugs have different characteristics, or pharmacokinetics, that

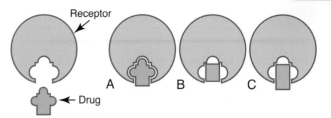

FIG. 3.1 Possible drug receptor actions. (A) Complete attachment as in an agonist. (B) An attachment that does not give a response or blocks a response as in an antagonist. (C) A small response as in a partial agonist. (From Clayton, B. D., & Willihnganz, M. J. (2017). *Basic pharmacology for nurses* (17th ed.). Elsevier.)

determine to what extent these processes will be used. To safely give and monitor how a drug works in a patient's body, it is important for you to understand each of these processes for the specific drug or drugs prescribed.

## ABSORPTION

**Absorption** is the way a drug enters the body and passes into the circulation to reach the part of the body it needs to affect. Absorption takes place through processes of diffusion, filtration, and osmosis (Box 3.1). These three mechanisms use passive transport to move molecules across a semipermeable membrane from an area of high concentration to an area of low concentration by way of kinetic energy (energy produced by the simple back-and-forth movement of the molecules). Many drugs pass into the circulation in this way.

Sometimes molecules must move up a gradient from an area of low concentration to an area of high concentration. Moving molecules up a gradient requires greater energy. This energy need is supplied by adenosine triphosphate (ATP) molecules, which store and provide energy to all the cells in the body. An example of active transport is the way in which the sodium-potassium pump functions in the heart. The heart uses electrical conductivity to produce a heartbeat in order for a cardiac contraction to occur. When the heart muscle is at rest, sodium ($Na^+$) stays on the outside of the cell and potassium ($K^+$) stays on the inside of the cell. When the heart contracts, the sodium-potassium pump moves $Na^+$ inside the cell and $K^+$ outside the cell. When the heart muscle relaxes again in order to fill the heart chambers with blood before the next contraction, the pump moves $Na^+$ back outside the cell and $K^+$ back inside the cell. A drug that affects this pump is the drug digoxin (Lanoxin). One action of digoxin is to decrease the activity of the ATP enzymes. When the ATP enzymes that give the pump energy are hindered, the movement of $Na^+$ and $K^+$ molecules across the cell membrane is inhibited, resulting in a slower heart rate. This is why it is so important to check the heart rate of patients who take digoxin.

| Box 3.1 | Mechanisms Involved in Absorption | |
|---|---|---|

| **DIFFUSION** | **OSMOSIS** | **FILTRATION** |
|---|---|---|
| Diffusion is the tendency of the molecules of a substance (gas, liquid, or solid) to move through a semipermeable membrane from an area of high concentration to one of lower concentration. A tea bag placed in hot water is an example of diffusion. | Osmosis is the diffusion of fluid through a semipermeable membrane; the flow is primarily from the thicker or more concentrated solution to the thinner or less concentrated solution. Dialysis removes waste products from the blood in this way. | Filtration is the passage of a substance through a filter or through a material that prevents passage of certain molecules. An example of filtration is brewing coffee using a filter containing coffee grounds. Water passes through the filter, but the grounds do not. |
| 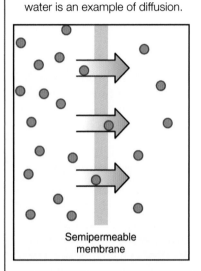 | 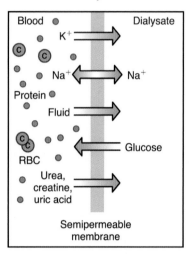 | 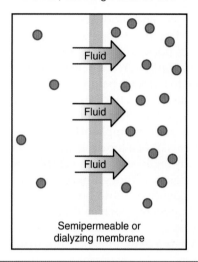 |
| Semipermeable membrane | Semipermeable membrane | Semipermeable or dialyzing membrane |

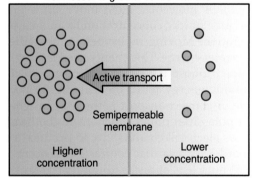

ActiveTransport
Moves molecules up the gradient
from lesser to greater concentrations

FIG. 3.2 Active transport moves molecules up the gradient from lesser to greater concentrations. This process is helped by enzymes and requires energy.

The mechanisms of absorption are illustrated and explained in Box 3.1 (passive transport) and Fig. 3.2 (active transport). How fast the drug is absorbed into the body through these processes depends on how easily the drug dissolves, how the drug is introduced into the body (by mouth or by injection), and whether there is good blood flow through the tissue where the drug is located.

All drugs must be dissolved in body fluid before they can enter body tissues. The ability of the drug to dissolve is called solubility. To achieve the best possible action, sometimes the drug must be dissolved quickly; at other times it should be dissolved slowly. Solubility is often controlled by the form of the drug. For example, liquids are more soluble than capsules or tablets because a liquid is absorbed faster than a tablet or capsule, which first must be dissolved. An injection with an oil base must be chemically changed before absorption can take place; this delay in absorption holds the drug in the tissues longer, which may be the desired action, especially if it is an antibiotic. When your patient takes water with a tablet, it not only helps in swallowing but also helps dissolve the drug. That is why a full glass of water should be given with oral drugs unless the patient has a health problem that requires fluid restriction.

The route of administration also influences absorption. Drugs can be given in many different ways: by an enteral route via the mouth (orally), through a nasogastric or feeding tube, or rectally; by a parenteral route via injection underneath the skin, into the fat (subcutaneous), into the muscle (intramuscular [IM]), into the cerebrospinal fluid (epidural), or into the bloodstream (intravenous [IV]); on top of the skin (topical or percutaneous); under the tongue (sublingual); against the cheek (buccal); or by way of breathing (inhalation).

In areas where the blood flow through tissues is very high, drugs are rapidly absorbed. The IV route delivers drugs directly into the bloodstream, and the drugs are immediately distributed to the tissues. Muscles (IM), under the tongue (sublingual), inside the nose (intranasal), and inside the lungs (inhalation) are areas that have very high blood flow, and drugs given by these routes begin to work very quickly. Fig. 3.3 shows the action of drugs in the body from the fastest to the slowest onset.

## DISTRIBUTION

After a drug enters the body's circulation, it must reach the organ or tissues where it will have its action. Movement of a drug in the body toward its site of action is its **distribution**. Distribution occurs by way of the blood and lymph systems. Distribution of the drug is usually uneven because of differences in how much blood is able to penetrate the tissue (perfusion), the type of tissue (bone, fat, or muscle), and how easy it is for the drug to penetrate the cell membranes. For example, tissues in the placenta and in the brain make it difficult for drug molecules to pass through. Some drugs can bind together with various blood substances and proteins such as albumin. This binding allows only "free" drug (that which is not bound) to penetrate the tissues.

Some drugs are attracted to tissues other than the target receptor sites. For example, drugs that dissolve easily in lipids (fats) prefer adipose tissue (fat tissue), and stores of the drug may build up in these areas. Eventually this buildup of the drug in the fat cells will be released, making the effect of the drug last a long time. Diazepam (Valium), an antianxiety agent, is a highly lipophilic (fat-loving) drug, and its sedative effects last much longer than those of lorazepam (Ativan), a less lipophilic antianxiety agent.

## METABOLISM

Once a drug is absorbed and distributed in the body, the body transforms or alters the drug into active or inactive chemicals. This process, known as **biotransformation**, happens in various sites in the body but mainly in the liver, where enzymes break down the chemicals that make up the drug into its usable and unusable parts. Drugs that are known as **prodrugs** have to be transformed and activated by these enzymes before they can be used by the body. Liver disease may impair the transformation of the inactive form of a prodrug into an active form of the drug.

Drugs move very quickly from the stomach or small intestines to the liver. Much of the drug is then inactivated on its **first pass** through the liver before it can be distributed to other parts of the body. That is why some drugs are given sublingually or intravenously; otherwise the drug would be inactivated and patients would not receive the amount of drug they require. How a drug is given may affect how much

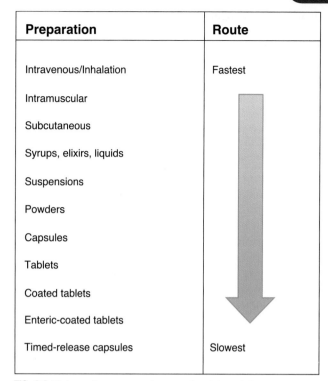

| Preparation | Route |
|---|---|
| Intravenous/Inhalation | Fastest |
| Intramuscular | |
| Subcutaneous | |
| Syrups, elixirs, liquids | |
| Suspensions | |
| Powders | |
| Capsules | |
| Tablets | |
| Coated tablets | |
| Enteric-coated tablets | |
| Timed-release capsules | Slowest |

**FIG. 3.3** Various drug preparations are listed from fastest to slowest onset based on drug absorption and availability.

of it is needed. (For example, only 1 mg of propranolol [Inderal] is required intravenously, but 40 mg is required when the drug is given by mouth because so much is inactivated during the first pass through the liver.)

Genetic differences in the enzyme pathways in the liver also explain why people respond differently to a drug. Some people grow tolerant to the drug and seem to need larger doses, but others are sensitive to the drug and need only a small dose. These liver enzyme pathways, known as the *cytochrome P-450 system*, are produced by the cytochrome P-450 genes and play an important role in adverse drug reactions (ADRs), especially when several drugs are taken at the same time or when there are drug–food interactions. Individual genetic differences in the enzyme pathways cause different patients to respond differently to the same drug. An example is abacavir (Ziagen)/lamivudine (Dovato), which is a drug used with other antiretrovirals when treating HIV infection. A percentage of patients taking abacavir suffer very severe side effects. Genetic testing can be done on individuals prior to prescribing this drug.

## EXCRETION OR ELIMINATION

All *metabolites*, including inactive chemicals, chemical by-products, and waste, finally break down through **metabolism** and are removed from the body through the process of **excretion**. Fibrous or insoluble waste is usually passed through the gastrointestinal (GI) tract and excreted as feces. Chemicals that can be made water-soluble are dissolved and filtered out as they pass through the kidneys and then are lost in the urine. Some chemicals are exhaled from the lungs through breathing or lost through evaporation from the skin during sweating. Very small amounts of drug may also escape in tears, saliva, or the milk of breast-feeding mothers. This process is why penicillin, asparagus, and nicotine can sometimes be smelled in the urine or alcohol can be smelled on the sweat and breath of someone who has consumed large amounts of beer or whiskey. If the patient has poorly functioning kidneys, water-soluble metabolites may build up in the body and become toxic if they cannot be excreted in the urine, which is why it is so important for you to monitor the urine function of very ill patients.

The major processes involved in drug utilization in the body are shown in Fig. 3.4. These four processes are basic to understanding how drugs are used in the body. If you understand these four processes well, you will be able to understand many of the ways in which drugs differ from each other. When you understand how drugs are used in the body, you will be better able to identify when patients experience toxic or ill effects of drugs on the body. You should watch a patient closely after he or she takes a drug to see the response to the drug. This is especially important the first time the patient takes the drug, whenever there are changes in the patient's condition or diet, or when other drugs are introduced into the medical regimen.

> **Memory Jogger**
>
> **PROCESS OF PHARMACOKINETICS**
> **A**bsorption
> **D**istribution
> **M**etabolism
> **E**xcretion

> **? Did You Know?**
>
> Grapefruit juice affects (usually reduces) the absorption of many drugs, such as antihistamines, cholesterol-lowering drugs, HIV drugs, and transplantation drugs.

Some drugs enter and leave the body very quickly; other drugs remain for a long time. The standard method of describing how long it takes to metabolize and excrete a drug is the **half-life**, or the time it takes for 50% of the drug to be removed from the body. Usually, patients have similar rates of metabolism and excretion for a given drug, so the half-life helps explain the dose (how much drug should be taken), the frequency (how often it should be taken), and the duration (how long it will last). If a drug has a long half-life, it may need to be taken only once a day. If a person takes too much drug with a long half-life, an adverse reaction may occur because the action of the drug lasts for such a long time. If the half-life of a drug is short, such as for many antibiotics, the person must take frequent doses to keep the correct level in the blood. If a person's liver or kidneys do not function correctly, a drug may not be properly metabolized or excreted and higher doses of the drug will circulate for a longer time and produce symptoms of overdosage. For this reason, drugs are often dosed based on kidney and liver function, which is why blood is drawn for kidney and liver function tests (blood work).

Some drugs such as narcotics and antihypertensive drugs come in an extended-release (ER) or long-acting (LA) form for ease of administration. Many of these drug names end in –*contin* or include the terms *ER* or *LA*.

> **Top Tip for Safety**
>
> Long-acting or extended-release drugs ***must never be crushed, chewed, opened (if a capsule), or cut*** because this will result in an overdosage.

## DRUG ACTIONS

When a drug is given to a patient, it is usually possible to predict the chemical reaction that will result. However, because each patient is different, some unexpected chemical reactions are also possible. With each patient, giving a drug is somewhat of an experiment, so watching patients closely to monitor their reaction to the drug is an important role of the nurse. This is most important the first time a patient is given a newly prescribed drug.

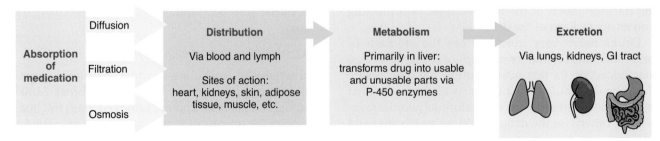

FIG. 3.4 Processes of absorption, distribution, metabolism, and excretion. *GI*, Gastrointestinal.

The expected response of the drug is called the **desired action**. This is when the drug does what is desired and the therapeutic goal is reached—for example, a fentanyl patch (Duragesic) relieves pain.

Because a drug may influence many body systems at the same time, the effect of the drug is often not restricted to the desired action. Other actions, called *side effects* or *adverse reactions*, may also take place. **Side effects** are usually seen as mild but annoying responses to the drug. Side effects are expected effects. For example, a drug used to relieve pain may make the patient very sleepy. Certain side effects, such as nausea, may be avoided if the dosage is reduced or the drug is given with food or a full glass of water. Some side effects are such a problem that the drug must be changed or stopped; examples are insomnia (inability to sleep) and fainting (syncope). Expected side effects that are very common are usually related to the GI system: nausea, constipation, and diarrhea.

**Adverse reactions**, or adverse effects, imply more severe symptoms or problems that develop because of the drug. Some adverse effects may require the patient to be hospitalized or may even be life-threatening. Examples include a necrotic skin condition called *Stevens-Johnson syndrome* and anaphylactic shock. If severe adverse effects such as damage to the kidney (**nephrotoxic** drug), damage to the liver (**hepatotoxic** drug), or bleeding develop, often the drug must be stopped. You, as a nurse, are on the front line to notice if and when an adverse reaction occurs, and you are responsible for the well-being of your patients.

Occasionally a patient has a drug reaction that is a surprise. Strange, unique, peculiar, or unpredicted responses to drugs are called **idiosyncratic responses**. These reactions may be the result of missing or defective metabolic enzymes caused by a genetic or hormonal variation in that individual. They often produce either an unexpected result, such as pain or bleeding, or an overresponse to the drug. These types of reactions are usually rare. One type of idiosyncratic response is called a *paradoxical effect*. In this situation, the patient's reaction may be just the opposite of what would be expected. For example, diphenhydramine (Benadryl) is an antihistamine with sedative (sleep-inducing) effects. This drug is in many over-the-counter (OTC) sleep aids such as Motrin PM. Instead of sedation, some people have a **paradoxical response** and remain awake and excited.

A second type of unexpected reaction is an increased reaction to a drug (**hypersensitivity**) or a sensitivity caused by an antibody response to a drug (**allergy**). Some drugs (sulfa products, aspirin, penicillin) and some conditions (asthma) are more likely to produce allergic reactions than others. Allergic reactions usually occur when an individual has taken a drug and the body has developed antibodies to it. When the patient takes the drug again, the antigen–antibody reaction produces hives, rash, itching, or swelling of the skin.

This type of allergic reaction is very common, so ask all patients about whether they have ever had a drug reaction. Patients with an allergy to one drug may be more likely to develop an allergy to another drug, but individuals may also develop a reaction to drugs they have taken before without problems or drugs they have been taking for a long time and only now show signs of an allergy.

**? Did You Know?**

Allergic reactions to antibiotics can happen even the first time a patient takes a drug because he or she may have been previously exposed to the antibiotic in milk or meat from livestock fed antibiotics.

Occasionally an allergic reaction is so severe that the patient has trouble breathing and the heart may stop. This life-threatening response is called an **anaphylactic reaction**. A patient who has a mild allergic reaction to a drug is much more likely to develop the more severe anaphylactic reaction if the drug is given again. An anaphylactic reaction is a true medical emergency because the patient may suffer severe breathing problems, including swelling of the lips, throat, and trachea, that prevent air from entering the lungs.

**Top Tip for Safety**

Always warn patients who have anaphylactic reactions about their allergy so they will not take the drug again. Teach them to wear a medical alert bracelet or necklace or carry identification about their allergy. Some patients may need to carry an adrenaline (epinephrine)-filled syringe that they can use to inject themselves to prevent anaphylaxis when symptoms begin.

Patients often confuse an allergy with side effects, both of which may produce unpleasant symptoms. If a patient reports an "allergy" to a drug, make sure you ask the right questions to understand the exact past reaction to the drug. If the patient had nausea or stomach pain when taking aspirin, that is a side effect but not an allergy. If the patient reported sedation when taking an antihypertensive drug, that also is not an allergy. Because patients often do not understand the difference between an allergy and a side effect, it is important for you to clarify the difference when patients say they have had an allergic reaction.

 **Memory Jogger**

The following are possible types of drug actions and responses:
- Desired effect
- Side effect
- Adverse effect or reaction
- Idiosyncratic response
- Paradoxical reaction
- Allergic (hypersensitivity) response
- Anaphylactic reaction

## BIOEQUIVALENCE

After a new drug enters the market, an exclusive patent protects the financial interests of the drug company for some time, usually 17 years, by limiting other companies from producing that drug. After the patent ends, other companies may make the same drug under a generic name. Brand name drugs are usually more expensive than generic drugs because the maker of the brand name drug is attempting to recover the huge sums of money spent on research and drug development. Generic products are often less expensive because they do not face those costs.

Drug products seen as identical with respect to their active ingredients are known as *generic equivalents*. However, slight differences in processing or formulation may mean that the action of the generic drug in the body is slightly different from that of the brand name product. These differences most commonly cause variations in absorption, distribution, or metabolism. The product called for in a prescription may vary according to what specific brand the pharmacist dispenses. Some generic-equivalent products are chemically the same or identical to the brand name product and are therefore bioequivalent. Bioequivalence may be particularly important for some cardiac or antiseizure drugs. An example is a prescription or an order written for Lanoxin, a trade name for digoxin. If the pharmacy dispenses a generic brand that is not considered bioequivalent, then the product may not have the same action as Lanoxin in the body.

## DRUG INTERACTIONS

When one drug changes the action of another drug, a drug interaction is present. These reactions often take place during the process of metabolism (or biotransformation) in the liver and are a result of the cytochrome P-450 enzyme pathways each person inherits genetically from his or her parents. The actions of a number of drugs may be altered when they are taken with other drugs; examples include some antidepressants, respiratory drugs, anticlotting drugs, antibiotics, and opiates. Some drugs are given together on purpose because the combination produces an additive effect. The drugs work as a team, so to speak. For example, probenecid (Probalan) is given with penicillin to increase the amount of penicillin that is absorbed. This is called an additive effect. Other drug interactions produce adverse effects. For example, many antibiotics make birth control tablets less effective, and this makes it more likely a woman will get pregnant if she is sexually active while taking both drugs.

If one drug interferes with the action of another drug, it has an *antagonistic effect*. At times, one drug may replace another drug at a receptor site, decreasing the effect of the first drug (displacement). For example, flumazenil (Romazicon) is a drug that can be given to displace the effects of a sedative such as diazepam (Valium). Sometimes *incompatibility* occurs when drugs do not mix well chemically. Attempts to mix them together, especially in a syringe or IV solution, may cause a chemical reaction so that neither of the drugs can be given. Heparin is an example of such a drug. If heparin is mixed together in a syringe or an IV line with many drugs, a white, hazy precipitate will occur.

If the effect of two drugs taken at the same time is greater than the sum of the effects of each drug given alone, the drugs have a synergistic effect. For example, acetaminophen (Tylenol) is often given with codeine for added pain relief.

### Food, Alcohol, and Drug Interactions

Food, alcohol, and most drugs taken by mouth must travel through the liver to undergo chemical changes before they can be used by the body. The risk for drug interaction with food or alcohol is high because all of these products go through the liver. When taken together, food or alcohol and drugs may alter the body's ability to handle a particular food or drug. Part of these interactions may be caused by activation of the P-450 enzyme system or competition for receptor sites. One class of antidepressant drugs, the *monoamine oxidase inhibitors*, is noted for drug–food interactions. They cannot be taken with aged cheese, red wine, or many processed foods. Information every patient should know about possible drug interactions includes the following:

1. Cigarette smoking can decrease the effect of drugs or create other problems with some drugs by increasing their metabolism. Some antipsychotics, antidepressants, hypnotics, and anxiolytics can be affected by cigarette smoking. Blood concentration of these drugs can be decreased with smoking.
2. Caffeine, which is found in coffee, tea, some soft drinks, chocolate, and some drugs, can also affect the action of some drugs. Caffeine has enzyme-inducting capabilities and can lower plasma levels of acetaminophen, for example. Caffeine also increases urination, which can affect the excretion of drugs.
3. Drugs should never be taken during pregnancy or by a patient trying to get pregnant without the advice of the healthcare provider.
4. If the patient has any problem related to drugs, the healthcare provider or a pharmacist should be contacted immediately.
5. Some drugs are blocked from being absorbed by the body by grapefruit juice, fatty meals, milk products, or other drugs.

Some drugs or foods increase or decrease the action of the anticlotting drug warfarin (Coumadin) by increasing or decreasing the blood clotting time and can therefore increase the risk for stroke or heart attack. Other drugs might raise the blood pressure, increase vasoconstriction in tissues, or cause other vascular changes that can be harmful to the patient. Almost every drug has the potential to have an effect on other drugs the patient is receiving, so you will need to be aware of potential drug interactions as you learn about different drug categories.

The amount of alcohol use is very high in the US population. It has been estimated that approximately 70% of adults consume alcohol at least occasionally. Many patients may not be aware that alcohol is one of the products that react most commonly with drugs. The extent to which a drug dose reaches its site of action is called *availability*. Alcohol can influence whether a drug is effective by changing its availability.

It is estimated that alcohol–drug interactions may be a factor in at least 25% of all emergency department admissions. According to the National Institute on Alcohol Abuse and Alcoholism (NIAAA), more than 150 drugs have harmful additive or interactive effects when combined with alcohol. Narcotics, antianxiety agents, antidepressants, antihistamines, antihypertensive agents, and antibiotics are just a few of the drugs that will cause problems when combined with alcohol.

Older adults are more likely to suffer drug side effects compared with younger persons, and these effects tend to be more severe with advancing age.

### Personal Factors That Influence Drug Therapy

Some personal factors affect how effective drugs are for any specific patient. All drug therapy requires adequate hydration and blood flow for drugs to be distributed to target tissues. Therefore any problem that interferes with blood flow decreases drug effectiveness. Such problems include dehydration, overhydration, low blood pressure, shock, heart failure, and reduced blood flow to one or more body areas.

In addition to alcohol intake, use of other prescribed, OTC, or illicit drugs can often increase the activity of metabolic enzyme systems. This change increases the rate at which some drugs are deactivated and eliminated, often requiring that the doses be increased and/or given more frequently to be effective. For example, opioid drugs for pain are metabolized and eliminated much faster in a person who drinks alcohol on a daily basis, so the dose may need to be higher for that person to obtain pain relief.

Any person who has problems involving the liver or the kidneys will retain a drug for a much longer time, increasing the risk for adverse and toxic effects. If a patient has either liver dysfunction or kidney problems, dosages usually need to be reduced and the drug given less frequently.

Body size and lean-to-fat ratios also affect drug therapy responses. For many drugs, bigger people (adults or children) require larger dosages. Drug dosages are based on kilograms of body weight or on body surface area for children, as are dosages of drugs that are considered dangerous (e.g., heparin, chemotherapy drugs).

Ethnicity and genetic makeup can change the expected drug response. For example, many people of Asian descent have a greater-than-usual response to the anticoagulant drug warfarin, which greatly increases their risk for excessive bleeding, hemorrhage, and stroke. As a result, the starting dosage of warfarin is lower for Asians and is increased at a slower rate until the individual patient's response is known.

There is great variation in the activity of the P-450 enzyme system from one person to the next as a result of genetic differences. A person may be a rapid metabolizer of drugs and require higher-than-expected dosages to achieve the same desired effect. Another person may be a slow metabolizer and have more problems with side effects, adverse reactions, and toxic effects even from what are considered "normal" drug dosages.

These personal differences in drug therapy require all healthcare professionals to be aware of the possibility of unexpected patient responses. One size does NOT fit all when it comes to drug therapy. This is especially true for drugs that have a narrow therapeutic range, which means that the dose that is effective is very close to the dose that causes adverse and toxic reactions. You are on the front line of drug therapy to prevent, as well as to recognize, unexpected patient responses.

## DRUG THERAPY AND SPECIAL POPULATIONS

People respond to drugs differently at various lifespan stages. These differences are based on body size, water content, organ maturity, and general organ health.

### PEDIATRIC DRUG THERAPY CONSIDERATIONS

#### Overview

Childhood extends from birth to adolescence. During these years the processes of drug absorption, distribution, metabolism, and elimination continue to change. As children grow, total body water decreases (but is still greater than in an adult), body size increases, and body fat stores increase. Overall, body metabolism is highest in infants and slowly decreases as the child ages. However, healthy children have a higher metabolism than do adults. These normal changes alter a child's responses to drug therapy.

#### Drug Absorption

In neonates (less than 1 month of age), oral drugs are absorbed poorly from the GI tract because no gastric acid is present to help break down drugs, no intestinal bacteria or enzyme function is present to metabolize a drug, and the speed at which a drug moves through the stomach and intestines is slow. The effectiveness of oral drugs in this age group is not very predictable. In later infancy and childhood these factors change, making oral drugs more effective.

Absorption of IM injections is based on muscle mass and muscle blood flow. Neonates and infants have relatively small muscle mass and blood flow, which reduces IM absorption. In older children, muscle size and circulation in the muscles affect how rapidly a drug is absorbed. There is more rapid absorption from the deltoid muscle (shoulder and upper arm) than from the vastus lateralis muscle (thigh), and the slowest absorption is from the gluteal (buttock) muscle.

### Drug Distribution

Distribution of water-soluble drugs is faster and more widespread in neonates, infants, and younger children because of their high percentages of total body water. For older children and adolescents, distribution is affected by the lean-to-fat body mass ratio in the same way that it is for adults.

### Drug Metabolism

In neonates and infants, the systems that metabolize drugs in the liver are immature. As a result, prodrugs (drugs that must be metabolized before they are active) are slower to be activated and to become effective. For drugs that are active when absorbed, deactivation takes longer and drug levels can build up more quickly. This increases the risk for side effects, toxic effects, and overdosages in this age group.

Older infants and young children have higher metabolic rates and a rapid turnover of body water. This often results in greater drug dosage requirements per kilogram of body weight than in the adolescent or adult. Often these young children require more frequent drug dosing to maintain blood drug levels. For example, the dosing of digoxin (Lanoxin), a heart drug that can become toxic very easily (narrow therapeutic index), is four times higher in the neonate than in the adult.

During adolescent growth spurts, metabolism increases along with body weight. Drug dosages often must be increased at this time, especially for drugs that control seizure disorders.

### Drug Elimination

As with metabolism, the growth and maturity of a child's organs have important effects on the child's ability to excrete drugs, which changes expected drug responses. Preterm infants, neonates, and infants younger than 6 months have less mature kidneys that may not excrete drugs effectively. Careful monitoring of responses and blood drug levels are needed to determine the most effective dosages and scheduling of drug therapy.

### OLDER ADULT DRUG THERAPY CONSIDERATIONS

Older adult patients also react differently to drugs than younger persons. Drugs are absorbed, metabolized, and excreted more slowly and less completely in older adults. In adults older than 65 years, problems with drugs are often due to a lack of understanding of the way drugs are processed in the aging body and the body's changed response to drugs. To further complicate matters, people age differently, and their individual body systems may also age at different rates.

Many older adults with chronic illnesses take drugs daily. These drugs are helpful in controlling disease, but they also present a very real hazard to older adult patients. ADRs are common in older adults. Issues such as falls, hypotension, delirium, kidney failure, and bleeding are common clinical manifestations. Many of these issues can also be attributed to aging, which leads to ADRs being frequently overlooked in this population. You are the person most likely to notice ADRs and alert the prescriber to the possibility of the problem.

Because many older adult patients take several drugs, interactions among these different drugs may also cause problems for them. These patients may see several specialists, each of whom may prescribe different drugs. This is called *polypharmacy*. If the specialists do not know about all the different drugs a patient may be taking at the same time, the patient is at risk for adverse interactions.

All drugs have some risk or hazard, but those most dangerous to older adults are tranquilizers, sedatives, and other drugs that alter the mind and change what the patient thinks he or she sees or cause the patient to become dizzy or lose balance. Diuretics and cardiac drugs pose special dangers and must be given with caution and careful observation of how the patient responds. Older adult patients may become dehydrated easily, allowing the amount of drug in the blood to increase. This places them at greater risk for side effects and toxicity with normal dosages. Diuretics lead to an increase in urination, and this can lead to loss of electrolytes. Electrolytes are important for electrical energy in regard to all body functions, such as muscle contraction and nerve impulses, but particularly for the proper electrical function of the heart. Electrolyte levels must be monitored by blood tests, and electrolytes may have to be replaced if they are low.

### Drug Absorption

The overall importance of changes in the absorption of drugs with aging is not completely clear. There may be some delay in the absorption process. Physiologic changes that affect the GI tract include a reduction in acid output. The result is a more alkaline environment, which may affect drugs that require an acid medium for absorption. Reductions in blood flow, enzyme activity, gastric emptying, and bowel motility may delay the absorption of some drugs. Compounds such as iron, calcium, and some vitamins that depend on active transport mechanisms for absorption may be affected by the decreased blood flow in the aging patient's GI tract.

### Drug Distribution

The distribution of drugs in the body may also be affected by the aging process and is linked to the chemical makeup of the agent. There is a decline in total body water and lean body mass with aging that may result in less movement or distribution of water-soluble drugs into some tissues. If the dose of these drugs is not decreased, the patient may develop higher serum concentrations, leading to an increased effect or toxicity. The usual rule is to use a low dose when starting a drug and then increase the dose slowly in older adult patients. You should be mindful of the distribution of the drug you are giving so you can be alert to possible toxic effects.

The distribution of fat-soluble drugs may also be changed by the aging process. With aging, there is usually a decrease in lean body mass and an increase in total body fat. Lipid-soluble drugs may be stored in larger amounts in fat tissues and remain in the body for a longer time. This can cause problems with drug toxicity as well as safety issues for a patient.

Another important concern for some older adults is a decrease in serum proteins. When serum proteins are low, greater amounts of unbound drug may circulate and cause adverse or toxic reactions.

## Drug Metabolism

Overall, a decrease in liver mass occurs with age, along with a reduction in liver blood flow. When blood flow is reduced, less of the drug is metabolized, so increased amounts of the active form may remain in the blood.

In an aging liver, there also may be changes in the phases of metabolism during which certain chemical and molecular changes occur to prepare the drug for use in the body. The drug may stay in the body too long and/or not be eliminated.

Drugs that are metabolized by the liver may have less or reduced metabolism because of other changes in the liver and also because of the influence of various diseases. The aging liver often gets smaller, has less blood flow, is affected by changes in nutritional status, and may become overloaded with fluid from diseases such as chronic heart failure or chronic renal failure. These factors may result in a loss of the liver's ability to handle all the different chemicals it must process. In this situation, the patient may have more risk for adverse effects when drugs are added to the existing treatment plan.

## Drug Elimination

Kidney (renal) function is an important factor that causes ADRs. Changes in the aging kidney include a decreased number of nephrons; decreases in blood flow, glomerular filtration, and tubular secretion rate; and kidney damage. In addition, damage to the arterial walls of blood vessels and lowered cardiac output reduce the amount of blood that flows to the kidneys by 40% to 50%. The creatinine clearance rate is an estimated measure of how well the kidney is functioning. This rate decreases with age, which allows drugs

to remain in an older adult's system longer, increasing the risk for adverse and toxic effects.

Important factors to remember when caring for older adults who are taking drugs that will be excreted by the kidneys is that each patient may respond a little differently to the drug. The dosage ordered is adjusted by the prescriber based on the best creatinine clearance estimates, and low doses or longer intervals between doses are used if kidney damage is present. Drugs that depend on the kidneys for elimination include many antibiotics, some antiviral agents, anticancer drugs, antifungals, analgesics, and many cardiac drugs.

## PATIENT TEACHING CONSIDERATIONS

Many older adults require special teaching about how to take their prescription drugs and about the danger of taking nonprescription drugs at the same time. Failure of older adults to follow their drug therapy plan may be related to the cost of a drug, difficulty in getting it from a pharmacy, poor memory, lack of desire to take the drug regularly, depression, and/or feeling overwhelmed by the responsibility of taking care of oneself. In some cases, arthritis or another disease that causes physical disability may make it difficult to open bottle lids or use an inhaler. Poor eyesight may make it hard to draw up insulin or read labels accurately. Some older adults share drugs, and some may cut pills in half or skip doses without realizing that this action can interfere with the effectiveness of the drug.

## DRUG THERAPY CONSIDERATIONS DURING PREGNANCY AND LACTATION

Pregnant and breast-feeding women may have chronic diseases and/or acute problems that require drug therapy. In pregnancy, the drug is really going to two individuals, so how the drug may affect the growing fetus is a consideration. The benefit of any drug to a pregnant patient must be carefully weighed against the possible (or potential) risk to the fetus. It is important for pregnant women to avoid as many drugs as possible, especially those drugs with *teratogenic* potential (i.e., likely to cause malformations or damage in the embryo or fetus).

Many drugs have been confirmed as teratogenic in humans. The US Food and Drug Administration (FDA) has new guidelines for drug use during pregnancy. The pregnancy letter categories assigned to prescription drugs are being replaced by content that will create awareness of the risks involved in taking drugs during pregnancy. The new guidelines can be found at https://www.drugs.com/pregnancy-categories.html.

Factors such as what drug the mother takes, how much is taken, and the age of the fetus when the drug is taken are related to different types of malformations. Taking a drug during the first 2 weeks after conception (before implantation) results in an all-or-nothing effect: The ovum either dies of exposure to a lethal dose of a teratogen or recovers completely with no adverse effects. The critical period for teratogenic effects in humans lasts from about 2 to 10 weeks after the last menstrual period. This period is the time of organ development (14–56 days), during which any teratogenic drug taken by the mother may produce major abnormalities in the embryo. Taking a teratogen later in the pregnancy, during the fetal period (57 days to term), may result in minor structural changes, but abnormalities are more likely to involve problems with growth, mental development, and reproductive organ abnormalities. Clearly it would be best if women would stop taking all drugs before they got pregnant and not resume them until the baby is born. Always ask about the possibility of pregnancy when giving a drug to a woman of childbearing age.

As the fetus grows, most drugs and foods can cross the placental barrier from the mother to the baby. However, the reaction of a fetus to a drug is different from that of the mother. The immature blood–brain barrier fails to prevent many drugs from passing into the brain of the fetus. Immaturity of the liver means that the fetus does not metabolize drugs well.

Many drugs can pass into human breast milk, and this is also a major concern for the baby. Nicotine, cocaine, heroin, marijuana, and angel dust are examples of illicit drugs that pass into the breast milk.

If a mother is given a prescription while she is nursing, she can lessen the infant's drug exposure by taking the drug just before the infant is due to have a lengthy sleep period or immediately after a feeding. A bottle can then be substituted for the next scheduled feeding, and the affected breast milk can be expressed and discarded. Nevertheless, the infant should be watched for emotional changes, altered feeding habits, sleepiness, or restlessness. If short-term drug therapy is required, the mother may need to consider stopping breast-feeding for a short time and instead pumping and discarding her milk to maintain lactation until drug therapy is finished.

## DRUG CARDS

According to the FDA, there are over 19,000 drugs on the market, and new drugs are approved by the FDA

every day. The most frequently prescribed classes of drugs are analgesics, antidepressants, and antihyperlipidemic agents. By now you have realized how important it is for you to understand everything you can about the patient and the drug that you will be giving.

A good way to learn and remember drugs is to write drug cards on the most popular drugs, as well as any and all drugs you will give to a patient. A drug card should include both the trade and generic names of the drug, the dosage range, the desired action, expected side effects, adverse effects, how to give the drug, and lastly, important information that you will need to know before giving the drug. The golden rule of drug administration is to never give a patient a drug with which you are not fully familiar.

As you progress through the drug card text, you will notice that many drugs belong to a classification and that part of the drug's generic name provides a hint. For example, what do you notice about the suffix (ending of a word) of each generic drug mentioned in the following list?
- acebutolol (Sectral)
- atenolol (Tenormin)
- bisoprolol (Zebeta)
- metoprolol (Lopressor, Toprol XL)
- nadolol (Corgard)
- nebivolol (Bystolic)
- propranolol (Inderal)

All of these drugs are examples of a classification of antihypertensives known as beta-blockers. They all have the suffix -olol, and the way they work in the body is similar: They block the action of epinephrine at the body's beta-receptor sites. Beta-blockers are antagonist drugs. If epinephrine, a neurotransmitter in the body, cannot connect with a beta-receptor, the result will be a decreased heart rate and relaxation of the veins and arteries (vasodilation). Thus the desired action is to decrease the blood pressure. The dosage range and specific information for each of these drugs may differ, but they all work in the same way. The nurse may want to make one "classification" drug card listing all of the drugs included in that group to become acquainted with the drugs that belong in that classification. Table 3.1 provides a list of common suffixes and prefixes.

### Table 3.1   Common Generic Drug Prefixes and Suffixes

| PREFIX, ROOT, SUFFIX | EXAMPLES (GENERIC NAMES) | DRUG CLASS OR DRUG CATEGORY |
| --- | --- | --- |
| -afil | avanafil; sildenafil; tadalafil; vardenafil | phosphodiesterase (PDE) inhibitor |
| -asone | betamethasone; dexamethasone; diflorasone; fluticasone; mometasone | corticosteroid |
| -bicin | doxorubicin; epirubicin; idarubicin; valrubicin | antineoplastic; cytotoxic agent |
| -bital | butabarbital; butalbital; phenobarbital; secobarbital | barbiturate (sedative) |
| -caine | bupivacaine; lidocaine; mepivacaine; prilocaine; proparacaine | local anesthetic |
| cef-, ceph- | cefaclor; cefdinir; cefixime; cefprozil; cephalexin | cephalosporin antibiotic |

## Table 3.1  Common Generic Drug Prefixes and Suffixes—cont'd

| PREFIX, ROOT, SUFFIX | EXAMPLES (GENERIC NAMES) | DRUG CLASS OR DRUG CATEGORY |
| --- | --- | --- |
| -cillin | amoxicillin; ampicillin; dicloxacillin; nafcillin; oxacillin | penicillin antibiotic |
| -cort- | clocortolone; fludrocortisone; hydrocortisone | corticosteroid |
| -cycline | demeclocycline; doxycycline; minocycline; tetracycline | tetracycline antibiotic |
| -dazole | albendazole; mebendazole; metronidazole; tinidazole | anthelmintic; antibiotic; antibacterial |
| -dipine | amlodipine; felodipine; nifedipine; nimodipine; nisoldipine | calcium channel blocker |
| -dronate | alendronate; etidronate; ibandronate; risedronate | bisphosphonate (bone resorption inhibitor) |
| -eprazole | esomeprazole; omeprazole; rabeprazole | proton pump inhibitor (PPI) |
| -fenac | bromfenac; diclofenac; nepafenac | NSAID (nonsteroidal) |
| -floxacin | besifloxacin; ciprofloxacin; levofloxacin; moxifloxacin; ofloxacin | quinolone antibiotic |
| -gliptin | saxagliptin; sitagliptin; linagliptin | antidiabetic; inhibitor of the DPP-4 enzyme |
| -glitazone | pioglitazone; rosiglitazone; troglitazone | antidiabetic; thiazolidinedione (insulin sensitizer) |
| -iramine | brompheniramine; chlorpheniramine; pheniramine | antihistamine |
| -lamide | acetazolamide; brinzolamide; dorzolamide; methazolamide | carbonic anhydrase inhibitor |
| -mab | adalimumab; daclizumab; infliximab; omalizumab; trastuzumab | monoclonal antibody |
| -mustine | carmustine; estramustine; lomustine; bendamustine | alkylating agent (antineoplastic) |
| -mycin | azithromycin; clarithromycin; clindamycin; erythromycin | antibiotic; antibacterial |
| -nacin | darifenacin; solifenacin | muscarinic antagonist (anticholinergic) |
| -nazole | fluconazole; ketoconazole; miconazole; terconazole; tioconazole | antifungal |
| -olol | atenolol; metoprolol; nadolol; pindolol; propranolol; timolol | beta-blocker |
| -olone | fluocinolone; fluorometholone; prednisolone; triamcinolone | corticosteroid |
| -olone | nandrolone; oxandrolone; oxymetholone | anabolic steroid |
| -onide | budesonide; ciclesonide; desonide; fluocinonide; halcinonide | corticosteroid |
| -oprazole | dexlansoprazole; lansoprazole; pantoprazole | proton pump inhibitor (PPI) |
| -parin-; -parin | dalteparin; enoxaparin; fondaparinux; heparin; tinzaparin | antithrombotic; anticoagulant (blood thinner) |
| -phylline | aminophylline; dyphylline; oxtriphylline; theophylline | xanthine derivative (bronchodilator) |
| -pramine | clomipramine; desipramine; imipramine; trimipramine | tricyclic antidepressant (TCA) |
| -pred-; pred- | loteprednol; prednicarbate; prednisolone; prednisone | corticosteroid |
| -pril | benazepril; captopril; enalapril; lisinopril; moexipril; ramipril | ACE (angiotensin-converting-enzyme) inhibitor |
| -profen | fenoprofen; flurbiprofen; ibuprofen; ketoprofen | NSAID |
| -ridone | iloperidone; paliperidone; risperidone | atypical antipsychotic |
| -sartan | candesartan; irbesartan; losartan; olmesartan; valsartan | angiotensin II receptor antagonist (ARB) |
| -semide | furosemide; torsemide | loop diuretic (water pill) |
| -setron | alosetron; dolasetron; granisetron; ondansetron; palonosetron | serotonin 5-HT3 receptor antagonist |
| -setron | dolasetron; granisetron; ondansetron; palonosetron | antiemetic and antinauseant |
| -statin | atorvastatin; lovastatin; pitavastatin; pravastatin; rosuvastatin; simvastatin | HMG-CoA reductase inhibitor; statin |
| sulfa- | sulfacetamide; sulfadiazine; sulfamethoxazole; sulfasalazine | antibiotic; anti-infective; anti-inflammatory |
| -tadine | alcaftadine; cyproheptadine; desloratadine; loratadine; olopatadine | antihistamine |
| -tadine | amantadine; rimantadine | antiviral; anti-influenza-A |

*Continued*

## Table 3.1    Common Generic Drug Prefixes and Suffixes—cont'd

| PREFIX, ROOT, SUFFIX | EXAMPLES (GENERIC NAMES) | DRUG CLASS OR DRUG CATEGORY |
|---|---|---|
| -terol | albuterol; arformoterol; formoterol; levalbuterol; salmeterol | beta agonist; bronchodilator |
| -thiazide | chlorothiazide; hydrochlorothiazide; methyclothiazide | thiazide diuretic (water pill) |
| -tinib | crizotinib; dasatinib; erlotinib; gefitinib; imatinib | antineoplastic (kinase inhibitor) |
| -trel | desogestrel; etonogestrel; levonorgestrel; norgestrel | female hormone (progestin) |
| tretin-; -tretin- | acitretin; alitretinoin; isotretinoin; tretinoin | retinoid; dermatologic agent; form of vitamin A |
| -triptan | almotriptan; eletriptan; rizatriptan; sumatriptan; zolmitriptan | antimigraine; selective 5-HT receptor agonist |
| -tyline | amitriptyline; nortriptyline; protriptyline | tricyclic antidepressant (TCA) |
| -vir-; -vir | abacavir; efavirenz; enfuvirtide; nevirapine; ritonavir; tenofovir | antiviral; anti-HIV |
| -vir-; -vir | adefovir; entecavir; ribavirin (along with interferon) | antiviral; anti-hepatitis |
| -vir | acyclovir; famciclovir; penciclovir; valacyclovir | antiviral; anti-herpes |
| -vir | cidofovir; ganciclovir; valganciclovir | antiviral; anti-cytomegalovirus (anti-CMV) |
| -vir | oseltamivir; zanamivir | antiviral; anti-flu |
| -vudine | lamivudine; stavudine; telbivudine; zidovudine | antiviral; nucleoside analogues |
| -zepam | clonazepam; diazepam; flurazepam; lorazepam; temazepam | benzodiazepine |
| -zodone | nefazodone, trazodone, vilazodone | antidepressant |
| -zolam | alprazolam; estazolam; midazolam; triazolam | benzodiazepine |
| -zosin | alfuzosin; doxazosin; prazosin; terazosin | alpha blocker |

# Get Ready for the Next-Generation NCLEX® Examination!

## Key Points

- An agonist drug increases a cell's or organ's activity, and an antagonist drug slows or stops the activity.
- Drug absorption and availability are fastest with the IV and other parenteral routes and slowest for extended-release oral drugs.
- *Do not crush or let the patient chew, open (if it is a capsule), or cut* long-acting or extended-release drugs because this will result in an overdosage.
- Most drugs are metabolized by the liver and eliminated by the kidneys.
- Patients with liver or kidney impairment often require drug dosages to be lower to prevent adverse effects.
- Side effects are common expected reactions to drugs and are usually mild, although they may be annoying.
- Adverse reactions or effects are serious and sometimes life-threatening patient responses to drug therapy that may require stopping the drug.
- Always warn patients who have anaphylactic reactions about their allergy so they will not take the drug again.
- Teach patients with a drug allergy to wear a medical alert bracelet or necklace or carry identification about their allergy.
- Special considerations are needed when giving drugs to pediatric patients, pregnant or breast-feeding women, and older adults.
- Distribution of water-soluble drugs is faster and more widespread in neonates, infants, and younger children because of their high percentage of total body water.

- The critical period for adverse drug effects during pregnancy is between conception and 57 days.
- Older adults taking many different drugs are at risk for serious drug interactions.
- Ethnicity and genetics can affect drug action in certain individuals.
- All drugs that belong to the same category work in the same way and often have similar side effects.
- Agonist drugs activate a receptor, and antagonists prevent the receptor from affecting a response.
- Alcohol can make a drug either more or less effective.
- Consider barriers to compliance in older adults who require special teaching regarding their drugs.
- Never give a drug with which you are not fully familiar.

## Clinical Judgment and Next-Generation NCLEX® Examination-Style Questions

### Case Study

Ms. Dayan is a member of the Women's Professional Golf Association (PGA). She is being seen in the clinic today for a urinary tract infection (UTI). She has an allergy to penicillin. Her medications include a birth control pill every morning and an antidepressant (amitriptyline) every evening. The healthcare provider (HCP) has prescribed the antibiotic cephalexin 250 mg every 6 hours for 7 days. Ms. Dayan tells the nurse she is worried she will forget to take the medication as her schedule is very busy and asks why she must take this drug every 6 hours instead of once a day.

1. **Which explanation given by the nurse is the most correct?**

   1. Cephalexin works quicker if taken every 6 hours.
   2. Cephalexin was prescribed because you are allergic to penicillin.
   3. Cephalexin's half-life is short, so it needs to be dosed more frequently.
   4. I can ask the HCP to change the dose and timing of the cephalexin.

2. **Ms. Dayan tells the nurse that her husband had to take an antibiotic for more than 3 weeks once to treat a bone infection and is concerned that 7 days may not be enough time to treat her UTI. Which explanation given by the nurse is most correct?**

   1. Cephalexin does not bind to the proteins in your blood, so more gets to the tissue.
   2. Antibiotics used for bone tissue work differently.
   3. Infections in the bone are usually resistant to antibiotics.
   4. Bone has less blood supply, so antibiotic penetration is more difficult.

3. **Ms. Dayan calls the clinic the next day and says she has developed a rash. What is the likeliest reason for the rash?**

   1. Ms. Dayan has developed an allergy to cephalexin.
   2. Ms. Dayan has developed an idiosyncratic response to cephalexin.
   3. The rash is a simple side effect.
   4. The rash is a response to the generic form of the drug.

4. **Complete the following sentence by choosing from the lists of options.**

   Once a drug is ____1____ and ____2____ in the body, the body transforms the drug. This process is called ____3____.

   | OPTIONS FOR 1 | OPTIONS FOR 2 | OPTIONS FOR 3 |
   |---|---|---|
   | Administered | Distributed | Elimination |
   | Absorbed | Diffused | First Pass |
   | Distributed | Metabolized | Biotransformation |

5. **Which responses after taking a drug are indicative of an adverse reaction? Select all or any that apply.**

   1. Nausea
   2. Double vision
   3. Diarrhea
   4. Rash
   5. Wheezing
   6. Headache
   7. Throat tightness
   8. Heart palpitations

6. **After eating a large bag of potato chips, a person becomes thirsty. Which mechanism involved in absorption causes thirst in this situation?**

   1. Filtration
   2. Diffusion
   3. Osmosis
   4. Active transport

7. **The patient is prescribed the prodrug codeine for a persistent postviral cough. Which patient condition should the nurse be most concerned about?**

   1. Asian ethnicity
   2. Liver cancer
   3. Past history of alcoholism
   4. Slightly below-normal creatine clearance level

8. **The most common route for excretion of drugs is through the renal system. How else are drugs excreted in the body? Select all or any that apply.**

   1. Tears
   2. Lungs
   3. Skin
   4. Feces
   5. Hair
   6. Saliva
   7. Breast milk
   8. Semen

9. **A patient is given sublingual nitroglycerin for acute chest pain instead of a nitroglycerin capsule. What is the advantage of administering the nitroglycerin sublingually?**

   1. Sublingual drug administration has a high first-pass effect, making it more effective.
   2. Sublingual drug administration is more effective for administering drugs that have a high potency
   3. Sublingual drug administration allows the drug to enter the bloodstream without causing side effects.
   4. Sublingual drug administration is faster because the drug is absorbed quickly by way of the blood vessels under the tongue.

10. **A 90-year-old patient in the nursing home is prescribed a diuretic for high blood pressure. What factors should the nurse consider before administering the drug? Select all or any that apply.**

    1. Other medications the patient takes
    2. Current blood pressure reading
    3. Ability to self-ambulate
    4. Fluid intake
    5. Arthritis
    6. Dementia
    7. Electrolyte levels
    8. Creatinine clearance rate

## Next-Generation NCLEX® (NGN) Examination–Style Question

A nurse is caring for the client on the medical-surgical unit and reviews the client's history and physical, flowsheet, and imaging studies.

### Yesterday 1200

A 68-year-old male is admitted to the medical-surgical unit after undergoing elective total right knee arthroplasty.
Physical Exam:
General: no acute distress
Respiratory: breath sounds clear bilaterally
Cardiovascular: S1, S2, no murmur
Skin: warm, dry

### Today 0900

Physical Exam:
General: anxious
Respiratory: tachypnea, bilateral crackles
Cardiovascular: S1, S2, tachycardia, increased JVD
Skin: cool, clammy

### Nurse's Notes
### Today 0900

The nurse is called to the client's bedside. The client reports an acute onset of chest pain and shortness of breath. Provider notified and EKG obtained.

### Today 0910

Provider at bedside evaluating the client. The provider states, "I'm going to put in an order for nitroglycerin and oxygen. This client will be going to the cath lab STAT."

### Flow Sheet
### Today 0900

Blood Pressure: 148/90 mm Hg
Heart Rate: 98/min
Respiratory Rate: 20/min
Temperature: 98.6°F (37°C)

### Imaging Studies
### Today 0900

ECG: ST elevation consistent with myocardial infarction
Drag one route of administration and one rationale to complete the sentence(s).

The nurse anticipates that the nitroglycerin will be ordered to be administered ____1____ because ____2____.

| OPTIONS FOR 1 | OPTIONS FOR 2 |
|---|---|
| Epidurally | The blood flow through tissues is very high |
| Sublingually | The delay in absorption holds the drug in the tissues longer |
| Subcutaneously | The drug has a long half-life |
| Orally | The distribution of water-soluble drugs is faster in this client's age group |

See answer on Evolve at http://evolve.elsevier.com/Visovsky/LPNpharmacology/.

# Drug Calculation: Preparing and Giving Drugs

http://evolve.elsevier.com/Visovsky/LPNpharmacology/

## Learning Outcomes

1. Apply the appropriate formula to accurately calculate drug dosages.
2. Select the correct equipment to prepare and give parenteral drugs, including insulin.
3. Explain the different types of parenteral drug delivery.
4. Identify anatomic landmarks used for giving parenteral drugs.
5. Apply the correct formula for calculating intravenous flow rates for infusions.
6. Correctly apply Clark's rule used to accurately calculate drug dosages for children.
7. Explain the principles and procedures to safely and accurately give drugs by the enteral, parenteral, and percutaneous routes.

## Key Terms

**ampule** Small, breakable glass container that contains one dose of drug for intramuscular or intravenous injection.

**aseptic technique** Manipulation that does not contaminate the sterility of the drug and drug delivery system.

**aspirate** The process of drawing back on the syringe after the needle is inserted to check for blood prior to giving an intramuscular injection.

**body surface area (BSA)** The total tissue area (based on height and weight) of a patient's body.

**buccal route** A drug that is given by being applied to or held in the cheek. The drug diffuses through the oral mucosa directly into the bloodstream.

**capsule** Gelatin container that holds powder or liquid drug.

**Clark's rule** A method for determining pediatric drug dosage calculated by ratio and proportion, based on the child's body weight.

**drop factor** The number of drops per milliliter of fluid.

**flow rate** The rate at which intravenous fluids are given.

**intradermal injections** Injection that is given into the dermis, just below the epidermis; most often used for allergy testing and tuberculosis testing.

**intramuscular (IM) route** Administration of a drug by injection past the dermis and subcutaneous tissue, deep into the muscle mass.

**intravenous (IV) route** The administration of drugs directly into the bloodstream.

**Mix-o-Vial** A two-compartment vial that contains a sterile solution in one compartment and the powdered drug in the second compartment, separated by a rubber stopper. The solution and drug powder are mixed together immediately before use.

**nasogastric (NG) tube** An enteral route of drug administration and oral feeding that bypasses the mouth by use of a tube going through the nose and esophagus into the stomach.

**nomogram** A chart that displays the relationships between two different types of data so that complex calculations are not necessary.

**parenteral route** Administration of a drug by injection directly into the dermal, subcutaneous, or intramuscular tissue; epidurally into cerebral spinal fluid; or through intravenous injection into the bloodstream.

**percutaneous route** Administration of a drug through topical (skin), sublingual (under the tongue), buccal (against the cheek), or inhalation (breathing) methods.

**piggyback infusion** A second or secondary intravenous fluid bag or bottle containing drugs or solution that is connected to the main intravenous line rather than directly to the patient.

**subcutaneous injections** Injection that places no more than 2 mL of drug solution into the loose connective tissue between the dermis of the skin and the muscle layer.

**sublingual route** Application of a drug to the mucous membranes under the tongue.

**tablet** Dried, powdered drugs compressed into small shapes.

**topical route** Application of a drug directly to the area of the skin requiring treatment; most common forms are creams, lotions, and ointments.

**transdermal** Refers to drugs applied to the skin for absorption into the bloodstream.

**vial** Small, single- or multiple-dose glass drug container.

**Z-track technique** A type of intramuscular injection technique used to prevent tracking (leakage) of the medication into the subcutaneous tissue (underneath the skin).

## INTRODUCTION

This chapter provides an explanation of dosage calculations, presents the basic principles of drug administration, and reviews the procedures enteral, parenteral, and percutaneous drug administration.

## CALCULATING DRUG DOSAGES

Ensuring the safety of patients by giving the correct drug dose during drug administration is one of the most important responsibilities of the licensed practical or vocational nurse (LPN/VN). Drugs that are prepackaged with the correct dose already prepared for the patient (known as unit-dose drugs) are becoming increasingly common. However, you will need to understand how to accurately calculate the correct drug dosage using basic mathematical formulas. Sometimes the specific dose the healthcare provider orders is not available. You will need to use a mathematical formula to figure out how much of the drug is to be given to the patient. Even a small error in drug dosage can have severe consequences for the patient.

The metric system is a system of measurement that uses the meter (distance), liter (volume), and gram (weight) as the units of measure. In nursing practice, the metric system is used to convert from one unit of measure to another (Fig. 4.1). For example, the metric system is used in the calculation of drug dosages, the conversion of Fahrenheit to Celsius when taking temperatures, and the conversion of pounds to kilograms when weighing patients. These number relationships form the basis of accurate drug dosage. In the following section we provide a brief review of essential information to master in calculating drug dosages. If you need a review of basic mathematics associated with drug calculations, read this section carefully and then use the Student Study Guide or Evolve resources to practice fractions, percentages, proportions, and ratios.

This section shows several methods to calculate drug dosages to achieve the prescribed dose of the drug (what you want to give) starting from the kind and amount of the drug that is available (what you have on hand). For example, the order may be for 200 mg of a drug (want), but all you have is 50-mg tablets (have). How do you calculate the correct number of tablets to give? In this case:

$$\frac{\text{Want}}{\text{Have}} = \text{number of tablets to give}$$

$$\frac{200\,\text{mg}}{50\,\text{mg}} = 4\,(\text{the number of tablets to give})$$

### FRACTION METHOD

When you are using fractions to compute drug dosages, write an equation consisting of two fractions. First, set up a fraction showing the number of units to be given as the numerator and the unknown number of tablets or milliliters to give ($x$) as the denominator. For example, if the healthcare provider's order states "ibuprofen 600 mg" and you have tablets, you would write $\frac{600\ \text{mg}}{x\ \text{tablets}}$ on the left-hand side of the equation. On the other side of the equation, write a fraction showing the amount of drug in each tablet, as listed on the drug label. For example, if the ibuprofen bottle label states

| Metric Measurements | | |
|---|---|---|
| Common Measure | Conversion Factor | Common Use |
| **Volume** | | |
| L = Liter | 1000 ml = 1 L | IV solutions orders |
| mL = milliliter | 1 mL = 1 cc = 1/1000 L | Parenteral and liquid oral medications |
| **Weight** | | |
| kg = kilogram | 1 kg = 1000 g = 2.2 lb | Measuring body weight |
| g = gram | 1 g = 1000 mg | Parenteral and oral medications |
| mg = milligram | 1 mg = 1/1000 g | Parenteral and oral medications |
| μg = microgram | 1 μg = 1/1000 mg<br>1 μg = one-millionth g | Pediatric medications |

Fig. *4.1* Metric conversion chart. *IV,* intravenous.

"200 mg per tablet," the second fraction would be $\frac{200 \text{ mg}}{x \text{ tablets}}$. The equation then reads:

$$\frac{600 \text{ mg}}{x \text{ tablets}} = \frac{200 \text{ mg}}{1 \text{ tablet}}$$

Notice that the same units of measure are in both numerators and the same units of measure are in both denominators. Now solve for $x$ by multiplying across the diagonal:

$$\frac{600 \text{ mg}}{x \text{ tablets}} = \frac{200 \text{ mg}}{1 \text{ tablet}}$$
$$\frac{600}{x} = \frac{200}{1}$$
$$200x = 600$$
$$x = 3$$

To give a dose of 600 mg, you would give 3 tablets, each containing 200 mg of the drug.

## RATIO AND PROPORTION METHOD

A fraction uses a division line to describe the mathematical relationship between two numbers; for example, $\frac{1}{4}$ or $1/_4$. Proportions describe the relationship between two sets of numbers. For example, $\frac{1}{2} = \frac{2}{4}$, so when you multiply across the diagonal, $1 \times 4$ equals $2 \times 2$.

When using the ratio method, first write the amount of the drug to be given and the quantity of the dosage ($x$) as a ratio. Using the previous example, you would write this as "600 mg : $x$ tablets." Next, complete the equation by forming a second ratio consisting of the number of units of the drug in the dosage form and the quantity of that dosage form as taken from the bottle. Using the previous example, the second ratio is 200 mg : 1 tablet. Expressed as a proportion, the relationship is:

$$600 \text{ mg} : x \text{ tablets} :: 200 \text{ mg} : 1 \text{ tablet}$$

Solving for $x$ determines the dose:

$$600 \times 1 = 200 \times x$$
$$600 = 200x$$
$$x = 600/200$$
$$x = 3$$

Using this method provides the correct answer, 3 tablets.

 **Memory Jogger**

Steps to Solving Drug Dosage Calculations
1. Change doses to the same unit of measurement if they are different.
2. Set up your equation to work step by step from what dose is ordered (want) and what dose you have on hand (have) toward what amount of the available formulation to give the patient.
3. Calculate the dose, using fractions or ratios and proportions.
4. Check your answer for correctness. Ask yourself, "Does this make sense knowing the dosage range for the drug?"

## DRUG CALCULATION USING UNITS

Insulin is an example of a parenteral drug that is not given by milligrams but by units. Great accuracy is important in preparing and giving insulin because the quantity given is very small, and even minor variations in dosage may result in severe consequences for the patient.

The preparation and calculation of insulin dosages are unique in three ways:
1. There are many kinds of insulin, including short- and long-acting forms. All types of insulin come in a standardized measure called an insulin unit. Insulin is available in 10-mL vials and in a specific strength (concentration), usually U-100 (100 units per 1 mL of solution) (Fig. 4.2).
2. Insulin should be drawn up in a special insulin syringe that is marked or calibrated in units (Fig. 4.3).
3. The insulin order, the insulin bottle, and the insulin as drawn up should always be rechecked by another nurse for maximum accuracy before the insulin is given.

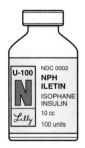

**Fig. 4.2** U-100 vial.

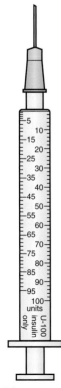

**Fig. 4.3** U-100 syringe.

To draw up a dose of U-100 insulin, use the corresponding 100-unit syringe. Draw up the number of units ordered. For example, if the order reads "48 units NPH insulin U-100 1 hour before breakfast," you would draw up 48 units of NPH insulin using a U-100 syringe.

Occasionally an order is written by the healthcare provider for two different types of insulin. In some cases, both types of insulin may be given at the same time in the same syringe. Usually one type of insulin has a cloudy appearance and one type appears clear. Some types of insulin cannot be mixed at all. For example, never mix Lantus or Levemir insulin with any other insulin preparation. Be sure to check with your healthcare provider, pharmacist, or diabetes educator before mixing. Chapter 20 has complete information on the processes used to give insulin. Be certain that you are using the correct type of insulin.

---

### 🔒 Top Tip for Safety

- Insulin is a high-alert drug that can cause serious harm to a patient if given at too high or too low a dose or if it is not given to the patient for whom it was prescribed.
- You must be very accurate in insulin calculations. A small error makes a big change in insulin dosage. Use the correct syringe, the correct insulin, and the correct dose.
- Check your calculations, insulin type, and dose with another nurse or licensed healthcare professional before giving the drug.

---

## CALCULATING DRUG DOSAGES FOR INFANTS AND CHILDREN

It is well known that drug administration errors can lead to patient harm. This is especially true in the pediatric setting, as drug errors by healthcare professionals and parents occur more frequently and have the potential for greater harm. Pharmaceutical companies list the recommended dosages of their drugs for a child or infant, and these dosages are much smaller than the recommended adult dosage. Although children's dosages were once frequently calculated, there remain only a few drugs that require the nurse to determine how much to give a child. In past years, several general rules were developed to calculate these special reduced dosages for infants and children. The Joint Commission, a nonprofit agency that credentials and certifies healthcare organizations, now recommends that all dosages for children be weight based, usually in kilograms.

One of the most widely accepted methods for determining a child's dosage based on the child's body weight is Clark's rule. This rule is used to calculate drug doses for children 2 to 17 years of age. Just as for adult drug dosage calculations, the method of ratios and proportions may be used to calculate the pediatric value. Assuming that an average adult weighs 150 lb and we know the adult dosage, it follows that if we know the child's weight, we can calculate the child's dosage. The formula for calculating pediatric drug doses based on Clark's rule is as follows:

$$\text{Pediatric child dose} = (\text{Weight of child} / 150 \,\text{lb}) \times \text{Adult dose}$$

Another way to calculate drug dosages for the pediatric patient is based on body surface area (BSA) of the child, which is the total tissue area (calculated from the child's height and weight). This is the most accurate method for determining pediatric dosages. The reason for using the BSA is that children have a greater surface area than adults in relation to their weight. For drugs that require careful dosage, charts known as nomograms are used to calculate the BSA in square meters. These nomograms (BSA charts) are constructed from height and weight data. Even with the use of standardized charts, the calculated dosages are more accurate for children than for very young infants. When giving drugs to infants or children, an important nursing responsibility is to double-check the original order and confirm that the correct dose was calculated before giving the drug. Most healthcare organizations require any dose calculations for this population to be double-checked by two individual nurses to prevent drug errors that can have severe consequences for the pediatric patient. Your agency pharmacist is also an invaluable resource for any questions or concerns that arise regarding infant or child drug dosage and administration.

## CALCULATIONS FOR INTRAVENOUS INFUSIONS

Drugs can also be given through the intravenous (IV) route, which delivers the drug directly into the circulatory system though a vein. IV therapy can be used to correct dehydration in a patient or to give drugs directly and immediately into the bloodstream. Some drugs cannot be taken by mouth or by subcutaneous or intramuscular (IM) injection into the skin because of issues with drug absorption. However, because IV fluids and drugs enter the bloodstream directly, the potential for adverse events such as fluid overload or an adverse drug reaction is a concern. Adverse drug reactions are unintended responses associated with the use of a drug in a patient. These can range from mild allergic reactions to severe problems resulting in tissue damage or death.

An IV fluid administration order has several components:
- The specific IV fluid to be infused
- The amount (volume) of fluid to be infused
- The duration of time for which the IV fluid should be infused
- The rate (how fast) the IV fluid should be infused

The flow rate of an IV fluid refers to how fast the IV fluid infuses. The flow rate is used to determine how many milliliters of the fluid are given to the patient in an hour. The diameter of the IV tubing determines the flow rate of the IV. IV tubing with a larger diameter will permit larger drops into the vein and therefore more fluid into the body for a given period of time. The number of drops used to make a milliliter of IV fluid is called the drop factor.

Regulating the IV infusion rate is a common nursing responsibility. Some institutions have automatic infusion pumps that make flow rate calculations easy. All nurses will learn to use the equipment available at their place of employment; however, they must learn to calculate infusion rates without relying on equipment in case of power or equipment failure or when working in agencies where no automatic pumps are available.

A completed IV infusion order specifies not only the type of solution and the volume to be infused (usually 500 or 1000 mL) but also the duration (length of time) over which the total volume of IV is to be infused. The flow rate needs to be calculated to determine how fast the drug will be infused. You can consult with the pharmacist or healthcare provider if the IV order is not clear, or not complete, or if you are infusing a high-alert drug such as heparin and wish to verify your calculations.

You must be familiar with two mathematical procedures regarding IV infusions:
- Calculating the flow rates for IV fluid administration
- Calculating total administration time for IV fluid

To calculate the flow rate for IV fluid administration, you must understand two concepts: the flow rate and the drop factor. The rate at which IV fluids are given is the flow rate, and this is measured in drops per minute. The drop factor is the number of drops per milliliter of liquid and is determined by the size of the drops. The drop factor is different for different manufacturers of IV infusion equipment, and it must be checked by reading it on the infusion set itself. Regular infusion sets (macrodrip) range between 10 and 20 drops/mL; these are called macrodrops. Other infusion sets (microdrip) produce a drop factor of 60 drops/mL, called microdrops; these sets are most commonly used with pediatric patients and in skilled nursing or home care settings.

## CALCULATING INTRAVENOUS FLOW RATE

After you know the drop factor for the equipment being used, you can calculate the flow rate by using the following formula:

$$\text{Drop factor}(\text{drops/mL}) \times \text{mL/min}$$
$$= \text{Flow rate}(\text{drops/mL})$$

Occasionally, you may see an order for an IV fluid to "keep vein open" (KVO) or "to keep open" (TKO). While this practice is very widespread, the lack of consistent guidelines for what flow rate is recommended for KVO can pose problems such as fluid overload for some patients. Therefore an IV flow rate must be specified in a KVO order, or institutions with a specific policy

that addresses the flow rate for a KVO order can be used to meet the criteria for safe drug administration. For example, a KVO IV order may equal 20 drops/min in one institution, but 30 drops/min at another institution. Either way, the flow rate must be clearly established by a healthcare provider's order or by institution policy.

Suppose an order reads "1000 mL normal saline (NS) to be given over 5 hours." The drop factor is 15 drops/mL. The total minutes required for the infusion is 5 h × 60 min/h, or 300 min. To calculate the flow rate, use the formula:

$$\frac{\text{Total amount of fluid to give}(\text{mL})}{\text{Total time}(\text{min})} \times \frac{\text{Drop factor}}{(\text{drops/mL})}$$
$$= \text{Flow rate}(\text{drops/min})$$

$$\frac{1000\,\text{mL}}{300\,\text{min}} \times 15\,\text{drops/mL} = \frac{15,000\,\text{drops}}{300\,\text{min}}$$
$$= 50\,\text{drops/min}$$

## CALCULATING TOTAL INTRAVENOUS INFUSION TIME

Calculating the total administration time for IV fluid when the flow rate is given depends on calculating the total number of drops to be infused. Using this information, plus the drop factor, you can easily determine the total infusion time. First, calculate the total number of drops to be infused by multiplying the prescribed dose (mL) by the drop factor (drops/mL). Then use the following formula to obtain the infusion time:

$$\frac{\text{Total drops to be infused}}{\text{Flow rate}(\text{drops/min})} \times 60\,\text{min/h}$$
$$= \text{Total infusion time}(\text{h})$$

To summarize, the total infusion time is calculated in two steps:
1. Determine the total number of drops ordered: The healthcare provider's order for the total amount of fluid to be infused is multiplied by the drop factor read from the infusion set to determine the total number of drops to be infused.
2. Determine the amount of time the IV is required to flow: The prescribed flow rate is multiplied by the conversion factor of 60 min/h to obtain the number of drops infused in 1 hour, then divided into the total number of drops to determine the time required for the IV infusion.

For example, if the order reads "1000 mL D5W [5% dextrose in water] to be given at 50 drops/min with a drop factor of 10 drops/mL," use these calculations:

$$1000\,\text{mL} \times 10\,\text{drops/mL} = 10,000\,\text{total drops}$$
$$50\,\text{drops/min} \times 60\,\text{min/h} = 3000\,\text{drops/h}$$
$$\frac{10,000\,\text{drops}}{3000\,\text{drops/h}} = 3.33\,\text{h, or 3 h and 20 min}$$

## FACTORS THAT INFLUENCE INTRAVENOUS FLOW RATES

Other factors may influence the flow rate of an infusion such as age, body size, and condition of the patient and the patient's veins. The size of the IV catheter needle, the needle's position in the vein, the height of the IV pump or pole, and the patient's position may be changed or altered to assist in infusion of IV fluids. If the fluid does not infuse at the calculated rate, the entire IV system should be carefully checked from the IV solution down to the IV catheter insertion site for problems with any of the following: level of fluid in the IV set drip chamber, air in the tubing that obstructs flow, patency of the IV, or signs of IV infiltration (e.g., redness or swelling of the area).

### FLOW RATES FOR INFANTS AND CHILDREN

Infants and small children are very sensitive to extra amounts, or volumes, of fluids. Large amounts of IV fluids can cause hypervolemia and potentially electrolyte imbalance. For infants and children, smaller total amounts of IV fluids are often ordered, and the infusions are given in microdrops to prevent accidental fluid overload and ensure patient safety. The drop factor used for infants is typically 60 microdrops/mL. As with adults, the drop factor must be determined from the infusion set. For calculating the flow rates in infants, the same formula is followed, but the microdrop drop factor must be used:

$$\frac{\text{Total amount of fluid to give (mL)}}{\text{Total time (min)}} \times \frac{\text{Drop factor}}{\text{(microdrops/mL)}}$$
$$= \text{Flow rate (microdrops/min)}$$

For example, if the IV infusion order reads "Give 50 mL D5W [5% dextrose in water] IV in 4 hours" and the drop factor is 60 microdrops/mL, calculate the flow rate as follows:

$$\frac{50 \text{ mL}}{240 \text{ min}} \times 60 \text{ microdrops/mL}$$
$$= 12.5 \text{ microdrops/min}$$

Modifications to the IV flow rate or IV drug dosage for an infant or child are strictly controlled and are ordered only by the healthcare provider.

---

 **Memory Jogger**

- The drop factor for infusions depends on the type of equipment and must be read from the IV set label.
- The flow rate is calculated by using the following formula:

    Drop factor × mL/min = Flow rate (drops/min)

- IV administration time is calculated using the following formula:

$$\frac{\text{Total fluid to be given}}{\text{Total time (min)}} \times \text{Drop factor (drops/mL)}$$
$$= \text{Flow rate (drops/min)}$$

- The total infusion time depends on the total number of drops to be infused:

$$\frac{\text{Total drops to be infused}}{\text{Flow rate (drops/min)}} \div 60 \text{ (min/h)}$$
$$= \text{Total infusion time (h)}$$

---

## GENERAL PRINCIPLES OF DRUG ADMINISTRATION

The process of oral drug administration involves several steps and safety measures to ensure that you have correctly adhered to the *9 Rights of Drug Administration* (see Chapter 1), the nursing process, and your institution's policies. In general, you are responsible for knowing the drug you are giving, the reason the drug is being given, side effects that can be expected, and the adverse effects for which the patient should be monitored. You must also know any specific allergies your patient may have and how these may relate to drugs ordered. Some drugs have specific limits on when and if they can be safely given. For example, you would not give a drug for hypertension (high blood pressure) if the patient's blood pressure was below a certain point. The healthcare provider may include these types of limits in the original order, or you may use your nursing judgement to hold (not give) a certain drug until you clarify the order with the prescriber.

The following steps are a general guide for giving drugs to your patient:

- Follow the *9 Rights of Drug Administration*.
- Minimize interruptions and distractions while preparing drugs (see Chapter 2).
- Wash your hands to avoid contamination of the drugs.
- Assemble necessary equipment such as medication cups and water for swallowing drugs.
- Follow the written drug order. Compare the written order with the medication administration record (MAR) and the drug label. Be alert to look-alike and sound-alike drug names, which are a significant source of drug error!
- Accurately identify the patient before giving any drugs by checking the patient's wristband and asking the patient to provide name and date of birth. For barcoded drug administration systems, scan the patient's wristband to confirm that the correct drug, dose, and route are given to the correct patient.
- Do not unwrap or remove the drug from the container until you are with the patient.
- Follow **aseptic technique** for oral drugs by not touching the drug or the inside of the drug container. Pour the oral liquid or pills into the appropriate medication cup. When measuring liquid drugs, hold the cup at eye level to avoid errors.
- Follow sterile technique when handling needles and syringes for giving subcutaneous, IM, or IV drugs. Dispose of needles and syringes properly immediately after giving the drug.
- Follow institution procedure for proper documentation (charting) after giving the drug or if the patient refuses the drug.

### ENTERAL DRUGS

Enteral drugs are given directly into the gastrointestinal (GI) tract, which extends from the mouth through the anus. Enteral drugs can be given by the oral (PO), nasogastric (NG), or rectal route.

## GIVING ORAL DRUGS

The most common way of giving drugs is by the oral route. Oral drugs come in several different forms, and each form serves a specific purpose. For example, different forms of oral drugs can promote increased absorption, delayed absorption, or reduced irritation to the stomach. Some oral drugs are available in tablet or capsule form; patients may call this type of drug form a "pill," but that is an outdated term for health professionals to use. Tablets may be covered with a special coating that resists the acidic pH of the stomach, but they will dissolve in the alkaline pH of the intestine.

Advantages of oral preparations are:

- Oral drugs are convenient, economical, and noninvasive.
- A variety of short- or long-acting formulations may be available, and some have an enteric coating to protect the stomach.

Disadvantages of oral preparations are:

- Oral drugs cannot be given to patients who are nauseated, vomiting, or unconscious.
- Oral drugs cannot be given to patients who cannot swallow.
- Older adult patients may need additional time to swallow oral tablets or capsules.
- Some drugs become ineffective when mixed with the acid and enzymes in the stomach and intestines.
- The onset of drug action may vary because the drug absorption in the GI tract varies among patients.

---

> **⚠ Safety Alert!**
>
> You are responsible for the following aspects of patient safety:
> - You have the responsibility to ensure that each patient safely takes the drugs given. Do not leave drugs at the bedside for patients to take later.
> - Never give a drug that has been poured or prepared by another nurse or healthcare provider to a patient. You may give only the drugs that you have prepared.

---

### Giving Oral Tablets or Capsules

Tablets and capsules are different forms of oral drugs. A **tablet** is made up of dried, powdered drugs that have been compressed into small, solid shapes; a **capsule** is a gelatin container that holds powder or liquid drug. Before you give oral drugs, you must make sure the patient can safely swallow any drug given. If the patient is unable to swallow the drug as ordered, notify the healthcare provider who ordered the drug. Be sure you have followed all the steps in the correct procedure for drug administration (see General Principles of Drug Administration) and have a glass of water ready for the patient. If the drug is in the form of a lozenge, it is meant to be sucked, not swallowed.

All oral drugs are brought to the patient's bedside unwrapped or in the original container and can be placed in a paper soufflé cup using aseptic technique before giving the drug.

Do not crush tablets or break capsules without checking with the pharmacist. Many drugs have special (enteric) coatings that are essential for proper absorption. If they are broken, cut, crushed, or chewed, drug absorption can be so rapid that adverse effects are more likely.

If a patient has difficulty swallowing the drug, have the patient take a few sips of water before placing the drug in the back of the mouth, then follow with more water. Help patients keep their head forward while swallowing, as they do when they eat. It is generally not helpful to tilt the head backward.

You are responsible for making sure the patient takes all drugs safely and on schedule. Do not leave drugs at the patient's bedside to be taken later or ask another person to give them for you.

### Giving Liquid-Form Oral Drugs

Liquids or solutions often must be shaken before they are poured to ensure that the drug is evenly distributed throughout the liquid. Check to make sure the lid on the bottle is tightly closed before shaking. Take the lid off the bottle and place the lid upside down (outer surface down) on a flat surface. This protects the inside of the lid from dirt or contamination. When pouring liquids from a bottle into a plastic medication cup, hold the bottle so the label is against your hand. This prevents the drug from running down onto the label so that it cannot be read. Hold the medication cup at eye level to read the proper dose (Fig 4.4). Read the level at the lowest point in the medication cup.

A liquid drug can also be drawn up from the bottle or medication cup with a syringe or a medicine dropper (Fig. 4.4). These methods are useful in helping you to be accurate when a small dose is ordered or when giving drugs to infants or small children. The syringe or medicine dropper is placed halfway back in the baby's

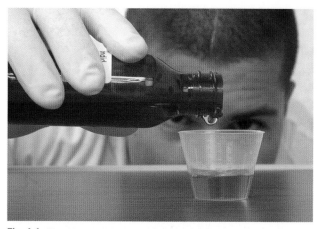

**Fig. 4.4** Checking the drug dose in a medication cup. (From Potter, P. A. (2017). *Fundamentals of nursing* (9th ed.). Elsevier.)

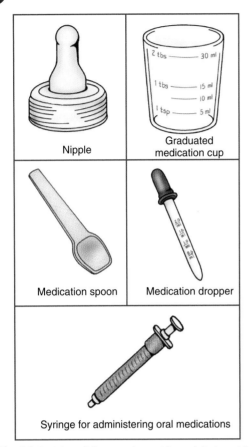

| Nipple | Graduated medication cup |
| Medication spoon | Medication dropper |
| Syringe for administering oral medications | |

Fig. 4.5 Oral drug delivery equipment for an infant or child.

mouth, between the cheek and gums, and slowly emptied, giving the baby time to swallow it. The drug in the syringe or medicine dropper can be emptied into a nipple for an infant to suck the dose (see Fig 4.5). Wipe any extra drug from the bottle top and replace the lid quickly to avoid contamination. Do not dilute a liquid drug unless ordered to do so by the prescriber.

### Lifespan Considerations

**Older Adults: Giving Drugs**

Allow extra time when giving drugs to older adult patients. These individuals often are slower to take a drug, slower in swallowing drugs and water, and slower in understanding the answers provided to questions about their drugs.

### GIVING DRUGS BY NASOGASTRIC OR PERCUTANEOUS ENDOSCOPIC GASTROSTOMY TUBE

Patients who cannot swallow, are nauseated, or have bowel obstruction may be able to take drugs through an NG tube or a percutaneous endoscopic gastrostomy (PEG) tube. A **nasogastric (NG) tube** is an enteral route of drug administration and oral feeding that bypasses the mouth by use of a tube going through the nose and esophagus into the stomach. The tubing and a clamp allow the nurse to easily give drugs in this way. The PEG tube is similar, but instead of going through the nose

it is placed by surgical endoscopy directly through the wall of the abdomen and into the stomach.

As with any other oral drug administration method, check with the pharmacist before crushing tablets or opening capsules. Some tablets may be crushed, mixed with 50 mL of water, and given through an NG or PEG tube. For drugs that cannot be crushed, a liquid formulation must be ordered. It is important to know that some drugs are not compatible with feeding formulas (e.g., phenytoin [Dilantin]) or are degraded more quickly after crushing, making them less effective (e.g., enteric-coated pantoprazole). Sustained-release drugs are meant to be delivered over a period of time, so crushing this type of tablet can release the drug too quickly, resulting in increased drug blood levels and toxicity.

### Top Tip for Safety

Do not open, cut, crush, or allow a patient to chew a sustained-release drug because these actions can release the drug too quickly and result in toxicity.

Follow the general procedure for preparing for drug administration (see General Principles of Drug Administration). Double-check the prescriber's order to make sure you are giving the drug by the correct route because all nonliquid drugs will need to be crushed or capsules opened before they are given through an NG or PEG tube. Wash your hands and use gloves as needed, following your agency's policies during this procedure. Place the patient in an upright position. For NG tube drug administration, check that the NG tube is in the stomach. Aspirate (remove) some stomach contents with a syringe and test the pH of the stomach contents. If the pH is 0 to 5, then the tube is most likely in the stomach. Auscultation over the area of the stomach and listening for a whooshing sound is no longer considered a reliable way to test NG tube placement.

The process for giving a drug through a PEG tube is very similar to that for the NG tube. In addition to the tubing, the PEG has a gastrostomy feeding button (a small, flexible silicone device with a mushroom-shaped dome at one end and two small wings at the other end) that can be used to close the tube between uses. Irrigate this button with sterile water or normal saline after the drug has been given and clean the area according to institution policy.

Avoid crushing tablets or capsules together; drugs should not be mixed together for administration through an NG or PEG tube. Each drug should be given separately because of possible incompatibilities, tube blockage, or changes in the pharmacodynamics of the drugs. Crushing enteric-coated drugs breaks them into small pieces that, when mixed with water, can result in clogging of the tube. Always rinse the tube with sterile water or sodium chloride before and after giving the drug or drugs.

### Patients Who Are Receiving Enteral Feedings

For patients who are receiving enteral feedings, after tube placement is checked, the residual (amount) of stomach contents must also be checked before a drug is given through an NG or PEG tube. Drug administration may be withheld if the residual amount of feeding exceeds the standards set by the institution. Clamp the NG tube and attach a syringe. Next, pour the drug mixed with water into the syringe, unclamp the NG tube, and let the drug run in by gravity. Add 50 mL of sterile water or normal saline, according to the institution's policy, to flush and clean out the tubing after all the drug has passed through the tube. Clamp the feeding tube for 30 minutes before and after drug administration to minimize interactions with the feeding formula, making sure to rinse the feeding tube well with sterile water or normal saline.

### Patients With Nasogastric Tube to Suction

If an NG tube is attached to suction, disconnect it and clamp the suction tube shut for 30 minutes before drug administration. Attach a syringe, pour the drug mixed with sterile water or normal saline into the syringe, unclamp the NG tube, and let the drug run in by gravity. Add 50 mL of sterile water or normal saline, according to the institution's policy, to flush and clean out the tubing after all of the drug has passed through the tube, making sure to rinse the feeding tube well. Keep the feeding tube clamped for 30 minutes before and after drug administration to minimize interactions with the feeding formula.

The tube remains clamped for at least 30 minutes before the suction tube is reattached so that there is time for the drug to be absorbed. For additional information on this procedure, refer to your nursing fundamentals textbook.

## PARENTERAL DRUGS

### GENERAL PRINCIPLES

The term parenteral is usually used for drugs given by injection or infusion, or by an intradermal or subcutaneous route. Drugs are given parenterally for the following reasons:
- The patient is unable take an oral drug.
- The patient needs a drug that can act quickly.
- The drug needed may be destroyed by gastric enzymes.
- A rapid or steady blood level of the drug is needed.

- The plasma drug level needs to be carefully adjusted to avoid over- or underdosing. An IV infusion allows the drug to be easily adjusted to achieve the desired effect.
- The drug is not available in an oral form.

For example, patients with severe, life-threatening infections may need IV antibiotics, or a patient may need to receive continuous IV heparin for anticoagulation.

IV drugs that are injected directly into the bloodstream act quickly, whereas drugs given by IM or subcutaneous injection require time for the drug to reach the bloodstream, thus the onset of drug action is slower than for drugs given IV. Some IV drugs are effective for only a short time, requiring frequent doses. If an overdose of an IV drug is accidentally infused, the consequences to the patient can be very serious because the effects are almost instantaneous. Once injected, the drug cannot be removed, so accurate administration of the correct drug and dose is essential. When giving subcutaneous or IM drugs, you must accurately locate the appropriate injection site to avoid pain or tissue damage. Aseptic (sterile) technique must be followed to prevent infection.

Potential exposure to blood or body fluids can occur when giving parenteral drugs. The Centers for Disease Control and Prevention (CDC) has issued standard precautions that include the wearing of gloves when there is risk for exposure to blood, body fluids, broken skin, or mucous membranes to prevent disease transmission. Always wear gloves when giving any parenteral drugs.

When giving parenteral drugs, it is important that you do not recap needles and that you dispose of them properly in a designated "sharps" container to prevent needlestick injury. Usually sharps containers are present within a patient's room or in other patient care areas. Many hospitals and clinics now use needleless systems, retractable needles, or needles with a plastic safeguard to protect healthcare workers from needlestick injuries (Fig. 4.6A–C). Needle-free syringes dispense the drug by using a highly pressurized air cartridge. Although the needleless syringe is not a sharp object, it may be contaminated with blood as the syringe tip contacts the injection site. Retractable needles have a spring-loaded syringe that immediately pulls the needle back inside after use. To dispose of potentially contaminated syringes in accordance with the Occupational Safety and Health Administration (OSHA) Bloodborne Pathogen recommendation, place the needleless syringe into a leakproof color-coded, labeled or sharps container, according to institution policy (see Fig. 4.6B).

### Syringes

Syringes come in a variety of sizes and are made up of three main parts. The tip is the portion that holds the needle. The needle screws onto the tip or fits tightly so

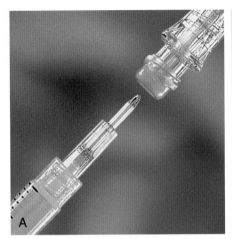
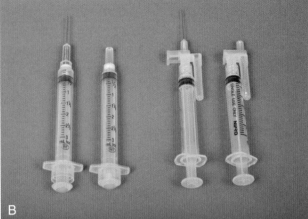
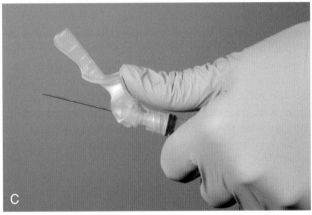

Fig. 4.6 (A) Needleless access for intravenous injection. (B) Retractable needle. (C) Syringe with plastic safeguard. (A, From Turner S. J. (2023). *Mulholland's the nurse, the math, the meds: Drug calculations using dimensional analysis* (5th ed.). Elsevier; B, Niedzwiecki, B., Shearer, M., Pepper, J., et al. (2023). *Kinn's the medical assistant: An applied learning approach* (15th ed.). Elsevier; C, Bonewit-West, K. (2024). *Clinical procedures for medical assistants* (11th ed.). Elsevier.)

it does not fall off. The barrel is the container for the drug. The calibrations are printed numbers on the barrel, and they indicate the amount or volume of drug in milliliters or units (Fig. 4.7). The plunger is the inner portion that fits into the barrel of the syringe. When the plunger is pushed into the barrel, the drug is forced out through the needle.

### Needles

The needle is made up of the hub, which attaches to the syringe; the shaft, which is the hollow part through which the drug passes; and the pointed or beveled tip, which pierces the skin (Fig. 4.8). The longer the pointed tip of the needle, the more easily the needle enters the skin. The diameter of the needle is called the gauge. The larger the number of the gauge, the smaller the hole (e.g., a 25-gauge needle is smaller than a 17-gauge needle). Thick solutions require larger diameters for injection. The needle gauge is written on the needle hub and on the package. Needles also come in varying lengths. Generally, the smaller the needle (larger the gauge), the shorter the needle. The smallest needles are used for intradermal or subcutaneous injections because they do not need to go very far into the skin and do not enter other tissues. Filter needles

are also available for use when a drug is drawn from an ampule or glass vial to prevent uptake and possible injection of glass shards.

The sizes of the needle and syringe are determined by how viscous (thick) the drug is and by the amount to be injected. For example, blood is very thick and requires a 15- to 18-gauge needle. Sometimes when the volume is very small and the dosage must be very accurate (as with heparin or insulin), a small-gauge needle (e.g., 27 gauge) is used so that no drug is lost. If more than 3 mL of drug is to be given IM, the drug must be divided and given in two injections so that a large pool of drug does not form in the tissue, which would irritate the tissue. A general guide for choosing the best syringe and needle size is presented in Table 4.1. Various needleless syringes are also used because they remove the risks associated with reuse or disposal of needles.

### PROCEDURE FOR PREPARING AND GIVING PARENTERAL DRUGS

The basic procedure for preparing and giving parenteral drugs is similar to that of oral drugs (Box 4.1). The type of parenteral injection and the specific drug to be given require selection of the appropriate equipment

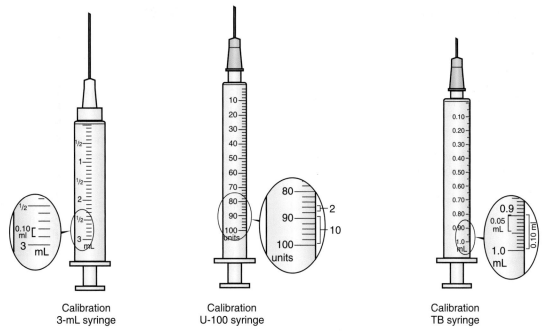

Fig. 4.7 Comparison of three different types of syringes.

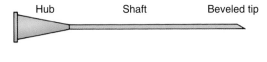

Hub        Shaft        Beveled tip

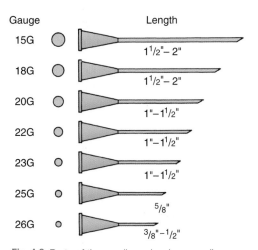

| Gauge | | Length |
| 15G | ○ | 1¹/₂"– 2" |
| 18G | ○ | 1¹/₂"– 2" |
| 20G | ○ | 1"–1¹/₂" |
| 22G | ○ | 1"–1¹/₂" |
| 23G | ○ | 1"–1¹/₂" |
| 25G | ○ | ⁵/₈" |
| 26G | ○ | ³/₈"–¹/₂" |

Fig. 4.8 Parts of the needle and various needle gauges.

| Table **4.1** | Suggested Guide for Selecting Syringe and Needles | | |
| --- | --- | --- | --- |
| **ROUTE** | **GAUGE (G)** | **LENGTH (INCHES)** | **VOLUME TO BE INJECTED (mL)** |
| Intradermal | 25–27 | 3/8–1/2 | 0.01–0.1 |
| Subcutaneous | 25–27 | 1/2–1 | 0.5–2 |
| Intramuscular | 20–22 | 1–2 | 0.5–2 |
| Intravenous | 15–22 | 1/2–2 | Unlimited |

and injection techniques. Inspect all syringe and needle packages to ensure that they are sealed and that the sterilization date has not expired. Any drug with a questionable seal that has changes in color or appearance or is expired is to be returned promptly to the pharmacy unused.

### Top Tip for Safety

- Check all equipment and drugs to ensure they are correct, sterile, and not expired before preparing the drug.
- Always wear gloves when giving parenteral drugs to avoid exposure to blood and body fluids.
- Clean the skin from the center outward, using a circular motion to minimize risk for infection.
- Do not recap needles! Recapping needles can result in needlestick injury and disease exposure.
- Immediately document that the drug was given to prevent drug errors.

### Preparation of Parenteral Drugs

Parenteral drugs are supplied in a variety of different forms. A **vial** is a small, single- or multiple-dose glass or plastic container of a drug. The top of the glass container is fitted with a rubber diaphragm and a small aluminum lid. To draw up a drug from a vial, the metal lid is removed, and the rubber diaphragm is cleansed with alcohol. An amount of air equal to the amount of solution to be withdrawn is injected with a syringe into the vial to assist the withdrawal of the drug (Fig 4.9). Needles are always inserted into the vial bevel up so you can inspect the needle as it goes into the rubber stopper. The vial may contain a solution, or it may contain a powder to which a liquid diluent is added to

## Box 4.1   Giving Parenteral Drugs

**STEP ONE: PREPARATION**

- Check the drug order as written for the patient, any drug allergies, and the time the drug is to be given.
- Wash hands well to avoid contaminating the drug and equipment.
- Assemble all the necessary equipment (needles, syringes, alcohol swabs, and drug ordered).
- Make certain the equipment is sterile and not expired.
- Compare the drug order with the drug label. Check for the right patient, drug, route, dosage, and time to be given.
- Attach the needle to the syringe, keeping the needle covered with a cap.
- Open the drug vial or ampule, cleansing the top of the drug container as appropriate.
- Insert the needle into the drug container and fill the syringe with the proper amount of drug. Remove any air bubbles.
- Do not mix more than one drug in a syringe unless they are compatible.
- Replace the needle with a new sterile needle after the drug has been drawn up through a rubber stopper, multidose vial, or glass ampule.

**STEP TWO: GIVING THE DRUG**

- Accurately identify the patient per institution policy.
- Explain what drug is being given, and answer any of the patient's questions.
- Examine previous injection sites for signs of necrosis, infection, or swelling. Examine the site to be injected.
- Don gloves. Clean the skin with alcohol. Follow the specific procedure for intradermal, subcutaneous, or intramuscular injection.
- Dispose of the syringe per institution policy and then wash your hands.
- Document that the drug was given as ordered per institution policy.
- Check the patient, noting the response or adverse effects that must be recorded and reported.

make a solution. Read the label carefully to determine the type and amount of diluent that is required. Roll the vial carefully to make certain all the powder is dissolved in the liquid. If the powder does not completely dissolve, do not give the drug and notify the pharmacy.

*Ampules.* An ampule contains one dose of a drug in a small, breakable glass container. The narrow neck of the base usually has a line (score) or ring around it, indicating a weakened area where the top can be broken off. Flick the top of the ampule lightly with a finger to ensure all of the drug is shifted to the bottom of the ampule. Grasp the top above the scored or ringed area with a small gauze pad and pull down quickly on the glass top, breaking the ampule at the level of the line or scored area, allowing insertion of the needle into the ampule to draw up the drug (Fig. 4.10). A filter needle is used to prevent any glass shards from being drawn up into the syringe.

*Mix-o-Vials.* Parenteral drugs may come in a two-compartment vial called a **Mix-o-Vial**. The top compartment contains a sterile liquid; the bottom compartment contains the drug powder. A rubber stopper separates the two areas. Pressure on the rubber plunger of the top compartment forces the stopper to fall below into the bottom compartment, letting in the liquid that dissolves the powder. Roll the vial gently between your palms to help dissolve the powder. When the powder has dissolved, insert the needle of the syringe to withdraw the solution (Fig. 4.11).

*Multiple-dose vials.* Any multiple-dose vial or newly mixed (reconstituted) powdered solution must be clearly labeled with the date, time, drug concentration and expiration time, and your initials. Once you withdraw a drug dose from a multiple-dose vial, change the needle before injecting the drug into the patient. Forcing the needle through the rubber stopper makes it dull and causes pain when injected into skin.

*Mixing two parenteral drugs.* Occasionally two drugs are ordered that may be given in the same syringe. For example, two compatible drugs are often given together as preoperative sedation before surgery, or two types of insulin (regular and NPH) may be ordered to be given together. In contrast, many antibiotics must be given in separate syringes because they will precipitate (form solid particles) or become inactive if mixed together. When drugs that are compatible are mixed together, inspect the syringe for precipitates, changes in color, or a cloudy appearance.

 **Memory Jogger**

It is important when mixing two drugs in one syringe to remember:

- The compatibility of the two drugs must be known: check with an up-to-date drug resource or your pharmacist.
- Air must be injected into both vials before any drug is withdrawn (to avoid accidental injection of a drug already in the syringe into the second vial).

*Prefilled syringes or cartridges.* Prefilled syringes and cartridges packaged this way are a convenient and reliable way of giving parenteral drugs. For patients, the advantages are ease of preparing and injecting drugs at home. Many opioids (narcotics) and emergency drugs (e.g., epinephrine) come in prefilled syringes and cartridges. These drug cartridges may be quickly slipped into a plastic holder and screwed into place (Fig. 4.12). The drug may then be quickly and accurately given.

### Giving Intradermal Drugs

**Intradermal injections** are used for several purposes such as allergy sensitivity testing, tuberculosis exposure testing, and some vaccinations. Intradermal

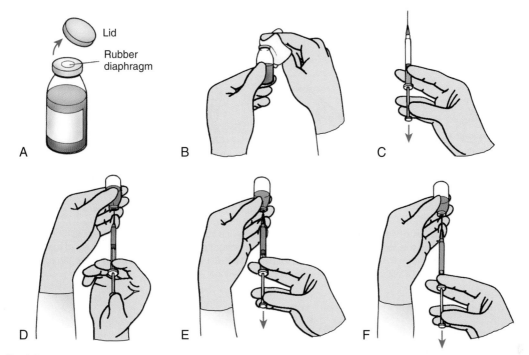

**Fig. 4.9** (A) Example of a vial. (B) Remove the metal lid and cleanse the diaphragm with an alcohol wipe. (C) Pull into the syringe an amount of air equal to the amount of solution to be withdrawn. (D) Insert the needle with the bevel up and inject the air into the space above the solution. (E) Begin withdrawing the drug. (F) Move the needle downward to allow the syringe to continue to fill to the correct amount.

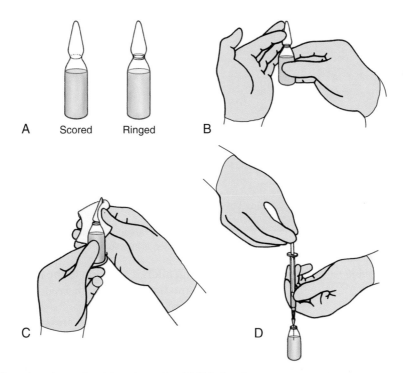

**Fig. 4.10** (A) Examples of scored and ringed ampules. (B) Shift drug from the top to the bottom portion of the ampule by flicking the top lightly with a finger. (C) Wrap a gauze pad around the neck of the ampule and use a snapping motion to break off the top of the ampule along prescored line at the neck. Always break away from the body by bending the top toward you. (D) Insert the filter needle into the ampule and draw up the drug.

injections consist of a drug injection into the intradermal space between the upper two layers of the skin—the epidermis and the dermis (Fig. 4.13). Injections are made into the inner aspect of the forearm, the scapular area of the back, and the upper chest if these areas are reasonably hairless. The blood supply to this area of the skin is less than that in other areas, thus there is very slow absorption from the intradermal layer. Usually just a small volume is injected, producing a small bump like a mosquito bite, called a bleb. Once

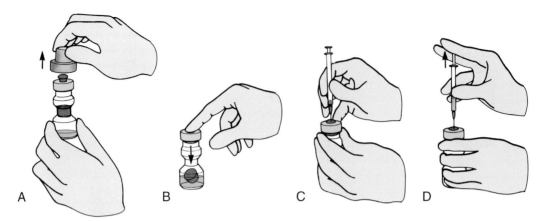

**Fig. 4.11** Example of a Mix-o-Vial. (A) Remove the protective sterile cap from the Mix-o-Vial. (B) Press the rubber plunger on the top compartment; this forces the rubber stopper into the bottom compartment and lets the liquid mix with and dissolve the powder. Gently roll the container to mix the solution well. (C) Insert the needle through the top rubber diaphragm into the solution. (D) Withdraw the required dose into the syringe.

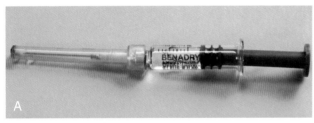

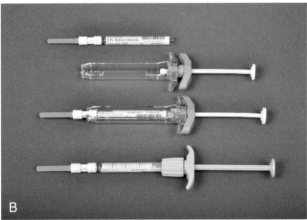

**Fig. 4.12** Examples of prefilled syringes. (A, From Bonewit-West, K. (2024). *Clinical procedures for medical assistants* (11th ed.). Elsevier; B, Niedzwiecki, B., Shearer, M., Pepper, J., et al. (2023). *Kinn's the medical assistant: An applied learning approach* (15th ed.). Elsevier.)

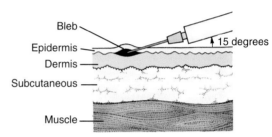

**Fig. 4.13** Anatomy of skin showing placement of the needle for intradermal injections.

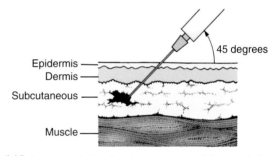

**Fig. 4.14** Anatomy of skin showing placement of the needle for subcutaneous injections.

the drug has been injected, instruct the patient not to wear tight clothing over the area.

For intradermal injections, choose a needle that is small (25 gauge) and short (3/8 inch). Wash your hands and don gloves. Cleanse the skin before giving the injection. After you draw up the drug, insert the needle firmly at a 15-degree angle with the bevel of the needle pointing upward. Do not aspirate (pull back) the syringe plunger before giving the drug. Inject the drug and then quickly remove the needle. The small bleb should be seen on the skin at the point where the drug was injected into the intradermal space. After giving the injection, check the patient's skin for sensitivity or

an allergic reaction to the injection. You may see an immediate reaction, or reactions may take hours to several days to develop.

Tuberculin tests are given intradermally and are checked for reactivity 48 to 72 hours after the injection. Making a circle mark around the injection site with a pen as soon as the drug is given can help you identify the site of the injection and the size of the reaction. Document any reaction noted and notify the healthcare provider.

### Giving Subcutaneous Drugs

Subcutaneous injections are given into the tissue between the dermis of the skin and the muscle layer (Fig. 4.14). With subcutaneous injections, there will be a slow but long duration of drug action because less blood is normally supplied to this area. Heparin and insulin are the drugs most frequently given by subcutaneous injection. See Chapters 16 and 20 for detailed information on these drugs. The drug volume given in a subcutaneous injection is usually between 0.5 and 1 mL per injection. When giving subcutaneous drugs daily over a long time period, you will need to rotate the injection sites to avoid irritating the tissue or causing changes in the tissue with repeated injections in the same area.

Subcutaneous injections require a small syringe and needle. Usually a 25- or 27-gauge needle with a 3/8-inch needle length is used. Subcutaneous injections may be given in the upper arms, upper back, scapular region, anterior thighs, and abdomen. Before giving the injection, wash your hands and don gloves, then cleanse the appropriate skin area with alcohol. To give a subcutaneous injection, take your thumb and index (pointer) finger and pinch the skin. Lift the skin away from the body. Pinching and pulling gently will pull the subcutaneous tissue away from the muscle. Insert the needle bevel up into the skin at a 45-degree angle. Do not aspirate before giving the drug, to prevent bruising and other tissue damage. Inject the drug and remove the needle. After the needle has been removed, apply slight pressure to prevent bleeding. Apply additional pressure or pressure of longer duration if the patient is at risk for bleeding. Document the injection site (location) and any skin or other reactions to the injection.

 **Top Tip for Safety**

To prevent bruising and other tissue damage, do not aspirate before giving a drug subcutaneously.

If a patient is to continue subcutaneous drug administration for any length of time at home, teach the patient about the drug, expected effects and adverse effects to report, and proper techniques for drug administration. Teach the patient and family to develop a plan for rotating injection sites. The front view in Fig. 4.15 shows areas usually used for subcutaneous self-injection. The back view shows less commonly used areas that may be accessed for injection by a family member.

### Giving Intramuscular Drugs

Drugs given by the intramuscular (IM) route are deposited deep into the muscle mass (Fig 4.16), where the rich blood supply allows for a more rapid drug absorption compared with the subcutaneous route. The muscles also contain large blood vessels and nerves, so it is important to place the needle correctly to avoid damage to these structures.

IM injections for adults typically range from 1 to 3 mL; infants and children rarely receive more than 1 mL. If more than 3 mL of drug is ordered for an adult patient, you will need to divide the total drug dose between two syringes, giving two injections at two different sites. To give an IM injection, choose a 20- to 22-gauge needle with a length of 1 to 1.5 inches

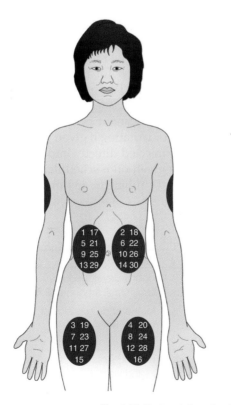
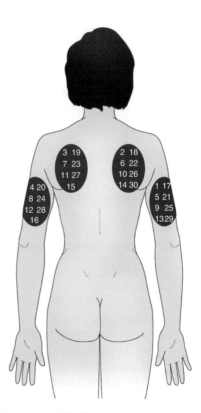

Fig. 4.15 Body rotation sites for subcutaneous injections.

to allow deeper placement into the muscle. You will need to make adjustments for very thin or very obese patients, who require a shorter or longer needle for proper drug placement.

The sites for IM injections include the deltoid, vastus lateralis, and ventrogluteal muscles. Each site has advantages and disadvantages, and you must be able to correctly identify each site for giving IM drugs safely. Table 4.2 describes the advantages and disadvantages of each IM injection site. The dorsogluteal site is not recommended because the presence of nerves and blood vessels in the area increases the risk for tissue damage.

### Top Tip for Safety

The dorsogluteal site is not recommended for IM injections because the nerves and blood vessels in the area increase the risk for tissue damage. If for some reason the dorsogluteal muscle is used for an IM injection, the close proximity of the gluteal artery requires you to aspirate prior to injecting the drug. Aspiration involves drawing back on the syringe after the needle is inserted to check for blood before injecting the drug. Aspirating before giving an IM injection is not required for any other site.

Before preparing the IM drug for injection, carefully select the site and identify the landmarks. Figs. 4.17 through 4.19 show how to identify sites for IM injections. Position the patient properly to access the injection site. Wash your hands and don gloves. Clean the injection area with alcohol. Insert the needle firmly, at a 90-degree angle, and inject the drug. Aspiration

is not recommended for IM injection of vaccines or immunizations. If aspiration is required for a certain drug, pull back the plunger after inserting the needle and check for the presence of blood being drawn into the syringe. If this occurs, remove the needle, then discard the drug and syringe properly. You will then need to prepare a new dose of the drug and inject into a different site.

After withdrawing the needle, apply gentle pressure to the site with a dry cotton ball. Avoid massaging the area of injection. Rotate the site of injection when repeated injections are needed. Note the time and site of the injection and be sure to check the patient for expected and adverse effects of the drug; document your findings.

The **Z-track technique** may be used for IM injections of drugs that can stain the skin or are known to be irritating to the tissues (Fig. 4.20). To give drugs using the Z-track technique, draw up the drug as usual, plus 0.1 to 0.2 mL of air. The injection of the air seals the injection site, preventing leakage of the drug. Drugs of the type that require the Z-track technique are injected into the ventrogluteal site. Once the injection site is prepared, pull the tissue downward and away from the injection site. Inject the drug and allow the skin to move back into place before you remove the needle. This action allows the tissue to make a seal over the injection site, sealing the drug in place. Do not massage the injection site.

### Giving Intravenous Drugs

Intravenous drugs are delivered by an IV "push" or bolus route, IV "piggyback" or intermittent infusion, or continuous IV infusion. The IV route injects a drug directly into the vein, where it enters the bloodstream immediately. The rate of absorption and onset of drug action are faster for the IV route than for oral or IM routes because IV drugs have not been exposed to other enzymes or tissues before reaching the bloodstream. Some drugs cannot be given orally and may be very painful or irritating if given IM. In emergencies, a drug may be injected directly into a vein, but usually the IV drug is given on a scheduled basis or infused slowly through IV tubing or an infusion line that is already in the vein.

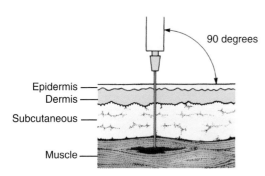

Fig. 4.16 Anatomy of skin showing placement of the needle for intramuscular injections.

| Table 4.2 | Intramuscular Injection Site Advantages and Disadvantages | |
| --- | --- | --- |
| **INJECTION SITE** | **ADVANTAGES** | **DISADVANTAGES** |
| Deltoid (upper arm) | Easily accessible<br>Useful for vaccinations in adolescents and adults | Poorly developed in young children<br>Only small amounts (0.5–1 mL) can be injected |
| Vastus lateralis (thigh) | Preferred site for infant injections<br>Relatively free of large blood vessels and nerves<br>Easily accessible | Intake of drug is slower than the arm but faster than buttocks |
| Ventrogluteal (hips) | Used for children 7 years or older and adults<br>Less likely to be inadvertently injected<br>    subcutaneously | Patient anxiety because of unfamiliarity with site<br>    and visibility of site during injection |

From Workman, M. L., & LaCharity, L. (2016). *Understanding pharmacology* (2nd ed.). Elsevier.

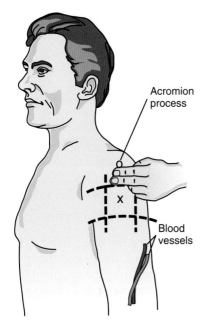

Fig. 4.17 Deltoid intramuscular injection site landmarks. (From Workman, M. L., & LaCharity, L. (2016). *Understanding pharmacology* (2nd ed.). Elsevier.)

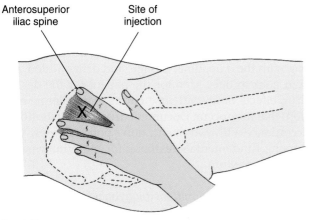

Fig. 4.18 Ventrogluteal intramuscular injection site landmarks. (From Potter, P. A. (2016). *Fundamentals of nursing* (9th ed.). Elsevier.)

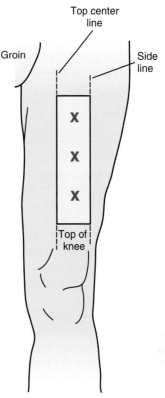

Fig. 4.19 Vastus lateralis (thigh) intramuscular injection site landmarks. (From Workman, M. L., & LaCharity, L. (2016). *Understanding pharmacology* (2nd ed.). Elsevier.)

### Top Tip for Safety

- Check the provider's IV drug order to ensure that it is complete and clear.
- The drug, dose, timing, and type of IV administration (IV push, intermittent, or continuous infusion) must be specified, along with the rate of infusion.
- A drug order that states to give an IV drug "slowly" is not acceptable because it leaves the timing open to interpretation and may prove harmful to the patient if done improperly.

Greater skill and drug knowledge are needed to give IV drugs, and care is needed to prevent infiltration and infection at the needle site. In addition, because the effect of the drug is immediate, drug overdosages, errors in dosage calculation, or failure to control the rate of administration may produce serious or fatal consequences for the patient. You have an increased responsibility for implementing and evaluating the IV drug given. Registered nurses are usually the nurses who will administer IV drugs, but an LPN/VN often assists in this procedure and may evaluate the IV site and patient response as directed by the RN. In some states the LPN/VN may give IV drugs into an already existing IV set up either by piggyback or as an IV push dose. Initiating the actual IV system is not within the LPN/VN scope of practice in many states. You are responsible for checking your state's Nurse Practice Act to determine your legal role in IV drug administration.

All IV drugs that are prepared directly in advance of administration must be clearly labeled and given only by the person who prepared it. All IV drugs that need to be reconstituted (powders to be mixed with liquid) must be mixed using the recommended liquid in the reconstitution process to prevent crystals or other harmful precipitates from forming. Before giving drugs into an existing IV connected to an IV pump, make sure you have been oriented to the proper use of the pump to prevent infusion errors.

Always use aseptic technique to prevent contamination to the drug and drug delivery system when giving IV drugs. You must wash your hands and don gloves in preparation for giving IV drugs. Make sure you disinfect the diaphragm of the drug vial and the injection portal before giving the IV drug or injecting it into a piggyback or IV solution. Make sure you use the proper personal protection equipment if you will be exposed to blood or body fluids. Use a filter needle

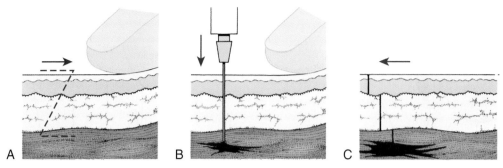

**Fig. 4.20** Z-track injection technique. (A) Pull the tissue laterally. (B) Insert the needle straight down into the muscle and inject the drug. (C) Release the tissue as the needle is withdrawn; this allows the skin to slide over the injection track and seal the drug inside.

to withdraw a drug from a glass vial, then change the needle before injecting the drug (or use a needleless syringe). Be sure to properly dispose of needles and syringes following IV drug administration.

*Giving intravenous push drugs.* Many IV drugs are commonly given by syringe through an IV infusion that is already running, as a push or bolus dose. In this way the drug directly enters the patient's bloodstream rather than the IV bottle or bag. In addition to the directions presented here, review your nursing fundamentals textbook for more information about this procedure.

Wash your hands and don gloves. Clean the drug injection portal with alcohol, then slowly inject the drug into the IV line using the portal closest to the patient and according to the prescribed rate of IV push infusion for that drug. There are specific guidelines for the length of time of IV push injection for all drugs that can be given in this manner. After all the drug has been injected, the needle is withdrawn and properly disposed of. The main IV solution is then restarted at the specified infusion rate. Document the IV injection, note whether the effects of the drug have been achieved (e.g., pain relief), and monitor the patient for any adverse effects.

*Giving drugs by peripheral intravenous lock.* A patient may have a butterfly or scalp vein needle inserted and left in place, without being attached to a primary IV solution, to serve as a means for giving drugs intermittently. These units may be referred to as peripheral IV or saline locks because normal saline is used to maintain the patency of these devices. Peripheral IV or saline locks are typically left in place for 72 hours and are flushed with saline every 8 hours or per institution policy. State practice regulations and institution policy regulate whether an LPN/VN may give drugs through these systems. Follow institution policy if you, as an LPN/VN, are permitted to give drugs in this manner.

To begin, wash your hands and don gloves. Use an alcohol wipe to cleanse the top of the rubber diaphragm at the end of the tubing. Follow the institution's policy and procedures for flushing the tubing

before and after giving the drug. Refer to your nursing fundamentals textbook to review this procedure. Be sure to inject the drug over the specified length of time recommended for that drug and observe for expected and adverse effects.

*Adding drugs to an intravenous solution container.* Make certain that the drug is compatible with the solution into which it will be injected. Wash your hands and don a pair of gloves. Identify the proper portal and cleanse it with an alcohol wipe. Fill the syringe with the drug and inject it slowly with a small needle through the portal into the IV container. Label the IV bottle or bag with the date, time, dosage, and drugs added, and sign your initials. Monitor the patient for the desired drug effects or any adverse effects (e.g., allergic reaction) that may occur. Document drug administration in accordance with your institution's policy. Review your nursing fundamentals textbook for more information on this procedure.

*Giving drugs by intermittent (piggyback) infusion.* While an existing IV infusion is running, it may be clamped off to allow a second IV infusion for giving drugs by intermittent infusion. Antibiotics are an example of drug types often given in this manner. The drug order will specify the time over which the piggyback IV solution containing the drug should be infused. Wash your hands and don gloves. The drug is added to a second, small IV bottle or bag connected to the drug portal. This second IV container, or piggyback infusion, is hung slightly higher than the primary IV solution, and the tubing to the primary IV is clamped off to allow the piggyback IV containing the prescribed drug to be infused. The piggyback IV is to be labeled with the time, date, drug and dosage, and your initials. Once the piggyback is infused, the setup is removed, the clamp on the primary IV is reopened, and the infusion is reset to the prescribed flow rate (drops/min).

*Intravenous infusions.* Giving IV fluids is considered another type of IV drug delivery system. Remember that whenever you infuse fluids or drugs directly into the vein, they immediately enter the bloodstream.

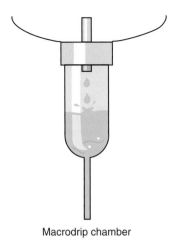

Macrodrip chamber

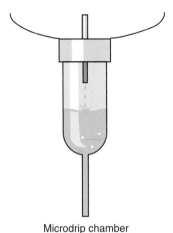

Microdrip chamber

**Fig. 4.21** Macrodrip chamber and microdrip chamber. (From Workman, M. L., & LaCharity, L. (2016). *Understanding pharmacology* (2nd ed.). Elsevier.)

When IV fluids are given, this is known as a continuous intravenous infusion. IV infusions may be given for the purpose of hydration or as another way to give parenteral drugs. When the healthcare provider orders IV fluids for hydration, the order must include the type of fluid, the amount to be infused, and the duration (time) over which the fluid should infuse.

The IV flow rate tells how fast the IV infusion should run. The healthcare provider's order must state the amount (in milliliters) over time. For example, the order may instruct you to give 250 mL of a solution over 1 hour. The size of the tubing influences the rate of the infusion. Thicker tubing will give more drops per minute as compared with smaller, thinner tubing. Each tubing has what is known as a drop factor, which is the number of drops needed to make a milliliter of fluid. Each manufacturer places the drop factor on each IV administration tubing set.

Remember that IV tubing is divided into two types: macrodrip and microdrip tubing. The actual drip chamber (the clear plastic cylinder attached to the IV tubing) of the IV tubing differs considerably. Fig. 4.21 shows the differences between the macrodrip and microdrip chambers.

When the IV tubing is primed to be ready for IV fluid administration, the drip chamber is filled only halfway so you can see the fluid dripping and count the number of drops per minute, if needed. Depending on the manufacturer, the drop factor for a macrodrip IV set is 10, 15, or 20 drops/mL. However, all microdrip tubing delivers 60 drops/mL. This information is important because you need to know the drop factor for every IV calculation. Fig. 4.22 shows the different parts of the IV infusion set.

*Intravenous fluid regulation.* To regulate the flow of IV fluids, you will need to calculate the flow rate, as described in the Calculations for Intravenous Infusions section earlier in this chapter. Recall that the flow rate is the number of drops per minute needed to have the IV infused in the amount of time ordered by the prescriber. There are essentially two ways to regulate IV fluids: You can use the roller clamp on the tubing to regulate the flow of the IV solution or, more commonly, you can use an IV pump. An IV pump is an electronic device that infuses the IV solution into the vein by pressure. The IV pump has buttons for specific settings that are involved in infusion of IV fluid and can be manually programmed.

The IV pump settings are:
- On/Off
- Start/Enter
- Stop
- Silence
- IV Lock (prevents tampering)
- Primary (controls main or primary IV solution infusion)
- IVPB (controls IV piggyback or secondary infusion)

IV pumps are made by different companies, so you will need to be oriented to the IV pumps used in your facility and follow the manufacturer's directions. Some IV pumps are set to deliver the IV solution in milliliters per hour and others in drops per minute.

 **Memory Jogger**

To infuse IV fluids properly, you will need to know these four items:
- The correct type of fluid ordered
- The volume to be infused (how much)
- The duration of the infusion (how long)
- The rate at which the IV solution is to be infused (how fast)

The healthcare provider's order must address the type of fluid to be infused, the amount (volume) to be infused, and the duration (length of time) over which the fluid should be infused. You will need to calculate the rate of the infusion. For example, the order may read "Infuse 1000 mL of 0.9% normal saline over 12 hours." You can use this information to program the IV pump. You will need to note the start and stop

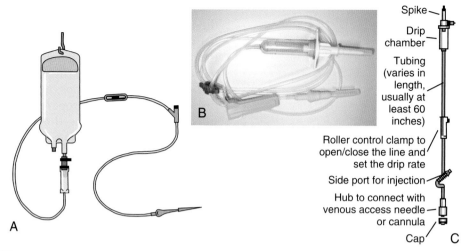

Fig. 4.22 Intravenous (IV) tubing administration sets. (A) Administration set connected to an IV solution bag. (B) Photograph of IV tubing administration set. (C) Details of IV tubing administration set. (From Workman, M. L., & LaCharity, L. (2016). *Understanding pharmacology* (2nd ed.). Elsevier.)

times of the infusion. Many factors influence the gravity flow, thus a solution may not necessarily continue to flow at the rate originally set. Therefore IV infusions must be monitored to verify that the fluid is flowing at the intended rate. Mark the IV bag or bottle with tape showing the start time of the infusion. The flow rate is calculated when the solution is originally hung and then rechecked at least hourly to ensure it is infusing on time.

**Calculating the intravenous flow rate.** The IV flow rate is the rate at which an IV fluid is given; it can be calculated from the IV tubing drop factor and the volume and duration of the IV infusion. The basic formula is:

$$\frac{\text{Volume}(\text{mL})}{\text{Time}(\text{min})} \times \text{Drop factor}(\text{drops}/\text{mL})$$
$$= \text{Flow rate}(\text{drops}/\text{min})$$

**Macrodrip calculation.** In the example, 1000 mL of normal saline is to be infused over 12 hours. The first step is to find out the number of milliliters to be infused in 1 hour (or 60 minutes):

$$\frac{1000\,\text{mL}}{12\,\text{h}} = 83\,\text{mL}/\text{h} = \frac{83\,\text{mL}}{60\,\text{min}}$$

A check of the IV administration set shows a drop factor of 10 drops/mL. To calculate the flow rate (drops/min) needed to infuse the IV fluid at 83 mL/hour, use the formula:

$$\frac{\text{Volume}(83\,\text{mL})}{\text{Time}(60\,\text{min})} \times \left(\frac{10\,\text{drops}}{1\,\text{mL}}\right)$$
$$= 1.38 \times 10 = 13.8\,\text{macrodrops}/\text{min}$$

You may round up to 14 drops/min.

**Microdrip calculation.** Recall that the drop factor for microdrip tubing is 60 drops/mL. Use the same formula as for the macrodrip set:

$$\frac{83\,\text{mL}}{60\,\text{min}} \times \frac{60\,\text{drops}}{1\,\text{mL}} = \frac{83}{1} = 83\,\text{microdrops}/\text{min}$$

Notice that the number of drops per milliliter (drop factor) in a microdrip IV set is the same as the number of minutes in 1 hour (i.e., 60), and they cancel each other out. Therefore the mL/h will always be the same as the drops/min (in this case, 83). In a microdrip set, calculation of the infusion rate in milliliters per hour automatically gives you the flow rate in drops per minute.

*Completing IV therapy.* When IV therapy is to be discontinued, clamp the tubing, loosen the adhesive tape, and don gloves. Holding a gauze pad in the nondominant hand, apply gentle pressure on the venipuncture site with the gauze pad and carefully withdraw the needle with the dominant hand. The area is then cleaned with an alcohol wipe and elevated, if possible, and direct pressure is applied to stop any bleeding at the site. Check for bleeding after 1 to 2 minutes. Follow institutional procedure for any additional steps regarding ointments or pressure dressings as needed. Dispose of all contaminated equipment per institution policy.

*Evaluation for complications of intravenous therapy.* There are six primary areas for evaluation of patients receiving IV therapy. Table 4.3 summarizes the problems and complications that may occur with an IV infusion and the appropriate nursing actions to take.

The first step for evaluating the situation if an IV fails to infuse properly is to check the patient for bending of the IV tubing or obstruction of flow (e.g., lying on the tubing). If the rate of infusion is very slow, a small clot may form at the end of the needle, blocking the flow. The IV container may have to be elevated to keep adequate pressure for infusion. Check every part

Table **4.3**   Complications of Intravenous Infusions

| PROBLEM | APPROPRIATE NURSING ACTION |
|---|---|
| Failure to infuse properly | Check for bent tubing, catheter against vein wall, or small clot at the end of the catheter; the intravenous (IV) pole may be too low or the needle may be out of the vein. Check for damage done from tissue infusion. Stop infusion and report problem to the registered nurse. |
| IV infiltration | Note the presence of redness, swelling, warmth at the IV insertion site, and failure for the fluid to infuse. Assess for signs of tissue damage. Notify healthcare provider of any necrosis or sloughing. Apply warm, wet compresses to the area to reduce pain. Stop infusion and report problem to the registered nurse (RN). |
| Signs of infection | Check for local (inflammation, pain) and systemic (fever) symptoms. Stop infusion and notify healthcare provider. Treat as recommended by institution policy or by orders of the healthcare provider. Save the solution for microbial testing. |
| Allergic reactions | Watch for symptoms of allergic or hypersensitivity reactions such as rash, hives, itching, swelling of the face, lips, or tongue. Stop infusion and notify the RN and healthcare provider immediately. Take vital signs. Remain with the patient until treatment (if needed) has been determined. |
| Circulatory problems | Watch for symptoms of pulmonary edema: shortness of breath, coughing, increased respiratory rate, poor color, anxiety, restlessness. Notify the RN and healthcare provider immediately. Remain with the patient. |
| Other | Watch for symptoms of pulmonary embolus: chest pain, shortness of breath, cough, poor color, and coughing up blood. Notify the RN and healthcare provider immediately. Monitor vital signs. Remain with the patient. |

of the infusion setup for any problems that could block infusion, including lack of blood return to the tubing, which would lead you to suspect that the catheter is out of place or blocked.

**Infiltration.** IV infiltration is complication of the intravenous therapy that occurs when the IV catheter becomes dislodged from the vein causing fluid to seep out or infiltrate into the surrounding tissues. Infiltration produces pain, swelling of the area, and redness. When the infiltrating fluid irritates or damages the surrounding tissue, it is known as extravasation. When an IV infiltration is discovered, inspect the infusion site carefully for signs of infection or injury. Discontinue the infusion and contact the healthcare provider who ordered the IV to report the infiltration and to determine if the IV needs to be reinserted. Report any swelling, redness, tissue loss, or necrosis. Warm, moist compresses may be ordered to be applied to the area. In the case of necrosis, more intensive treatment would be needed; promptly notify the pharmacist as well as the healthcare provider.

**Infection.** Signs of infection from an existing IV or of inflammation of the vein (phlebitis) include redness, swelling, warmth, and burning along the course of the vein. Inflammation and infection can be associated with irritating solutions or certain drugs such as potassium, antibiotics, or anticancer drugs. In these cases, stop the IV and notify the healthcare provider. Warm, moist compresses may be applied to the area.

**Allergic reactions.** Because IV infusions directly enter the vein and bloodstream, there is a greater risk of potential allergic reaction to the drug. Monitor the patient receiving IV drugs for shortness of breath, temperature elevation, facial swelling, or rash. Reactions to blood or blood products are not common, but they can be harmful to the lungs and kidneys and can cause itching, shaking chills, temperature elevations, back pain, dark urine, and shortness of breath. Stop the drug infusion or blood transfusion immediately, obtain vital signs, and remain with the patient while another colleague immediately notifies the healthcare provider.

**Fluid overload.** The potential for fluid overload is a concern for older adult patients, infants, and children because they are more sensitive to the amount of fluid infused. These individuals may have heart, lung, or kidney problems that decrease their ability to handle extra fluid. Fluid overload may develop when fluids are infused too rapidly or when the volume to be infused is too great. Signs of fluid overload include shortness of breath (dyspnea), weakness, lethargy, reduced urine output, edema of the extremities, sacral edema, a weak but rapid pulse, and shallow, rapid respirations. If the excess fluid accumulates primarily in the lungs, producing coughing, difficulty breathing, crackles in the lung sounds, and frothy sputum, slow the infusion immediately, monitor the patient's vital signs, and notify the healthcare provider.

---

### Top Tip for Safety

- Check IV patency flow rates hourly.
- Observe the patient for signs of fluid overload (shortness of breath, edema).
- Monitor the patient's urinary output. Urinary output should be at least 30 mL/hour.
- Observe the IV site for redness or swelling that may indicate infiltration.
- Monitor the patient for signs of allergic reactions to any IV drug.

## PERCUTANEOUS DRUGS

The **percutaneous route** is the delivery of drugs by application to the skin or mucous membranes. Using this route makes it difficult to predict how well the drug will be absorbed. The amount of drug absorbed through the skin or mucous membranes depends on several factors:

- The size of the area covered by the drug
- The concentration or strength of the drug
- The length of time the drug stays in contact with the area
- The general condition of the skin, including any areas of skin irritation or breakdown, skin thickness, and the general hydration, nutrition, and tone of the skin

Methods of percutaneous administration include:

- Giving drugs into the mucous membranes of the ear, eye, nose, mouth, or vagina
- Applying topical creams, powders, ointments, or lotions
- Giving aerosolized liquids or gases by inhalation to carry drugs to the nasal passages, sinuses, and lungs
- Applying transdermal patches or topical gel systems

Follow the same general procedures and patient safety considerations outlined for other routes of administration when applying drugs to the skin or mucous membranes. The general method for giving percutaneous drugs is outlined in Box 4.2.

### GIVING TOPICAL AND TRANSDERMAL DRUGS

Drugs given by the **topical route** are applied directly to the area of skin that requires treatment. There are many forms of topical drugs, the most common being creams, lotions, and ointments. Each form of topical application has specific advantages and characteristics. **Transdermal drugs** are semipermeable membranes and adhesive patches that are applied to the skin, through which the drug is absorbed into the bloodstream. Drugs using a transdermal delivery system include fentanyl, nitroglycerin, birth control pills, scopolamine, testosterone, and clonidine. Various antismoking programs also use nicotine patches.

### Topical Drugs

1. Choose the skin site carefully in accordance with the drug manufacturer's instructions. Avoid skin that has been tattooed, skin that has lesions, and broken skin, all of which can affect absorption.
2. Clean the skin before applying topical drugs to reduce the risk for infection and remove remaining drug from the previous application to prevent drug buildup.
3. Wear gloves for protection because the drug you are giving can also be absorbed through your skin.

Apply a thin layer of the topical drug with a tongue depressor, a cotton-tipped applicator, or a gloved finger. The topical drug may also be applied directly onto a gauze pad and placed on the skin if the site requires a dressing (Fig 4.23). Anchor the dressing as ordered by the healthcare provider.

### Transdermal Patches

1. Follow steps 1 through 3 for giving topical drugs.
2. To apply transdermal patches, carefully pick up the patch and remove the clear plastic backing (Fig. 4.24).
3. Firmly press the patch drug side down onto the skin. The adhesive on the edges will hold the patch tightly to the skin.
4. Transdermal patches are changed on a regular schedule, as indicated by the provider's order. Transderm-Nitro, fentanyl patches, Nitro-Dur, and birth control patches may be worn while showering; all other drug patches are to be applied after bathing.

### Topical and Transdermal Drugs

Many topical and transdermal drugs are continued after the patient leaves the hospital. Teach the patient how to clean the area, apply the drug, and dress the area as needed. Note the site where the ointment or patch is placed, along with the date and time. Also teach the patient to remove the drug or patch before applying a new dose.

Document all drugs given; note the site for any drug (e.g., patch) that requires the site to be rotated and the condition of the skin where topical drugs are placed. Document the expected actions and any adverse effects experienced.

| Box 4.2 | Giving Percutaneous Drugs |

**STEP ONE: PREPARATION**
- Check the drug order as written for the patient, allergies, and the time to be given.
- Wash your hands well to avoid contaminating the drug or equipment used.
- Assemble all the necessary equipment (drug, gloves, and plastic wrap).
- Compare the drug order with the label on the container. Check for the right patient, drug, route, dosage, and time to be given.

**STEP TWO: GIVING THE DRUG**
- Accurately identify the patient per institution policy.
- Explain what drug is being given, and answer any of the patient's questions.
- Apply the drug as ordered to the appropriate area.
- When the procedure is complete, discard all used dressings and gloves. Wash your hands.
- Document that the drug was given as ordered per institution policy.
- Check the patient, noting the response or adverse effects that must be recorded and reported.

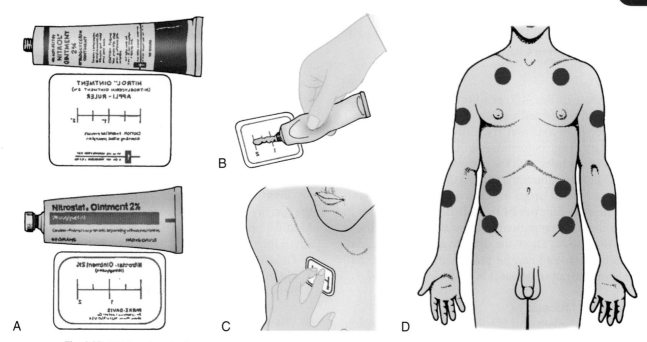

Fig. 4.23 (A) Nitroglycerin ointment and special application papers. Notice that the papers are printed backward. (B) The correct amount of ointment is squeezed onto the paper. (C) The paper is applied to the patient's skin at one of the sites shown in (D). Clear plastic wrap may be applied over the paper to increase absorption and protect clothing from staining.

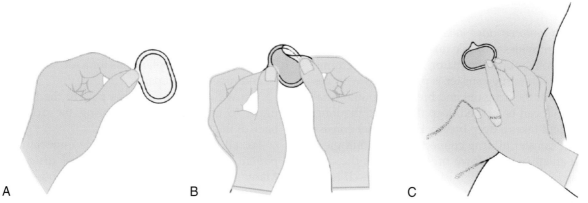

Fig. 4.24 (A) Nitroglycerin patch. (B) Remove the plastic backing, being careful not to touch the drug inside. (C) Place the side with drug on the patient's skin and press the adhesive edges into place.

### Top Tip for Safety

Avoid touching topical or transdermal drugs with your bare hands or fingers to prevent absorbing the drug through the skin into your system.

## GIVING DRUGS THROUGH MUCOUS MEMBRANES

The mucous membranes are the other major route of percutaneous drug administration. Drugs can be given by the **sublingual route** (under the tongue); by the **buccal route** (against the cheek); in the mucous membranes of the eye, nose, or ear; or through aerosol inhalation into the lungs. Vaginal suppositories or creams and drugs given rectally also represent treatment through mucosal membranes. Drugs for mucous membranes may be formulated as small tablets, drops, ointments, creams, suppositories, or aerosols.

Before giving drugs through the mucous membranes, follow all the general steps noted earlier in this chapter for safe drug administration, wash your hands, and don gloves.

### Sublingual and Buccal Drugs

Place sublingual drugs, such as nitroglycerin tablets or spray, under the tongue. There is a rich blood supply in this area, so the drug is absorbed quickly. Teach the patient not to chew or swallow the drug because drugs meant for the sublingual route are less effective if absorbed by the GI tract. Teach the patient to avoid food or drink until the drug is completely dissolved.

To give drugs by the buccal route, place the drug between the cheek and teeth of the upper jaw. Lozenges are often given by this route.

## Eye Drops and Ointments

Detailed information about giving eye drops and ointments is provided in Chapter 22.

## Eardrops

As described in Box 4.3, position the patient on one side, with the affected ear up. You will need to pull the earlobe (pinna) down in children who are younger than 3 years of age before instilling the drops. For older children and adults, pull the earlobe up and out. These actions help straighten the ear canal. Now place the required number of drops into the ear canal. Avoid contaminating the dropper by not touching the dropper to the ear. Instruct the patient to remain in position for at least 5 minutes to allow the drug to coat the ear canal. A small cotton ball can be placed into the ear canal. Repeat on the opposite ear if both ears are affected.

## Respiratory Mucosa

Drugs can be given and inhaled through the respiratory mucosa. Common types of aerosol devices used for inhaled drug delivery are the pressurized metered-dose inhaler (MDI), the dry-powder inhaler (DPI), and continuous aerosol therapy. Table 4.4 lists the advantages and disadvantages of inhaled drug delivery.

*Pressurized metered-dose inhaler.* A MDI is a portable device that provides multiple doses of a drug, typically a corticosteroid or bronchodilator, by a specialized (metered) valve. The drug canister is pressurized with gas, which propels the drug out and breaks it up into small particles that can be carried deep down into the lungs as the patient takes a deep breath. Each inhaler consists of a small canister of drug connected to a mouthpiece. As the patient presses down on the canister, the drug is released in the form of a mist into the lungs. It is important to teach the patient to use the inhaler correctly or the correct dose may not be delivered. This type of device must be primed by pressing the device to expel the drug into the air before the first use and periodically thereafter, especially if there are long periods between use. Otherwise the drug and propellant may fail to combine, and the correct dose may not be delivered.

Patient instructions for using the pressurized MDI are as follows:
- Remove the cap over the mouthpiece and hold the inhaler upright.
- Stand or sit up straight.
- Shake the inhaler.
- Tilt your head back slightly and breathe out all the way.
- Put the inhaler in your mouth making a seal with your lips.
- Press down on the inhaler quickly to release the medicine as you start to breathe in slowly.
- Breathe in slowly for 3 to 5 seconds.
- Hold your breath for 10 seconds to allow medicine to go deeply into your lungs.

- Breathe out slowly.
- Repeat puffs as directed by the prescription. Wait 1 minute before taking the second puff.

Some inhalers (such as steroid inhalers) also recommend rinsing your mouth out with water and gargling with water (spit out the water) after use.

*Dry-powder inhaler.* A DPI is an aerosol device that delivers the drug in a powdered form when the patient takes a deep breath. DPIs do not require the hand-breath coordination of a pressurized MDI. DPIs are breath activated, meaning the drug is released to the airway when the patient takes a deep, fast breath. Medication particles in DPIs are powdered and are so small they can reach the tiniest airways.

Patient instructions for using a DPI are as follows:
1. Do not shake the DPI.
2. Stand or sit up straight and breathe out completely to empty the lungs.
3. With most DPIs, the mouthpiece should be pointed up or held horizontal when using it.
4. Place the mouthpiece into your mouth, close your lips tightly around it, and breathe in quickly and forcefully.
5. Remove the DPI from your mouth, holding your breath for 5 to 10 seconds. This action allows the drug to settle before another puff is taken as ordered.
6. Exhale slowly.
7. If your treatment plan calls for a second dose, reload and repeat the steps.

You will need to teach the patient the proper technique to avoid simply delivering the drug into the back of the throat or nose.

For all prescribed inhalers, it is important that the patient keep an adequate supply of drug on hand. Many metered-dose canisters click and count each spray (Fig. 4.25). For those that do not, teach the patient to count every spray.

*Continuous aerosol therapy.* Continuous aerosol therapy is used to treat an acute respiratory illness such as an asthma attack. The drug typically comes in a small, disposable container that is opened and placed in the nebulizer chamber. Oxygen is used to deliver the drug while the patient uses the mouthpiece to inhale in and out slowly and deeply while in an upright position. The nebulizer treatment is continued in this way until the drug is completely gone from the nebulizer chamber, about 10 to 20 minutes. The nebulizer must be cleaned with water after each use. All patients have their own nebulizer equipment, and to avoid contamination these are not shared between patients (Fig. 4.26).

## Vaginal Drugs

Vaginal drugs are typically given to treat infection in the area. Vaginal creams, jellies, tablets, foams, and suppositories are examples of the types of vaginal drugs used. These drugs are kept at room temperature. Before giving

## Box **4.3**   Instructions for Giving Buccal, Sublingual, Ear, and Eye Drugs

### STEP 1: PREPARATION
- Always follow the *9 Rights of Drug Administration*.
- Check the drug label.
- Gather the necessary equipment, including gloves, cotton ball (if needed), and the correct drug. Wash your hands before giving any drug.
- Correctly identify the patient. Explain the procedure to the patient.
- For optic or otic drugs, identify the correct eye or ear to be treated.

### STEP 2: GIVING THE DRUGS
#### Giving Buccal Area Drugs
- Place the drug into the patient's mouth using a gloved hand.
- Instruct the patient to hold the drug between the cheek and molar teeth.

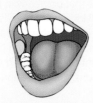

- Dispose of gloves and then wash your hands.
- Drugs given by the buccal route are rapidly absorbed into the bloodstream, reaching the systemic circulation without metabolism by the liver.

#### Giving Sublingual Drugs
- Using a gloved hand, instruct the patient to lift the tongue. Place the tablet under the tongue, where it will dissolve. Dispose of gloves and then wash your hands.

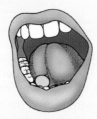

- Drugs given sublingually are rapidly absorbed through the blood vessels. This site is used for nitroglycerin tablets to relieve chest pain.

#### Giving Drugs for the Ear
- Localized infection or inflammation of the ear is treated by dropping a small amount of a sterile drug solution into the ear. Be sure the drug label indicates that it is for otic (ear) usage.
- Instruct the patient to lie on the side with the affected ear up. Shake the drug container well and then draw up the drug into the dropper. Instill the ear drops, being sure not touch the dropper to the ear.
- For children younger than 3 years, gently pull the earlobe down and back.

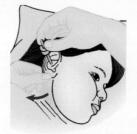
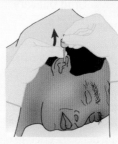

- For adults, gently pull the earlobe up and out. This will straighten the external canal for proper drug placement.
- Keep the patient in the same position for 5 min to allow the drug to coat the inner canal.
- A cotton ball may be ordered for insertion to keep the drug in place.
- Repeat in the other ear if indicated.
- Dispose of gloves and then wash your hands.

#### Giving Drugs for the Eye
- Sterile drops or ointments may be used to treat inflammation or infection of the eye.
- Be sure that the drug is specifically labeled for ophthalmic (eye) use.
- Any discharge from the eye may be removed with a cotton ball saturated with normal saline, wiping from the inner canthus out to prevent contamination of the eye. Use one cotton ball per stroke.
- Instruct the patient to look up, then pull out the lower lid to show the conjunctival sac. Instil the prescribed drops or ointment into the eye.

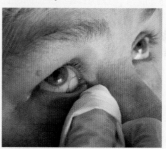

- Do not touch the eye with the dropper or the ointment tip. Drop the drug or squeeze the ointment into the conjunctival sac, not onto the eye itself.
- Apply gentle external pressure with a tissue to the inner corner of the eyelid on the bone for 1–2 min to ensure adequate concentration of drug and prevent the drug from draining rapidly into the nose.
- Apply a sterile dressing, if ordered.
- Dispose of gloves, and then wash your hands.
- Instruct the patient to move the eyes around with eyelids closed to spread the ointment over the surface of the eye.
- Sterile dressings may be ordered to cover the eye at the conclusion of treatment.

#### For All of the Above Categories
- Document drug administration in accordance with institution policy.
- Assess the patient's response to the drug.

Photograph from Workman, M. L., & LaCharity, L. (2016). *Understanding pharmacology* (2nd ed.). Elsevier.

| Table **4.4** | Advantages and Disadvantages of Inhaled Drug Delivery |
|---|---|

**Advantages**

Drug dose is reproducible when used correctly.
A smaller drug dose can be delivered with fewer side effects.
The drug has a faster effect when delivered directly to the respiratory mucosa.

**Disadvantages**

It may be difficult for patients to coordinate the hand and breath action needed to dispense the drug.
The equipment/mouthpiece may become contaminated, providing a source for infection if not cleaned properly.

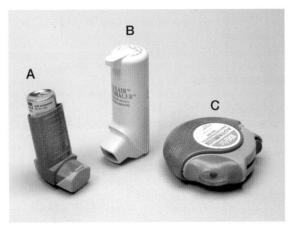

**Fig. 4.25** Types of inhalers. (A) Metered-dose inhaler (MDI). (B) Breath-activated inhaler. (C) Dry-powder inhaler (DPI). (From Lilley, L. L., Collins, S. R., & Snyder, J. (2015). *Pharmacology and the nursing process* (8th ed.). Mosby.)

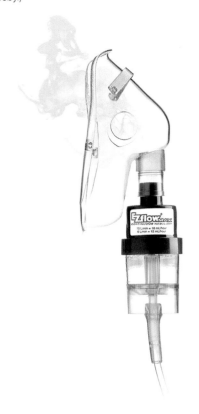

**Fig. 4.26** EZflow and EZflow MAX continuous nebulizers. (Courtesy Mercury Medical.)

| Box **4.4** | Giving Vaginal Drugs |
|---|---|

Drugs to treat local vaginal infections or irritation include creams, jellies, tablets, foams, suppositories, and irrigations (douches).

**STEP 1: PREPARATION**
- Always follow the *9 Rights of Drug Administration*.
- Check the drug order and drug label.
- Gather the necessary equipment, including gloves, lubricant (if needed), and the correct drug. Wash your hands and apply gloves before giving vaginal drugs.
- Correctly identify the patient. Explain the procedure to the patient.

**STEP TWO: GIVING VAGINAL DRUGS**
- Room-temperature suppositories are inserted into the vagina with a gloved hand, much like a rectal suppository is inserted.
- Creams, jellies, tablets, and foams are inserted with a special applicator that comes with the drug.
- With the patient lying down, the filled vaginal applicator is inserted as far into the vaginal canal as possible and the plunger is pushed, depositing the drug.
- Instruct the patient to remain lying down for 10–15 min so that all of the drug can melt and coat the vaginal walls.
- Offer the patient a perineal pad to catch any drainage or prevent staining.

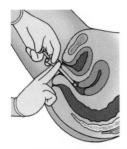

vaginal drugs, ask the patient to empty her bladder. As described in Box 4.4, wash your hands and don gloves. Instruct the patient to lie down. Suppositories may be lubricated before insertion into the vagina. Creams, jellies, and foams typically have their own specialized applicators and are placed into the vagina as far as possible. There is a plunger-type applicator that is used to give the drug. Instruct the patient to lie down for 15 minutes after insertion of a vaginal drug to prevent drug loss.

**Rectal Drugs**

Rectal drugs are used for local or systemic therapy when the oral route is not possible. Rectal drugs, such as suppositories, are typically used for short-term treatment. The rectal route is preferred in nausea or vomiting, for reducing fever in children, for pain relief, and for promoting bowel movements in patients who are constipated. Rectal suppositories should be refrigerated to keep them from melting. As described in Box 4.5, prepare for rectal drug administration by first washing your hands. Place the patient in the modified left prone recumbent position. Don nonsterile gloves and use a

## Box 4.5   Giving Rectal Drugs

### STEP ONE: PREPARATION

- Always follow the *9 Rights of Drug Administration*.
- Check the drug order and label.
- Gather the necessary equipment, including gloves, lubricant (if needed), and the correct drug. Wash your hands before giving any rectal drug.
- Correctly identify the patient per institution policy. Explain the procedure to the patient.
- Assemble the drug and the necessary equipment (lubricant and rubber gloves).

### STEP TWO: GIVING THE DRUG

- Explain what drug is being given and answer any of the patient's questions.
- Turn the patient onto the side with one leg bent over the other in the modified left prone recumbent position. Protect the patient's modesty as much as possible.
- Don gloves. Remove the rectal suppository from the foil packet; place a small amount of water-soluble lubricant on the tip of the suppository and on the inserting finger. Instruct the patient to take a deep breath and to bear down slightly. This will relax the sphincter so that the suppository may be pushed into the rectum about 1 inch.
- Instruct the patient to remain on the side for about 20 min. With children it may be necessary to hold the buttocks together to prevent release of the suppository.
- If the drug is being given by disposable enema, follow the same procedure preparation; insert the lubricated tip into the rectum and slowly squeeze the 50–150 mL of drug from the disposable container.
- Dispose of equipment and gloves.
- Wash your hands.
- Document your actions per institution policy.
- Check the patient and note any response or adverse effects that should be documented and/or reported.

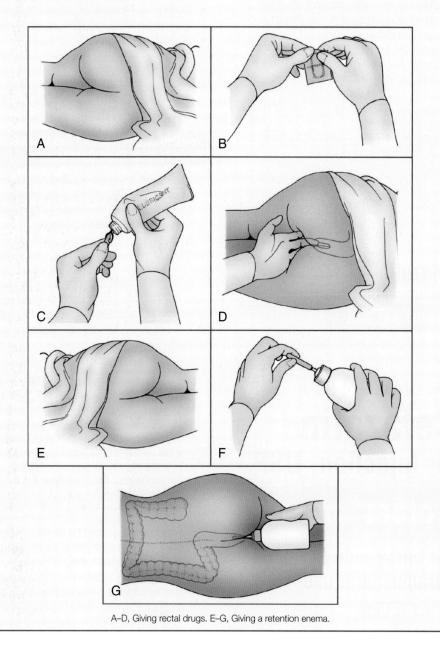

A–D, Giving rectal drugs. E–G, Giving a retention enema.

water-soluble lubricant on the tip of the suppository for easy insertion. Insert the drug past the internal anal sphincter. If the suppository is inserted improperly, the patient might expel it before the drug can dissolve and be absorbed. Have the patient remain in a supine position for about 5 minutes after insertion of a rectal drug to ensure drug absorption.

The procedure for giving drugs by rectal enema is similar: Insert the lubricated tip of the enema into the rectum and squeeze the enema liquid into the rectum. Instruct the patient to use the anal sphincter muscles to "hold" the enema as long as possible. Remain nearby but provide the patient privacy. Offer a bedpan or escort the patient to the toilet when needed. Record the results of the enema.

## Get Ready for the Next-Generation NCLEX® Examination!

### Key Points

- Always wash your hands before preparing to give a drug, regardless of route.
- Never give a drug you have not prepared, nor leave a drug at the bedside for a patient to take later. You will not be able to verify whether the drug was correct or actually taken.
- The drop factor for IV infusions depends on the type of equipment and must be read from the IV setup label.
- Allow extra time when giving drugs to older adult patients because physical changes due to aging may make handling and swallowing the drug more difficult.
- Never open, cut, crush, or allow a patient to chew an oral sustained-release drug or a drug capsule because this can result in a too rapid release or absorption of the drug resulting in overdose or drug toxicity.
- Shake oral liquid drugs and solutions well before pouring to ensure that the drug is evenly distributed.
- When reading the dose of a liquid drug poured into a medication cup, hold the cup at eye level to ensure the correct amount is present.
- Use puncture-resistant containers for disposing all needles and sharps to avoid accidental needlestick injuries.

- Never recap needles used to give parenteral drugs to avoid accidentally sticking yourself or someone else.
- Always don gloves when giving any parenteral drug to avoid exposure to blood or body fluids.
- The dorsogluteal site is not recommended for IM injections because the presence of nerves and blood vessels in the area increases the risk for tissue damage.
- Do not aspirate before giving a drug subcutaneously to prevent bruising and other tissue damage.
- Avoid applying topical or transdermal drugs for systemic use to skin that has been tattooed, skin that has lesions, or broken skin because absorption can be affected.
- Avoid touching topical or transdermal drugs with your bare hands or fingers to prevent absorbing the drug through the skin into your system.

### Clinical Judgment and Next-Generation NCLEX® Examination-Style Questions

1. The healthcare provider has ordered cefazolin 500 mg IM for a patient. Your institution has the following formulation on hand: cefazolin 1 g/vial in a powdered form that needs to be diluted before administration (see label).

**Cefazolin**
**for Injection, USP**
**1 gram\* per vial**

To open - Cut seal along dotted line.

PLB132-WES/2
Rx only

NDC 0143-9924-90

**Cefazolin**
**for Injection, USP**

**1 gram\* per vial**

**For Intravenous or Intramuscular use**

25 x 1 g Vials

NDC 0143-9924-90

\*Each vial contains sterile cefazolin sodium equivalent to 1 gram cefazolin. The sodium content is 48 mg.
**Usual Adult Dosage:** 250 mg to 1 gram every 6 to 8 hours. For more information see package insert.
**For Intramuscular Administration:** Add 2.5 mL of Sterile Water for Injection. SHAKE WELL to dissolve. Withdraw entire contents. Provides an approximate volume of 3.0 mL (330 mg/mL).
**For Intravenous Administration:** See package insert. Reconstituted solution is stable for 24 hours at room temperature or for 10 days under refrigeration (5°C or 41°F). Reconstituted solutions may range in color from pale yellow to yellow without a change in potency.
**Store at 20° to 25°C (68° to 77°F) [See USP Controlled Room Temperature]. Protect from light.**
Mfd. by HIKMA FARMACÊUTICA (PORTUGAL). S.A.
Dist. by Hikma, Berkeley Heights, NJ 07922

**hikma.**

1. How much sterile water should you use to reconstitute this drug before it is given?
2. How many milliliters will you give to the patient?

2. A patient with diabetes has an order for 40 units of NPH insulin to be given subcutaneously each morning. The vial contains 100 units per 1 mL. How much insulin must be given?

   1. 0.4 mL
   2. 40 mL
   3. 1.4 mL
   4. 0.45 mL

3. A patient preparing for surgery has an order for cefazolin sulfate (Ancef) 500 mg IV. The drug is available in a vial of powder and is labeled with the following instructions: "Add 2.0 mL of sterile water for injection. This will provide 250 mg/mL." How many milliliters of solution should you prepare?

   1. 2 mL
   2. 0.2 mL
   3. 4 mL
   4. 0.4 mL

4. A patient is to receive 1000 mL of normal saline infused IV over 24 hours. The drop factor is 10 drops = 1 mL. What is the flow rate in milliliters per hour of this infusion?

   1. 84 mL/h
   2. 24 mL/h
   3. 42 mL/h
   4. 60 mL/h

5. A patient who requires anticoagulation has an order for heparin 7500 units subcutaneously daily. The pharmacy has provided an ampule that contains 5000 units per 1 mL. How many milliliters should you prepare for this injection?

   1. 0.15 mL
   2. 0.75 mL
   3. 0.50 mL
   4. 1.5 mL

6. As part of preoperative care, the surgeon has ordered atropine 0.2 mg IM. The multidose vial reads "1 mL = 0.1 mg." How many milliliters will be given to this patient?

   1. 0.1 mL
   2. 2 mL
   3. 0.2 mL
   4. 1 mL

7. You are preparing to give metoprolol 50 mg orally twice daily for a patient with hypertension. The pharmacy has provided you with scored tablets of 100 mg each. How many tablets of this drug should you give to the patient?

   1. ½ tablet
   2. 1 tablet
   3. 2 tablets
   4. 1½ tablets

8. Which patient(s) would be the best candidate to receive drugs by IM or IV route? **Select all or any that apply.**

   1. The older patient who has difficulty swallowing
   2. The patient who is experiencing an episode of prolonged weakness
   3. The patient who requires a steady blood level of the drug
   4. The patient who is experiencing vomiting after surgery
   5. The patient who needs an antibiotic for bronchitis
   6. The patient who is a child younger than 1 year

9. You are preparing to give an intradermal injection for allergy testing to your patient. Which of the following reactions should you expect to see from this injection?

   1. Blister
   2. Bleb
   3. Bruise
   4. Contusion

10. The nurse is taking care of a patient receiving an IV infusion. During rounds, the nurse discovers that the IV infusion is failing to flow properly.

   Place an X for the nursing action that is indicated (appropriate or necessary), contraindicated (could be harmful), or nonessential (makes no difference or not necessary) for the patient's care at this time.

| NURSING ACTION | INDICATED | CONTRA-INDICATED | NON-ESSENTIAL |
|---|---|---|---|
| Change the IV tubing | | | |
| Lower the IV pole height | | | |
| Check the IV tubing for kinks | | | |
| Check the position of the needle | | | |
| Examine IV site for infiltration | | | |
| Check the IV solution type | | | |
| Reposition the patient's wrist and elbow | | | |

## Next-Generation NCLEX® (NGN) Examination–Style Question

**Nurses' Notes**
**0800**

The laboratory department calls with a report of a critical calcium level on the client. Provider notified and orders received.

**0830**

Infusion initiated as prescribed via peripheral IV catheter in the client's left forearm. The nurse notes the client's IV access site is clean, dry, and nontender with an occlusive dressing in place.

**0930**

The nurse is called to the client's room because "the IV is beeping." The nurse notes that the client's IV site is red, tender, swollen, and warm.

**Laboratory Results**
**0700**

| TEST/PANEL | RESULT | NORMAL |
|---|---|---|
| Calcium | 6 mg/dL | 9–10.5 mg/dL (2.25–2.62 mmol/L) |

**Flow Sheet**
**0800**

Blood pressure: 128/80 mm Hg
Heart rate: 78/min
Respiratory rate: 16/min
Temperature: 98.6°F (37°C)

**Orders**
**0800**

Calcium gluconate in 250 mL of 0.9% sodium chloride

A nurse is caring for the client and reviews the client's nurses' notes, laboratory results, flowsheet, and orders.

For each assessment finding, click to indicate whether the nursing action is indicated, contraindicated, or nonessential for the client's care at this time.

*Each row must have only one response option selected.*

| NURSING ACTION | INDICATED | CONTRA-INDICATED | NON-ESSENTIAL |
|---|---|---|---|
| Increase the rate of infusion | | | |
| Check the tubing for kinks | | | |
| Stop the infusion | | | |
| Place the client on left side, preferably with head of bed raised | | | |
| Assess the skin for necrosis | | | |
| Apply a warm, wet compress to the IV site | | | |
| Assess the client's breath sounds | | | |

See answer on Evolve at http://evolve.elsevier.com/Visovsky/LPNpharmacology/.

# Drugs for Bacterial Infections

# 5

http://evolve.elsevier.com/Visovsky/LPNpharmacology

## Learning Outcomes

1. Explain how infections, pathogens, drug spectrum, drug resistance, and drug generation affect antibiotic drug therapy.
2. List the names, actions, possible side effects, and adverse effects of the penicillins and cephalosporins.
3. Explain what to teach patients and families about penicillins and cephalosporins.
4. List the names, actions, possible side effects, and adverse effects of the common tetracyclines, macrolides, and aminoglycosides.
5. Explain what to teach patients and families about tetracyclines, macrolides, and aminoglycosides.
6. List the names, actions, possible side effects, and adverse effects of the common sulfonamides and fluoroquinolones.
7. Explain what to teach patients and families about sulfonamides and fluoroquinolones.

## Key Terms

**antibacterials** Antimicrobial drugs that kill or slow the reproduction of bacteria only; often used interchangeably with antibiotics.

**antibiotic** Any drug that has the ability to destroy or interfere with the development of a living organism; often used interchangeably with the term *antibacterial*.

**antimicrobial drug** A general term for any drug that has the purpose of killing or inhibiting the growth of pathogenic microorganisms.

**antimicrobial resistance** The ability of an organism to resist the killing or growth-suppressing effects of anti-infective drugs.

**bacteria** Microscopic living organisms that exist everywhere and are both beneficial and dangerous and are capable of preventing and causing infection.

**bactericidal** Drugs with mechanisms of action that kill bacteria.

**bacteriostatic** Drugs with mechanisms of action that only suppress or slow bacterial growth.

**drug generation** A new group of drugs developed from other similar drugs. Each new generation of antibiotics manufactured from the original generation has significantly greater antimicrobial properties than the preceding generation.

**normal flora** Organisms of many different types that are usually present on the skin and in the mouth, intestinal tract, and vagina of a healthy individual and do not cause infection unless the person has reduced immunity or the organisms are located in the wrong body area.

**pathogen** An organism that is expected to cause infection even among people with strong immune systems.

**pseudomembranous colitis** An abnormal intestinal reaction to a strong antibiotic that causes excessive watery, bloody diarrhea, abdominal cramps, and low-grade fever; it can lead to dehydration and damage the walls of the intestinal tract.

**spectrum** The number of specific organisms the drug is effective against.

## INFECTION

An infection is an invasion of body tissue by disease-producing pathogens that multiply and produce toxins that react in a dangerous way and produce illness in a host organism. Infections can be caused by bacteria, viruses, parasites, fungi, and insects. Anti-infective drugs are some of the most commonly given drugs because of the many types of infections they have been developed to treat. These drugs are most effective and have fewer side effects when taken correctly. It is therefore important for you to learn as much as possible about these drugs and about what to teach patients who are taking them.

### NORMAL FLORA

Many types of organisms are always present on or in the skin, mouth, intestinal tract, and vagina of a healthy person. These organisms are collectively known as **normal flora** and are considered *nonpathogens* because they usually do not cause infection. Normal flora can cause infection when a person has very low immunity, when the organisms are present in excessive amounts and overwhelm the body, or when they are located in the wrong place. For example, if *Escherichia coli*, which are part of the normal flora in the bowel, are present in the bladder or other parts of the renal/urinary system, they can cause an infection in the urinary tract. If skin flora enter a surgical incision, a wound infection can develop. Infants, young children, people with AIDS, anyone receiving cancer chemotherapy, anyone who is taking a drug that suppresses the immune system, and older adults have the greatest risk of infection. Other factors that increase the risk of infection include poor circulation, poor nutritional status, and chronic diseases.

Antibiotic use can upset the balance of the normal flora in the body and cause yeast or fungal infections to occur. *Candida* is a common body yeast that often overgrows to cause a fungal infection. When a person is given antibiotics to kill infectious bacteria, normal flora also are killed. The gut, mouth, and vaginal mucosa have bacterial floras that act as barriers against fungal infections. When the barrier weakens, yeast infections can occur. If a yeast infection occurs after antibiotic therapy, it is known as a *secondary infection* or a *superinfection*.

Some evidence supports using probiotic bacteria with an antibiotic as a strategy to prevent yeast infections. Probiotic (beneficial) bacteria can be found in many foods that can easily be added to a diet—for example, yogurt, dark chocolate, miso soup, pickles, and sauerkraut—and in capsule form. The healthcare provider can prescribe probiotics in capsule form and recommend any necessary dietary changes.

## PATHOGENS

An organism that is expected to cause infection even among people with a strong immune system is a **pathogen**. A variety of pathogenic organisms exist, and they can cause disease in different ways. For example, they may be able to divide rapidly and overwhelm the immune system or produce toxins.

**Bacteria** are a large domain of single-celled microorganisms that exist everywhere. Bacteria can be both beneficial and dangerous. For example, *E. coli* bacteria in the intestines benefit digestion but become infective if overgrowth occurs.

Bacteria have different shapes and characteristics. They are shaped as rods, spheres, or spirals, and they can survive with oxygen (*aerobic*) or without oxygen (*anaerobic*). When stained with a Gram solution, they can stain violet (*gram-positive*) or red (*gram-negative*). Gram-positive bacteria have a thick cell wall and outer capsule. The cell wall of gram-negative bacteria is much more complex, with an outer capsule and two

cell wall membranes. This complex cell wall makes gram-negative bacterial infections more difficult to treat. It is harder for an antibiotic to penetrate the gram-negative bacterial wall.

A *fungus* is a member of a large group of microorganisms that includes yeasts and molds, which have cell features similar to those of human cells. Fungi are everywhere and exist by absorbing nutrients from a host organism. A fungal infection is called a *mycosis*. Fungi are discussed in Chapter 6.

A *virus* is a small infectious agent that can replicate (reproduce itself) only inside the living cells of organisms. Viral infections and antiviral drugs are discussed in Chapter 7.

A *parasite* is an organism that lives on or in a human and relies on the human for its food and other functions. Common human parasites include worms (helminths), amoebas, and protozoa. Parasites are discussed in Chapter 6.

 **Memory Jogger**

Antibiotics have a difficult time penetrating the cell walls of gram-negative bacteria, which makes these infections more difficult to treat.

## DETERMINATION OF INFECTION

Some infections are diagnosed by healthcare providers based on the patient's symptoms and the type of organism that commonly causes a specific infection in that community. In this situation, healthcare providers usually know what the most likely organism is and which drug or drugs are effective against it. Prescribing a drug without identification of the specific organism is called *empiric treatment* or *empiric therapy*, and it is based on experience and clinical expertise.

Sometimes the cause of the infection is not known, and it must be evaluated to identify the specific pathogenic organism and the drug that will be most effective against it. Bacteria are often stained, cultured, and tested to determine which drugs are effective against them (*antimicrobial sensitivity*). A specimen of the infective material is taken for culture and sensitivity testing, which are performed before anti-infective therapy is begun. Learning the correct identity of the organism allows the healthcare provider to order the correct drugs to kill it or stop its reproduction before the illness worsens.

## ANTI-INFECTIVES

Anti-infective agents are drugs that can kill or inhibit the spread of infectious agents such as bacteria, viruses, fungi, or protozoans. It is a general term used synonymously with the term *antimicrobial*. Examples of **antimicrobial drugs** are antibacterials, antivirals, antifungals, and anthelmintics. These drugs are classified by their chemical structures, mechanisms of action, and the types of organism they effectively combat. For example, antimicrobials that kill or slow the reproduction of bacteria are called antibacterials. An antibiotic is any drug that has the ability to destroy or interfere with the development of a living organism. In anti-infective therapy, *antibiotic* is used interchangeably with *antibacterial*.

## DRUG SUSCEPTIBILITY AND RESISTANCE

Overuse or unnecessary use of antibiotics has led to problems in infection management. When antibacterials are overused, prescribed for conditions that are not responsive to these drugs, or taken improperly, drug-resistant strains of bacteria develop. Antimicrobial resistance is the ability of an organism to resist the killing or growth-suppressing effects of anti-infective drugs. Organisms that can be killed or have their reproduction suppressed by anti-infective drugs are *susceptible*. Those that are neither killed nor suppressed by anti-infective drugs are *resistant* organisms. Many organisms, especially bacteria, that were once susceptible to a variety of anti-infective drugs have become resistant to most types. When an organism is resistant to three or more different types of drugs to which it was once susceptible, it is termed a *superbug* or a *multidrug-resistant (MDR) organism*.

Each year, more organisms become resistant to standard anti-infective drugs. Infections caused by resistant organisms cost more to treat, increase the length of hospital stays, and lead to higher mortality rates. The drugs used against MDR organisms often are more powerful and have more side effects than standard anti-infective drugs. Drug resistance has developed in many disease-causing bacteria, viruses, retroviruses, fungi, and some parasites, and the problem is worsening. It has been 35 years since the last class of antibiotics was discovered in 1987. Antibiotics discovered since then are variations of current classes. For this reason, resistance to them may develop faster.

The Centers for Disease Control and Prevention (CDC) has identified 18 drug-resistant threats in the United States. Of those threats, five are considered urgent: *Clostridium difficile* (C-diff), carbapenem-resistant Enterobacterales (CRE), *Neisseria gonorrhoeae, Candida auris*, and carbapenem-resistant Acinetobacter.

 Bookmark This!

Bacterial resistance to antibiotics is a constant threat. To keep current on bacterial resistance and treatment options, check out the CDC Web site at https://www.cdc.gov/drugre sistance/index.html.

Beta-lactamases (penicillinases) are enzymes produced by some bacteria that give them resistance to beta-lactam antibiotics, which include penicillins, cephalosporins, monobactams, and carbapenems. Inhibitor agents are added to the primary antibiotic (e.g., amoxicillin/clavulanate potassium) to make the antibiotics less resistant to beta-lactamases.

## GENERAL CONSIDERATIONS FOR ANTI-INFECTIVE (ANTIMICROBIAL) DRUG THERAPY

Drug management for infection is very common and usually short term. Although there are many types of antimicrobial drugs, some nursing interventions are the same for all of them. Many of the points to teach patients and families about these drugs are the same. Box 5.1 describes these common nursing interventions, and Box 5.2 describes general patient teaching points. Specific interventions and patient teaching issues are listed in the individual drug categories.

 Lifespan Considerations

**Breast-feeding**

Breast-feeding should be avoided during antimicrobial therapy because most of these drugs are excreted in breast milk, exposing the infant (who may not have an infection) to the actions, side effects, and adverse effects of the chosen drug.

## ANTIBIOTICS

Antibiotics work in different ways to affect pathogenic bacteria (Fig. 5.1). They may attack a bacterium's internal cellular processes, which are vital to its existence, or they may destroy the external cell wall, making it weaker or unable to reproduce; in some cases, they kill the organism. Drugs that are bactericidal kill the bacteria; those that are bacteriostatic limit or slow the growth of the bacteria, weakening or eventually leading to the death of the bacteria.

 Memory Jogger

The *-cidal* or *-static* part of the word describing an antibiotic gives a hint about its activity.
- Bactericidal drugs kill the bacteria (think about the word *homicide*).
- Bacteriostatic drugs only limit or slow the growth of bacteria, relying on the patient's immune system to kill the organism.

Bacteria are often classified as gram-positive or gram-negative organisms. The number of specific organisms the drug is effective against is its spectrum. Some antibiotics are effective against only a few types of bacteria and are called *narrow-spectrum drugs*. Drugs that are effective against more types of bacteria, including both gram-negative and gram-positive bacteria, are known as *broad-spectrum drugs*.

Some drugs have become more refined, purified, and sensitive as a result of long-term testing. Each new group of drugs developed from other, similar drugs is called a drug generation. The original drugs are referred to as *first-generation drugs*, and later groups are called *second-generation drugs, third-generation drugs*, and so on.

Each new generation of drugs usually has certain advantages over older-generation drugs. For example, the newer drugs may have improved effectiveness,

## Box 5.1  General Nursing Implications for Antimicrobial Drug Therapy

### ASSESSMENT
- Obtain a complete drug history from the patient to prevent possible drug interactions.
- If ordered and before starting antibiotic therapy, obtain specimens for culture and sensitivity to ensure drug sensitivity.
- Do a focused assessment to include the current condition of the infectious site, vital signs, white blood cell (WBC) count, and other baseline laboratory data that may be ordered before therapy to establish a baseline, such as liver enzymes, kidney function, and drug levels.
- A patient can have an allergy to any anti-infective drug. Always ask patients about specific drug allergies and what specific type of problem occurred as part of the allergy before starting any new antimicrobial drug.
- Have emergency drugs and equipment (e.g., diphenhydramine, epinephrine, crash cart) available to treat allergic reactions or anaphylaxis.
- If a female patient is on oral contraceptives and does not wish to be pregnant, an alternative or additional method of contraception should be recommended while taking antibiotic therapy.

### PLANNING AND INTERVENTION
- If the patient develops a rash or itching while on an antimicrobial drug, immediately report the problem to the healthcare provider. If the patient has difficulty breathing, a lump in the throat, or a sudden, severe drop in blood pressure, call the emergency team.
- A common and expected side effect of anti-infective therapy, especially of antibacterial drugs, is diarrhea. This response occurs because the drug reduces the numbers of bacteria in the intestinal tract that normally help digestion. With fewer intestinal flora, diarrhea results. This is *not* an allergy.
- Some very strong antibiotics can cause severe and damaging inflammation of the colon when there is overgrowth of *Clostridium difficile*. This serious and abnormal complication is **pseudomembranous colitis**, which presents with symptoms that include excessive, watery, bloody diarrhea; abdominal cramps; and low-grade fever.
- Many antibiotics allow yeast to overgrow when normal flora are reduced in the mouth and vagina. In the mouth, white patches (thrush) appear, especially on the tongue and roof. In the vagina, an itchy discharge may occur. Both problems may require antifungal therapy.
- Antimicrobials work best against infection when blood drug levels remain consistent, and it is best to give them on an even, around-the-clock schedule. If an antibiotic

is ordered to be given four times a day, the schedule is every 6 hours. Remind the prescriber or the person making the schedule to use 6:00 a.m., noon, 6:00 p.m., and midnight instead of 9:00 a.m., 1:00 p.m., 5:00 p.m., and 9:00 p.m. If the drugs were given on the 9, 1, 5, and 9 schedule, during the 12 hours the drugs were not given, the blood level would be so low that the organisms would start growing again.
- Many antimicrobials given parenterally have interactions with other drugs. Be sure to consult a pharmacist or drug reference to determine whether a specific drug can be given in the same IV line used for other drugs.
- Most parenteral antimicrobial drugs must be given slowly, over 30 to 60 minutes. Consult a pharmacist or drug reference to determine the time needed to give a specific drug intravenously.
- Some antimicrobial drugs have toxic side effects, and their use has a time limit. For example, the aminoglycoside antibiotics can damage the nerves of the ear and cause hearing loss. Typically, these drugs are used for only 5 days. You must know the start and stop dates of antimicrobial drugs to prevent accidental excessive exposure to the drug.
- The usual duration of antibiotic therapy is 10 to 14 days, but the duration of antimicrobial therapy varies for different types of infections. For example, some uncomplicated bladder infections (e.g., cystitis) may require only 3 days of a specific antibacterial drug for complete therapy; in contrast, tuberculosis (TB) usually requires at least 6 months of four different types of drugs to suppress the infection.

### EVALUATION
- A major nursing responsibility with antimicrobial therapy is evaluating the effectiveness of the drug prescribed for the infection. It is therefore important to know the patient's infection symptoms and monitor them daily to assess whether the drug therapy is reducing them.
- If symptoms continue at the same intensity or become worse after 72 hours, notify the prescriber.
- Whatever duration is prescribed, it is important for the patient to receive all of the therapy. Stopping antimicrobial therapy after infection symptoms are no longer present but before the prescribed duration of treatment is completed increases the risk of infection recurrence and development of drug-resistant organisms.
- Re-evaluate laboratory work that has been ordered to prevent adverse effects such as liver and kidney damage or altered drug levels.

fewer side effects, or a faster onset of action. Some newer-generation drugs have a narrower spectrum of bacteria that are susceptible to them but are more powerful than previous generations against the susceptible bacteria.

## PENICILLINS

All bacteria have plasma membranes just as human cells do (Fig. 5.1 [2]). In addition to a plasma membrane, some bacteria also have the extra protection of cell walls that surround the bacterium outside of the plasma membrane (see Fig. 5.1 [1]). Cell walls are much tougher than plasma membranes. Like a brick wall, the cell wall needs to be continuously maintained and repaired to prevent damage and protect the bacterial cell inside. A variety of substances work like bricks and mortar to hold the cell wall together. Different enzymes help make the "mortar,"

## Box 5.2   General Teaching Points for Patients and Families During Antimicrobial Drug Therapy

- Explain to patients that ordinary diarrhea is an expected side effect and not an allergic response to antimicrobial drugs. It is not usually a reason to stop the drug. However, excessive watery and bloody diarrhea with severe abdominal pain and fever is a complication that needs to be reported to the prescriber immediately.
- Instruct patients to call 911 immediately if they develop a lump in the throat, difficulty breathing, or swelling of the lips, tongue, or throat.
- Instruct patients to take their prescribed antimicrobial drugs exactly as prescribed and for as long as prescribed to prevent infection recurrence and drug resistance.
- Instruct patients to stop taking the antimicrobial drug and notify the healthcare provider if a rash or hives develop.

A drug allergy can develop at any time after the patient begins treatment.
- Remind patients to report to the healthcare provider any new symptoms that occur while taking antimicrobial therapy because they may represent an adverse reaction.
- Tell patients that even though it may be inconvenient to take a drug in the middle of the night, it is important to space the drug's doses evenly during the 24 hours for best results.
- Instruct patients not to save antimicrobial drugs because many expired drugs deteriorate and become less effective.

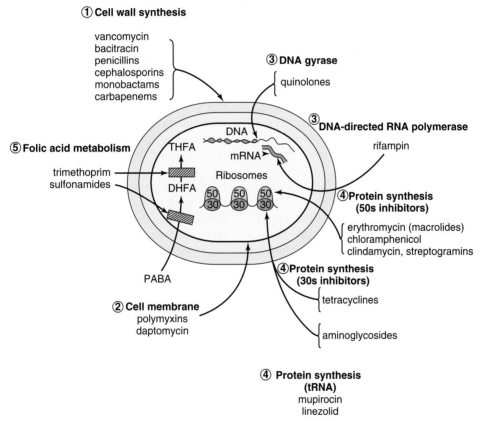

FIG. 5.1 Sites of antimicrobial bactericidal or bacteriostatic action on bacterial pathogens. Five general actions include (1) inhibition of synthesis or building of the cell wall, (2) damage to the cell membrane, (3) modification of nucleic acid synthesis, (4) modification of protein synthesis (at ribosomes), and (5) modification of energy metabolism within the cytoplasm (at the folate cycle). *DHFA*, dihydrofolic acid; *mRNA*, messenger RNA; *PABA*, *para*-aminobenzoic acid; *THFA*, tetrahydrofolic acid; *tRNA*, transfer RNA. (From Wecker, L. (2010). *Brody's human pharmacology* (5th ed.), Elsevier.)

replace old or crumbling "bricks," and keep the cell wall intact.

### Action

Penicillins are one type of a class of drugs known as *cell wall synthesis inhibitors*. They interfere with the creation and repair of bacterial cell walls. They also bind or stick to specific enzymes that the bacteria need so that the bacteria cannot use them. This process makes the bacterial cell weak and allows it to break down more easily. This action is bactericidal for bacteria susceptible to penicillin's actions. Pure penicillin may be combined with other ingredients to make the drug stay in the body longer or to prevent the drug from being destroyed by bacterial enzymes. Penicillin and other cell wall synthesis inhibitors are effective only against bacteria that have cells walls, and they have no action against bacteria without cells walls. Although penicillin can be very effective, many organisms have become resistant to its killing effects over time.

## Uses

Alexander Fleming created penicillin in 1929 from a fungus. It was used as an antibiotic throughout World War II. Since that time, five generations of synthetic penicillins have been developed. Sadly, bacterial resistance to many penicillin drugs has developed. Regardless of the increased resistance, penicillin G remains the drug of choice for many infections, including syphilis and certain types of endocarditis. Penicillins are used for infections that occur in the mouth, throat, skin, other soft tissues, heart, lungs, and ears. Penicillin is also used for *prophylactic* (preventive) treatment against bacterial endocarditis in patients with rheumatic or heart disease before they have dental procedures or surgery of the upper respiratory tract, genitourinary tract, or gastrointestinal (GI) tract. Some penicillins may be used for treating exposure to agents of biological warfare. Penicillins are still considered the safest antibiotics and are the broad-spectrum drugs of choice for susceptible gram-negative and gram-positive organisms.

Many penicillin products are available in a variety of forms, ranging from oral drugs to parenteral drugs. There are five generations of penicillins:

1. *Natural penicillins* (e.g., penicillin G, penicillin V) combat non-beta-lactamase–producing gram-positive cocci, including *Streptococcus viridans*, group A streptococci, *Streptococcus pneumoniae*, and anaerobic streptococci.
2. *Penicillinase-resistant penicillins* (e.g., dicloxacillin, nafcillin, oxacillin) combat *Staphylococcus* but are not effective against methicillin-resistant *Staphylococcus aureus* (MRSA) or methicillin-resistant *Staphylococcus epidermidis* (MRSE). Methicillin is no longer manufactured.
3. *Aminopenicillins* (e.g., ampicillin, amoxicillin) combat the same bacteria as the natural penicillins but have improved activity against some gram-negative bacteria. Combining an aminopenicillin with a beta-lactamase inhibitor (clavulanic acid or sulbactam) treats infections caused by beta-lactamase–producing organisms.
4. *Carboxypenicillins* (e.g., carbenicillin, ticarcillin) have increased activity to penetrate the cell wall, and they are used against gram-negative bacteria such as *Pseudomonas aeruginosa* and *Proteus*.
5. *Ureidopenicillins* and *piperazine penicillin* (e.g., piperacillin) are the latest class of penicillin antibiotics that combat gram-negative bacteria such as *Klebsiella*. When a beta-lactamase inhibitor is added (e.g., piperacillin and tazobactam), it becomes a very powerful broad-spectrum antibiotic against many gram-positive and gram-negative bacteria, and it is used only in cases in which other antibiotics have been ineffective to prevent resistance. These penicillins and the carboxypenicillins are used only intravenously.

Table 5.1 lists examples of common penicillins with their dosages and nursing implications. Always consult a drug reference book or a pharmacist for information about a specific penicillin.

## Expected Side Effects

Penicillin has fewer side effects and fewer drug interactions than other antibiotics. The most common side effect of penicillin (and many other antibiotics) is simple diarrhea of two to four loose stools daily. This is not an allergy; it happens because the drug has killed some of the normal flora of the GI tract that help digest food. If the diarrhea is severe, the healthcare provider needs to be notified about additions or changes that need to occur with therapy. Other common and expected side effects include nausea, vomiting, and epigastric distress.

C-diff is an infectious form of diarrhea caused by antibiotic use, particularly with amoxicillin/clavulanate potassium. If C-diff is suspected, notify the healthcare provider, and obtain a stool culture before treatment with another antibiotic.

## Adverse Reactions

Allergy to penicillin occurs in no greater than 5% of the population, producing rash, *erythema* (redness or inflammation), *urticaria* (hives), *angioedema* (swelling of the skin and mucous membranes), *laryngeal edema* (swelling of the larynx), and *anaphylaxis* (shock). These allergic reactions may occur suddenly, within an hour, or after the patient has been taking the drug for some time, and it may cause life-threatening anaphylactic shock. Penicillin is the most common cause of anaphylactic shock, causing an estimated 40% to 50% of all anaphylactic deaths in the United States. Approximately 6% of people with an allergy to penicillin may also have an allergy to cephalosporins due to cross-sensitivity.

Penicillin allergies decrease with time. Tend to decrease by 10% each year. Most are no longer allergic after 10 years Joint Task Force on Practice Parameters. Ann Allergy Asthma Immunol. 2010 Puchner TC, et al. Ann Alllergy Asthma Immunol. 2002

## Drug Interactions

Other bacteriostatic antibiotics such as tetracycline (Panmycin) and erythromycin (E.E.S.) may decrease the bactericidal effect of penicillin. Probenecid (Benemid) blocks the excretion of penicillin, prolonging blood levels and making the antibiotic more effective. Ampicillin (Ampi) reduces the effectiveness of oral contraceptives, which can lead to an unplanned pregnancy. Indomethacin (Indocin), phenylbutazone (Butazolidin), or aspirin may increase serum penicillin levels. Antacids may decrease the absorption of penicillin. Penicillin may change the results of some laboratory tests.

 **Top Tip for Safety**

Teach women who are taking oral birth control pills to use another reliable method of pregnancy protection while taking penicillin or any antibiotic and for 1 month after completing antibiotic therapy to prevent an unplanned pregnancy.

## Table **5.1**   Common Penicillins and Cephalosporins

*Penicillins* and *cephalosporins* are cell wall synthesis inhibitors that kill susceptible bacteria by preventing their cell walls from being made and maintained. Vancomycin and carbapenems also are powerful cell wall synthesis inhibitors.

| DRUG/ADULT DOSAGE | NURSING IMPLICATIONS |
|---|---|
| **Penicillins** | |
| amoxicillin (Moxatag) 500 mg orally every 12 hours *or* 775 mg to 1 g orally once daily<br><br>amoxicillin/clavulanate potassium (Augmentin) 875/125 mg combination orally every 12 hours (immediate-release formula)<br><br>penicillin G benzathine (Bicillin L-A) 1.2 million units IM as a single injection<br><br>penicillin G procaine 600,000 to 1.2 million units intramuscular (IM) once daily for 10 days<br><br>penicillin V potassium (Veetids) 250–500 mg orally every 6 hours | • Shake liquid suspension drugs thoroughly before giving because this drug form separates.<br>• Give amoxicillin (Moxatag) within 1 hour after the patient completes a meal for best absorption and fewer gastrointestinal (GI) side effects.<br>• Remind patients not to chew the extended-release forms to avoid counteracting the slow-release feature.<br>• Penicillin G procaine is never injected into a blood vessel because the procaine it contains can cause severe neurovascular complications.<br>• With penicillin G, use the Z-track method of IM injection deep into the muscle to prevent the drug from leaking through the tissues and causing pain or damage.<br>• Aspirate before injecting the IM dose to ensure that the drug is not injected into the bloodstream.<br>• Do not interchange the various suspensions of amoxicillin/clavulanate potassium because they contain different amounts of clavulanic acid.<br>• Concentrations of penicillin V potassium are higher when taken on an empty stomach, but if GI upset occurs, it can be taken with food. |
| **Cephalosporins**<br><br>**First Generation**<br>cefazolin (Kefzol) 250–1000 mg IM or intravenous (IV) every 8 hours<br>cephalexin (Keflex) 500 mg orally every 12 hours<br>**Second Generation**<br>cefaclor (Ceclor) 250–500 mg orally every 8 hours<br>cefuroxime (Ceftin) 250–500 mg orally every 12 hours *or* 750 mg IM or IV every 8 hours<br>**Third Generation**<br>cefdinir (Omnicef) 300 mg orally every 12 hours *or* 600 mg orally once daily<br>ceftriaxone (Rocephin) 1–2 g IM or IV every 12–24 hours<br>**Fourth Generation**<br>cefepime (Maxipime) 0.5–2 g IM or IV every 8–12 hours | • Make sure to check for a penicillin allergy before giving a cephalosporin because patients may have a cross-sensitivity to the drug.<br>• Do not give oral cephalosporins within 1 hour before or after antacids because they interfere with absorption of cephalosporins.<br>• Give IM cefazolin, cefuroxime, ceftriaxone, and cefepime using the Z-track method of IM injection deep into the muscle to prevent drug from leaking through the tissues and causing pain or damage.<br>• Aspirate before injecting the IM dose to ensure that the drug is not injected into the bloodstream.<br>• Cefuroxime tablets and suspension cannot be substituted milligram for milligram because they are not bioequivalent.<br>• Cefuroxime suspension must be given with food to ensure a consistent blood drug level.<br>• IV ceftriaxone cannot be given with Ringer lactate because Ringer lactate contains calcium that precipitates the drug.<br>• IV ceftriaxone and cefepime cannot be given by IV push and must be infused over 30 minutes to reduce the risk of immediate cardiac side effects.<br>• Warn patients not to drink alcohol while taking cephalosporins to reduce the side effects of copious vomiting, hypotension, dyspnea, and chest pain. |

*Continued*

Table **5.1**   Common Penicillins and Cephalosporins—cont'd

| DRUG/ADULT DOSAGE | NURSING IMPLICATIONS |
|---|---|
| **Vancomycin** | |
| vancomycin (Vancocin) 500 mg IV every 6 hours *or* 1 g IV every 12 hours; 125 mg orally every 6 hours for pseudomembranous colitis caused by *Clostridium difficile* | <ul><li>Vancomycin solutions containing dextrose may be contraindicated in patients who have a history of an allergy or a hypersensitivity to corn.</li><li>Vancomycin tablets must be swallowed whole, not crushed, to avoid altered dosing.</li><li>Regularly assess hearing and monitor urine; assess blood urea nitrogen (BUN)/creatinine intermittently; notify the healthcare provider about outlying values because this drug is toxic to the ears and kidneys and accumulates in the body.</li><li>IV vancomycin must be infused over *at least* 60 minutes and at a rate of no more than 10 mg/min to avoid *red man syndrome*, a histamine response. Stopping or slowing the infusion decreases the histamine response.</li><li>Parenteral doses of vancomycin must be monitored using serum vancomycin concentration peak and trough levels because the drug can accumulate to toxic levels quickly. Make sure that the trough level is drawn 30 minutes before the next dose is to be given (so it accurately reflects the drug's lowest level) and that the peak level is drawn 1–2 hours after the dose has infused to accurately reflect the drug's highest level.</li><li>Monitor urine output and renal blood tests very closely when vancomycin is given with other renal-toxic drugs (e.g., aminoglycosides) because renal toxicity occurs faster with the combination.</li><li>Administration of vancomycin with cidofovir (Vistide) is contraindicated because these drugs together cause severe renal toxicity.</li></ul> |
| **Carbapenems** | |
| imipenem (Primaxin) 500–1000 mg IV every 6–8 hours *or* 500–750 mg IM every 12 hours<br>meropenem (Merrem) 1–2 g IV every 6–8 hours<br>ertapenem (Invanz) 1 g IM or IV once daily | <ul><li>Do not use the IM formulation of imipenem or ertapenem for IV administration because it contains lidocaine (Xylocaine), which can cause severe cardiac side effects.</li><li>Give IM injections of the carbapenems using the Z-track method of IM injection deep into the muscle to prevent the drug from leaking through the tissues and causing pain or damage.</li><li>Aspirate before injecting the IM dose to ensure that the drug is not injected into the bloodstream.</li><li>Monitor patients receiving carbapenems closely for confusion and seizure activity because these drugs can cause central nervous system changes.</li><li>Carbapenem use with ganciclovir (Cytovene) or valproic acid (Depakote) can cause seizures because simultaneous use increases the risk of seizure activity.</li><li>Monitor patients receiving carbapenems with warfarin (Coumadin) for bleeding abnormalities and changes in the international normalized ratio levels because carbapenems increase warfarin action, which increases the risk of bleeding.</li><li>When carbapenems are used along with other antibiotics, monitor urine and laboratory tests closely and report abnormal results to the healthcare provider because the combination greatly increases the risk of kidney damage.</li></ul> |

## Nursing Implications and Patient Teaching

In addition to the general nursing implications and teaching points for all antimicrobial drugs, specific ones for the penicillins are listed in Table 5.1.

**Top Tip for Safety**

Using the Z-track method for all intramuscular (IM) injections seals the needle track, thus preventing leakage in the subcutaneous tissue. This action seals the drug in the muscle and minimizes skin irritation.

Take the patient's vital signs before giving IM penicillin injections to have baseline information. In an office or clinic setting, keep the patient for 30 minutes after giving the first dose orally or IM to observe for signs of adverse or allergic reactions.

### CEPHALOSPORINS

#### Action

Cephalosporins are cell wall synthesis inhibitors that are chemically similar to penicillin and work in the same way to kill bacteria. Over the years, five generations of cephalosporins have been developed, all of which have broad-spectrum activity (see Table 5.1).

#### Uses

The first generation of cephalosporins (e.g., cefazolin, cephalexin) supplies mostly gram-positive coverage and limited coverage against gram-negative bacteria. The second-generation drugs (e.g., cefoxitin, cefotetan) have the same gram-positive coverage as the first generation and are more effective against gram-negative and anaerobic organisms. Third-generation drugs (e.g., ceftriaxone, ceftazidime) are more potent against gram-negative bacteria than the earlier generations but are less active against gram-positive bacteria. The fourth-generation cephalosporin (cefepime) has increased activity against both gram-negative and gram-positive bacteria and is available only intravenously. The fifth-generation drug (ceftaroline) is also available only in IV form and has the broadest spectrum against both gram-negative and gram-positive bacteria. It is the only cephalosporin that can treat MRSA. In November 2019 the US Food and Drug Administration (FDA) approved cefiderocol (Fetroja) for intravenous use. It is primarily used for the treatment of complicated urinary tract infections, including pyelonephritis caused by susceptible Gram-negative bacteria, in patients with no other treatment option.

**Memory Jogger**

Most cephalosporin drugs have *ceph*, *cef*, or *kef* in their names.

Cephalosporins are used for uncomplicated skin and soft tissue infections; for infections of the lower respiratory tract, central nervous system (CNS), genitourinary system, joints, and bones; and for serious infections, such as bacteremia and septicemia (infections of the blood).

#### Expected Side Effects

Common side effects of cephalosporins are similar to those of penicillin. Nausea, vomiting, and diarrhea frequently occur but are usually mild.

#### Adverse Reactions

The most common adverse effect is acute *hypersensitivity* (allergy). Although some patients have only a minor rash and itching, a major event with anaphylaxis is possible. Patients who are allergic to penicillins have a risk of allergic reactions to cephalosporins because cephalosporins are structurally similar to penicillins. This is known as *cross-sensitivity*, and if a cephalosporin must be used, it is used with caution. Never give cephalosporins to a patient who had an anaphylactic reaction to penicillin in the past.

*Nephrotoxicity* (adverse kidney effects) has been reported with some cephalosporins, and the incidence is greater among older adult patients and those with poor renal function. There may also be severe pain at the injection site.

#### Drug Interactions

Alcohol taken with cephalosporins may produce a disulfiram reaction. (Disulfiram is a drug used to prevent alcohol use by producing a severe sensitivity to alcohol.) The reaction results in severe flushing, copious vomiting, throbbing headache, dyspnea, tachycardia, hypotension, and chest pain.

Antacids and iron can cause decreased absorption of some cephalosporins, and probenecid (Probalan) can decrease elimination of the drug.

## Nursing Implications and Patient Teaching

In addition to the general nursing implications and teaching points for all antimicrobial drugs, those specific for the cephalosporins are listed in Table 5.1.

**Top Tip for Safety**

Patients who are allergic to penicillin are often also allergic to the cephalosporins because the chemical structures are similar. Inform the prescriber about a penicillin allergy.

Many cephalosporins are given by the IV or IM route because some formulations are not absorbed from the GI tract. Table 5.1 summarizes the names, dosages, and nursing implications of common cephalosporins. Always consult a drug reference book or a pharmacist for information about a specific cephalosporin.

### OTHER CELL WALL SYNTHESIS INHIBITORS

Two other powerful cell wall synthesis inhibitors are vancomycin (Vancocin) and a group of drugs known as carbapenems (see Table 5.1). The carbapenems (imipenem/cilastatin [Primaxin], meropenem [Merem], ertapenem [Invanz], and doripenem [Doribax]) have the broadest spectrum of antibacterial activity against gram-positive and gram-negative bacteria. These drugs typically are used for infections caused by MDR bacteria in hospitalized patients. Side effects and adverse effects are severe, and the use of these drugs is usually limited to treatment of severe and life-threatening bacterial infections.

Vancomycin (Vancocin) is used to treat MRSA and other drug-resistant infections. Vancomycin-resistant enterococci (VRE) and CRE exist. Enterococci are bacteria found in the intestines and in the female genital tract, and Enterobacteriaceae such as *E. coli* and *Klebsiella* are normally present in the intestines. Usually, patients in hospitals or nursing homes who are critically ill and taking numerous antibiotics are susceptible to these resistant bacteria.

These drugs are given by IV push or infusion over an hour or more in an acute care setting. Dosages and schedules are based on the patient's weight, their organ health, and the severity of the infection. Vancomycin has an oral form that is used to combat the pseudomembranous colitis caused by C-diff. Imipenem/cilastatin (Primaxin) comes in an IM form that contains lidocaine (Xylocaine).

### Expected Side Effects and Adverse Reactions

Nausea, vomiting, diarrhea, headache, rash, fever, and chills can occur with these powerful drugs. Vancomycin often causes flushing and hypotension. An unusual response is a deep red rash on the upper body known as *red man syndrome*. The reaction is a response to histamine release. Slowing the infusion rate and pretreating the patient with antihistamines and an $H_2$-receptor blocker offer protection against red man syndrome.

Carbapenems can cause adverse CNS effects such as confusion and seizures. Vancomycin and carbapenems in high doses can produce nephrotoxicity and ototoxicity.

### Drug Interactions

Carbapenem drugs compete with probenecid (Probalan), and these drugs should not be given at the same time. The drug may reduce the activity of valproic acid, which is given to prevent seizures. Simultaneous use of carbapenems with ganciclovir (Cytovene) increases the risk of seizures.

Vancomycin adds to the toxicity of antibiotics such as the aminoglycosides and other drugs that are ototoxic or nephrotoxic. Cholestyramine (Prevalite) and colestipol (Colestid) decrease the absorption of the oral form of the drug.

 **Memory Jogger**

When a drug is nephrotoxic (i.e., damages the kidneys), it is also ototoxic (i.e., damages the ears) because ear and kidney tissue are immunologically and biologically related.

## TETRACYCLINES

### Action

Tetracyclines are a group of antibacterial drugs classified as *protein synthesis inhibitors* (e.g., tetracyclines, macrolides, aminoglycosides). All protein synthesis inhibitors (not to be confused with cell wall synthesis inhibitors) enter the bacterium and interfere with the bacterial processes used to make important proteins needed for growth. If the bacteria cannot make protein, it will not be able to reproduce, or it will die. Tetracyclines usually have only bacteriostatic action against susceptible organisms. This means that bacterial reproduction is reduced and the patient's immune system must rid the body of the organism.

### Uses

The tetracyclines are broad-spectrum drugs that are similar to penicillins in that they are effective against many gram-negative and gram-positive organisms. Many other drugs are more effective against those organisms, and tetracyclines are therefore the first choice for treating only a few diseases, such as acne, urinary tract infections, infections of the skin and respiratory tract, Lyme disease, stomach ulcers caused by *Helicobacter pylori*, *Chlamydia*, Rocky Mountain spotted fever, typhoid fever, sexually transmitted diseases (e.g., chlamydia, syphilis, gonorrhea), and inhalation anthrax exposure. Tetracyclines are also used for malaria prophylaxis.

### Expected Side Effects

Tetracyclines commonly produce mild episodes of nausea, vomiting, and diarrhea that may require stopping the drug. These effects are often dose related, and they result from irritation of the GI tract, changes in the normal bacteria in the bowel, and overgrowth of yeast. Tetracyclines increase the sensitivity of the skin to the sun, and severe sunburns are possible, even among people with dark complexions. Yeast infections of the mouth (thrush) and the vagina are more common with lengthy tetracycline therapy and in patients who are immunosuppressed or have diabetes. Yeast infections can be treated topically or orally with antifungal drugs.

### Adverse Effects

Use of tetracyclines is contraindicated in women who are pregnant or breast-feeding and in children younger than 12 years. These drugs may cause inadequate bone or tooth development, produce permanent yellow-brown tooth discoloration, or cause permanent damage (skeletal retardation) in a developing fetus.

Tetracyclines should be used with caution in patients with poor liver function because the drug may cause liver toxicity. In high doses, tetracyclines can decrease kidney function. Persistent dizziness, blurred vision, ringing in the ears, confusion, and headache can occur and may indicate increased pressure inside the brain.

**Lifespan Considerations**

Tetracyclines should not be taken by pregnant or breast-feeding women, or by children under 12 years old. Tetracyclines discolor growing teeth and may cause permanent teeth to be malformed. Staining of permanent teeth is usually temporary but can be lifelong.

## Drug Interactions

Food, dairy products, aluminum, magnesium, and calcium interfere with the intestinal absorption of tetracyclines. For this reason, tetracyclines are best taken with water on an empty stomach 1 hour before eating or 2 hours after eating. In addition to the general nursing implications and teaching points for all antimicrobial drugs, those specific for the tetracyclines are listed in Table 5.2.

## MACROLIDES

### Actions

Macrolides are protein synthesis inhibitors that work in the same way as tetracyclines. Macrolides are either bactericidal or bacteriostatic, depending on the organisms and the dose used. Azithromycin (Zithromax) and clarithromycin (Klaricid) are considered advanced-generation macrolides compared with erythromycin (E.E.S.), which was the first macrolide antibiotic. The later macrolides have a longer duration of action than erythromycin, have fewer side effects, and can penetrate the tissues better, making them more effective at destroying bacteria. Blood levels of drug remain higher for longer periods, reducing the number of required doses and the duration of therapy. Macrolides, in particular azithromycin, also have anti-inflammatory and immunomodulatory effects by interfering with inflammatory cytokines.

### Uses

The macrolides are effective against many of the same infectious organisms that are sensitive to penicillin, such as pneumonia, sinusitis, pharyngitis, and tonsillitis. Macrolides are used as alternatives to penicillin for patients who have a penicillin allergy and for infections caused by organisms that are resistant to penicillin. These drugs are effective against aerobic and anaerobic gram-positive cocci. They are not effective against MRSA or some other staphylococcal bacteria and some types of streptococci.

Additional uses of macrolides include *Mycoplasma pneumoniae* and *Chlamydia* infections. They are also used in Legionnaires' disease and in the treatment of pertussis (whooping cough). Using a triple therapy protocol, clarithromycin (Klaricid) is used to treat *Helicobacter pylori* infection, a cause of gastrointestinal ulcers. Macrolides are essential in treating chronic obstructive pulmonary disease (COPD) exacerbations because of their anti-inflammatory and immunomodulating features.

### Expected Side Effects

The most common side effects of macrolides are associated with the GI tract and include mild abdominal pain, nausea, flatulence, and diarrhea. These drugs increase the sensitivity of the skin to sunlight. Severe sunburns are possible, even among people with darker skin.

### Adverse Effects

Macrolides can impair the liver and cause jaundice. When macrolides are given intravenously, phlebitis and other types of vein irritation are common.

### Drug Interactions

Macrolides, which are protein bound and metabolized by the liver, can have numerous drug interactions. Macrolides enhance the actions of digoxin (Lanoxin), theophylline (Elixophyllin), warfarin (Coumadin), cyclosporine (Gengraf), and carbamazepine (Tegretol). These drugs can have toxic effects if levels are not followed closely. The combination of a macrolide with other drugs, such as ergotamine (Cafergot) for migraines or pimozide (Orap) for Tourette syndrome, can precipitate life-threatening cardiac dysrhythmias. Anesthetic agents and anticonvulsant drugs may interact to cause high serum drug levels and toxicity. Macrolides can also prolong the QT interval, which can cause life-threatening dysrhythmias such as ventricular tachycardia and ventricular fibrillation. Erythromycin (E.E.S.) has the uppermost tendency to cause these dysrhythmias. Consult a drug reference book or a pharmacist for information when other drugs are prescribed during macrolide therapy.

### ❖ Nursing Implications and Patient Teaching

The major differences between erythromycin (E.E.S.) and the newer macrolides are better GI tolerability, a broader spectrum of activity, and reduced dosing frequency for the newer products. The strength of erythromycin varies by product. Stomach acid inactivates erythromycin. This is the reason erythromycin is prepared as an enteric-coated drug combined with other products to form different drugs such as erythromycin base (Pediazole), erythromycin estolate (Ilosone), erythromycin ethylsuccinate (EryPed), and erythromycin stearate (Erythrocin Stearate). Different erythromycin preparations have different dosages. One type of erythromycin tablet should never be substituted for another type unless advised to do so by the pharmacist or healthcare provider.

Many macrolides may be given orally or parenterally. Topical application should be avoided to prevent sensitization. Keep the patient well hydrated (supplied with fluids). Drinking extra fluids to ensure a minimum urine output of 1500 mL/day decreases the odds of renal toxicity. In addition to the general nursing implications and teaching points for all antimicrobial

**Table 5.2** Examples of Common Tetracyclines, Macrolides, and Aminoglycosides

*Tetracyclines*, *macrolides*, and *aminoglycosides* are protein synthesis inhibitors that can enter the bacterium and prevent it from making important life-cycle proteins. Most are bacteriostatic rather than bactericidal and depend on the patient's immune system to fully rid the body of the infectious organisms.

| DRUG/ADULT DOSAGE | NURSING IMPLICATIONS |
|---|---|
| **Tetracyclines** | |
| doxycycline (Vibramycin) 100 mg orally every 12 hours<br>minocycline hydrochloride (Minocin) 100–200 mg orally or intravenously every 12 hours<br>tetracycline (Panmycin) 250–500 mg orally every 6–12 hours | • Remind patients taking tetracyclines to wear sun-protective clothing and sunscreen when going outdoors because these drugs increase skin sun sensitivity and can cause severe sunburns.<br>• Instruct patients to take these drugs 1 hour before a meal or drinking milk or 2 hours after eating a meal or drinking milk because food and milk inhibit intestinal absorption.<br>• Ask patients if they are using retinoids (isotretinoin [Absorica] or acitretin [Soriatane]) for acne because using these drugs with tetracyclines can cause a severe rise in intracranial pressure and is contraindicated. Topical retinol (Renova) may be used but will increase the chances for sunburn if a sunscreen is not used. |
| **Macrolides** | |
| azithromycin (Zithromax) 500 mg orally for one dose, then 250 mg orally once daily for 4 days<br>clarithromycin (Biaxin) 250–500 mg orally every 12 hours<br>clarithromycin extended release (Biaxin XL) 1000 mg orally once daily<br>erythromycin (E.E.S.) 250–500 mg orally every 6–12 hours | • Consult with the healthcare provider and the pharmacist for patients taking other drugs with macrolides because they interact with many drugs.<br>• Clarithromycin and erythromycin should not be used with moxifloxacin (Avelox), pimozide (Orap), thioridazine (Mellaril), or other drugs that may prolong the QT interval because life-threatening dysrhythmias can occur.<br>• Tell patients that palpitations and chest pain can occur while taking clarithromycin or erythromycin, and instruct them to seek emergency help immediately because these drugs can cause cardiac dysrhythmias.<br>• Instruct patients to take erythromycin with food or milk because the drug is not absorbed as well when taken on an empty stomach.<br>• Monitor liver enzymes and assess for jaundice in patients taking a macrolide because these drugs can cause liver damage, especially in older people. |
| **Aminoglycosides** | |
| amikacin (Amikin) 15–30 mg/kg intravenous (IV) every 8–12 hours<br>gentamicin (Garamycin) 3–5 mg/kg per day IV or intramuscular (IM)<br>streptomycin (Streptomycin) 1–2 g IM every 6 or 12 hours | • Give these drugs only for as long as prescribed because they can cause kidney damage and hearing loss.<br>• When giving these drugs intravenously, be sure to dilute them well and give over 30–60 minutes to reduce vein irritation and prevent cardiac side effects.<br>• Assess patients for confusion, weakness, sleep disorders, or eye disorders because these drugs, especially streptomycin, can induce nervous system toxicities. If adverse effects appear, notify the healthcare provider immediately to prevent severe complications. |
| **Other Protein Synthesis Inhibitors** | |
| clindamycin (Cleocin) 150–450 mg orally every 6 hours | • Give with food or a full glass of water to minimize gastrointestinal irritation. |
| linezolid (Zyvox) 600 mg orally or IV every 12 hours | • Monitor blood pressure and heart rate of patients who are taking a selective serotonin reuptake inhibitor antidepressant because the risk of serotonin syndrome is increased.<br>• Ask patients if they are on monoamine oxidase inhibitor antidepressants because use with linezolid can cause severe cardiac problems and is contraindicated.<br>• Tell patients to notify their healthcare provider if unusual bruising or bleeding occurs because these may be signs of a low platelet count.<br>• Tell patients to avoid alcohol and tyramine-containing foods to avoid severe hypertension. |
| dalfopristin/quinupristin (Synercid) 7.5 mg/kg IV every 12 hours | • Mix the drug according to the manufacturer's instructions and give the infusion over 60 minutes to reduce vein irritation and injection-site reactions.<br>• Consult with the pharmacist about patients taking other IV drugs with macrolides because some drug combinations are not compatible.<br>• Consult with the healthcare provider and the pharmacist about patients taking other drugs with dalfopristin/quinupristin because it interacts with many drugs. |

drugs, those specific for the macrolides are listed in Table 5.2.

## AMINOGLYCOSIDES

### Action
Like other protein synthesis inhibitors, aminoglycosides weaken bacteria by limiting the production of protein, which is essential for life.

### Uses
Aminoglycosides, such as gentamicin (Garamycin) and amikacin (Amikin), are used in the treatment of serious aerobic gram-negative infections, including those caused by *E. coli*, *Serratia*, *Proteus*, *Klebsiella*, and *Pseudomonas*; aerobic gram-negative bacteria; mycobacteria; and some protozoans. Some drugs are used to sterilize the bowel before intestinal surgery and to treat hepatic encephalopathy.

### Expected Side Effects
When given intravenously, aminoglycosides irritate the veins. Additional common side effects include nausea, vomiting, rash, lethargy, and fever.

### Adverse Reactions
Aminoglycosides can cause serious adverse effects, including damage to the kidney (*nephrotoxicity*) that is usually reversible if the drug is stopped quickly. They can also produce permanent damage to the inner ear (*ototoxicity*), hearing impairment, dizziness, loss of balance, ringing in the ears, and persistent headache or other types of neurotoxicity, particularly with drugs such as gentamicin (Gentamicin).

Aminoglycosides have a narrow therapeutic range (the lowest and highest acceptable drug levels are not far apart). This requires that the sample for the antibiotic blood level be drawn just before the next scheduled dose is given. This sample shows the lowest blood level of the antibiotic (*trough*), rather than a blood level at a higher range (*peak*). The lowest blood level determines whether the dosage needs to be adjusted to stay within the therapeutic range and not reach the toxic level or go below the effective level. Aminoglycoside dosage is calculated on the basis of the patient's weight. The dosage is adjusted according to creatinine clearance (based on creatinine blood levels) so that a therapeutic level is maintained without nephrotoxicity. Blood urea nitrogen (BUN) and glomerular filtration rates are also closely monitored.

### Drug Interactions
Using aminoglycosides with many other drugs, particularly vancomycin (Vancocin), increases the risk of nephrotoxicity. Ototoxicity is increased with aspirin, furosemide, ethacrynic acid, and many other drugs. Consult a drug reference book or a pharmacist for information when other drugs are prescribed during aminoglycoside therapy.

### ❖ Nursing Implications and Patient Teaching
In addition to the general nursing implications and teaching points for all antimicrobial drugs, those specific for the aminoglycosides are listed in Table 5.2. Aminoglycosides are given parenterally for systemic bacterial infections because they are poorly absorbed from the GI tract.

Patients should have frequent hearing and urine tests to monitor for ototoxicity and nephrotoxicity, respectively. Nurses monitor the blood levels of aminoglycosides, particularly for patients in the hospital. The drug levels peak and trough (go up and down), and close monitoring is important.

 **Top Tip for Safety**

Monitor patients for ototoxicity symptoms, which include dizziness, unsteady gait, loss of coordination, wavering vision, feelings of something stuffed in the ear, and ringing in the ear.

## MISCELLANEOUS PROTEIN SYNTHESIS INHIBITORS

Three classifications of protein synthesis inhibitors do not fit into other categories and are not used commonly: lincosamides, oxazolidinones, and streptogramins. They are usually given intravenously to treat bacterial infections that have not responded to other antibiotics, and their use is limited to life-threatening infections such as MRSA and vancomycin-resistant *Staphylococcus aureus* (VRSA). Clindamycin (Cleocin) is a lincosamide that can be given orally for skin infections such as impetigo and cellulitis and for complicated skin and soft tissue infections such as diabetic foot ulcers. It is used intravenously for bone infections, intraabdominal abscess, peritonitis, cellulitis, septicemia, bacteremia, and anaerobic pneumonia. Clindamycin is an older drug, and more organisms are resistant to it. It is also more likely than other antibiotics to cause antibiotic-associated diarrhea, including C-diff colitis.

Linezolid (Zyvox) is an oxazolidinone that can be given orally or intravenously. It is used for MRSA, VRE, and sepsis after treatment with vancomycin has failed. Dalfopristin/quinupristin (Synercid) can be given only intravenously and is reserved for patients with bacteremia or sepsis. Table 5.2 describes specific implications of giving these drugs.

 **Safety Alert!**

Do not confuse Zyvox with Zovirax or Zyban. Zyvox is an antibiotic, Zovirax is an antiviral, and Zyban is a drug used for smoking cessation.

**Bookmark This!**

For a full list of soundalike drugs, you can download a PDF file from the Institute for Safe Medical Practices (ISMP) at https://www.ismp.org/Tools/confuseddrugnames.pdf.

## SULFONAMIDES

### Action

Sulfonamides are antibacterial drugs from a class known as *metabolism inhibitors*. They enter the bacteria and prevent them from making the final form of folic acid, which is needed for bacterial growth and function. Sulfonamides are bacteriostatic rather than bactericidal because they do not kill bacteria.

### Uses

Sulfonamides have a broad spectrum of activity. They are eliminated by the kidneys and have a high concentration of activity in the kidneys. This makes sulfonamides a good choice for treating acute and chronic urinary tract infections, particularly cystitis, pyelitis, and pyelonephritis. The drug sulfamethoxazole is combined with trimethoprim (Bactrim or Septra) and is the most commonly used sulfonamide. It is effective for infections caused by *E. coli*, *Klebsiella*, *Proteus mirabilis*, and *S. aureus*. However, resistant strains of these bacteria are developing because sulfonamides have been used for many years.

Other indications for sulfonamide use include respiratory infections from susceptible organisms, and prevention and treatment of pneumocystis pneumonia in patients with HIV. Additional uses include treatment of otitis media from *Haemophilus influenzae*, community-acquired MRSA in children, toxoplasmosis, CNS infections, and MRSA infections of the skin and joints.

### Expected Side Effects

Common side effects of sulfonamides include many minor but irritating problems such as headache, drowsiness, fatigue, dizziness, *insomnia* (inability to sleep), *anorexia* (lack of appetite), nausea, vomiting, and abdominal pain. More problematic effects include *vertigo* (feeling of dizziness or spinning), *tinnitus* (ringing in the ears), hearing loss, and *stomatitis* (inflammation of the mouth).

### Adverse Reactions

Sulfonamides can crystalize in the kidney and cause kidney damage. Allergic reactions to sulfonamides are relatively common, including anaphylaxis. Typically, sulfonamides cause skin reactions, such as a rash that begins with a fever. Increased sun sensitivity (photosensitivity) reactions are common and can result in a severe sunburn. These drugs can suppress bone marrow function, increasing the risk of anemia, bleeding, and reduced immunity during and for several weeks after therapy is completed.

### Drug Interactions

Sulfonamides may increase the effect of sulfonylureas that are used to treat diabetes type 2 and cause hypoglycemia. They may increase the neurotoxic effects of phenytoin (Epanutin) and increase warfarin (Coumadin) drug levels, which lead to excess bleeding. If other drugs eliminated by the kidneys are taken at the same time, sulfonamides can increase the risk of nephrotoxicity. The effect of sulfonamides may be decreased by local anesthetics. Use of sulfonamides with some phenothiazine antipsychotic drugs can cause lethal cardiac dysrhythmias. Patients with an allergy or sensitivity to thiazide diuretics, oral sulfonylureas, or carbonic anhydrase inhibitors may exhibit the same allergy or sensitivity to sulfonamides. Consult a drug reference book or a pharmacist for information when other drugs are prescribed during sulfonamide therapy.

### ❖ Nursing Implications and Patient Teaching

In addition to the general nursing implications and teaching points for all antimicrobial drugs, those specific for the sulfonamides are listed in Table 5.3. Warn the patient to stay out of the sun because severe photosensitivity (abnormal response to exposure to sunlight) can occur if the patient's skin is exposed to excessive amounts of sunlight or ultraviolet light.

Sulfonamide dosage depends on the severity of the infection being treated, the drug used, and the patient's response to and tolerance of the drug. Short-acting sulfonamides usually require a special first dose (initial loading dose) that is larger than the dose that will then be taken regularly.

Sulfonamides should be taken with food, milk, or a full glass of water to minimize stomach irritation. To prevent formation of crystals in the urine, the patient must drink at least 1.5 L/day unless this is contraindicated.

## FLUOROQUINOLONES

### Action

Fluoroquinolones destroy bacteria by inhibiting two enzymes needed for DNA synthesis and reproduction. They are a type of bactericidal DNA synthesis inhibitor.

### Uses

All four generations of fluoroquinolones are effective against gram-negative pathogens. The newer ones are significantly more effective against gram-positive microbes. They are primarily excreted by the kidneys, making them a good choice for treating complicated urinary tract infections. These drugs are also used in the treatment of respiratory, GI, gynecologic, skin, soft tissue, bone, and joint infections. Ciprofloxacin (Cipro) is the drug of choice for anthrax exposure in a bioterrorist attack.

### Expected Side Effects

Nausea, vomiting, diarrhea, abdominal pain, and headache are the most common side effects of fluoroquinolones. These drugs concentrate in the urine, making them more irritating. For patients who dribble urine or who are incontinent, the skin in the genital area can become red and sore. This problem is reduced by having the patient increase his or her fluid intake to dilute the urine.

**Table 5.3   Examples of Common Sulfonamides and Fluoroquinolones**

*Sulfonamide* drugs are metabolism inhibitors that work by entering bacteria and preventing them from making the final form of folic acid, which is needed for bacterial growth and function. *Fluoroquinolone* drugs are DNA synthesis inhibitors that prevent bacterial reproduction and induce bacterial death by suppressing enzymes needed for DNA synthesis and important life-cycle activities.

| DRUG/ADULT DOSAGE | NURSING IMPLICATIONS |
|---|---|
| **Sulfonamides** | |
| sulfamethoxazole/trimethoprim (Bactrim, Septra) 400 mg/80 mg orally every 12 hours<br>sulfamethoxazole/trimethoprim (Bactrim DS, Septra DS) 800 mg/160 mg orally once daily | • If there are no fluid restrictions, have the patient drink a full glass of water when taking the drug and increase fluids to 1.5 L/day to prevent crystals from forming in the kidney and causing kidney damage.<br>• Remind patients to stay out of the sun while taking sulfonamide drugs to prevent severe sunburn.<br>• Warn patients who are on sulfonylureas (drugs for diabetes type 2) that fatigue, shakiness, anxiety, and irritability (hypoglycemia) may occur. |
| **Fluoroquinolones** | |
| ciprofloxacin (Cipro, Cipro XR) 250–750 mg orally every 12 hours or 1 g orally once daily *or* 200–400 mg intravenous (IV) every 12 hours<br>levofloxacin (Levaquin) 250–750 mg orally or IV once daily<br>moxifloxacin (Avelox 400 mg every day orally or IV) | • Give with food (no dairy) to ensure absorption.<br>• These drugs are not used for children younger than 18 years because they interfere with the growth of bones, muscles, and tendons.<br>• Because these drugs can cause tendon rupture, teach patients to stop the drug and call their healthcare provider if they develop joint pain or inflammation.<br>• IV doses should be mixed according to manufacturer's directions and given over 60–90 minutes to reduce vein irritation and injection-site reactions.<br>• Teach patients to drink increased fluids to dilute urine to prevent crystallization of urine.<br>• Teach patients to avoid sunlight to prevent severe sunburn.<br>• Teach patients with diabetes to check blood glucose levels frequently because fluctuations in glucose levels can occur and cause hyperglycemia or hypoglycemia.<br>• To avoid complications from peripheral neuropathy, teach patients to notify their healthcare provider if numbness, tingling, or pain occurs in hands or feet.<br>• Teach patients to notify their healthcare provider about tendonitis symptoms that may occur (ache, pain, redness, and swelling in a joint or area where a tendon attaches to a bone).<br>• Moxifloxacin is eliminated hepatically making it a good option for patients with renal failure. |

## Adverse Reactions

*Arthropathy* (joint pain and disease) can occur, especially in children who are receiving fluoroquinolones. Life-threatening heart rhythm changes can occur if fluoroquinolones are used with antidysrhythmic drugs such as quinidine (Cardioquin), sotalol (Sotacor), or amiodarone (Pacerone). Fluoroquinolones are generally contraindicated for patients on an antidysrhythmic. Tingling, burning, and numbness in the feet and hands (*peripheral neuropathy*) can occur. Rupture of a tendon in the shoulder, hand, arm, wrist, legs, or heel can occur, especially in patients with decreased renal function, older patients, and those taking prednisone (Deltasone). There is an increased risk of rupture or dissection of aortic aneurysm, exacerbation of myasthenia gravis, and retinal detachment associated with the use of fluroquinolones. The FDA has also warned against mental health side effects, hypoglycemia, and hyperglycemia. In addition, the FDA is advising that the serious side effects associated with fluoroquinolones generally outweigh the benefits for patients with sinusitis, bronchitis, and uncomplicated urinary tract infections (UTIs) who have other treatment options. For patients with these conditions, fluoroquinolones should be reserved for those who do not have alternative treatment options. Fluoroquinolones should be taken 2 hours before or 4 hours after multivitamins, minerals, antacids, and iron because these agents reduce the absorption of the antibiotic by as much as 90%. Fluoroquinolones increase the anticoagulant effects of warfarin (Coumadin) when taken with it. Dairy products and enteral tube feedings reduce the absorption of fluoroquinolones. In patients taking antidiabetic drugs, hyperglycemia or hypoglycemia may occur. Consult a drug reference book or a pharmacist for information when other drugs are prescribed during fluoroquinolone therapy. Fluoroquinolones also have been associated with an increased risk of tendon rupture that may result in disability and/or require surgical repair.

 **Black Box Warning: Fluoroquinolones**

Cardiac dysrhythmias, mental health side effects, hypoglycemia, hyperglycemia, increased risk of rupture or dissection of aortic aneurysm, exacerbation of myasthenia gravis, and retinal detachment can occur.

❖ **Nursing Implications and Patient Teaching**

In addition to the general nursing implications and teaching points for all antimicrobial drugs, those specific for the fluoroquinolones are listed in Table 5.3. Fluoroquinolones are to be taken with food, but not dairy products, to decrease adverse GI effects. Keep older patients well hydrated to prevent decreased renal function.

# Get Ready for the Next-Generation NCLEX® Examination!

## Key Points

- Before giving a patient the first dose of an anti-infective drug, be sure to ask the patient about previous allergic reactions to anti-infective drugs.
- Antibiotics should be given on an even around-the-clock schedule to maintain a consistent blood level.
- An increased risk for recurrence of infection and drug-resistant organism development may occur when antimicrobial therapy is discontinued before the prescribed duration.
- Bactericidal drugs kill bacteria, and bacteriostatic drugs limit or slow the growth of (inhibit) bacteria.
- Breast-feeding should be avoided during antimicrobial therapy because most drugs are excreted into breast milk, leaving the infant vulnerable to drug side effects and adverse reactions.
- Patients who are allergic to penicillin are often allergic to the cephalosporins due to the similar chemical structure of both drugs. The prescriber should be informed about a penicillin allergy.

## Clinical Judgment and Next-Generation NCLEX® Examination-Style Questions

### Case Study

Jean M. is a 16-year-old female who is being seen in the dermatology clinic for alleviation of facial acne. She has no known drug allergies. The healthcare provider has prescribed tetracycline 500 mg by mouth twice a day for 6 weeks and a benzoyl peroxide face wash twice a day.

1. Jean asks the nurse, "How does tetracycline work"? Which answer by the nurse is the most correct?

    1. Tetracycline is a protein synthesis inhibitor.
    2. Tetracycline is a broad-spectrum antibiotic used for acne.
    3. Tetracycline is a bacteriostatic antibiotic; it doesn't kill bacteria.
    4. Tetracycline makes it difficult for the bacteria to make enough protein to grow.

2. The nurse is teaching Jean about side effects she may experience while taking tetracycline.

    Instructions: Complete the sentences below by choosing the best option for the missing information that corresponds with the numbered list of options provided below.

    Tetracycline's expected side effects commonly result from irritation to the_____. A significant side effect is ____ due to heightened sensitivity of the _____.

| OPTION 1 | OPTION 2 | OPTION 3 |
|---|---|---|
| Integumentary system | Diarrhea | Skin |
| Central Nervous system | Sunburn | Intestines |
| GI system | Yeast | Genitals |
| Cardiovascular system | Dizziness | Inner ear |

3. Instructions: Highlight or circle each aspect of data collection the nurse will perform when considering the nursing implications related to tetracycline.

    1. Ask if Jane is on birth control.
    2. Ask if Jane is pregnant.
    3. Ask if Jane is breast-feeding.
    4. Advise taking probiotics to prevent yeast infection.
    5. Instruct Jane to wear sunscreen when outdoors.
    6. Record all prescription/OTC drugs Jane is taking.
    7. Advise not to take with dairy products or antacids.
    8. Advise to take with food.
    9. Tell the patient not to use topical retinol serum.

4. Order: gentamicin 3 mg/kg Intramuscular (IM) every 8 hours.

    On hand: Gentamicin 40 mg/mL.
    Patient weighed 176 lbs.
    1. How many kg does the patient weigh?
    2. How many mg of gentamicin will the nurse administer?
    3. How many mL of gentamicin will the nurse administer?

5. The nurse is preparing to administer gentamicin 240 mg/6 mL IM every 8 hours. Which action will the nurse take?

   1. Administer 6 mL of gentamicin intramuscularly in the left ventrogluteal muscle.
   2. Administer 3 mL of gentamicin intramuscularly in the right and left ventrogluteal muscle.
   3. Administer 6 mL of gentamicin intramuscularly in the right dorsogluteal muscle.
   4. Administer 3 mL of gentamicin intramuscularly in the right and left dorsogluteal muscle.

6. Which actions will the nurse take when administering gentamicin? Select all or any that apply.

   1. Monitor creatinine clearance, BUN, and glomerular filtration
   2. Monitor the patient for ringing in the ears, headache, and dizziness
   3. Monitor the peak and trough levels of gentamicin.
   4. Alert the healthcare provider the patient is taking aspirin.
   5. Tell the patient that chest pain and palpitations can occur after administration.
   6. Increase fluid intake if not contraindicated.
   7. Administer the gentamicin immediately before the peak level is drawn.
   8. Ensure that urine output is at least 40 mL/hr.
   9. Administer the IM injection though Z-track method only.

7. Which precautions should be taken when administering fluoroquinolones. Select all or any that apply.

   1. Administer on an empty stomach 1 hour before meals or 2 hours after.
   2. Stop the drug and call the healthcare provider if joint pain or inflammation occurs.
   3. Increase fluids to ensure urine output is at least 1500 mL a day.
   4. Check blood sugars frequently in diabetic patients.
   5. Monitor mental health changes in patients taking fluoroquinolones.
   6. Do not administer to patients that are on antidysrhythmic drugs.
   7. Do not administer with dairy products or enteral tube feedings.
   8. Monitor for an inflamed and sore mouth (stomatitis).
   9. Do not administer to children under 2.

8. A patient who has been taking antibiotics for 2 weeks to treat *Heliobacter pylori* asks the nurse what she should do to prevent a yeast infection. What is the best response from the nurse?

   1. "I will ask the healthcare provider to order a dose of fluconazole for you to take."
   2. "You can treat a yeast infection yourself with OTC Monistat cream."
   3. "*Lactobacillus acidophilus* probiotic capsules work well to prevent yeast infections".
   4. "Start eating Greek yogurt every day and call the healthcare provider if you begin having discharge."

9. Aminoglycosides can be used for infections by which pathogen? Select all or any that apply.

   1. *Staphylococcus*
   2. *Klebsiella*
   3. *E. coli*
   4. *Streptococcus*
   5. MRSA
   6. *Clostridium difficile*

10. Which antibiotics can be safely used for a patient who has an anaphylactic reaction to penicillin? Select all or any that apply.

    1. Penicillin VK
    2. Gentamicin
    3. Augmentin
    4. Erythromycin
    5. Ceftriaxone
    6. Amoxicillin
    7. Clarithromycin
    8. Cephalexin
    9. Vancomycin

**History and Physical**
**Two Days Ago, 0800**

An elderly client is admitted to the medical-surgical unit for evaluation and treatment of lower-extremity cellulitis.
Physical Exam:
General: no acute distress
HEENT: mucous membranes moist
Respiratory: breath sounds clear bilaterally
Cardiovascular: S1, S2, no murmur
GI: soft, nondistended, nontender, bowel sounds active x 4 quadrants.

**Today, 0600**

Physical Exam:
General: no acute distress
HEENT: oropharynx clear, mucous membranes dry
Respiratory: breath sounds clear bilaterally
Cardiovascular: S1, S2, no murmur
GI: no rebound or guarding, hyperactive bowel sounds

**Nurse's Notes**
**Today, 0600**

The client states that they have "not been able to stay out of the bathroom all night." The client states that abdominal cramping and pain started yesterday evening. The client states "my stool may even have had some blood in it."

**Flow Sheet**
**Two Days Ago, 0800**

Blood Pressure: 139/89 mm Hg

Heart Rate: 85/min
Respiratory Rate: 18/min
Temperature: 99.4°F (37.4°C)

**Today, 0600**

Blood Pressure: 104/68 mm Hg
Heart Rate: 92/min
Respiratory Rate: 18/min
Temperature: 101.0°F (38.3°C)

**Orders**
**Two Days Ago, 0800**

Clindamycin 300 mg PO every 6 hours
   A nurse is caring for the client on a medical-surgical unit and reviews the client's history and physical, nurse's notes, flowsheet, and orders.
   **Which of the following nursing actions are indicated? Select all or any that apply.**

- Advise the client that this is considered an allergic reaction to their antibiotic.
- Notify the provider.
- Collect a stool specimen for culture.
- Anticipate the administration of oral vancomycin.
- Advise the client that this is an expected side effect of clindamycin administration.
- Educate the client that they may have inflammation of the colon due to overgrowth of intestinal bacteria.
- Anticipate that the provider will increase the dose of clindamycin.
- Initiate an IV in anticipation of transition to IV antibiotics.

See answer on Evolve at http://evolve.elsevier.com/Visovsky/LPNpharmacology/.

# Drugs for Tuberculosis, Fungal, and Parasitic Infections

**6**

## Learning Outcomes

1. List the names, actions, possible side effects, and adverse effects of first-line antitubercular drugs.
2. Explain what to teach patients and families about first-line antitubercular drugs.
3. List the names, actions, possible side effects, and adverse effects of antifungal drugs.
4. Explain what to teach patients and families about antifungal drugs.
5. List the names, actions, possible side effects, and adverse effects of antiparasitic drugs.
6. Explain what to teach patients and families about antiparasitic drugs.

## Key Terms

**antibacterial** Antimicrobial drugs that kill or slow the reproduction of bacteria only; often used interchangeably with the term *antibiotic*.

**antifungal drug** Any drug used to treat a fungal infection; also called a fungicide or fungistatic drug.

**antimicrobial drug** A general term for any drug that kills or inhibits the growth of pathogenic microorganisms.

**antimicrobial resistance** The ability of an organism to resist the killing or growth-suppressing effects of anti-infective drugs.

**antitubercular** A drug or treatment that is effective against tuberculosis.

**fungi** A group of microorganisms that are everywhere in the environment and exist by absorbing nutrients from a host organism; includes yeasts and molds. A fungal infection is called a mycosis.

**helminths** Parasitic worms.

**parasite** An organism that lives on or in a human and relies on the human for its food and other functions.

## TUBERCULOSIS

Tuberculosis (TB) is a common lung infection found in the United States and around the world. In fact, the World Health Organization (WHO) reports that over 10 million people worldwide are diagnosed with TB annually and nearly 1.5 million people die each year. Although the overall incidence of TB cases in the US has decreased since 1992, there are still as many as 13 million people in the US with latent TB. For nurses caring for patients who may be immunosuppressed or have diabetes, the risk of TB increases. Furthermore, the Centers for Disease Control and Prevention (CDC) recommends that TB screening programs be in place for anyone working or volunteering in any healthcare setting.

TB is caused by a type of slow-growing aerobic bacteria known as *Mycobacterium tuberculosis*. It is primarily a disease of the lungs but may also be seen in bones, bladder, kidneys, and other parts of the body. TB can be transmitted to human hosts by other infected humans and, uncommonly, by cows (bovine TB) or birds (avian TB). Droplets ejected during coughing or sneezing are inhaled by an uninfected host. Once the bacterium is inhaled, it rapidly multiplies in the oxygen-rich lung tissue. The lesion that is formed is inflamed and filled with bacteria. If the person's immune system is intact, the bacillus is encased in a granuloma, which is a collection of macrophages that walls off the bacteria to stop its growth. The person will not become sick, but the TB test will remain positive because the immune system continues to recognize the exposure. A person who has acquired the TB infection but has no disease symptoms is said to have *latent or inactive TB*. Patients with latent TB can still develop *active TB* (called secondary TB) at a later time if they become immunocompromised (Fig. 6.1). Often the healthcare provider will decide that treatment for a particular patient is warranted to kill the encased bacterium.

The immune response takes between 2 and 10 weeks after exposure and is confirmed by an intradermal TB skin test that shows a 10-mm or larger induration (hardened red area). If the person does not have resistance to the disease because of reduced immunity from advanced age, disease, or repeated exposure, the bacteria will multiply, grow, and spread into more places in the lungs. The bacterium can also enter the bloodstream, which is how other organs become infected.

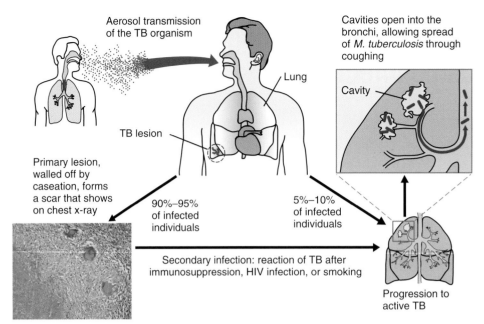

**Fig. 6.1** Primary tuberculosis *(TB)* infection with progression to secondary infection and active disease. (From Kumar, V., Abbas, A., Fausto, N., & Aster, J. (2009). *Robbins and Cotran pathologic basis of disease* (8th ed.). Saunders. Photograph courtesy of Dominick Cavuoti, D.O., Dallas, Texas.)

 **Memory Jogger**

**SYMPTOMS OF ACTIVE TB INFECTION**
Symptoms of active TB infection include productive cough, bloody sputum, poor appetite, unplanned weight loss, night sweats, low-grade fever, and chills.

Far more adults have latent infection than actually experience development of active TB. Even when a person is heavily exposed to the organism and inhales it deeply and often, if the immune system is functioning well, no actual disease will develop. Active TB is more commonly seen in underdeveloped nations, where living conditions are crowded and unsanitary. However, it is also increasingly found in the United States among patients who are immunocompromised (such as those with HIV, diabetes, or substance use disorder) or persons who have been recently exposed (such as people who have immigrated from areas with high rates of TB or people who work closely with patients with TB). According to the CDC, about 5% to 10% of patients who have latent TB will go on to have active TB disease if not treated.

 **Bookmark This!**

The Centers for Disease Control and Prevention provides up-to-date information on tuberculosis in the United States, including testing, treatment, and a wide range of patient teaching information at https://www.cdc.gov/tb/default.htm. For the impact of tuberculosis globally, check out https://www.who.int/health-topics/tuberculosis#tab=tab_1.

## ANTITUBERCULAR DRUGS

The TB organism is slow growing, and standard antibacterial drugs are not effective in controlling it. Select antitubercular drugs taken as a combination are used as first-line treatment to control uncomplicated active TB and prevent its transmission. Therapy continues until the disease is under control. The combination multiple-drug regimen controls the TB organisms as quickly as possible and reduces the development of drug-resistant organisms. Treatment usually last 4 to 9 months but may last longer for more complicated cases. People with TB are generally thought to no longer be infectious to others after they have been receiving drug therapy for several weeks, are feeling better, and are symptom free.

Recent guidelines from the CDC recommend several options as first-line treatment of TB. These can be either 4-, 6-, or 9-month regimens. The 4-month option consists of rifapentine (RPT), moxifloxacin (MOX), isoniazid (INH), and pyrazinamide (PZA) for the first 8 weeks, which is the intensive phase of treatment. The continuation phase lasts another 9 weeks, during which the patient takes RPT, MOX, and INH daily. The 6- and 9-month phases are slightly different using INH, PZA, as well as rifampin (RIF) and ethambutol (EMB) for the intensive phase and INH and RIF for the continuation phase. The CDC guidelines include additional treatment regimen guidelines that may be used for patients with HIV/AIDS or when treatment is difficult. The same drugs are used to prevent TB in people who were living with TB patients before being diagnosed and starting treatment (Table 6.1).

Although less common in the United States, some patients with TB are infected with *multidrug-resistant (MDR)* organisms that require susceptibility tests and alternative methods of treatment to control infection. The cause of MDR TB is usually due to TB drugs being misused or mismanaged (e.g., not taken regularly, treatment not available, or wrong treatment prescribed). TB is said to be MDR if the disease is resistant to at least two of the first-line drugs. In that case, second-line oral drugs are introduced. Examples include amikacin (see Chapter 5), kanamycin, and capreomycin (Table 6.2).

There is an *extensively drug-resistant tuberculosis (XDR-TB)* that is rare and resistant to isoniazid, rifampin, any fluoroquinolone, and at least one of the three injectable second-line drugs: amikacin, kanamycin, and capreomycin. Patients who have XDR-TB have a poor prognosis.

## Table 6.1   Drug Therapy for Tuberculosis*

*Rifapentine (RPT)* inhibits the ability of the TB bacteria to reproduce and causes cell death.

*Moxifloxacin (MOX)* is a fluoroquinolone antibiotic (see Chapter 5) that is bactericidal by inhibiting DNA synthesis.

*Isoniazid (INH)* kills mycobacteria actively growing outside the cell and inhibits the growth of dormant bacteria inside macrophages and granulomas.

*Rifampin (RIF)* kills slower-growing organisms, even those that reside inside macrophages and granulomas.

*Pyrazinamide (PZA)* kills organisms residing within the very acidic environment of macrophages, which is where the tubercle bacillus isolates itself. This drug is used in combination with other anti-TB drugs.

*Ethambutol* inhibits bacterial RNA synthesis, suppressing bacterial growth. It is slow acting, and because it is bacteriostatic rather than bactericidal, it must be used in combination with other anti-TB drugs.

| DRUG/ADULT DOSAGE | NURSING IMPLICATIONS |
|---|---|
| **Rifapentine** | |
| *For uncomplicated TB*<br>rifapentine (Priftin) for adults weighing 40 kg or more: 1200 mg orally once daily for 17 weeks as part of the 4-month regimen<br>*For prophylaxis or treatment of latent TB in combination with INH*<br>rifapentine for adults weighing 50 kg or more, 900 mg once weekly orally for 3 months. For adults weighing 32.1 kg to 49.9 kg, 750 mg orally once weekly for 3 months. | • Remind patients to avoid drinking alcoholic beverages while taking this drug due to its effects on the liver. Acetaminophen should also be avoided for the same reason.<br>• Teach patients to watch for signs of liver toxicity such as darkening of the urine, a yellow appearance to the skin or whites of the eyes, or an increased tendency to bruise or bleed.<br>• A common side effect is a reddish-orange staining of the skin, urine, and all other secretions, including tears and saliva. Although this is harmless, it may cause staining of clothing. Staining of soft contact lenses and dentures may be permanent.<br>• Rifapentine has multiple drug interactions. Teach patients to avoid taking herbal or OTC medications while taking it. |
| **Moxifloxacin** | |
| *For uncomplicated TB*<br>moxifloxacin (Avelox) for adults weighing 40 kg or more: 400 mg orally once daily for 17 weeks as part of the 4-month regimen | • Encourage patients to drink plenty of fluids while taking moxifloxacin.<br>• In older adults or patients with diabetes, monitor blood sugar because this drug can cause hyperglycemia or hypoglycemia.<br>• Avoid excessive sunlight as moxifloxacin can cause photosensitivity.<br>• Teach patients to report any watery diarrhea as this may be a sign of pseudomembranous colitis.<br>• Teach patients to avoid alcoholic beverages while taking moxifloxacin.<br>• Although rare, moxifloxacin may cause tendinopathy or tendon rupture. Report any shoulder, ankle, or other joint pain to the healthcare provider.<br>• Avoid taking any products with magnesium, iron, aluminum, or zinc, such as antacids or multivitamins by a least 4 hours before or 8 hours after taking moxifloxacin. |
| **Isoniazid** | |
| *For Uncomplicated TB*<br>Doses may be different as part of combination therapy isoniazid (INH) 5 mg/kg/dose (max: 300 mg/dose) orally 5–7 days/week for guideline-directed duration<br>*For Prophylaxis*<br>5 mg/kg/dose (Max: 300 mg/dose) by mouth once daily or 15 mg/kg/dose (Max: 900 mg/dose) by mouth twice weekly for 6–9 months. Doses may be different if as part of combination therapy<br>Or Isoniazid (INH) 5 mg/kg (maximum dose 300 mg) IM once daily or 15mg/kg/dose (maximum dose 900 mg) twice weekly for 6–9 months | • Instruct patients to avoid antacids and to take the drug on an empty stomach (1 hour before or 2 hours after a meal) to prevent slowing of drug absorption in the GI tract.<br>• Teach patients to take a daily multivitamin that contains the B-complex vitamins or vitamin $B_6$ (pyridoxine) while taking this drug because the drug can deplete the body of vitamin $B_6$ (pyridoxine), causing numbness and tingling in feet and hands (peripheral neuropathy).<br>• Remind patients to avoid drinking alcoholic beverages while taking this drug because the liver-damaging effects of the drug are potentiated by drinking alcohol. Acetaminophen should also be avoided for the same reason.<br>• Tell patients to report to the healthcare provider darkening of the urine, a yellow appearance to the skin or whites of the eyes, or an increased tendency to bruise or bleed because these are signs and symptoms of liver toxicity or failure.<br>• Ask patients about all drugs they are taking because many drugs can interact with INH.<br>• The IM route can be used only if the patient has difficulty with oral therapy. |

*Continued*

| Table 6.1 | Drug Therapy for Tuberculosis—cont'd |
|---|---|
| **DRUG/ADULT DOSAGE** | **NURSING IMPLICATIONS** |
| **Rifampin** | |
| *For Uncomplicated TB*<br>rifampin (Rifadin) 10 mg/kg/dose (maximum 600 mg/dose) orally 5–7 days per week for 6–9 months; in combination with other antitubercular drugs as directed | • Instruct patients to avoid antacids and to take the drug on an empty stomach (1 hour before or 2 hours after a meal) to prevent slowing of drug absorption in the GI tract.<br>• Warn patients to expect a reddish-orange staining of the skin, urine, and all other secretions.<br>• Tell patients not to wear soft contact lenses while taking this drug because they will become permanently stained.<br>• Remind patients to avoid alcoholic beverages and acetaminophen while taking this drug because its liver-damaging effects are potentiated by alcohol or acetaminophen use.<br>• Tell patients to report darkening of the urine, a yellow appearance to the skin or whites of the eyes, and an increased tendency to bruise or bleed, which are signs and symptoms of liver toxicity or failure.<br>• Teach patients with diabetes to check blood glucose levels frequently because fluctuations in levels can occur and cause hyperglycemia or hypoglycemia.<br>• Ask the patient about all other drugs in use because this drug interacts with many other drugs.<br>• The IV route can be used only if oral therapy is not practical.<br>• Mix IV doses according to the manufacturer's instructions and give over 30 minutes to 3 hours to reduce the chances for shocklike reactions and CNS symptoms. |
| **Pyrazinamide** | |
| *For Uncomplicated TB*<br>pyrazinamide weight-based doses of 1.5–maximum 3 g orally 5–7 days/week as part of 2-month intensive phase | • Ask whether the patient has ever had gout because the drug increases uric acid formation and will make gout symptoms worse.<br>• Confirm dose with healthcare provider as doses are weight based.<br>• Instruct patients to drink at least 8 ounces of water when taking this tablet and to increase fluid intake to prevent uric acid precipitation, which makes gout or kidney problems worse.<br>• Teach patients to wear protective clothing, a hat, and sunscreen when going outdoors in the sunlight because this drug causes photosensitivity and greatly increases the risk of sunburn.<br>• Remind patients to avoid alcoholic beverages while taking this drug because the liver-damaging effects of the drug are potentiated by drinking alcohol.<br>• Tell patients to report darkening of the urine, a yellow appearance to the skin or whites of the eyes, and an increased tendency to bruise or bleed, which are signs and symptoms of liver toxicity or failure. |
| **Ethambutol** | |
| *For Uncomplicated TB*<br>ethambutol (EMB) weight based dosing 15 mg/kg per dose (maximum 1.5 g) orally 5–7 days per week daily for 2 months | • Teach patients to take this drug with food to prevent or minimize stomach irritation.<br>• Instruct patients to immediately report to the healthcare provider any changes in vision, such as reduced color vision, blurred vision, or reduced visual fields, because the drug can cause optic neuritis, especially at high doses, and can lead to blindness. Minor eye problems are usually reversed when the drug is stopped.<br>• Remind patients to avoid drinking alcoholic beverages while taking this drug because the drug induces severe nausea and vomiting when alcohol is ingested.<br>• Ask whether the patient has ever had gout because this drug increases uric acid formation and will make gout worse.<br>• Instruct patients to drink at least 8 ounces of water when taking this drug and to increase fluid intake to prevent uric acid precipitation because ethambutol can make gout or kidney problems worse. |

*Always check current guidelines to determine drug doses for treatment of TB.

Note: Doses of common TB drugs may be weight based, so always confirm the dosage with the healthcare provider.

*CNS,* central nervous system; *GI,* gastrointestinal; *IM,* intramuscular; *IV,* intravenous; *OTC,* over the counter; *TB,* tuberculosis.

| Table **6.2** | Parenteral Drug Therapy for Tuberculosis |
|---|---|
| *Aminoglycosides* weaken bacteria by limiting the production of protein by binding to the ribosomes, which are vital for protein synthesis and life. | |
| **DRUG/ADULT DOSAGE** | **NURSING IMPLICATIONS** |
| capreomycin (Capastat) 15 mg/kg/dose IV or IM once daily or 5 days/week. Maximum 1 g IV or IM daily for 60–120 days. Followed by 1 g IV or IM 2–3 times per week for 12–24 months.<br>amikacin 15–20 mg/kg/dose IV or IM once daily or 5 days/week, duration will be determined based on location of the infection. | • Length of treatment and dosages may vary depending on weight, age, and specific resistance patterns.<br>• Nephrotoxic and ototoxic, so administration of an audiometry test and creatinine, BUN, and CBC tests should be done as a baseline parameter and repeated throughout duration of treatment. Periodic liver function tests should be performed.<br>• May cause respiratory depression and paralysis with IV use.<br>• Interference with metabolism and absorption of vitamins $B_6$ (pyridoxine) and $B_{12}$ (cobalamin) can lead to deficiency. Consider vitamin supplementation with extended treatment.<br>• Obtain kanamycin levels with peak and trough.<br>• Safety of these drugs in pregnant women has not been fully established, so the healthcare provider will consider the risks and the benefits of prescribing. |

*BUN,* blood urea nitrogen; *CBC,* complete blood count; *IM,* intramuscular; *IV,* intravenous; *IVPB,* intravenous piggyback.

## Action and Uses

The primary actions of first-line antitubercular drugs take place within and outside the cell walls of *M. tuberculosis* and slow down bacterial reproduction. The drugs used to treat TB are both bactericidal and bacteriostatic. Antitubercular drugs are used to control the active disease and prevent its spread to various organ systems in the infected patient or to other people. Drug therapy is used for direct treatment of TB infection and for prophylaxis in people who have been heavily exposed to the organism but have no symptoms of the disease.

Isoniazid (INH) inhibits the enzymes of the TB organism that are needed for reproduction and growth. It is a bactericidal drug. INH can inhibit the enzymes of TB bacteria whether they are in an infectious or a dormant state. It is metabolized by the liver and is available in oral and IM forms.

Both rifapentine and rifampin inhibit a TB enzyme that is needed for making DNA and proteins. These drugs are effective in preventing reproduction of the TB organism in infected tissues and in macrophages and TB granulomas. They can be bactericidal if the concentration of the drug is high enough in infected tissues.

Pyrazinamide appears to work by making the pH of infected cells lower (more acidic) than what the TB organism needs to reproduce and grow. It is especially effective at slowing the growth of TB organisms that are inside macrophages and in granulomas.

Rifater is a combination drug of isoniazid, rifampin, and pyrazinamide available for use. For information about each specific agent, refer to Table 6.1.

Ethambutol appears to interfere with RNA and protein synthesis in the TB organism, which reduces bacterial reproduction. It is bacteriostatic and is always used in combination with other drugs. Fig. 6.2 shows the sites of drug activity on the TB organism.

Moxifloxacin, a fluoroquinolone antibiotic (see Chapter 5), works by interfering with an enzyme essential for replication and repair of bacterial DNA. It is

part of the 4-month regimen in combination with RPT, INH, and PZA.

 **Lifespan Considerations**

### Pediatric Care

Children who have latent TB or who have active disease should be evaluated by an expert in pediatric TB. It is important to understand that children who are infected with TB typically become sick more quickly than adults and may have more severe illness. As a nurse, identification of children at risk is very important. For example, if you know of an adult who has been infected, make sure that any family members are identified and referred for screening and possible treatment. Drug therapy is typically weight based and may be similar to the therapy for adults. Make sure that there are adequate resources for the child to complete the full treatment. Ethambutol is not prescribed for infants or young children because they are unable to report visual changes that indicate a complication that could lead to permanent blindness.

## Pregnant and Breast-Feeding Women

In general, treatment for women with latent TB is delayed until several months after delivery. On the other hand, pregnant women with active disease will most likely need to begin therapy right away. Drugs, including INH, RIF, and EMB, may be safely given. For women with MDR TB, treatment may be more dangerous to the fetus, so the CDC recommends careful discussion with the patient regarding risks and benefits. Options for breastfeeding will vary according to the drug therapy prescribed, so it will be important to follow up with the healthcare provider.

## Expected Side Effects

Most of the first-line drugs against TB cause nausea, vomiting, diarrhea, headache, and sleeplessness. INH causes pyridoxine (vitamin $B_6$) deficiency, so supplements of vitamin $B_6$ are given during treatment. Rifampin and rifapentine cause a reddish-orange

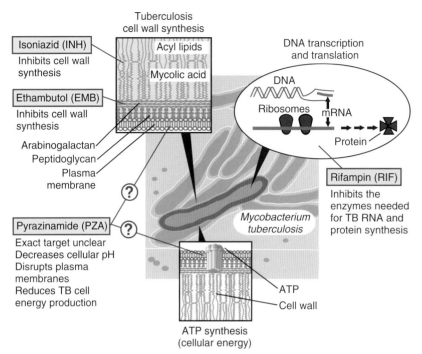

Fig. 6.2 Probable sites of drug activity against the tuberculosis *(TB)* organism. *ATP,* adenosine triphosphate; *mRNA,* messenger RNA. (From Workman, M. L., & LaCharity, L. A. (2016). *Understanding pharmacology* (2nd ed.). Elsevier.)

discoloration of urine and other body fluids. They both may stain soft contact lenses and dentures. Pyrazinamide increases sun sensitivity and causes muscle aches and acne. Pyrazinamide and ethambutol increase the formation of uric acid, which causes gout or makes its symptoms worse. Moxifloxacin can cause constipation in some patients.

## Adverse Reactions

The most common drugs for TB treatment are toxic to the liver. The toxicity is worsened if patients drink alcohol or use other liver-toxic drugs, such as acetaminophen, during TB therapy. INH, because it causes a deficiency in vitamin $B_6$, causes peripheral neuropathy with loss of sensation in the hands and feet. Ethambutol may cause confusion and optic neuritis that can lead to vision loss if the drug is not stopped. Pyrazinamide may interfere with blood clotting time and cause anemia. INH and ethambutol may cause psychological changes in some patients. Moxifloxacin can cause tendinopathy and even tendon rupture, as well as cardiac dysrhythmias.

Contraindications for the use of TB drugs are severe drug allergy and major renal or liver dysfunction. However, because of the fatal nature of TB, the risks may outweigh the benefits in these patients, and these drugs may be used very cautiously. Patients can be given supportive therapy such as antihistamines and steroids during treatment if drug allergies exist. Dosages may be adjusted for patients with renal or liver dysfunction.

## Drug Interactions

The drug treatment plan for TB is often complicated. No other drugs should be taken at the same time or immediately after antitubercular drugs are swallowed. Even topical agents on the skin are avoided while the patient is receiving anti-TB therapy. This is because other drugs may increase the significant risk for neurotoxicity and nephrotoxicity. All drugs taken by the patient should be checked closely for drug interactions, which are common among the antitubercular drugs. Consult a drug reference book or a pharmacist for information when other drugs are prescribed during antitubercular therapy.

## ❖ Nursing Implications and Patient Teaching

◆ *Assessment.* Assess the patient for signs and symptoms of active TB (productive cough with thick and often bloody sputum, low-grade fever, night sweats, anorexia, unplanned weight loss, and fatigue). It is important that the patient be a full partner in TB treatment because the drug therapy lasts for many months and is critical in controlling the disease. Assess whether the patient understands the importance of correctly taking the drugs every day. Also check whether he or she understands how to prevent infection spread.

Laboratory values are obtained before therapy begins, to establish baseline levels and to decrease the risk of adverse effects. These usually include a complete blood count (CBC) to assess for anemia, blood urea nitrogen (BUN) and creatinine to assess kidney function, liver enzymes to assess liver function, and a uric acid level to assess for gout. Any abnormal values may require adjusting doses or switching drug protocols prior to beginning treatment.

Antimicrobial resistance is likely to develop if only one drug is used for active TB or the patient does not take the drugs as prescribed. Assess the patient's ability to access the drugs from the pharmacy or local health department. If patients are homeless, outreach services and community clinics can be enlisted to ensure treatment success.

◆ *Planning and implementation.* Drug toxicity is a special problem because of the long-term nature of the required treatment. Ask patients receiving TB therapy about any severe side effects or signs and symptoms of adverse reactions. If you suspect any adverse reactions, hold the drugs and notify the healthcare provider immediately for further evaluation and to revise the plan of care. It is very important to continue drug treatment to avoid drug resistance, so timely notification of the healthcare provider is important.

Check for yellowing of the skin and eyes, light-colored stools, and darkening of the urine, which would indicate liver toxicity. Ask about any numbness, tingling, or pain in hands and feet that could indicate peripheral neuropathy due to vitamin $B_6$ deficiency. Symptoms of urinary retention, such as low abdominal discomfort, inability to urinate, painful urination, and bladder distention, may indicate urinary retention. Ask patients about joint pain and swelling that may indicate gout. Assess vision frequently, especially for patients taking ethambutol. Ask whether patients have noticed any changes in reading or driving and whether they have any pain or blurring of vision; these symptoms can indicate optic neuritis. Look for any changes in personality such as anxiety, withdrawal, or depression. Report all changes and unusual symptoms to the healthcare provider because all of these changes indicate possible adverse reactions to the drugs.

All drugs, unless stated otherwise, should be taken at the same time each day, preferably in the morning. If parenteral administration is required, the injection sites should be rotated and each site inspected for signs of tenderness, swelling, or redness.

Rifampin and isoniazid are best absorbed on an empty stomach. They should be taken 1 hour before or 2 hours after a meal.

If the patient cannot be relied on to take the drugs exactly as prescribed, he or she may need to be enrolled in a program of directly observed therapy (DOT), in which the drugs are given by an authorized person who watches to ensure that the patient actually swallows the drugs. Your local or state public health department, hospital, or pharmacy can provide more information on DOT programs.

◆ *Evaluation.* The positive skin test for TB does not change during therapy. Patients are assessed on a monthly basis for improvement of TB symptoms and the presence of active organisms in sputum cultures. Vital signs and new symptoms should be monitored for recurrence of acute infection. Weigh patients at each visit to monitor their general health status. Report weight loss to the healthcare provider because it may indicate worsening of the disease. Diet changes and nutritional supplements may be indicated.

◆ *Patient and family teaching.* In addition to the general nursing implications and teaching points for all antimicrobial drugs, those specific for first-line antitubercular therapy are listed in Table 6.1. Patients must take their drugs for a long time, so it is important to give clear instructions at the scheduled visits about the importance of continuing to take the drugs as ordered and the problems that should be reported to the healthcare provider. Stress the following important instructions:

- Do not drink alcohol for the entire duration of your TB treatment because these drugs can damage your liver and the damage is worse when alcohol is consumed.
- Set a regular time each day to take your anti-TB drugs to help you remember to take them.
- Take these drugs exactly as directed. If a dose is missed, take it as soon as you remember it, unless it is almost time for the next dose. Then do not take the missed dose, just follow the regular dosing schedule.
- Report any new symptoms promptly to your healthcare provider. Symptoms to report include any episodes of easy bruising, fever, sore throat, unusual bleeding, rashes, mental confusion, headache, tremors, severe nausea, vomiting, diarrhea, malaise, yellowish discoloration of the skin, visual changes, excessive drowsiness, changes in personality or affect (seems not to respond to stimuli), and severe pain in knees, feet, or wrists.
- Remember that while taking rifampin, your urine will be reddish orange. Although it can stain underwear and toilet, this is a normal side effect.
- Do not wear soft contact lenses while taking the combination drugs for TB because rifampin can permanently stain contact lenses.
- Do not take other drugs without the knowledge and permission of your healthcare provider.
- Take rifampin and isoniazid 1 hour before or 2 hours after eating or taking an antacid because food and antacids delay absorption of the drugs and may reduce their effects.
- Take ethambutol with food to reduce stomach irritation.
- Keep all appointments with your healthcare provider, and undergo laboratory tests so that progress can be measured.
- If you need assistance remembering to take your drugs, do not hesitate to contact your local public health department. There may be resources to help you remember to take them. It is better to ask for assistance early than to risk increasing drug resistance.

## FUNGAL INFECTIONS

A fungus is a member of a plant kingdom (Fungi) that includes yeasts and molds. Fungi are found everywhere in the environment and thrive in dark, moist places. Most of the time, these microorganisms exist in harmony with humans; however, they can become pathogens and cause infection. A fungal infection is called a mycosis or a mycotic infection. Fungi can be ingested or inhaled, and they easily grow on skin and nails. Some fungal infections, such as athlete's foot, are localized (kept to a specific area), whereas others, such as an invasive candidiasis (caused by Candida yeast), can become systemic and spread throughout the patient's whole body.

When fungi come into contact with a person who has reduced immunity, they take advantage of the weakened immune system and cause infection. For this reason, they are called opportunistic infections. Patients at increased risk for developing a fungal infection include patients with diabetes, pregnant women, women taking birth control drugs, patients taking corticosteroids, persons who are taking antibiotics (particularly women), and newborns. Transplant patients who are taking immunosuppressive drugs, cancer patients on chemotherapy, and patients with HIV infection are at risk for developing severe systemic fungal infections.

Fungi are more complex organisms than bacteria and more closely resemble human cells. They require drugs that act in a different way than antibacterials. In addition, because antifungal drugs often target the same structures that human cells have, they usually have more adverse effects when taken systemically.

### ANTIFUNGAL DRUGS

### Action and Uses

Antifungal drugs can be used orally, topically, vaginally, intravenously and even in shampoos to treat a variety of fungal or mycotic infections. Antifungal drugs have six classifications: azoles, polyenes, allylamines, antifungal antibiotics, antimetabolites, and echinocandins. Azoles, polyenes, and allylamines all prevent the production of a lipidlike substance that forms the fungal cell membrane. Without the cell membrane, the fungus becomes damaged and cannot reproduce (fungistatic effect) or dies (fungicidal effect). The antifungal drug griseofulvin stops the fungus from reproducing. Antimetabolites (flucytosine) disrupt the metabolic pathway of the fungal cell and interfere with reproduction and growth of the fungus. Echinocandins damage the cell wall of the fungus, killing it; they are the newest class of antifungals and are given only by the intravenous route for the treatment of invasive candidiasis, especially in critically ill patients.

The actions and specific uses of common systemic antifungal drugs are described in Table 6.3. Instructions for patients using topical antifungal agents for superficial fungal infections are presented in Box 6.1.

 **Memory Jogger**

Fluconazole, ketoconazole, itraconazole, posaconazole, and voriconazole all have the suffix -azole. They are all fungistatic and fungicidal at higher doses.

### Expected Side Effects and Adverse Reactions

Nausea, vomiting, and diarrhea are the most common expected side effects of antifungal drugs. Adverse reactions are associated with more severe problems, such as neurologic, cardiac, hematologic, liver, and renal toxicity. Skin reactions, rashes, and a rare serious rash such as Stevens-Johnson syndrome can occur. Stevens-Johnson syndrome begins with a painful red or purple rash, blisters, and flu symptoms, and it is a medical emergency.

Amphotericin B in particular, which is given intravenously, is associated with numerous adverse reactions, and to prevent them patients are premedicated with antihistamines, antipyretics, corticosteroids, and opiates. Amphotericin B is associated with serious adverse effects, and these patients must be closely monitored. Increased sun sensitivity (photosensitivity) can cause severe sunburn in patients taking ketoconazole, voriconazole, or griseofulvin. Griseofulvin can cause liver toxicity and numbness and tingling of the hands and feet (paresthesia). Terbinafine (Lamisil) and flucytosine (Ancobon) can increase the risk for infection because they can reduce the white blood cell (WBC) count. Terbinafine is also associated with hair loss in some individuals. Azoles at high doses given intravenously can cause life-threatening cardiac dysrhythmias.

 **Top Tip for Safety**

Adverse reactions to systemic antifungals, such as peeling, blistering, itching, burning, and redness of the skin, are similar to the symptoms of the diseases they are intended to cure. It is therefore sometimes difficult to determine whether the patient needs more or less drug.

### Drug Interactions

Superinfections can result when antifungals are given together with corticosteroid therapy because corticosteroids reduce the immunity response, making the person more vulnerable to a fungal infection. The activity of oral anticoagulants is decreased when used at the same time as griseofulvin. Fluconazole and itraconazole increase the effects of anticoagulants, causing patients to bleed, and can cause hypoglycemia when used with an oral hypoglycemic. Voriconazole interferes with many antidysrhythmic drugs and can cause life-threatening dysrhythmias. Antacids, anticholinergics, and H$_2$ blockers (e.g., famotidine [Pepcid] and nizatidine [Axid]) change gastrointestinal pH and interfere with drug absorption.

Toxicity can result when flucytosine is used together with other drugs that depress bone marrow or during radiation therapy. Use of flucytosine with hepatotoxic or nephrotoxic drugs should be avoided. The use of flucytosine also decreases leukocyte and platelet counts and hemoglobin levels. Consult a drug reference book or a pharmacist for information when other drugs are prescribed during antifungal therapy.

| Table 6.3 | Examples of Common Antifungal Drugs |
|---|---|

*Azoles* alter the cellular membrane of the fungus by depleting a lipidlike substance (ergosterol), which damages the fungus and keeps it from reproducing. At higher doses, azoles kill the fungus. They provide prophylaxis for high-risk patients and are used to treat topical and systemic infections caused by Candida and other fungi susceptible to their action.

*Polyenes* bind to fungal cell membranes and can increase cell permeability. They can be fungistatic or fungicidal depending on the organism and dosage. They can be used to treat many types of fungal infection, even some that are life-threatening.

| DRUG/ADULT DOSAGE | NURSING IMPLICATIONS |
|---|---|
| **Azoles** | |
| fluconazole (Diflucan) For oral candidiasis 100–200 mg orally once daily for 7–14 days; 150 mg orally for treatment of vaginal candidiasis. Dosage varies according to location of infection.<br><br>ketoconazole (Nizoral, Extina) 200–400 mg orally once a day (ketoconazole can also be applied topically)<br><br>miconazole nitrate 2% cream, powder, ointment, solution, vaginal suppository, apply as directed | • Length of treatment depends on the nature of the infection. Tell patients to take the drugs as prescribed for as long as they are prescribed to ensure adequate protection against infection or adequate treatment of infection.<br>• Instruct patients to monitor for rash, redness, or blistering because this could indicate Stevens-Johnson syndrome, a serious medical emergency. If these symptoms occur, they must notify the healthcare provider immediately.<br>• Instruct patients taking oral antidiabetic drugs to monitor glucose levels closely because these drugs can cause fluctuations in glucose control.<br>• Monitor blood urea nitrogen (BUN), serum creatinine, and liver function studies because these drugs can cause kidney and liver damage.<br>• Tell patients to report yellow skin, light-colored stools, dark urine, or yellowing of the eye sclera to the healthcare provider because these are indications of adverse liver reactions.<br>• Mix IV doses of fluconazole according to the manufacturer's direction and give no faster than 200 mg/hour to reduce the risk for cardiac dysrhythmias.<br>• Teach patients how to take their pulse daily, and to report to the healthcare provider a pulse greater than 100 beats per minute or lower than 60 beats per minute, or a newly irregular heart rate because these drugs can cause cardiac rhythm problems.<br>• Instruct patients to take ketoconazole with an acidic beverage such as cola to increase its absorption.<br>• Teach sexually active women to use effective birth control while taking azoles because these drugs may cause birth defects.<br>• Miconazole should not be used intravaginally for longer than 7 days. The healthcare provider should be contacted if there is no improvement in symptoms after 3 days. Topical application for athlete's foot (tinea pedis) or ringworm (dermatomycosis) should not exceed 4 weeks, and application for jock itch (tinea cruris) should not exceed 2 weeks. |
| **Polyenes** | |
| nystatin (Bio-Statin, Nyamyc) 400,000–600,000 units oral suspension orally times daily for 7–14 days; divide dose so that one-half of each dose is placed in each side of the mouth<br><br>Note: nystatin is also available as a tablet, cream, lozenge ointment or powder.<br><br>amphotericin B (Amphocin, Fungizone) 0.25–0.3 mg/kg/dose IV piggyback (IVPB) every 24 hours with doses increased by 5–10 mg/day to reach a full dose of 0.5–0.7 mg/kg/dose IV every 24 hours. Doses up to 1 mg/kg/day or 1.5 mg/kg/dose given every other day<br><br>Note: For amphotericin B, test doses of 1 mg (in 20 mL of 5% dextrose solution) administered over 20–30 minutes may be prescribed 2–4 hours prior to administration of the full dose. This is to evaluate for hypersensitivity reaction. | • Teach patients to prepare only a single dose of the nystatin powder for suspension because it does not contain preservatives and will not stay fresh.<br>• Teach patients to shake the suspension liquid well before taking it because the drug separates quickly.<br>• Teach patients to take one-half of the dose in each side of the mouth to completely cover the oral tissues.<br>• Teach patients to retain the suspension in the mouth for several minutes before swallowing to ensure that the drug comes into contact with any oral fungus.<br>• Warn patients who have diabetes and are taking nystatin suspension that it may increase their blood glucose levels because it contains sucrose.<br>• Always read infusion directions very carefully prior to administration. Typically, doses are given over 4–6 hours.<br>• Premedication of an antipyretic, an antihistamine, a steroid, and/or meperidine may be prescribed to reduce side effects of fever, chills, or rigor.<br>• Monitor BUN and creatinine as this drug may be toxic to the kidneys.<br>• Discontinue immediately if any shortness of breath and contact the healthcare provider.<br>• Report to the healthcare provider any skin reactions such as rash, itching, or blisters immediately as these may be an indicator or a severe adverse effect. |

*Continued*

## Table 6.3 Examples of Common Antifungal Drugs—cont'd

| DRUG/ADULT DOSAGE | NURSING IMPLICATIONS |
| --- | --- |
| **Other** | |
| griseofulvin (Gris-PEG, Grifulvin) 500–1000 mg orally once daily or in divided doses 2–4 times per day (microsize) or 375–750 mg once daily or in 2–3 divided doses per day (ultramicrosize). Dosage and duration vary according to the site of infection | • Teach patients to take the drug with a fatty meal to increase absorption.<br>• Teach patients to check for numbness and/or tingling of the feet and report these to their healthcare provider because these drugs can cause peripheral neuropathy.<br>• Tell patients to wear sunscreen and protective clothing when outdoors to prevent a severe sunburn because this drug increases sun sensitivity.<br>• Teach patients to alert their healthcare provider if symptoms such as rash or hives develop because these may indicate an allergy (hypersensitivity) to the drug.<br>• Tell patients to report to the healthcare provider yellow skin, light-colored stools, dark urine, or yellowing of the eye sclera because these drugs can damage the liver.<br>• Advise patients to avoid alcoholic beverages while taking griseofulvin because they may experience a rapid heart rate, sweating, and flushing.<br>• Teach sexually active women to use effective birth control because these drugs can cause birth defects. |

## Box 6.1 Teaching Points for Patients Using Topical Antifungal Drugs

### GENERAL PRINCIPLES
• Report any indication of an allergic reaction (new redness, swelling, blisters, skin peeling, or drainage) to the prescriber.
• Wash your hands to remove all traces of the drug immediately after applying it.
• Avoid getting an antifungal drug in your eye. If the drug does get into your eye, wash it with large amounts of warm, running tap water, and notify the prescriber.
• Use the drug exactly as prescribed and for as long as prescribed to ensure that the infection is cured.

### POWDERS
• Ensure that the skin area is clean and completely dry before applying the powder to prevent it from caking.
• Hold your breath while applying a powder to avoid inhaling the drug.
• For the foot area, be sure to get the powder between and under your toes. Wear clean cotton socks (night and day). Change the socks at least twice daily.
• For the groin area, wear clean, close-fitting (but not tight) cotton underwear (briefs or panties) to keep the drug in contact with the areas that are infected.

### DERMAL LOTIONS, CREAMS, AND OINTMENTS
• Ensure that the skin area is clean and dry before applying the drug to ensure best contact with the affected area.
• Be careful to apply the drug only to the skin that has the infection. Keep it off the surrounding skin to prevent healthy skin from reacting to the drug.
• Apply a thin coating as often as prescribed.
• Wash the area and dry it immediately before applying the next dose to ensure that the fresh drug is able to come into contact with the affected area.
• Loosely cover the area to prevent spreading the drug to other body areas, clothing, or furniture.

### ORAL LOZENGES
• Brush your teeth and tongue before using the tablet or troche to remove as much of the organism as possible so that the drug can come into direct contact with the affected area.
• Let the tablet or troche completely dissolve in your mouth for maximum release of the drug.
• Clean your toothbrush daily by running it through the dishwasher or soaking it in a solution of 1 part household bleach with 9 parts water. After using bleach, rinse the toothbrush thoroughly. Cleaning keeps the infection from recurring.

### VAGINAL CREAMS AND SUPPOSITORIES
• Vaginal creams or suppositories should be placed just before going to bed to help keep them longer within the vagina.
• Wash your hands before inserting the drug to avoid transferring other organisms into the vagina.
• Insert a suppository (rounded end first) into the vagina as far as you can reach with your finger so that the drug reaches all affected areas.
• Insert an applicator full of the cream as far into the vagina as is comfortable so that the drug reaches all affected areas.
• Wash the applicator and your hands with warm, soapy water; rinse well; and dry to prevent re-infecting yourself with organisms left on the applicator.
• A sanitary napkin can be worn to protect your clothing and bed from drug leakage.
• Avoid sexual intercourse during the treatment period. If you do have intercourse, the drug can make holes in a condom or damage a diaphragm and increase your risk for an unplanned pregnancy. You could also spread the infection or get re-infected with the yeast.

Adapted from Workman, M. L., LaCharity, L. A. (2016). *Understanding pharmacology* (2nd ed.). Elsevier.

### ❖ Nursing Implications and Patient Teaching
◆ *Assessment.* Ask patients prescribed an antifungal about any allergy, bone marrow depression, use of alcohol or other drugs that may produce drug interactions (particularly corticosteroids), and the possibility of pregnancy. Some antifungal drugs can be teratogenic (cause birth defects).

The patient may have a history of fever and chills at the onset of infection. Many patients report itching if they have a fungal infection. A history of recent antibiotic therapy is common. Inspect the mouth for the classic signs of thick, white, nonmovable plaques that coat the tongue and for erythema (redness or irritation) associated with thrush (Candida infection). The patient may also have a history of multiple scaly or blistered red patches on the skin, itching and soreness of infected areas, or brittle nails with yellow discoloration and separation from the nail bed. Check current laboratory work for CBC, platelet count, BUN, creatinine, and liver enzyme values to establish a baseline and to prevent kidney, liver, or hematologic damage. Check and document vital signs, accurate height and weight measurements, and culture and sensitivity reports.

 **Top Tip for Safety**

Closely monitor renal and hepatic functioning when giving ketoconazole or fluconazole. Closely monitor hematologic, renal, and hepatic status when giving flucytosine.

◆ *Planning and implementation.* Observe the patient for any signs of allergic reactions, such as hives, swelling of the lips and face, rapid pulse, or lower blood pressure. Alert the rapid response team immediately if any of these symptoms occur because they indicate an anaphylactic reaction.

- Check the skin for rashes, blisters, or increased itching that may indicate an adverse reaction or worsening of the fungal infection.
- Assess the site of infection daily for any changes, and document your findings. Assess vital signs daily as ordered, and alert the healthcare provider to any changes, particularly changes in temperature and pulse rate.
- Check the patient daily for signs of jaundice that may indicate hepatotoxicity: yellow skin, yellowing of the eye sclera, dark urine, clay-colored stool, and abdominal pain.
- Check the ongoing ordered laboratory work for any abnormalities that could indicate an adverse reaction or worsening of disease symptoms. Alert the healthcare provider as soon as possible if there are changes from baseline levels.

◆ *Evaluation.* Observe the patient for therapeutic effects: Chills or fever associated with some infections should disappear, and signs and symptoms should improve. Also watch for development of adverse effects and signs of GI distress. Remind the patient to continue taking the drug for the prescribed length of time and/or until the laboratory tests show that normal function has returned.

 **Top Tip for Safety**

If you are monitoring a patient who is receiving amphotericin B, give prescribed drugs to prevent adverse effects before the start of the infusion, and avoid giving any other drugs during the infusion. Monitor vital signs closely, and watch for reactions such as fever, chills, abdominal pain, cramping, diarrhea, nausea, vomiting, headache, flushing, and decreased blood pressure. Monitor for pain and inflammation at the infusion site.

◆ *Patient and family teaching.* Stress the following important instructions to the patient and family:

- Do not take any over-the-counter drugs, and let your healthcare provider know of all drugs you are currently taking or any drugs that another practitioner may prescribe for you during treatment because antifungals have many possible drug interactions.
- Take griseofulvin with high-fat foods or meals like cheeseburgers, whole milk, or ice cream. This causes more of the drug to be absorbed and reduces possible stomach upset.
- When taking ketoconazole, voriconazole, or griseofulvin, avoid direct sunlight and wear sunscreen and protective clothing while outside to prevent severe sunburn.
- Notify your healthcare provider if you have dark urine, light-colored stool, or yellowing of the whites of the eyes because these are signs of liver problems.
- Notify your healthcare provider if you have increased fatigue and shortness of breath, which may indicate an anemia.
- Be alert to flu symptoms, rash, or blisters and notify your healthcare provider immediately because these symptoms can indicate a severe adverse reaction to the drug and require hospitalization.
- Notify your healthcare provider about any skin rash or worsening nausea, vomiting, or diarrhea.
- When taking more than one capsule per dose, spacing them at least 15 minutes apart can reduce the likelihood of GI upset.
- If symptoms do not resolve within 2 to 3 days, notify your healthcare provider.
- Finish all of the drugs you were given, even if your symptoms improve, so that the infection does not return and resistance to the antifungal does not develop.
- If you take an azole, do not take the drug with grapefruit juice, and limit the amount of grapefruit juice you drink daily because it increases the potency of the drug, increasing the risk for adverse effects.

## PARASITIC INFECTIONS

A parasite is an organism that can survive only by living in or on a host organism. Billions of people worldwide and millions of people in the United States are affected by parasites that cause serious illnesses and can even cause death, especially in immunocompromised individuals. Parasites can be picked up from food, water, or insects and can be transmitted from person to person. Three main classes of parasites can cause disease in humans: protozoa, helminths, and ectoparasites (fleas and lice).

### PROTOZOA

Amebiasis and giardiasis are usually contracted from food and water contaminated by feces or from unwashed hands after using the bathroom or changing a diaper. These infections reside in the intestinal tract, and common symptoms are diarrhea, abdominal pain, vomiting, and foul-smelling stools. Amoebas are able to invade other parts of the body if they reach the bloodstream, and they can cause liver abscesses.

Toxoplasmosis is usually asymptomatic in a healthy individual but can cause serious illness in people with chronic disease. It is contracted from contaminated raw food and water or by handling contaminated soil, cat litter, or raw meat and then touching the mouth, nose, or eyes.

Trichomoniasis is transmitted through sexual exposure. Symptoms of trichomoniasis include burning, itching, redness, and vaginal or penile discharge.

Malaria is common in southeast Asia and Africa. It is spread through the bites of mosquitoes that have been infected by malaria-causing parasites (Plasmodium). The parasite migrates to the liver, where it matures and then enters the bloodstream. It lives and reproduces in the blood, using the hemoglobin and nutrients inside the red blood cell (RBC) until the blood cell ruptures and causes anemia. Treatment for malaria is guided by the CDC and depends on where the person contracted the disease. The CDC also has a prophylactic treatment guide for persons traveling to areas where malaria is prevalent. Malaria signs and symptoms include fever, chills, sweating, headaches, extreme fatigue, body aches, nausea, and vomiting. Even after treatment the disease is able to relapse.

 Bookmark This!

For information on the malarial disease process and up-to-date prophylaxis and treatment options, visit the CDC at www.cdc.gov/malaria.

## ANTIPROTOZOAL DRUGS

### Action and Uses

Antiprotozoal drugs work in several different ways inside the cell, affecting the function of DNA and/or RNA to kill the protozoan parasites. Antiprotozoals used to treat amebiasis, giardiasis, toxoplasmosis, and trichomoniasis are metronidazole (Flagyl) and iodoquinol (Yodoxin). Metronidazole is also used to treat bacterial vaginitis in conjunction with antibiotics used for the treatment of pelvic inflammatory disease.

Drugs used to prevent or treat malaria include quinine, chloroquine (Aralen), hydroxychloroquine (Plaquenil), mefloquine (Lariam), and primaquine. Chloroquine, hydroxychloroquine, quinine, and mefloquine inhibit the DNA and RNA enzymes necessary for the parasite to reproduce and live. They also raise the pH inside the parasite so that it is unable to use the hemoglobin in the human RBC to live and reproduce. All of these actions cause damage to the parasite. Pyrimethamine inhibits enzymes necessary for the parasite to produce substances necessary for

its survival. The malarial drugs are used in combination to kill the malarial parasite in different stages of its life cycle. Antimalarial drugs are sometimes used to treat other parasitic diseases as well. Table 6.4 provides a summary of antiprotozoal and antimalarial drugs.

### Expected Side Effects and Adverse Reactions

All drugs used to treat parasitic infections can cause nausea, vomiting, headache, anorexia, diarrhea, or GI distress. Additional drugs may be warranted to minimize these side effects. Iodoquinol (Yodoxin) is an iodine-based drug, so patients may experience hypothyroidism or hyperthyroidism, and thyroid function tests may be altered. Iodoquinol may also cause a yellow-brown nail, hair and skin discoloration, as well as discolored sweat. Optic neuritis can occur with symptoms of eye pain or vision changes. Permanent vision loss can occur if the drug is not stopped quickly. Peripheral neuropathy symptoms such as numbness and tingling of the fingers can occur with prolonged therapy. Metronidazole (Flagyl) can cause peripheral neuropathy as well as confusion. Fungal superinfections may occur with the use of metronidazole.

Common side effects of drugs used to treat malaria are similar to those used to treat other parasitic conditions: diarrhea, nausea, vomiting, headache, and GI distress. Primaquine can cause hemolytic anemia, leukopenia, and life-threatening dysrhythmias. Hydroxychloroquine can cause visual defects and possible loss of vision. Chloroquine and hydroxychloroquine can cause CNS changes such as personality changes, anxiety, and depression.

### Drug Interactions

There are no significant drug interactions with the use of iodoquinol. Metronidazole increases the effects of warfarin, and serious bleeding can occur when the two drugs are taken together. Alcohol-containing drinks, food, or mouthwash taken with or used during metronidazole can result in severe nausea, vomiting, headache, shortness of breath, and hypotension (disulfiram-like reaction). Chloroquine can decrease levels of valproic acid and increase levels of digoxin. Mefloquine and primaquine interact with many antidysrhythmic drugs like quinidine, beta-blockers, and calcium channel blockers and can increase the risk for life-threatening dysrhythmias. Consult a drug reference book or a pharmacist for information when other drugs are prescribed during drug therapy for parasitic infestations.

### ❖ Nursing Implications and Patient Teaching

◆ *Assessment.* Ask the patient about any allergy to drugs, current use of alcohol or disulfiram, the possibility of pregnancy, and the existence of chronic renal, hematologic, cardiac, thyroid, or liver disease. These conditions are contraindications or precautions to the use of

**Table 6.4     Examples of Common Antiparasitic Drugs**

*Antiparasitics* (not used for malaria) work in several ways on DNA and RNA to kill protozoal parasites.

*Antimalarials* inhibit the DNA and RNA enzymes necessary for the parasite Plasmodium to live and reproduce.

*Anthelmintics* destroy worms by paralyzing the parasite, killing it, and disrupting its adherence to the host site.

| DRUG/ADULT DOSAGE | NURSING IMPLICATIONS |
|---|---|
| **Antiparasitics** | |
| Dosage and route may vary depending on site of infection. Also is available as extended release tablet, cream, lotion or gel.<br>metronidazole (Flagyl) 500 or 750 mg orally every 8 hours for 5–10 days<br>iodoquinol (Yodoxin) 650 mg every 8 hours daily | • Teach patients to swallow metronidazole extended-release tablets whole; do not crush, break, or chew them because that releases drug too rapidly, leading to adverse effects.<br>• Give metronidazole at least 1 hour before or 2 hours after a meal to ensure best absorption.<br>• Give iodoquinol with a meal or directly after a meal to minimize stomach upset.<br>• Advise patients to take metronidazole or iodoquinol with a full glass of water to support excretion by the kidney.<br>• Check the patient's baseline liver and kidney function laboratory test results, and alert the healthcare provider if there are abnormalities because these drugs are metabolized by the liver and excreted by the kidney and can cause damage in compromised individuals.<br>• Remind patients taking metronidazole to avoid alcohol and products that contain alcohol because severe side effects can occur.<br>• Consult with the healthcare provider and the pharmacist about patients taking other drugs with metronidazole because it interacts with many drugs, leading to life-threatening dysrhythmias.<br>• Tell patients taking iodoquinol to contact their healthcare provider for any visual changes because the drug can cause optic neuritis and permanent vision loss.<br>• Advise patients taking iodoquinol to contact their healthcare provider about worsening symptoms of thyroid problems because the drug can interfere with drugs used for thyroid disorders. |
| **Antimalarials** | |
| **For Malaria Treatment**<br>chloroquine (Aralen) 1000 mg orally, then 500 mg orally in 6–8 hours, then 500 mg orally once daily for 2 days<br>primaquine 52.6 mg orally daily for 14 days in combination with chloroquine<br>atovaquone 250 mg/proguanil 100 mg (Malarone) 4 adult-strength tablets orally once daily for 3 consecutive days for malaria resistant to chloroquine (also for children and adolescents over 40 kg)<br>**For Malaria Prophylaxis**<br>chloroquine (Aralen) 500 mg orally weekly on the same day of each week, starting 2 weeks before entering the endemic area and continuing for 8 weeks after leaving the area<br>atovaquone 250 mg/proguanil 100 mg (Malarone) 1 tablet orally once daily. Begin 1 to 2 days before entering the endemic area and continue during the stay and for 7 days after leaving the area. (Dose may also be given to children and adolescents weighing more than 40 kg.) | • Give chloroquine and primaquine with meals to minimize stomach upset.<br>• Observe patients for corneal opacities and changes in vision because chloroquine can cause retinopathy, especially in older adults. If visual changes occur, contact the healthcare provider immediately because retinal changes can be permanent if the drug is not stopped.<br>• Warn patients with psoriasis that chloroquine may worsen psoriasis symptoms of red, scaly skin patches.<br>• Teach family members to watch for any changes in personality and to notify the healthcare provider if they occur because these drugs can affect the central nervous system.<br>• Tell patients taking chloroquine who also take valproic acid or digoxin that they may need drug levels measured more frequently. Chloroquine decreases valproic acid levels, increasing the risk of seizures, and increases digoxin levels, increasing the risk of digoxin toxicity.<br>• Teach patients taking primaquine to observe for increased fatigue, darkening of the urine, and a feeling of fullness in the stomach area that may indicate an enlarged liver because this drug may impair liver function. If these signs and symptoms occur, the healthcare provider should be notified immediately.<br>• Consult with the healthcare provider and the pharmacist about patients taking other drugs with primaquine because it interacts with many drugs, increasing the risk of life-threatening dysrhythmias.<br>• Atovaquone, proguanil may be given in areas where the malaria organism is resistant to chloroquine |

*Continued*

| Table **6.4** Examples of Common Antiparasitic Drugs—cont'd | |
|---|---|
| **DRUG/ADULT DOSAGE** | **NURSING IMPLICATIONS** |
| **Anthelmintics** | |
| praziquantel (Biltricide) 20–25 mg/kg orally three times daily for 1 or 2 days. Separate doses by 4–6 hours | • Tell patients to take tablets with food and a full glass of water to minimize stomach upset.<br>• Warn patients to check for yellowing of the eyes, darkening of the urine, or light-colored stools and to report these symptoms to their healthcare provider because this drug can damage the liver.<br>• Tell patients with a history of cardiac dysrhythmia to contact their healthcare provider if dizziness or irregular heart rate occurs and to call 911 if chest pain occurs because this drug can cause cardiac dysrhythmias. |

antiparasitics and antimalarial drugs. Baseline laboratory tests should be completed before therapy begins.

◆ *Planning and implementation.* Observe the patient for any signs of allergic reactions such as hives, swelling of the lips and face, rapid pulse, or lower blood pressure. Alert the rapid response team immediately if any of these symptoms occur because they indicate an anaphylactic reaction.

• Monitor nutritional status and encourage adequate food and fluid intake to help fight infection.
• Monitor for superinfections, and notify the healthcare provider of any changes. Assess vital signs as ordered daily, and alert the healthcare provider of any changes, particularly in temperature.
• Check the patient daily for signs of jaundice that may indicate hepatotoxicity: yellow skin, yellowing of the sclerae, dark urine, clay-colored stool, and abdominal pain.
• Check the ongoing laboratory work as it is ordered for any abnormalities that can indicate an adverse reaction or worsening of disease symptoms. Alert the healthcare provider as soon as possible if there are any changes from baseline levels.

◆ *Evaluation.* After drug therapy, periodic laboratory blood and stool tests are required to make certain the disease has been controlled or eliminated. These tests may be needed monthly for up to 1 year after therapy. Be alert to signs of drug toxicity. If severe symptoms appear, the drug may have to be stopped.

◆ *Patient and family teaching.* Stress the following important instructions to the patient and family:

• Take antiparasitics with or after meals to decrease the chances of stomach upset.
• Take antiparasitics with a full glass of water to prevent stomach upset.
• Report worsening symptoms of infection such as increased fever, increasing fatigue, or anorexia.
• Take the entire course of drug, even if symptoms improve, to prevent relapse or worsening infection.
• If taking metronidazole, avoid all forms of alcohol so that severe adverse effects do not occur.

• When traveling to areas where malaria is common, take prophylactic doses as prescribed.
• Notify your healthcare provider if expected side effects of nausea, vomiting, diarrhea, or abdominal pain cannot be controlled or if they worsen.
• When taking metronidazole for trichomoniasis or other sexually transmitted disease, refrain from sexual intercourse as ordered by your healthcare provider to prevent spreading the infection to others.

## HELMINTHS

When a patient has helminths (worms), the infestation is called helminthiasis. The condition is usually caused by flatworms, roundworms, tapeworms, or flukes. The worm gains entrance to the body through unclean food or water, unwashed hands, or the skin. Anthelmintic drugs are specific for the worms they can kill, and accurate identification of the worm is necessary. Identification is done by analyzing the stool, urine, blood, sputum, or tissue from the host to look for the larvae or eggs of the parasitic worm.

## ANTHELMINTIC DRUGS

### Action and Uses

Albendazole (Albenza), ivermectin (Stromectol), pyrantel pamoate (Nemex), and praziquantel (Biltricide) are examples of anthelmintic drugs that are currently being used. Albendazole is used to treat certain types of tapeworms, flatworms, and roundworms. Albendazole kills the larvae by destroying the cytoplasm of the worm (not the host cells); this disrupts the cellular function necessary for the survival of the worm. Ivermectin paralyzes certain kinds of roundworms. Praziquantel kills certain types of flukes and tapeworms by moving calcium into the cell membrane, which causes contraction and paralysis of the worm, dislodging it from the host site and killing it. Pyrantel pamoate also causes paralysis of the worm, which dislodges it from the intestines and allows it to be expelled through the stool. It is used for certain types of roundworm infestations (e.g., pinworms) and is available without a prescription. Table 6.3 provides a summary of anthelmintics.

## Expected Side Effects and Adverse Reactions

Nausea, vomiting, headache, abdominal pain, and drowsiness are common side effects of anthelmintic drugs. Praziquantel can worsen symptoms of asthma. The number of side effects increases with higher doses and longer length of treatment.

## Drug Interactions

If given together, anthelmintic drugs work against each other (are antagonistic). The drugs also may interfere with a number of specific drugs and a variety of laboratory tests. Consult a drug reference book or a pharmacist for information when other drugs are prescribed during drug therapy for helmintic infestations.

### ❖ Nursing Implications and Patient Teaching

◆ *Assessment.* Obtain a history and physical examination from the patient, including any history of liver disease or drug allergies. Ask about a history of any foods eaten and how they were prepared that may indicate the source of the infection. Obtain the patient's diet history, height, weight, appetite, and energy level. Other family members may also be infected and require assessment and treatment.

◆ *Planning and implementation.* Severe pruritus (itching) may occur during the treatment of a type of hookworm (cutaneous larva migrans), and the patient may need an anti-inflammatory agent for comfort.

To prevent a relapse, patients with a recent history of malaria should be treated with an antimalarial agent before they are given anthelmintics.

Patients may develop allergic reactions to the dead microfilaria and may need treatment for symptoms. Antihistamines or corticosteroids may be necessary to reduce allergic effects.

◆ *Evaluation.* Determine whether the patient is taking the prescribed drug as ordered and performing other actions that are prescribed parts of the therapy. Re-evaluate weight, energy level, and appetite to evaluate therapeutic results. Collect laboratory specimens after treatment and as ordered to make sure the worms are gone.

◆ *Patient and family teaching.* Stress the following important instructions to the patient and family:
- Take this drug as prescribed. Therapy usually involves an initial treatment that should kill all worms, but in some cases a second course of the drug must be taken.
- Report any symptoms that do not disappear after treatment.
- Worms passed in bowel movements are still alive and capable of infecting others. Use good techniques of hand washing and cleanliness to avoid transmission to others.
- Some people have diarrhea and abdominal discomfort while taking anthelmintics.
- You may need iron supplements and an iron-rich diet to counteract anemia during hookworm treatment.

### ECTOPARASITES

Head lice, body lice, and pubic lice are the most common ectoparasites that affect humans. One-percent (1%) permethrin or a mousse that contains pyrethrins and piperonyl butoxide can be used to treat both head lice and pubic lice. These drugs are available over the counter and are readily available for use without adverse effects. Body lice can be treated by washing the body and any contaminated items with hot soap and water.

## Get Ready for the Next-Generation NCLEX® Examination!

### Key Points

- Instruct patients taking drug therapy for TB not to drink alcohol for the entire duration of the treatment because these drugs are all toxic to the liver and alcohol increases the risk for liver damage.
- Antifungal drugs have many adverse effects, the most common of which is anemia.
- Azoles should not be given with grapefruit juice, and grapefruit juice should be limited to less than 24 ounces a day because this food increases the blood level of the drugs, which can lead to adverse reactions.
- Amphotericin B has numerous expected side effects, and patients must be premedicated with antihistamines, antipyretics, corticosteroids, and opiates to maintain comfort and prevent adverse effects.
- Superinfections can result from giving antifungals and corticosteroids together.
- Rash, flu symptoms, and blisters can indicate severe reactions to antifungals and are considered a medical emergency.
- Advise patients to take antiparasitics with or after meals and with a full glass of water to decrease the chance of stomach upset.
- Patients who are taking metronidazole for trichomoniasis or other sexually transmitted disease should refrain from sexual intercourse, as prescribed by the healthcare provider, to prevent transmitting the infection to others.
- Worms passed in bowel movements are still alive and capable of infecting others. Teach patients the importance of good hand washing and cleanliness to avoid transmission.

1. Which method is best for the nurse to instruct a patient with forgetfulness to adhere to first-line drug therapy for tuberculosis?

   1. Having a family member responsible for giving the drugs and watching the patient swallow them
   2. Setting up the patient's drugs using a daily pill dispenser that has alarms to remind the patient it is time to take a drug
   3. Having a family member ask the patient every night whether he or she has remembered to take the drugs
   4. Crushing all the drugs together so the patient only needs to take them once

2. Which precautions are important to teach a woman using a vaginal cream form of an antifungal drug? Select all or any that apply.

   1. Wear gloves to insert the cream.
   2. Wash the applicator with soap and water.
   3. Do not take baths until treatment is completed.
   4. Avoid sexual intercourse during the treatment period.
   5. The cream can make holes in a condom or diaphragm.
   6. Stop the drug immediately if you think you are pregnant.
   7. Stop the drug when symptoms have disappeared to avoid unnecessary exposure to it.

3. A patient who was infected with TB 15 years ago but never developed the disease has now been diagnosed with HIV infection. The patient recently developed a cough and night sweats and tested positive for TB. Which statement by the patient indicates the need for more teaching?

   1. "My HIV medications should be effective in treating the TB infection."
   2. "I need to make sure that I take the drugs exactly as prescribed."
   3. "I need to avoid alcohol and acetaminophen while taking my TB drugs."
   4. "After several weeks of taking my TB drugs, I will no longer be infectious."

4. Which response is the best response from the nurse when a patient beginning drug therapy for TB complains of reddish-orange color of their urine?

   1. "The red dye used in INH can cause this reaction."
   2. "Your hemoglobin may be low. I will call the healthcare provider for orders."
   3. "This is a common reaction to the rifampin and is nothing to worry about."
   4. "I will make an appointment for you to see the healthcare provider immediately."

5. A patient who is taking isoniazid is complaining of numbness and tingling in his hands and feet. What is the best response of the nurse?

   1. "You will need to change your position more frequently."
   2. "This is a common side effect of the drug you are taking."
   3. "I will call the prescriber and ask for a vitamin $B_6$ (pyridoxine) supplement."
   4. "I will call the prescriber and ask for the drug dosage to be decreased."

6. The nurse is developing a teaching plan for a patient recently diagnosed with TB who will complete the 4-month protocol using rifapentine, moxifloxacin, isoniazid, and pyrazinamide. Which of the following statements should be included?

   1. Reinforce the need to avoid alcohol while on drug therapy.
   2. Watch for any signs of liver toxicity, such as yellow coloring of the eyes or skin, dark urine, or easy bruising.
   3. Take acetaminophen for any fever or body aches.
   4. It is best to take the isoniazid with a full stomach.
   5. Make sure to include a multivitamin that contains vitamin $B_6$ (pyridoxine) daily.
   6. Notify your healthcare provider if you have any difficulty adhering to your drug therapy.

7. A patient prescribed fluconazole for a fungal infection calls the outpatient clinic and reports she developed a red, blistery rash after taking her second dose. Which of the following would be the best response?

   1. "I will contact your healthcare provider to get a prescription for hydrocortisone cream."
   2. "This is a side effect of your fluconazole, and it will improve in the next few days."
   3. "Come into the clinic for evaluation today as this may be an adverse effect of the drug."
   4. "Is this from a burn or new laundry detergent?"

8. A patient is prescribed metronidazole for giardiasis. Which instruction is most important for the nurse to reinforce?

   1. Contact the healthcare provider if you are prescribed thyroid medications.
   2. Do not drink alcohol or use products that contain alcohol.
   3. Contact the healthcare provider if you develop worsening nausea, vomiting, or diarrhea.
   4. If you develop constipation, increase fluids.

9. What instruction should the nurse give to a patient with oral thrush who is prescribed nystatin suspension?

   1. Once you have swallowed the drug, follow it with a glass of water.
   2. This drug may decrease your blood sugar, so it should be mixed with orange juice.
   3. Swish the drug around the mouth and hold it there for a few minutes before swallowing.
   4. You can stop using this drug once the white patches in your mouth have subsided.

10. Which breakfast menu should not be given to a patient who is prescribed fluconazole?

   1. Scrambled eggs, bacon, orange juice, and coffee
   2. Oatmeal with milk, grape juice, and tea
   3. Pancakes with maple syrup, coffee, and grapefruit juice
   4. Bagel with butter, poached egg, coffee, and apple juice

## Case Study

Mary Baker is a 32-year-old, moderately obese woman who is taking birth control pills and has a history of diabetes type 2. She has recently completed a 2-week course of cephalosporin for the treatment of pyelonephritis caused by *E. coli*. She is complaining of vaginal itching, painful urination (dysuria), and a thick white vaginal discharge. Choose the **most likely** options for the information missing from the statements below by selecting from the lists of options provided.

Factors that could have caused Mary's vaginitis are ____1____, ____1____, and ____1____. After examination, the healthcare provider has diagnosed a vaginitis. The most likely cause of Mary's vaginitis is ____2____. The nurse expects the healthcare provider to order ____3____ to treat Mary's vaginitis.

| OPTIONS FOR 1 | OPTIONS FOR 2 | OPTIONS FOR 3 |
|---|---|---|
| Antibiotic treatment for pyelonephritis<br>Moderate obesity<br>Birth control pills<br>Diabetes type 2<br>Wiping genital area from back to front when defecating | *E. coli*<br>Candida<br>Trichomoniasis<br>Plasmodium | fluconazole 150 mg<br>griseofulvin 300 mg<br>metronidazole 500 mg<br>iodoquinol 650 mg |

## Drug Calculation Review

1. After verifying that the patient weighs at least 40 kg, the nurse prepares to administer 1200 mg of rifapentine by mouth once daily. Rifapentine is supplied as 150 mg tablets. How many tablets will the patient require at each dose?

2. A patient weighing 85 kg is to receive 7.5 mg/kg kanamycin IM every 12 hours. It is available as 333 mg/mL How many mg will the patient receive with each dose? _____mg. How many mL will be given with each dose? ___mL

## Learning Outcomes

1. Describe the pathophysiology of viruses and retroviruses and how they cause infections.
2. List the names, actions, possible side effects, and adverse effects of common antiviral drugs for herpes simplex and influenza infections.
3. Explain what to teach patients and families about the common antiviral drugs for herpes simplex and influenza infections.
4. List the names, actions, possible side effects, and adverse effects of antiviral drugs for cytomegalovirus, respiratory syncytial virus, and COVID-19 infections.
5. Explain what to teach patients and families about antiviral drugs for cytomegalovirus, respiratory syncytial virus, and COVID-19 infections.
6. List the names, actions, possible side effects, and adverse effects of antiviral drugs for hepatitis B and C.
7. Explain what to teach patients and families about antiviral drugs for hepatitis B and C.
8. List the names, actions, possible side effects, and adverse effects of the common reverse transcriptase inhibitors and protease inhibitors.
9. Explain what to teach patients and families about reverse transcriptase inhibitors and protease inhibitors.
10. List the names, actions, possible side effects, and adverse effects of the common entry inhibitors, fusion inhibitors, integrase inhibitors, and postattachment inhibitors.
11. Explain what to teach patients and families about entry inhibitors, fusion inhibitors, and integrase inhibitors.
12. List the seven categories of antiretroviral therapy drugs.

## Key Terms

**acquired immunodeficiency syndrome (AIDS)** The late stage of HIV disease that causes a breakdown in the immune system, leaving the patient unable to fight infection.

**antiretrovirals** A subset of antiviral drugs that specifically suppress the reproduction of retroviruses.

**antiretroviral therapy (ART)** A combination of antiretroviral drugs that must be taken every day to combat the progression of HIV disease to AIDS or to prevent HIV infection after exposure.

**antivirals** Drugs that interfere with the ability of a virus to carry out its reproductive functions.

**entry inhibitor** Antiretroviral drug that prevents cellular infection with HIV by blocking the CCR5 receptor on CD4⁺ T cells; also known as a *CCR5 antagonist*.

**fusion inhibitor** Antiretroviral drug that prevents cellular infection with HIV by blocking the ability of the HIV surface protein gp41 to bind or fuse with the host cell's CD4 receptor.

**human immunodeficiency virus (HIV)** The specific retrovirus responsible for the immune system problems associated with destruction of helper T cells (CD4⁺ cells); infection results in HIV disease, which progresses to AIDS.

**integrase inhibitor** Antiretroviral drug that inhibits the HIV enzyme integrase, which the virus uses to insert the viral DNA into the human host cell's DNA.

**non-nucleoside reverse transcriptase inhibitor (NNRTI)** Antiretroviral drug that binds directly to the HIV-1 enzyme reverse transcriptase, preventing viral cell DNA replication, RNA replication, and protein synthesis.

**nucleoside reverse transcriptase inhibitor (NRTI)** Antiretroviral drug that has a structure similar to those of the four nucleoside bases of DNA; such drugs are referred to as counterfeit bases. When the counterfeit bases are used by the HIV enzyme reverse transcriptase, viral DNA synthesis and reproduction are suppressed.

**opportunistic infections** Result from viruses, bacteria, protozoa, or fungi that take the opportunity to cause an infection in an immunocompromised host.

**postattachment inhibitor** An antiretroviral drug that prevents the HIV virus from attaching to the CD4, CCR5, and CXCR4 coreceptors.

**protease inhibitor (PI)** An antiretroviral drug that suppresses the formation of infectious virions by inhibiting the retroviral protease enzyme.

**retrovirus** A viral organism that carries special enzymes (reverse transcriptase, integrase, and protease) and uses RNA instead of DNA as its genes to reproduce.

**virions** New viral particles reproduced in cells infected with retroviruses that can leave the cell and infect more human body cells.

**virus** A small infectious agent that can reproduce only inside other living cells, including human cells.

# VIRUS

A **virus** is a small infectious agent that can reproduce only inside other living cells of a host organism, including human cells. Viruses consist of RNA or DNA genetic material that is surrounded by a protein or fatty (or combination) coating, known as a *capsid*. The virus inserts its own genetic information into the host cell's nucleus and hijacks the cell's operations. This causes the host cell to produce and release more virus particles (virions), and the infection spreads. Damage, breakdown, and eventual death of infected cells occur with a viral infection.

Viruses cannot survive or reproduce without the host. Viral infections are not killed or suppressed by antibiotics. Drugs that interfere with the ability of a virus to carry out its reproductive functions are called **antivirals**.

# ANTIVIRALS

Antiviral drugs are used to treat a variety of common conditions caused by viruses, such as herpes zoster, herpes simplex, genital herpes, varicella, some influenza infections, COVID-19, and hepatitis B and C.

Antiviral drugs must enter the infected cell and act at the site of infection to be effective. Antivirals do not kill the virus but rather stop viral reproduction. This action means that all antivirals are virustatic but not virucidal. The antiviral drugs work in a variety of ways: by blocking the virus from entering the host cell, by targeting the enzymes and proteins inside the host cell that allow the viruses to replicate and then leave to infect additional cells, or by helping the host's immune system fight the viral infection.

## ANTIVIRAL DRUGS FOR HERPES SIMPLEX VIRUS INFECTIONS

Herpes simplex virus type 1 (HSV-1) is responsible for common cold sores of the mouth. This infection can become widespread in newborns and in anyone whose immune system is not functioning well. Herpes simplex virus type 2 (HSV-2) is responsible for genital herpes infections and lesions.

As with all other viruses, after a person becomes infected, HSV always remains in some tissues. However, symptoms come and go in patterns called *outbreaks*. An infected person is more likely to spread the virus to other people just before symptoms occur and during outbreaks. Outbreaks are uncomfortable and have other consequences. The goal of HSV antiviral therapy is to prevent outbreaks (or reduce the frequency and intensity of symptoms), which also helps reduce spread of the disease.

## Actions

The common antiviral drugs used to treat HSV infections are acyclovir (Zovirax), famciclovir (Famvir),

and valacyclovir (Valtrex) (Table 7.1). They are viral DNA polymerase inhibitors that form counterfeit molecules in the infected cell that block the virus and its enzymes from making more genetic material and virions. Without the genetic material, the virus cannot reproduce.

## Uses

Drugs in this class are most often used to prevent and control HSV infections. However, they can also help to control the symptoms of varicella zoster virus (VSV) infection, which causes chickenpox and shingles. This is because VZV and HSV have similar enzymes.

## ANTIVIRAL DRUGS FOR INFLUENZA

### Actions

For influenza viruses to infect cells, they must first open their outer coats to be able to fuse with the host's cell membranes. Most viruses that cause common influenza (flu) use a special viral enzyme on their surfaces, known as neuraminidase, to help the process of infection. This enzyme helps the virus burrow its way into cells that line the respiratory tract. The enzyme also helps the new viral particles (**virions**) made in cells infected with retroviruses to leave the cell, spread throughout the respiratory system, and infect more cells.

Three neuraminidase inhibitors used to treat influenza are oseltamivir (Tamiflu), zanamivir (Relenza), and intravenous peramivir (Rapivab). Neuraminidase inhibitors stop the release of the flu virus from infected cells.

Baloxavir (Xofluza), an endonuclease inhibitor, prevents viral replication by inhibiting nucleoproteins from binding to the viral RNA, thus stopping the virus from making copies of itself. Baloxavir is a prodrug with a half-life of 50 to 90 hours, making it an oral single-dose drug for people 12 years and older.

Amantadine (Symmetrel) and rimantadine (Flumadine) are no longer widely used due to increased resistance to influenza, their limitation in treating influenza A viruses, and their side effects.

According to the Centers for Disease Control and Prevention (CDC) 2021–2022 guidelines, the recommended treatment course for uncomplicated influenza is two doses per day of oral oseltamivir or inhaled zanamivir for 5 days, or one dose of intravenous peramivir or oral baloxavir for 1 day.

### Uses

All of the antiviral drugs used for influenza work to prevent infection in a patient who has been exposed to the virus or to reduce the symptoms of an existing influenza infection. They work best when given after exposure and before symptoms start or within 48 hours of the onset of symptoms. Both classes of drugs are effective in treating influenza A and influenza B.

Flu viruses are constantly changing, making some antiviral drugs work less well or not work at all.

| Table **7.1** | Antiviral Drugs for Influenza and Herpes Simplex Virus |

*Neuraminidase inhibitors* prevent influenza spread and reduce symptoms by suppressing the viral enzyme neuraminidase. The influenza virus cannot enter uninfected cells, and the virions in infected cells are not released for further spread.

*Uncoating inhibitors* prevent initial influenza infection and its spread by interfering with viral uncoating, which is needed for fusion of the virus with host cells, which is the first step in infection.

*Viral DNA polymerase inhibitors* reduce viral reproduction by forming counterfeit molecules that block the virus and its enzymes from making new virions in an infected host cell.

| DRUG/ADULT DOSAGE | NURSING IMPLICATIONS |
| --- | --- |
| **Neuraminidase Inhibitors** | |
| oseltamivir (Tamiflu) 75 mg orally twice daily for 5 days<br>zanamivir (Relenza) 2 oral inhalations of a 5-mg blister Diskhaler (total of 10 mg) twice daily for 5 days in a person with an active influenza infection *or* for 10 days in an uninfected adult living in the same household as an infected person.<br>peramivir (Rapivab) adults 600 mg IV as a single dose within 48 hours of symptom onset<br>12mg/kg/dose (IV as a single dose within 48 hours of symptom onset)<br>Used for patients 6 months and older who have been symptomatic for no more than 48 hours who are unable to take oseltamivir | • Before giving zanamivir, ask patients whether they have asthma because this orally inhaled drug can cause bronchospasms.<br>• Before giving zanamivir, ask patients whether they have a true milk allergy because it is a contraindication to zanamivir therapy due to cross-reactivity of the antibodies.<br>• Observe patients for confusion, hallucinations, nightmares, and depression because these drugs cross the blood–brain barrier and can cause CNS side effects.<br>• Gastrointestinal side effects are most common.<br>• Monitor for CNS effect because peramivir may cause psychosis in older individuals.<br>• Monitor BUN and kidney function.<br>• Do not administer the intranasal live attenuated influenza vaccine (LAIV) 2 weeks before or 5 days after administration of peramivir, unless medically indicated |
| **Endonuclease Inhibitor** | |
| baloxavir (Xofluza) 80 mg orally as a single dose administered as soon as possible after contact with an individual who has influenza *or* within 48 hours of symptoms<br>Children and adolescents 12 to 17 years weighing less than 80 kg, 40 mg orally as a single dose administered as soon as possible after contact with an individual who has influenza | • Gastrointestinal side effects are common.<br>• Do not administer with products containing aluminum hydroxide, calcium, chlorpheniramine, pseudoephedrine, selenium, vitamin $B_6$ (pyridoxine), or zinc because they interfere with its absorption.<br>• Do not administer the intranasal LAIV 2 weeks before or 5 days after administration of peramivir, unless medically indicated. |
| **Viral DNA Polymerase Inhibitors** | |
| acyclovir (Zovirax) 5 mg/kg IV for 7 days initially; 400 mg orally twice daily to decrease frequency of outbreaks<br>famciclovir (Famvir) 500 mg orally twice daily for 7 days (HSV-2)<br>penciclovir (Denavir) apply 1% cream every 2 hours while awake for 4 days when lesions appear<br>valacyclovir (Valtrex) 1 g orally twice daily for 10 days at first sign of outbreak; 500 mg orally once daily continually to prevent a person with herpes from spreading it to an uninfected sexual partner | • Before giving any of these drugs, ask the patient about all other drugs he or she takes, and check with a pharmacist because of the numerous possible drug interactions.<br>• Assess urine output and teach patients to stay hydrated because these drugs can damage the kidneys.<br>• Assess patients for fatigue and excessive bruising because these drugs decrease bone marrow production of red blood cells and platelets.<br>• For patients taking acyclovir or famciclovir, assess for yellowing of the skin and sclerae and for elevated liver enzymes because these drugs are hepatotoxic.<br>• Tell families to watch for confusion or behavioral changes because the systemic drugs can affect the CNS.<br>• To reduce anxiety should this symptom appear, warn patients that the skin may become red where the topical cream is applied.<br>• Warn patients that excessive use of the topical cream can cause systemic side effects and adverse effects because of skin absorption of the drug.<br>• Before giving acyclovir, ask patients whether they have a true milk allergy because it is a contraindication to acyclovir therapy due to cross-reactivity of the antibodies. |

*BUN,* blood urea nitrogen; *CNS,* central nervous system; *IV,* intravenous.

The CDC tests influenza viruses routinely for decreased susceptibility to antiviral drugs as it may suggest the potential for antiviral resistance. Oseltamivir, zanamivir, and peramivir are all recommended for use in children. Baloxavir is recommended for children over 12 years of age.

## ANTIVIRAL DRUGS FOR CYTOMEGALOVIRUS AND RESPIRATORY SYNCYTIAL VIRUS

Cytomegalovirus (CMV) is a virus of the herpes family that can infect human cells. In people with fully functioning immune systems, CMV infection causes few problems and may even go unnoticed. However, in those whose immune systems are not functioning well, such as people with AIDS, newborns, transplant recipients, and people who are immunosuppressed due to chemotherapy, CMV infection can cause serious problems, including brain infection (encephalitis), which can lead to brain damage and death, and serious eye infections (retinitis), which can lead to blindness. Treatment approaches are based on CMV status and comorbidities. Prophylaxis is given to prevent the infection, and proactive therapy can be given to people who are asymptomatic but test positive. The drugs of choice for treatment of CMV are ganciclovir and valganciclovir. Primary CMV infection and or reactivation of the disease are associated with increased morbidity and mortality in an immunosuppressed patient. Cidofovir (Vistide) can be used to treat refractory CMV retinitis, and foscarnet (Foscavir) is used to treat ganciclovir-resistant viruses.

Respiratory syncytial virus (RSV) is a common respiratory virus that infects the lungs and the bronchial tubes. It is a common cause of chest colds, croup, and pneumonia in children. For healthy people who have good immune function, the diseases it causes are mild, and most people recover in 5 to 7 days without treatment. However, in premature infants, newborns, small children with chronic illnesses, and older adults with weakened immune systems, the respiratory infection can be severe and lead to death. RSV in the United States ordinarily begins in the fall and continues through spring with peak activity occurring in February. Regional differences may occur. The American Academy of Pediatrics (AAP) supports the prophylactic use of palivizumab in pediatric patients who are at high risk during the RSV season. A new preventive drug for RSV, *nirsevimab*, is FDA approved for prevention of RSV and lower respiratory disease in infants and children. Its use reduces the incidence of lower respiratory tract infections caused by RSV by 74.5% with a single intramuscular (IM) injection given before RSV season.

## Actions and Uses

Ganciclovir is a nucleoside analogue that inhibits DNA synthesis. Valganciclovir is a prodrug of ganciclovir and is used for CMV infections that are not considered severe. Cidofovir (Vistide) and foscarnet (Foscavir) are used to treat resistant CMV infection. They are nucleoside analogues that inhibit the viral enzyme's ability to make more DNA for viral reproduction. As a result, fewer virions are made, and the infection symptoms subside.

The only drug approved for treatment of RSV infection is ribavirin (Virazole). It is very toxic, even when given in aerosol form, and requires careful handling (see Table 7.2). It also has some efficacy for treatment of infection caused by the hepatitis C virus (HCV).

For treating RSV, it is used only short term as an aerosol. For hepatitis C, it is taken orally along with other drugs for years. Palivizumab is given at the start and throughout the RSV season as a prophylactic for children who are immunosuppressed or at severe risk for RSV.

 **Black Box Warning: Ganciclovir and Valganciclovir**
Carcinogenic, Teratogenic, and Mutagenic

## ANTIVIRAL DRUGS FOR HEPATITIS B AND HEPATITIS C VIRUSES

Hepatitis B virus (HBV) and HCV are hardy viruses that can live in a variety of environments. In the United States and Canada, these viruses cause infection most commonly by the bloodborne route and by sexual transmission. Both have a long incubation period (2–26 weeks) after infection, followed by an acute illness and then often a chronic illness.

The acute phase of HBV disease may produce a noticeable illness in about 30% of infected people. The acute phase in others is so mild that there are no obvious symptoms. For HCV, few infected individuals have any symptoms during the acute phase. In HBV and HCV disease, active virus remains in the blood forever. Some people with hepatitis B have a chronic recurrence of symptoms from time to time. With hepatitis C, the disease remains dormant for years (although it can be transmitted) and then causes profound liver damage with cirrhosis.

The major drugs used to treat hepatitis B fall into three classes: nucleoside reverse transcriptase inhibitors (NRTIs), DNA polymerase inhibitors, and interferon. NRTIs are used as part of treatment for HIV infection and AIDS (see Antiretrovirals for the actions and nursing implications of this drug). The NRTI oral drug lamivudine works in the same way against HBV infection (although HBV is not a true retrovirus); a lower dosage is needed than for HIV infection.

The DNA polymerase inhibitors are adefovir (Hepsera), entecavir (Baraclude), lamivudine (Epivir), and telbivudine (Tyzeka). This class of drugs is used to treat chronic hepatitis B infection; they are given orally, once daily, for a long-term course (Table 7.3).

Interferon, specifically peginterferon alfa-2b, is a synthetic injected drug similar to the interferon the human body makes to fight viral infections. Interferon is a subcutaneous injection given three times a week for 1 year. Alfa-2a interferon therapy was discontinued in 2020 due to poor efficacy and a high rate of life threatening adverse effects.

Additional drugs are listed in Table 7.3. The six identified HCV strains are genetically different and do not change over time. After HCV infection is confirmed, testing for the specific genotype determines the medication and length of treatment.

The drug Harvoni, a combination of ledipasvir and sofosbuvir, is used to treat four of the genotypes of chronic hepatitis C infection. It suppresses HCV replication and viral concentration in the blood to such an extent that it is thought to result in a complete remission. However, the extreme cost of this drug for 12 weeks of treatment (about $95,000 in 2020) prohibits many patients from using it, and they instead continue with more standard therapy.

The U.S. Food and Drug Administration (FDA) released Mavyret in 2017. It combines glecaprevir, a protease inhibitor, and pibrentasvir, an inhibitor of the

---

**Table 7.2**    **Antiviral Drugs for Cytomegalovirus and Respiratory Syncytial Virus**

*Anticytomegalovirus drugs/DNA polymerase inhibitors* block the enzyme polymerase, which is needed to make DNA for viral replication. As fewer virions are made, the symptoms of acute infection stop.

The only *anti-RSV drug* is ribavirin, which directly damages genetic material (RNA and DNA), causing mutations that prevent virions from reproducing.

| DRUG/ADULT DOSAGE | NURSING IMPLICATIONS |
|---|---|
| **Anticytomegalovirus Drugs** | |
| ganciclovir 5 mg/kg/dose IV every 12 hours for 10–15 days depending on disease process<br>valganciclovir 900 mg PO every 12 hours for 14–21 days as an initial therapy<br>cidofovir (Vistide) 5 mg/kg intravenously once weekly for 2 weeks<br>foscarnet (Foscavir) 40 mg/kg intravenously every 8–12 hours for 14–21 days | • Do not mix with other drugs because incompatibility will occur.<br>• Monitor complete blood count (CBC) and BUN because anemia and nephrotoxicity can occur.<br>• Ganciclovir is associated with reproductive risk. The drug can be teratogenic if taken by the father near the time of conception.<br>• Monitor for adverse CNS effects: depression, dizziness, confusion, etc.<br>• Contraindicated in acyclovir or famciclovir hypersensitivity.<br>• Monitor for infection as bone marrow suppression may occur.<br>• Tell patient to avoid direct contact of skin or mucous membranes.<br>• Tell patient not to break or crush tablets or come in skin contact with oral solution because these actions can be carcinogenic.<br>• Tell patient to drink fluids and to avoid dehydration.<br>• Be sure the patient receives adequate hydration during therapy because these drugs are very toxic to the kidneys.<br>• Do not mix these drugs with other drugs because they are incompatible with most of them.<br>• These drugs should not be given to women who are pregnant unless the infection is life-threatening, because the risk for birth defects is high.<br>• Ask patients whether they have a seizure disorder because these drugs increase the likelihood for seizures.<br>• Assess patients frequently for signs of infection because bone marrow production of white blood cells is suppressed, increasing the risk of infections.<br>• Give drugs by slow infusion to reduce the risk of immediate adverse reactions.<br>• Frequently assess the patient's red blood cell count because these drugs suppress the bone marrow and can cause severe anemia.<br>• Assess the patient's heart rate, heart rhythm, and respiratory system frequently because these drugs can cause heart and respiratory adverse events.<br>• Use gloves and masks when giving these drugs because both are classified as hazardous drugs, and precautions are needed to avoid exposure of anyone except the patient.<br>• For patients receiving foscarnet, check the serum electrolytes whenever they are drawn because this drug causes many electrolyte imbalances.<br>• Before giving cidofovir, ask about allergies to sulfonamides or probenecid because cross-reactivity can result in a similar cidofovir allergic reaction. |
| **Anti-RSV Drugs** | |
| ribavirin (Virazole) aerosol or nasal inhalant of 190 mcg/L air or oxygen (for children and adults) *or* 600 mg orally twice daily for adults receiving therapy for hepatitis C<br>palivizumab, for RSV infection prophylaxis for pediatric patients at high risk of RSV disease 15 mg/kg/dose IM once monthly starting with commencement of RSV season and throughout the season | *Avoid all contact with this drug because it is very hazardous. Use these precautions when giving the aerosol form:*<br>• Wear gloves, a mask, and a gown during administration.<br>• Close the door to the patient's room to prevent the drug from entering the hallway and endangering others.<br>• If you are pregnant, *do not give* this drug because it can cause severe birth defects or fetal death.<br>• Assess the patient's red blood cell count frequently because these drugs suppress the bone marrow and can cause severe anemia.<br>• Assess patients frequently for signs of infection because bone marrow production of white blood cells is suppressed, increasing the risk of infections.<br>• There are no contraindications or drug interactions.<br>• Have epinephrine readily available as anaphylaxis has been known to occur. |

*BUN,* blood urea nitrogen; *CNS,* central nervous system; *IM,* intramuscular; *IV,* intravenous; *PO,* by mouth; *RSV,* respiratory syncytial virus.

bacterial protein NS5A, which is essential for replication. It covers all six genotypes and results in a 92% to 100% cure rate for hepatitis C. The cost is approximately $26,000 for an 8-week treatment. Epclusa (sofosbuvir/velpatasvir) is the first oral antiviral agent approved to treat all six major forms of hepatitis C virus. The cost is approximately $26,000 for a 12-week treatment. Sofosbuvir/velpatasvir is now generic, and most major insurers cover the cost of the generic drug.

## EXPECTED SIDE EFFECTS, ADVERSE REACTIONS, AND DRUG INTERACTIONS WITH ANTIVIRALS

Expected side effects of antivirals include vomiting, nausea, diarrhea, and headache. Adverse reactions are reported for some antivirals, and you should read current information before giving these drugs. Tables 7.1 through 7.3 provide specific adverse reactions and nursing implications for antiviral drugs.

All drugs can cause hypersensitivity and/or anaphylactic shock. Be aware of rashes, hives, difficulty breathing, and facial swelling. If hypersensitivity reactions occur, the drug should be discontinued and the prescriber alerted. If an anaphylactic event occurs, as indicated by difficulty breathing, swelling of the mouth and tongue, and unstable vital signs, emergency measures must be taken immediately.

Many antivirals also have drug interactions. As antivirals become more widely used, these interactions may be seen more often. To be prudent, always look up current information. Some antivirals can be applied topically; this avoids the systemic interactions they would have if they were taken orally or by injection.

## NURSING IMPLICATIONS AND PATIENT TEACHING FOR ANTIVIRALS

Table 7.1 describes the antivirals used to treat herpes infections and influenza infection or provide influenza prophylaxis. Notice that the antivirals have a common suffix of -vir or -dine.

Table 7.2 lists some very toxic intravenous antivirals used for the more serious problems of CMV retinitis and RSV infection. You may not be giving these drugs, but you may be responsible for caring for patients

### Table 7.3   Drugs for Hepatitis B and Hepatitis C

*DNA polymerase inhibitors* block the synthesis of the enzyme polymerase, which is needed to make DNA for viral replication. Fewer virions are made, and blood levels of the virus decline.

*Protease inhibitors* competitively block the viral enzyme protease, preventing viral replication and the release of viral particles.

*Combination agents*, which are reported to cure hepatitis C, include ledipasvir/sofosbuvir (viral protein inhibitor plus viral DNA polymerase inhibitor) and glecaprevir/pibrentasvir (protease inhibitor plus NS5A [bacterial protein] inhibitor).

| DRUG/ADULT DOSAGE | NURSING IMPLICATIONS |
|---|---|
| **DNA Polymerase Inhibitors** | |
| adefovir (Hepsera) 10 mg orally once daily<br>entecavir (Baraclude) 1 mg orally once daily<br>telbivudine (Tyzeka) 600 mg orally once daily | • Assess patients for yellowing of the skin and sclerae and for elevated liver enzymes because these drugs are toxic to the liver.<br>• Assess patients for nausea, vomiting, and severe epigastric pain because these drugs increase the risk of pancreatitis.<br>• Ask patients taking adefovir about bone pain because this drug can cause bone thinning and increased risk for fractures.<br>• Give entecavir on an empty stomach because stomach contents interfere with its absorption. |
| **Protease Inhibitors** | |
| simeprevir (Olysio) 150 mg orally daily along with other antiviral drugs | • Assess patients for yellowing of the skin and sclerae and for elevated liver enzymes because this drug is toxic to the liver.<br>• Teach patients to protect themselves from the sun with clothing, hats, and sunscreen because this drug increases sun sensitivity and can result in severe sunburn.<br>• Teach patients to take this drug with food to prevent gastrointestinal side effects. |
| **Combination Agents** | |
| ledipasvir 90 mg/sofosbuvir 400 mg (Harvoni); one tablet orally daily for 8–12 weeks<br>glecaprevir 100 mg/pibrentasvir 40 mg (Mavyret); three tablets orally daily for 8 weeks<br>sofosbuvir/velpatasvir (Epclusa); 400 mg sofosbuvir, 100 mg velpatasvir orally once daily for 12 weeks | • Assess patients for yellowing of the skin and sclerae and for elevated liver enzymes because these drugs are toxic to the liver.<br>• Ask the patient and family about any changes in mood or increase in depression because a higher incidence of suicide ideation has been seen with the use of ledipasvir/sofosbuvir.<br>• Glecaprevir/pibrentasvir and sofosbuvir/velpatasvir can interfere with international normalized ratio (INR) levels when used with warfarin, and INR levels must be monitored consistently. Hepatitis B exacerbation can also occur with the use of this drug. |

receiving them. All of these drugs carry serious warnings for patients and black box warnings for healthcare providers, and caution should be taken.

## COVID-19

COVID-19 is an infectious disease caused by a new coronavirus called Sars-CoV-2 or novel coronavirus. The World Health Organization (WHO) identified the virus in January 2020, and the virus has spread worldwide. The majority of people infected with COVID-19 will have mild to moderate respiratory illness and other flulike symptoms that last for 1 to 2 weeks. Older adults and others with chronic medical problems such as cancer, chronic obstructive pulmonary disease (COPD), diabetes, and cardiovascular disease are most likely to develop serious illness. According to the CDC, as of May 31, 2022, over 1 million deaths in the United States have been attributed to COVID-19. Mutant variants of the virus emerge and disappear while others persist. According to the CDC, as of May 2022, COVID-19 remains responsible for over 300 deaths a day in the United States despite 82.9% of the US population having had at least one vaccination.

Experts predict that infections will rise in fall and winter months and become endemic rather than pandemic—*endemic* meaning the virus will mostly be found among particular persons within certain areas. Endemic levels of the virus may be high or low depending on the effort taken with testing, vaccination, and quarantining.

The COVID-19 virus spreads primarily through droplets of saliva or discharge from the nose when an infected person coughs or sneezes. The droplets can land in the mouth or nose and be inhaled by people who are nearby. COVID-19 is most likely to be spread if people are closer than 6 feet apart. Because COVID-19 is easily spread, it is highly advisable to wear a well-fitting mask and stay away from crowded settings to

prevent infection if a person is immunocompromised or unvaccinated. Frequent handwashing, the use of alcohol-based hand sanitizer, and avoiding touching the face or eyes also prevent spread of the virus. For people who are at low or medium risk, it is personal preference whether or not to wear a mask. See Chapter 15 for COVID-19 vaccination information.

Clinical management of the virus incorporates infection prevention and control measures, supplemental oxygen, and mechanical ventilation when indicated. Therapeutic management of adults and children for COVID-19 is based on disease severity and is quite comprehensive. The National Institutes of Health (NIH) profiles a range of clinical manifestations and treatment protocols for five presentations of COVID-19: asymptomatic or presymptomatic, mild, moderate, severe, and critical. This information can be found at https://www.covid19treatmentguidelines.nih.gov/overview/clinical-spectrum. COVID-19 is constantly changing, so keeping up with the manifestations of disease, treatments, and protocols is constant, so it is important to survey the CDC or NIH Web site frequently for changes.

Some drug options are now available for treating nonhospitalized adults with mild to moderate COVID-19 who are at high risk of disease progression. Nirmatrelvir/ritonavir (Paxlovid) is a protease inhibitor that is active against a protease that is responsible for viral replication. It has antiviral activity for all human coronaviruses. Paxlovid is FDA approved for emergency use. It is authorized for use as a treatment for mild to moderate COVID-19 in patients 12 years and older with positive SARS-CoV-2 viral testing who are at high risk for progressing to severe COVID-19. The FDA has authorized state-licensed pharmacists to prescribe Paxlovid to patients who test positive for COVID-19. At this time it is the only highly effective oral antiviral for the treatment of COVID-19. See Table 7.4 for COVID-19 treatments.

| Table **7.4**  Drugs for COVID-19 | |
|---|---|
| Nirmatrelvir/ritonavir (Paxlovid) 300 mg nirmatrelvir (two 150 mg tablets) and 100 mg ritonavir (one 100 mg tablet) with all three tablets taken together by mouth twice daily for 5 days | • Monitor patient for yellow skin and yellow sclerae as liver dysfunction can occur.<br>• Do not administer to patients who have liver impairment or severe renal disease.<br>• Monitor for skin rash, dyspnea, hives, or other signs of an allergic or hypersensitive reaction.<br>• Consider drug interactions as this is a new drug under investigational use.<br>• Contraindicated for use in patients on CYP3A inducers such as the glucocorticoids, rifampin, carbamazepine, phenobarbital, phenytoin, and St. John's wort.<br>• Mild diarrhea and altered taste can occur (dysgeusia).<br>• **Reports of rebound COVID-19 symptoms have been reported.** |
| Remdesivir is used for hospitalized patients with severe disease. 200 mg intravenous (IV) once on day 1, followed by 100 mg IV once daily for 2 days | • Monitor patients during and for at least 1 hour after drug administration for hypotension, hypertension, sinus tachycardia, bradycardia, hypoxia, fever, dyspnea, wheezing, angioedema, rash, nauseous feeling, diaphoresis, and shivering.<br>• Contraindicated in severe renal disease.<br>• Monitor hepatic enzymes in all patients. |

**Patient and Family Teaching**

Tell the patient and family the following:

- When using topical drugs for treatment of herpes simplex virus (HSV)-1 (cold sores) or HSV-2 (genital herpes), use gloves and wash your hands thoroughly to prevent spread of the infection.
- There is no cure for herpes. Antivirals can treat herpes only prophylactically or symptomatically.
- To be effective, oral drugs should be started at the first sign of infection or re-infection.
- The drugs must be used daily for suppression of the herpesvirus.
- When using antivirals for flu, it is best to begin within 2 days of becoming ill; however, starting them later may still help prevent serious flu symptoms.
- Antivirals do not cure the flu, and there is still a need to reduce symptoms such as fever, cough, and pain.
- Check yourself daily for worsening symptoms that may indicate pneumonia or bacterial infection. If they are present, notify your healthcare provider immediately so that antibiotics can be started instead of antivirals.
- Antivirals can be used for prevention or prophylaxis of the flu in unvaccinated persons who have been exposed to the disease. Prevention works best if the drugs are taken before flu symptoms occur or within the first 24 to 48 hours after they appear.
- Follow the specific storage instructions listed on the package for the drug.

 **Top Tip for Safety**

COVID-19 is always changing. These changes occur constantly, and mutations occur creating new variants. Some come and go, and others persist. To learn more about variants and how to protect yourself and the public, see https://www.cdc.gov/coronavirus/2019-ncov/variants/about-variants.html.

 **Bookmark This**

https://www.covid19treatmentguidelines.nih.gov/overview/clinical-spectrum

## RETROVIRUSES

A retrovirus differs from a virus in that instead of merely hijacking a cell's DNA or RNA to reproduce, it transmits its own information into the cell's DNA. In a normal human cell, cellular DNA is unzipped by the enzyme *transcriptase*. The resulting DNA template is converted to an RNA sequence (transcription), which then conveys the instructions to the ribosome (translation), where proteins are synthesized. In this way, proteins, which are the building blocks of all tissues, are formed from the DNA information of genes.

A retrovirus is a viral organism that carries special enzymes (reverse transcriptase, integrase, and protease) and uses RNA instead of DNA as its genes to reproduce. The retrovirus inserts its genetic material into the host cell's DNA. The retrovirus uses the host cell's metabolic systems to make new virions (viral particles) that leave the cell and infect more cells.

The human immunodeficiency virus (HIV) is the specific retrovirus responsible for the immune system problems associated with destruction of helper T cells (CD4$^+$ cells); infection results in HIV disease, which progresses to acquired immunodeficiency syndrome (AIDS). After a person becomes infected with HIV, he or she will have the virus for life. HIV attacks the body's CD4$^+$ T cells (helper T cells) that are responsible for helping the immune system fight infections.

If HIV infection is left untreated, the decreased number of CD4$^+$ cells in the body (CD4 count) makes the person highly susceptible to infections such as tuberculosis, viruses such as CMV, and cancers such as non-Hodgkin lymphoma. These opportunistic infections signal the development of AIDS, which is the late stage of HIV disease. It is characterized by a breakdown in the immune system that leaves the patient unable to fight infections. The patient is diagnosed with AIDS when the CD4 count falls below 200 cells/mm$^3$. The normal CD4 count is between 500 and 1500 cells/mm$^3$.

In the United States, the groups at highest risk for development of AIDS include homosexual and bisexual men, although the fastest-growing group is minority heterosexual women. Compared with other racial and ethnic groups, HIV most often affects black and Hispanic individuals. Transgender women who have sex with men are among the groups at highest risk for HIV infection. Intravenous drug users remain at significant risk, and other high-risk groups are children born to HIV-positive women and individuals whose sexual partners have HIV/AIDS.

In 2019, according to the CDC, 1.2 million people age 13 and older who live in the United States are infected with HIV. There were 34,000 new HIV infections reported, the highest percentage being in the southern states. The percentage of people with HIV virally suppressed is estimated at 57%, and approximately 13% of people who live in the United States are infected with HIV but do not know it.

The HIV life cycle has seven stages, and HIV drugs are designed to attack the virus at different stages. The stages in the HIV life cycle and in which each category of HIV drugs works are described in the following section and in Fig. 7.1.

## ANTIRETROVIRALS

Antiretrovirals are an important group of drugs that slow the growth or prevent the duplication of retroviruses. They are used to limit or slow the advance of HIV disease and its progression to AIDS. Antiretroviral drugs are used in treating patients infected with HIV or adults and children at risk for HIV and AIDS. They do not cure HIV or AIDS, but they do help patients live healthier, longer lives by interfering with the ability of the retrovirus to replicate (reproduce) and slowing

# The HIV Life Cycle

**HIV medicines in seven drug classes stop (🛑) HIV at different stages in the HIV life cycle.**

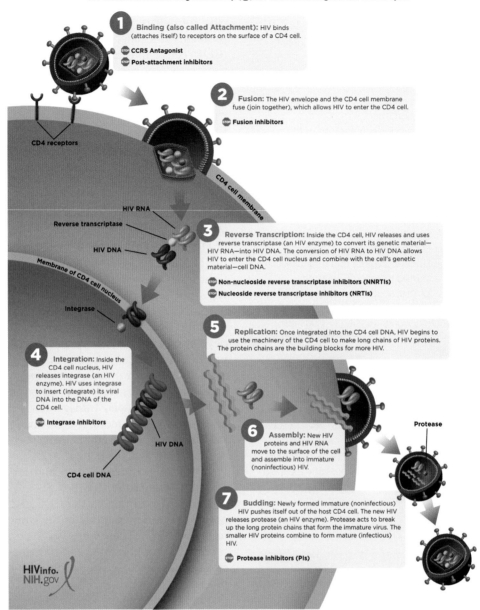

Fig. 7.1 The HIV replication cycle. (Courtesy National Institutes of Health, Bethesda, MD.)

the production of new retroviruses. All antiretroviral drugs are virustatic rather than virucidal. *None of these drugs kills the virus.*

Therapy for HIV infection and AIDS works best when several types of antiretroviral drugs are used together daily. This type of therapy is known as combination **antiretroviral therapy (ART)**. The seven categories of antiretroviral therapy drugs are NRTIs, non-nucleoside reverse transcriptase inhibitors (NNRTIs), protease inhibitors, integrase inhibitors, fusion inhibitors, entry inhibitors (CCR5 antagonists), and postattachment inhibitors. They are all called *inhibitors* because, rather than killing the virus, they suppress retroviral reproduction by preventing HIV from infecting host cells or by obstructing various steps in the HIV life

cycle. None of these drugs is effective against HIV when used alone.

Table 7.5 lists the common drugs in each category and their nursing implications. Fig. 7.1 shows where in the HIV infection process different categories of antiretroviral drugs inhibit retroviral reproduction. These drugs are used only for the management of HIV disease.

A big treatment advance occurred in 2021 when the FDA approved Cabenuva (cabotegravir/rilpivirine), the first long-acting HIV treatment, which requires a monthly injection at a healthcare provider's office. It is currently not being covered most by insurance companies, and the cost is about $4,500 per month. Also in 2021 the FDA approved Rukobia (fostemsavir), which

| Table 7.5 | Examples of Antiretroviral Drug Therapy for HIV Infection |
|---|---|

*Nucleoside reverse transcriptase inhibitors* (NRTIs) have structures similar to those of the four nucleoside bases of DNA and are referred to as counterfeit bases. When counterfeit bases are used by the HIV enzyme reverse transcriptase, viral DNA synthesis and replication are suppressed. All NRTIs are oral drugs.

*Non-nucleoside reverse transcriptase inhibitors* (NNRTIs) bind the HIV-1 enzyme reverse transcriptase, preventing viral cell DNA replication, RNA replication, and protein synthesis. This suppresses replication of the HIV-1 virus but not HIV-2. All NNRTIs are oral drugs.

*Protease inhibitors* (PIs) competitively block the HIV protease enzyme, preventing synthesis of functional proteins, viral replication, and release of viral particles. All PIs are oral drugs.

*Entry inhibitors/CCR5 antagonists* prevent HIV infection by blocking virus from binding to CCR5 receptors on CD4+ T cells, thereby prohibiting entry into host cells. These are all oral drugs.

*Fusion inhibitors* prevent infection of new cells by not allowing the HIV surface protein gp41 to bind to the host cell's CD4 receptor. Without fusion, HIV cannot enter and infect new cells.

*Integrase inhibitors* block the HIV enzyme integrase, which allows insertion of viral DNA into the host cell's DNA. Without a functional enzyme, viral proteins are not made, and viral replication is inhibited.

*Postattachment inhibitors* bind to the CD4 receptor on a host CD4 cell, blocking HIV from attaching to the CCR5 and CXCR4 coreceptors and entering the cell.

| DRUG/ADULT DOSAGES | NURSING IMPLICATIONS |
|---|---|
| **Nucleoside Reverse Transcriptase Inhibitors** | |
| abacavir (Ziagen) 300 mg orally twice daily *or* 600 mg orally once daily<br>didanosine (Videx EC) 125–200 mg orally twice daily<br>emtricitabine (Emtriva) 200 mg orally once daily<br>lamivudine (Epivir) 300 mg orally once daily<br>stavudine (Zerit) 40 mg orally twice daily<br>tenofovir (Viread) 300 mg orally once daily<br>zidovudine (Retrovir) 300 mg orally twice daily | • Remind patients to avoid fatty and fried foods because NRTI's can cause digestive upsets and may lead to pancreatitis.<br>• Teach patients to use precautions to prevent injury because these drugs induce peripheral neuropathy.<br>• Teach patients taking abacavir to report flulike symptoms to the provider immediately because they may indicate a hypersensitivity reaction that requires discontinuing the drug.<br>• Instruct patients to avoid or severely limit alcoholic beverages to reduce the risk of liver damage while taking these drugs.<br>• Do not give abacavir to patients who test positive for the HLA-B*57:01 tissue type because fatal allergic responses are likely.<br>• Tell patients that the solution form and capsule form of emtricitabine (Emtriva) are not interchangeable on a milligram-per-milligram basis.<br>• Tenofovir can cause renal insufficiency or Fanconi syndrome. |
| **Non-Nucleoside Reverse Transcriptase Inhibitors** | |
| efavirenz (Sustiva) 600 mg orally once daily at bedtime<br>etravirine (Intelence) 200 mg orally twice daily<br>rilpivirine (Edurant) 25 mg once daily with a meal | • Check laboratory values for increases in liver enzymes and decreased red blood cell counts because the most common side effects of these drugs are anemia and liver toxicity.<br>• Teach patients to take these drugs at least 1 hour before or 2 hours after taking an antacid to avoid inhibiting gastrointestinal (GI) absorption.<br>• Instruct patients to notify the prescriber if a sore throat, fever, various types of rashes, blisters, or multiple bruises develop because these are indications of a serious adverse drug effect. |
| **Protease Inhibitors** | |
| atazanavir (Reyataz) 300 mg orally daily<br>darunavir (Prezista) 800 mg orally twice daily<br>fosamprenavir (Lexiva) 700 mg orally twice daily<br>indinavir (Crixivan) 800 mg orally every 8 hours<br>lopinavir/ritonavir (Kaletra) 400 mg/100 mg orally twice daily<br>nelfinavir (Viracept) 1250 mg orally twice daily with a meal<br>saquinavir (Fortovase, Invirase) 500 mg orally twice daily<br>tipranavir (Aptivus) 500 mg orally twice daily | • Instruct patients not to chew or crush these drugs because this action may cause the drug to be absorbed too rapidly and thereby increase the risk of side effects.<br>• Teach patients to report jaundice, nausea, vomiting, or severe abdominal pain because these drugs can cause liver toxicity.<br>• Instruct patients to keep all appointments for laboratory work because these drugs increase blood lipid levels and increase the risk of atherosclerosis and pancreatitis.<br>• Remind patients to avoid St. John's wort while taking these drugs because the supplement reduces the effectiveness of all PIs.<br>• Teach patients taking atazanavir or ritonavir to check their pulse daily and report low heart rate to the prescriber because these two drugs can impair electrical conduction and lead to heart block.<br>• Do not give darunavir or fosamprenavir to patients who have a known sulfa allergy because these two drugs contain sulfa. |

*Continued*

**Table 7.5** Examples of Antiretroviral Drug Therapy for HIV Infection—cont'd

| DRUG/ADULT DOSAGES | NURSING IMPLICATIONS |
|---|---|
| **Entry Inhibitors/CCR5 Antagonists** | |
| maraviroc (Selzentry) 150–600 mg orally twice daily | • Instruct patients not to chew or crush this drug because this action may cause the drug to be absorbed too rapidly and thereby increase the risk of side effects.<br>• Teach patients to change positions slowly because hypotension is a common side effect, especially orthostatic hypotension.<br>• Teach patients to report jaundice, nausea, vomiting, or severe abdominal pain because these drugs can induce liver toxicity.<br>• Instruct patients to report pain or numbness in the hands or feet because this drug can induce peripheral neuropathy. |
| **Fusion Inhibitors** | |
| enfuvirtide (Fuzeon) 90 mg subcutaneously twice daily | • Teach patients how to prepare and inject the drug subcutaneously to ensure correct dosage and effectiveness.<br>• Assess injection sites for warmth, swelling, redness, skin hardening, or bump formation because these are indications of injection-site reactions.<br>• Instruct patients to report pain or numbness in the hands or feet because this drug can induce peripheral neuropathy.<br>• Teach patients to report jaundice, nausea, vomiting, or severe abdominal pain because this drug can induce liver toxicity.<br>• Teach patients to observe for and report cough, shortness of breath, fever, and purulent mucus because this drug increases the risk for severe respiratory infections, including pneumonia. |
| **Integrase Inhibitors** | |
| dolutegravir (Tivicay) 50 mg orally once or twice daily<br>elvitegravir (Vitekta) 85–150 mg orally once daily<br>raltegravir (Isentress) 400 mg orally twice daily | • Because knowing the expected side effects decreases anxiety when they appear, warn patients that diarrhea, nausea, rash, insomnia, and abdominal pain are common side effects of these drugs.<br>• Suggest that patients take the drug with food to reduce the GI side effects.<br>• Instruct patients not to chew or crush these drugs because this action may cause the drug to be absorbed too rapidly and increase the risk for side effects.<br>• Instruct patients to report new-onset muscle pain or weakness because these drugs can cause muscle breakdown (rhabdomyolysis), especially in adults taking a statin type of lipid-lowering drug.<br>• Teach patients with diabetes to closely monitor blood glucose levels because these drugs increase the likelihood of hyperglycemia.<br>• Do not give raltegravir to pregnant women because this drug is associated with an increased risk of birth defects. |
| **Combination Products** | |
| emtricitabine, tenofovir, and efavirenz (Atripla)<br>bictegravir sodium/emtricitabine/ tenofovir alafenamide (Biktarvy)<br>cabotegravir and rilpivirine (Cabenuva)<br>lamivudine and zidovudine (Combivir)<br>emtricitabine, rilpivirine, and tenofovir (Complera)<br>lamivudine and abacavir (Epzicom)<br>elvitegravir, cobicistat,[a] emtricitabine, and tenofovir (Genvoya)<br>elvitegravir, cobicistat,[a] emtricitabine, and tenofovir (Stribild)<br>dolutegravir, abacavir, and lamivudine (Triumeq)<br>emtricitabine and tenofovir (Truvada) | • Each ingredient has the same mechanism of action and nursing implications as the parent drug class. |
| **Postattachment Inhibitor** | |
| fostemsavir (Rukobia) 600 mg PO twice daily with or without food | • Check laboratory values for increases in liver enzymes and decreased red blood cell counts because the most common side effects of these drugs are anemia and liver toxicity.<br>• Warn patients that diarrhea, nausea, rash, insomnia, and abdominal pain are common side effects, with nausea being the most common.<br>• Check laboratory values for lipid panels as this drug can cause hypercholesterolemia. |

[a]Cobicistat is a metabolizing enzyme inhibitor that allows other drugs in the combination to remain active longer, thereby boosting their antiretroviral action.

is a postattachment inhibitor indicated for patients with heavily treatment-resistant HIV.

Although ART is usually started and managed by healthcare providers in special settings and clinics for immune disorders, this drug therapy must continue for the rest of the patient's life. Therapy is effective only if the patient takes the prescribed drugs correctly and on time at least 90% of the time. An HIV-positive person who is taking ART may be a patient or resident in any healthcare setting. Regardless of the setting, he or she must continue the prescribed therapy.

> ### Memory Jogger
>
> There are seven categories of antiretroviral therapy drugs:
> - Non-nucleoside reverse transcriptase inhibitors (NNRTIs)
> - Nucleoside reverse transcriptase inhibitors (NRTIs)
> - Protease inhibitors (PIs)
> - Fusion inhibitors
> - CCR5 antagonists
> - Integrase strand transfer inhibitors (INSTIs)
> - Postattachment inhibitors

> ### Lifespan Considerations
>
> **Pregnant Patients and Pediatric Patients**
>
> With the exception of delavirdine and efavirenz, the NRTI, NNRTI, and PI classes of antiretroviral drugs are commonly given throughout pregnancy for HIV-infected women and for children who are HIV positive. Taking this combination of drugs during pregnancy greatly reduces the risk of transmitting HIV to the unborn child. The other classes of antiretroviral drugs are not approved for use in children or pregnant women.

## ACTIONS OF DRUGS USED FOR ANTIRETROVIRAL THERAPY

### Nucleoside Reverse Transcriptase Inhibitors

**Nucleoside reverse transcriptase inhibitors (NRTIs)** are antiretroviral drugs that have a structure similar to those of the four nucleoside bases of DNA; these drugs are referred to as *counterfeit bases*. When the counterfeit bases are used by the HIV enzyme reverse transcriptase (see Fig. 7.1), viral DNA synthesis and reproduction are suppressed. Without reverse transcriptase, HIV cannot make new copies of itself. These drugs work early in the HIV life cycle.

### Non-nucleoside Reverse Transcriptase Inhibitors

A **non-nucleoside reverse transcriptase inhibitor (NNRTI)** is an antiretroviral drug that binds directly to the HIV-1 enzyme reverse transcriptase, preventing viral cell DNA replication, RNA replication, and protein synthesis. With these actions interrupted, HIV reproduction is slowed or stopped. These drugs work fairly early in the HIV life cycle (see Fig. 7.1).

> ### Memory Jogger
>
> Remember the class of NNRTIs by the letters *-vir-* in the middle of the generic drug names.

### Protease Inhibitors

A **protease inhibitor (PI)** is an antiretroviral drug that suppresses the formation of infectious virions by inhibiting the retroviral protease enzyme. They act later in the life cycle of the virus (see Fig. 7.1). In one of the final stages of the HIV life cycle, a single large protein is produced. It is then separated by protease (which acts like chemical scissors) into the smaller activated proteins needed for the production of infectious virions. PIs block the HIV enzyme protease and prevent these important proteins from being activated. As a result, infectious HIV virions are not produced and released.

> ### Memory Jogger
>
> Remember the PI class of drugs by the suffix *-navir* at the end of the generic drug names.

### Entry Inhibitors

An **entry inhibitor**, also known as a CCR5 antagonist, is an antiretroviral drug that prevents cellular infection with HIV by blocking the CCR5 receptor on CD4$^+$ T cells. The virus's gp120 protein must bind to the CD4 receptor and its gp41 to the CCR5 or CXCR4 receptor to achieve entry into the host cell. Entry inhibitors protect uninfected cells from HIV infection (see Fig. 7.1).

### Fusion Inhibitors

A **fusion inhibitor** is an antiretroviral drug that prevents cellular infection with HIV by blocking the ability of the HIV surface protein gp41 to bind or fuse with the host cell's CD4 receptor. Without fusion, infection of new cells does not occur. Like the entry inhibitors, fusion inhibitors protect uninfected host cells from becoming infected with HIV (see Fig. 7.1).

### Integrase Inhibitors

An **integrase inhibitor** is an antiretroviral drug that inhibits the HIV enzyme integrase, which the virus uses to insert the viral DNA into the host cell's DNA. Without this action, viral proteins are not made and viral replication is inhibited. Integrase inhibitors work early in the life cycle of HIV infection (see Fig. 7.1).

### Postattachment Inhibitors

**Postattachment inhibitors** are antiretroviral drugs that block the first step (binding step) in the viral process. They prevent HIV from attaching and getting into its target cell to replicate by blocking HIV from attaching to the CCR5 and CXCR4 coreceptors and entering the cell. They are part of the group called *entry inhibitors*.

## EXPECTED SIDE EFFECTS, ADVERSE REACTIONS, AND PRE-EXPOSURE PROPHYLAXIS WITH ANTIRETROVIRALS

Most antiretroviral drugs are taken in combination, and determining which drug is causing side effects can be difficult. Some of the side effects caused by HIV disease are also caused by the drugs used to treat it. Common expected side effects of all antiretroviral drugs include mouth ulcers, nausea, and diarrhea. Rashes and headaches are also common. Many patients report vivid dreams or nightmares while taking these drugs. Table 7.4 lists many of the common side effects of the drugs.

Antiretrovirals often cause severe toxic reactions. Most of these drugs can damage the liver (hepatotoxicity) or kidneys (nephrotoxicity). Many also cause inflammation of the pancreas, known as pancreatitis. Other possible adverse effects include lactic acidosis, peripheral neuropathy (loss of nerve function, especially in the hands and feet), and diseases that affect the blood.

Pre-exposure prophylaxis (PrEP) can prevent HIV transmission to the uninfected sex partners of people who are HIV positive and are using ART. The drug approved for this purpose is tenofovir disoproxil fumarate 300 mg/emtricitabine 200 mg (Truvada), which is an oral tablet taken once daily for as long as the person remains at risk for infection. It is taken only by people who are HIV negative but who are at high risk for becoming infected. The person taking Truvada must have his or her HIV status checked every 3 months. The person must take the drug as prescribed for at least 4 days before Truvada can begin to effectively protect against HIV infection. Descovy, a drug similar to Truvada, contains emtricitabine 200 mg/tenofovir alafenamide 25 mg. Descovy was released in late 2019 and contains a different form of tenofovir that is thought to be less toxic to the kidneys. The parameters of use remain the same for both drugs. PrEP drugs are highly effective and reduce the risk of getting HIV from sexual contact by about 99%, and they reduce the risk from injection drug use by 74%.

### Lifespan Considerations

**Older Adults**

- Immunocompromised older adult patients may have other chronic diseases and may be taking 8 or 10 drugs at a time. These patients often need encouragement to continue taking all of their drugs.
- Monitoring for the adverse effects of some drugs used to treat patients with HIV is more difficult for older adult patients. It is sometimes difficult to know which drugs are causing the adverse reactions because older adults have other health problems and take other drugs.

### Safety Alert!

**SIGNS AND SYMPTOMS OF PANCREATITIS**
Upper abdominal pain and/or pain that radiates to the back, pain that worsens after eating, fever, rapid pulse, increased nausea, and vomiting may indicate pancreatitis, which is a medical emergency.

### Safety Alert!

**SIGNS AND SYMPTOMS OF LACTIC ACIDOSIS**
Weakness, fatigue, unexplained muscle pain, nausea, vomiting, dizziness, cold arms and legs, irregular heart rate, and difficulty breathing are signs and symptoms of lactic acidosis.

## ❖ NURSING IMPLICATIONS AND PATIENT TEACHING FOR ANTIRETROVIRALS

### ◆ Patient and Family Teaching

The patient taking ART has probably been doing so for some time and may know more about these drugs than you do. However, it is important to remind the patient and his or her family about adhering to the following:

- Take the drugs exactly as ordered every day to ensure that the drugs work properly and your disease does not become resistant to them.
- Do not take too little of the drugs or skip doses because that leads to drug resistance and disease progression. It is imperative not to skip doses or decrease the dosage.
- Use pillboxes, pill reminders, and/or diaries to maintain strict compliance.
- Take the drugs at the same time every day, and use a cell phone reminder for time alerts. In this way, drug levels remain steady and viral suppression is ideal.
- Alert your healthcare provider immediately about specific symptoms that may indicate adverse reactions.
- Do not cut down or stop the drugs until told to do so by your healthcare provider.
- Safer sexual practice and standard precautions must be taken to prevent disease transmission.
- Impaired immunity makes it easier to contract diseases. Avoid eating raw meats or fish and avoid fruits or vegetables that cannot be peeled or scrubbed.
- If you are lactating, stop breast-feeding your baby because there is a high risk of HIV transmission in breast milk.
- Report to your prescriber any new over-the-counter drugs, herbs, vitamins, illegal drugs, and nutritional supplements because they could cause increased adverse reactions.
- Do not miss clinic or laboratory appointments. CD4 counts guide treatment. These drugs are highly toxic to the liver, and liver enzymes must be measured

frequently. Complete blood counts are used to monitor infections and adverse effects. Amylase and lipase levels are measured to monitor pancreatitis. Lactic acid levels are measured to monitor lactic acidosis because symptoms of lactic acidosis are nonspecific.

- Avoid alcohol and recreational drugs because of the increased risk of liver damage associated with these drugs.

- Report signs of neuropathy: numbness; tingling in the feet or hands that spreads to legs or arms; sharp, jabbing, throbbing, or burning pain in arms and legs; and decreased coordination and falling.
- If you have symptoms of pancreatitis (upper abdominal pain that may radiate to your back, pain that worsens after eating, increased nausea and vomiting), notify your healthcare provider immediately so that treatment can begin early.

## Get Ready for the Next-Generation NCLEX® Examination!

### Key Points

- Viruses are organisms that cannot self-reproduce, and they hijack a cell and use it to reproduce.
- Retroviruses do not just hijack a cell; they actually become a part of the cell and therefore are highly efficient at spreading their infection.
- All antiviral drugs are virustatic; they suppress viral reproduction but do not kill the virus.
- Nirmatrelvir/ritonavir (Paxlovid) is now available under investigational use for the treatment of COVID-19.
- Antiretroviral drugs are most effective when combinations of drugs from several categories are given daily. This type of therapy is known as combination antiretroviral therapy (ART).
- Teach patients to take antiviral drugs exactly as prescribed and not to stop unless ordered to do so by the prescriber.
- To be most effective in preventing HIV infection and slowing HIV reproduction, ART drugs must be taken correctly and on time at least 90% of the time.
- Except for the fusion inhibitor enfuvirtide (Fuzeon), antiretroviral drugs are given orally.
- Antivirals used for CMV retinitis and RSV infection (ganciclovir, valganciclovir, ribavirin, and cidofovir) carry a black box warning and are never to be used, or even *touched*, by anyone who is pregnant or breast-feeding.
- Antivirals have many interactions with other drugs. Always check for interactions using a drug handbook before giving these drugs.
- Antiretroviral drugs are highly toxic to the liver, kidney, and pancreas. Teach patients to be alert for signs and symptoms of toxicity.
- Some antiretroviral drugs must be taken together on an empty stomach or with food. Teach patients the importance of taking the drugs exactly as they were prescribed.

### Clinical Judgment and Next-Generation NCLEX® Examination-Style Questions

#### Case Study on RSV

Nick S is a healthy 2-year-old child who came to the emergency room with a cough, a runny nose, and difficulty breathing for 2 days. His mother has been treating him with saline nose drops and Vicks VapoRub. Vital signs: Temperature 102°F (38.8°C), Pulse 130/min, Respirations 34/min, Blood Pressure 110/63 mm Hg, SpO$_2$ 91% on room air. The child is awake but lethargic.

1. **Which action should be taken first?**

   1. Inquire how the child is eating.
   2. Inquire about any drug allergies.
   3. Administer oxygen per emergency department protocol.
   4. Administer acetaminophen per emergency department protocol.

The mother, who is pregnant, states that the child has not been eating or playing for the last day. She said that Nick was born premature and required oxygen in the nursery for several days before he was sent home. Chest sounds: bilateral wheezing and nasal flaring are present. He has tenting of his skin and has only wet his diaper once since he was admitted 6 hours ago.

2. **Which healthcare provider order should be initiated first?**

   1. Albuterol nebulizer
   2. Viral laboratory panel
   3. Chest x-ray
   4. Insertion of a peripheral intravenous line

The viral panel came back positive for respiratory syncytial virus (RSV), and Nick was admitted to the pediatric ward. Temperature 101°F (38.3°C), Pulse 128/min, Respirations 32/min, Blood Pressure 110/63 mm Hg, SpO$_2$ 93% on 2 liters of oxygen nasal cannula. Ribavirin inhalant of 190mcg/L via aerosol was ordered for 18 hours a day inside an oxygen tent for 4 days.

3. **Which of the following measures should the nurse take to ensure patient and staff safety? Select all or any that apply.**

   1. Assess the complete blood count daily.
   2. Keep the patient door open to observe Nick.
   3. Place an airborne precautions sign at Nick's room.
   4. Allow the mother to stay in the room at all times.
   5. Assign only male nurses to care for Nick.
   6. Monitor for yellow sclerae and skin.

4. **The licensed practical nurse (LPN) is team nursing with an infusion registered nurse (RN) who is preparing to administer intravenous ganciclovir to a female liver transplant patient who has cytomegalovirus. What data collected by the LPN will be reported to the RN prior to administration? Select all or any that apply.**

   1. Blood urea nitrogen of 18 mg/dL
   2. Liver enzyme results: alanine transaminase 70 U/L, aspartate aminotransferase 60U/L
   3. White blood cell (WBC) count of 7 WBCs per microliter (7 × 109/L)
   4. Red blood cell count of 4.4 million cells/mcL
   5. Patient on total parenteral nutrition
   6. Allergy to acyclovir (Zovirax)
   7. Patient's future reproductive plan
   8. Patient on birth control pills

5. A 6-year-old child is being seen in the clinic for a cough, sore throat, stuffy nose, and body aches. He has a fever of 103°F (39.4°C). Which drugs will the nurse anticipate the healthcare provider might order? **Select all or any that apply.**

   1. baloxavir (Xofluza)
   2. oseltamivir (Tamiflu)
   3. zanamivir (Relenza) disk inhaler
   4. rimantadine (Flumadine)
   5. amantadine (Symmetrel)
   6. peramivir (Rapivab)

6. **Instructions:** Drugs are listed in the left-hand column. In the right-hand column, in the space provided, write the letter for the drug that best fits the nursing implication associated with it. Each drug can be used only once.

| DRUG | NURSING IMPLICATION |
|---|---|
| A. nirmatrelvir/ritonavir (Paxlovid) <br> B. peramivir (Rapivab) <br> C. acyclovir (Zovirax) <br> D. fostemsavir (Rukobia) <br> E. sofosbuvir/velpatasvir <br> F. abacavir (Ziagen) <br> G. emtricitabine/tenofovir (Epclusa) <br> H. famciclovir (Famvir) <br> I. zanamivir (Relenza) <br> J. ribavirin (Virazole) | 1. _____Do not administer intranasal live flu vaccine 2 weeks before or 5 days after administration. <br> 2. _____Contraindicated in a true milk allergy. <br> 3. _____Contraindicated for use with CYP3A inducers like rifampin. <br> 4. _____Eating fatty foods can lead to pancreatitis. <br> 5. _____Interferes with INR levels if on warfarin. <br> 6. _____Causes hypercholesterolemia, need baseline lipid panel. <br> 7. _____Can cause bronchospasms in patients with asthma. <br> 8. _____Must wear gloves, mask, and gown during administration. |

7. Order: palivizumab 15mg/kg IM for a 10-month-old patient weighing 20 lbs. Available: 100mg/mL sterile solution for injection.

   A. How many mL will be administered?
   B. How will the medication be administered?
      1. 1.4 ml intramuscular using the vastus lateralis
      2. 0.7 ml intramuscular using both the right and left vastus lateralis muscle
      3. 0.7 ml intramuscular using both the right and left dorsogluteal muscle
      4. 1.4 ml intramuscular in the ventrogluteal muscle

8. **Instructions:** For the following, underline or highlight the risk factors and symptoms that indicate the patient may have COVID-19.

   John H is an overweight 67-year-old Hispanic male who presents to the clinic with a fever of 101°F (38.3°C) and an oxygen saturation of 90% on room air. He has a cough productive of yellowish-green sputum. He is visibly short of breath and states he has body aches and fatigue. His medical history is positive for diabetes type 2 and rheumatoid arthritis.

9. Which healthcare provider prescription would the nurse anticipate for an at-risk patient who is currently HIV negative?

   1. lamivudine and zidovudine
   2. lamivudine and abacavir
   3. enfuvirtide
   4. emtricitabine/tenofovir alafenamide

10. Which drug prescribed by the healthcare provider for a patient who is positive for hepatitis C would the nurse question prior to administering?

    1. adefovir
    2. entecavir
    3. sofosbuvir/velpatasvir
    4. peginterferon alfa-2b
    5. glecaprevir/pibrentasvir
    6. ledipasvir/sofosbuvir

11. **Instructions:** Complete the following sentences below by choosing the most probable option for the missing information that corresponds with the same numbered list of options provided.

    **Scenario:** The COVID-19 virus spreads primarily through ____1____. An oral investigational drug that patients may be prescribed to lessen the symptoms of COVID-19 is ____2____. This medication is contraindicated for use in patients who are currently on ____3____. The nurse must not administer this medication to patients with ____4____.

| OPTIONS FOR 1 | OPTIONS FOR 2 |
|---|---|
| Skin-to-skin contact | remdesivir |
| Contaminated surfaces | nirmatrelvir/ritonavir |
| Droplet transmission | emtricitabine, tenofovir, and efavirenz |
| Sexual transmission | tipranavir |

| OPTIONS FOR 3 | OPTIONS FOR 4 |
|---|---|
| phenytoin | Rheumatoid arthritis |
| voriconazole | Asthma |
| ritonavir | Stage 4 renal disease |
| indinavir | Elevated liver enzymes |

## Next-Generation NCLEX® (NGN) Examination–Style Question

### History and Physical
### 2 Months Ago, 1000

CC: "I'm having night sweats."

HPI: A 39-year-old female client reports night sweats and a recent unintentional weight loss of approximately 8 pounds over the last 2 months.

Past Medical History: none

Social History: client reports drinking three glasses wine/day, uses intravenous heroin "for fun," and uses a nicotine vape pen. Client reports "a few" sexual partners and "sometimes" uses condoms.

Physical Exam:

General: no acute distress, flushed

Respiratory: breath sounds clear bilaterally

Cardiovascular: S1, S2 no murmur

Extremities: diffuse lymphadenopathy

Skin: dry skin

### Nurse's Notes
### 2 Months Ago, 1000

Medication and lifestyle education provided.

### Today, 0800

The client returns for scheduled follow-up visit. The client reports burning, itching, and a thick, cottage cheese–like vaginal discharge for a week. The nurse discusses the client's medication compliance and lifestyle changes since their last visit.

### Laboratory Results
### 2 Months Ago, 1030

| TEST/PANEL | RESULT | NORMAL |
|---|---|---|
| Rapid HIV | Positive | negative |
| CD4+ | 180 cells/mm$^3$ | 800–2500 cells/mm$^3$ |
| WBC | 3,000/mm$^3$ | 5000–10,000/mm$^3$ or 5–10 × 109/L |

### Today, 0830

| TEST/PANEL | RESULT | NORMAL |
|---|---|---|
| Vaginal culture | *Candida albicans* | negative |

### Flow Sheet
### 2 Months Ago, 1000

Blood Pressure: 120/88 mm Hg
Respiratory Rate: 18/min
Heart Rate: 78/min
Temperature: 99.4°F (37.2°C)

### Today, 0800

Blood Pressure: 154/92 mm Hg
Respiratory Rate: 20/min
Heart Rate: 76/min
Temperature: 98.6°F (37°C)

### Orders
### 2 Months Ago

emtricitabine 200 mg orally once daily
tenofovir 300 mg orally once daily
efavirenz 600 mg orally once daily at bedtime
fluconazole 150 mg orally for one dose

A nurse is caring for the client in an outpatient provider's office. The nurse is reviewing the education provided during previous visits.

**Which of the following statements indicate that further teaching is needed today?**

### Select all or any that apply.

- "I will need a hemoglobin checked today because anemia is a potential side effect of my medication."
- "I have noticed some bruising on my legs, but this is an expected side effect of my medication."
- "I have been eating high-fat meals to promote medication absorption."
- "I have been monitoring for numbness and tingling in my feet."
- "I have limited my alcohol intake to reduce the risk of liver damage."
- "I will have my renal function monitored."
- "Today's symptoms and laboratory results are a common medication side effect."
- "The change in my blood pressure is due to my medications."

See answer on Evolve at http://evolve.elsevier.com/Visovsky/LPNpharmacology/.

## Learning Outcomes

1. Describe the causes and symptoms of allergy, asthma, and chronic obstructive pulmonary disease.
2. List the names, actions, possible side effects, and adverse effects of antihistamines, leukotriene inhibitors, and decongestant drugs.
3. Explain what to teach patients and families about antihistamines, leukotriene inhibitors, and decongestant drugs.
4. List the names, actions, possible side effects, and adverse effects of beta-adrenergic agonists and anticholinergic antagonists for asthma and chronic obstructive pulmonary disease.
5. Explain what to teach patients and families about beta-adrenergic agonists and anticholinergic antagonists for asthma and chronic obstructive pulmonary disease.
6. Explain what to teach patients for correct use of drugs delivered by aerosol inhalers and dry-powder inhalers.
7. Explain how asthma controller (prevention) drugs are different from asthma reliever (rescue) drugs.
8. List the names, actions, possible side effects, and adverse effects of mucolytic and antitussive drugs.
9. Explain what to teach patients and families about mucolytic and antitussive drugs.

## Key Terms

**allergy** An excessive reaction that leads to an inflammatory response when a person comes into contact with a substance (allergen) to which he or she is sensitive. It is a common immune response to substances such as pollen, animal dander, food, or dust. Also known as *hypersensitivity*.

**antihistamine** Drug that stops histamines from attaching to histamine receptors on cells and producing inflammatory and allergic symptoms. This action counteracts the response of histamine in causing smooth muscle contraction and dilation and leakage of capillaries.

**antitussive** Drug that works to relieve or suppress coughing.

**asthma controller drugs** Drugs that have the main purpose of preventing an asthma attack. These drugs must be taken daily even when no asthma symptoms are present. Also known as *asthma prevention drugs.*

**asthma reliever drugs** Drugs that have the main purpose of stopping an asthma attack after it has started. Also known as *asthma rescue drugs.*

**bronchodilator** Drug that relaxes the airway smooth muscles, allowing the lumens of the airways to widen.

**cholinergic antagonist** Drug that blocks the action of acetylcholine, thereby inhibiting the parasympathetic nervous system response. Also known as a *cholinergic blocker, parasympatholytic,* or *anticholinergic drug*. Also called *long-acting muscarinic antagonists*.

**corticosteroid** Drug built on the structure of cholesterol that is able to prevent or limit inflammation and allergy by slowing or stopping production of the mediators histamine and leukotriene.

**decongestant** Drug that reduces the swelling of nasal passages by shrinking the small blood vessels in the nose, throat, and sinuses so that breathing is easier.

**leukotriene receptor antagonist (LTRA)** Drug that blocks the leukotriene response and lessens or prevents the symptoms of allergy and asthma.

**long-acting beta$_2$-adrenergic agonist (LABA)** Orally inhaled drug that binds over time to beta$_2$-adrenergic receptors and is used as an asthma controller drug; it must be taken on a daily schedule to prevent bronchospasms and asthma attacks even when symptoms are not present.

**long-acting muscarinic antagonist (LAMA)** Orally inhaled drug that relaxes muscles around the airways to open wider by blocking acetylcholine. Also called *cholinergic antagonists*.

**mast cell stabilizer (cromone)** Drug that works on the surface of mast cells and prevents them from opening to release the inflammatory mediators.

**mucolytic** Drug that decreases the thickness of respiratory secretions and aids in their removal. Also called an *expectorant*.

**short-acting beta$_2$-adrenergic agonist (SABA)** Orally inhaled drug that binds rapidly to beta$_2$-adrenergic receptors and can start smooth muscle relaxation within seconds to minutes. Also known as an *asthma reliever* or *asthma rescue drug*.

**sympathomimetic** Drug that mimics the sympathetic nervous system and has the same actions as the body's own adrenaline. Also known as a *beta-* and/or *alpha-adrenergic agonist*.

## ALLERGY

When a person comes into contact with a substance or allergen to which he or she is sensitive, an excessive reaction that leads to an inflammatory response can occur. This is known as an **allergy**. It is estimated that one of every five people in the United States suffer from allergies. Allergens are usually harmless substances and include things people are surrounded with every day such as dust mites, plant pollen, pet dander, food, and insect bites. These substances cause allergic reactions only in people who are overly sensitive to them. Allergies, also known as *hypersensitivities*, occur when the immune system overacts and develops a response to substances in the environment. When the immune system overreacts to an allergen, symptoms appear where the allergen entered or touched the body, usually in the nose, lungs, or throat or on the skin.

The purpose of the immune system is to protect the body from living substances that cause infections, such as bacteria, viruses, and fungi. The immune system also protects the body from nonliving substances it views as dangerous, such as drugs, toxins, and chemicals. These "invaders" are known as *antigens* because they are not part of the body and can trigger the immune system to take protective actions. These protective actions occur when the immune system produces an antibody directed against the offending antigen. The antibodies are produced in the bloodstream by specific immune system cells known as *lymphocytes*. The action of an antibody is to neutralize the offending antigen or cause it to be destroyed and eliminated from the body. The lymphocytes make five different antibodies or immunoglobulins (Igs) for protection: IgA, IgD, IgE, IgG, and IgM. The IgE class of antibody is the body's defense against allergens.

After antibodies are released in response to the allergen, they trigger other immune system cells and mast cells to produce internal chemicals, known as *mediators*, to start and continue inflammation. The important mediators released by white blood cells (WBCs) when antibodies react with allergens are *histamine* and *leukotriene*. Histamine starts the inflammation, and leukotriene works with histamine to keep the inflammatory response going after it has started. These mediators initiate actions in tissues and blood vessels that result in inflammation and its symptoms. These mediators, especially histamine, cause contraction of smooth muscle and dilation and leakage of capillaries, which explains the symptoms of swelling, redness, tissue irritation, and mucus production.

Think about the person who has an allergy to pollens and develops hay fever. The symptoms include red, itchy eyes that produce tears to flush out the invader. The nasal passages swell, the nose is stuffed up to prevent entrance of more antigens, and the sinuses drain to get rid of the offender. Sneezing expels the invader from the airway passages. Contraction of the smooth muscle of the bronchioles (bronchoconstriction) caused by histamine and by leukotriene release prevents entry of air into the lungs and causes breathing difficulties. Unfortunately, as the body attempts to protect itself from the invaders, oxygen is also prevented from entering the body.

Air must be able to move from the upper respiratory system (oral and nasal cavities, sinuses, pharynx, larynx, and trachea) to the lower respiratory system (bronchi and lungs) for gas exchange to take place. The alveoli in the base of the lungs exchange life-giving oxygen entering on inspiration for the waste product of carbon dioxide leaving on expiration. Anything that interrupts this passage of air from the airway to the alveoli can cause death (Fig. 8.1). Disruptions that create problems include bronchospasm (a narrow or constricted opening), pulmonary edema (blockage caused by mucus, infection, or edema in the bases of the lungs), and collapse of the bronchioles and the alveoli themselves.

## DRUG THERAPY FOR ALLERGY

Drugs used to treat allergies are those that interfere with inflammation: antihistamines, leukotriene blockers, and corticosteroids. Leukotriene blockers are also used to treat asthma because allergies often trigger asthma attacks. Decongestants are other drugs that can help lessen the symptoms of allergy but do not interfere with inflammation. Drugs used for allergies may be taken orally, used as a nasal spray, or inhaled into the lungs when inflammation triggers asthma. They can also be applied topically to the skin when allergic reactions are present in the skin. Table 8.1 lists the common drugs for allergy together with the nursing implications.

 Bookmark This!

Research is always expanding treatment and drug options. For more patient and healthcare professional education regarding allergens and asthma, visit the American Academy of Allergy, Asthma & Immunology Web site at https://www.aaaai.org.

### ANTIHISTAMINES

#### Actions

An **antihistamine** is a drug that stops histamines from attaching to histamine receptors on cells and producing inflammatory and allergic symptoms. Allergens activate mast cells, which are the chief controllers of the immune system. They are manufactured in the bone marrow and are present in all tissues of the body. When the mast cells are activated, they release histamine. There are two types of histamine: $H_1$ and $H_2$. Antihistamines do not prevent histamine from being released; they block the receptors on the tissues. Blocking $H_1$ receptors limits blood vessel vasodilation,

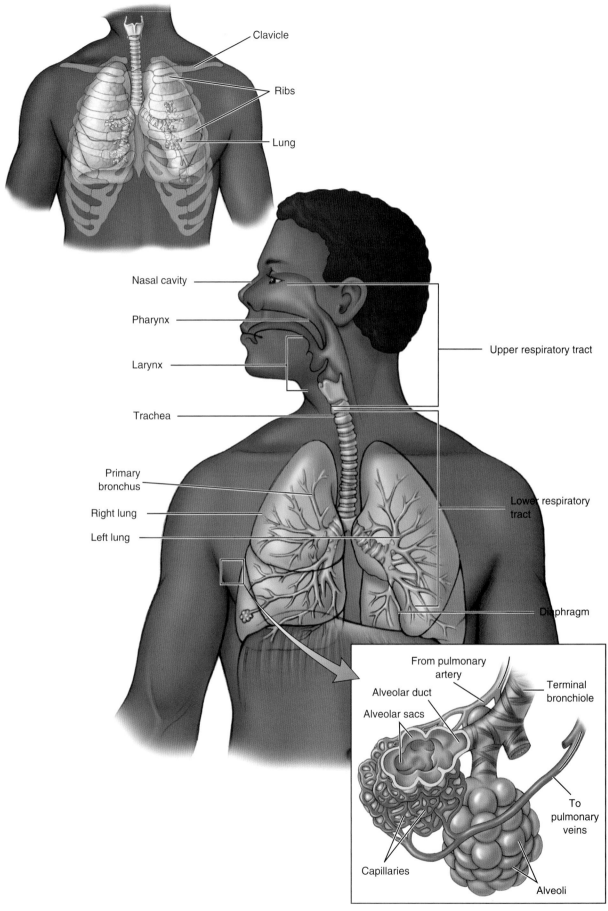

Fig. 8.1 The respiratory system. (From Herlihy, B. (2018). *The human body in health and illness* (6th ed.). Elsevier.)

| Table **8.1** | **Examples of Common Antihistamines, Leukotriene Inhibitors, and Mast Cell Stabilizers** |
|---|---|

*First-generation antihistamines* prevent histamine from attaching to the tissue receptor sites, decreasing allergic symptoms. These drugs can cause CNS depression.

*Second-generation antihistamines* prevent histamine from attaching to the tissue receptor sites, decreasing allergic symptoms. The incidence of CNS depression is much less with these antihistamines.

*Leukotriene receptor antagonists (LTRA):* Zileuton blocks production of leukotriene in WBCs, and montelukast and zafirlukast block the leukotriene receptors on tissues. Both actions stop allergy symptoms and prevent bronchoconstriction in asthma.

*Mast cell stabilizers (cromones)* prevent mast cell membranes from opening and releasing histamine and leukotriene.

| DRUG/ADULT DOSAGE | NURSING IMPLICATIONS |
|---|---|
| **First-Generation Antihistamines** | |
| diphenhydramine (Benadryl) 25–50 mg orally three to four times a day *or* 10–50 mg slow IM or slow IV over 10 minutes every 4–6 hours as needed<br><br>diphenhydramine cream (topical agent) 0.5%, 1%, or 2%; apply to affected area three to four times daily<br><br>brompheniramine (Dimetapp) 12–24 mg orally once daily (oral) *or* 10 mg IV slowly, IM, or subcutaneously every 6–12 hours as needed | • Warn patients not to drive or operate hazardous equipment because these drugs usually cause drowsiness.<br>• Warn patients about taking this medication with other anticholinergics (tricyclic antidepressants) as it will show additive symptoms.<br>• Check the urine output of patients who have an enlarged prostate gland because a side effect of these drugs is urinary retention.<br>• Avoid giving these drugs to patients with glaucoma because the action can increase intraocular pressure.<br>• Warn patients that many over-the-counter sleep aids contain first-generation antihistamines and taking them with an antihistamine could lead to overdose.<br>• Watch for hyperexcitability and restlessness in children or older adults because they are more likely to have a paradoxical reaction to these drugs.<br>• Tell patients who are breast-feeding to avoid brompheniramine because it enters breast milk and will produce side effects in the infant.<br>• Warn patients not to take these drugs with sedatives, opioids, anticholinergic drugs, or drugs that cause CNS depression because the CNS side effects will be more severe.<br>• Warn patients to take these drugs for 2 weeks or less to avoid tolerance and long-term side effects. |
| **Second-Generation Antihistamines** | |
| fexofenadine (Allegra) 60 mg orally twice daily *or* 180 mg orally once daily<br><br>loratadine (Claritin) 10 mg orally once daily<br><br>levocetirizine (Xyzal) 2.5–5 mg orally once daily in the evening<br><br>cetirizine (Zyrtec) 5–10 mg orally once daily in the evening | • Instruct patients taking the quick-dissolve tablets to place them under the tongue and not to eat or drink until they have dissolved to promote best absorption.<br>• Ask whether the patient has any kidney problems before giving fexofenadine or levocetirizine because poor kidney function allows the drug to remain in the system longer, which can lead to overdoses.<br>• Check the urine output of patients who have an enlarged prostate gland because a side effect of these drugs is urinary retention.<br>• Use cautiously with other drugs that cause sedation or CNS depression because, although these drugs have fewer CNS side effects, they may worsen the CNS depression of other drugs.<br>• Give levocetirizine and cetirizine in the evening because it has more sedating effects than other second-generation antihistamines.<br>• Tell patients to avoid grapefruit if taking fexofenadine as it will decrease the effectiveness of the drug. |
| **Leukotriene Inhibitors (Modifiers)** | |
| montelukast (Singulair) 10 mg orally once a day at the same time<br><br>zafirlukast (Accolate) 20 mg orally twice a day<br><br>zileuton (Zyflo) 1200 mg orally twice daily, within 1 hour after morning and evening meals | • Teach patients to report any yellowing of the skin or eyes, darkening of the urine, or white/gray stools because these drugs can impair the liver.<br>• Warn patients and families to observe for changes in behavior or mood because all of these drugs can cause these problems in some patients.<br>• These drugs are not to be used during an acute asthma attack because they require a long time to get to peak action. They are prevention, rather than reliever, drugs.<br>• Teach patients to take zafirlukast 1 hour before or 2 hours after a meal because the drug is best absorbed on an empty stomach. |

*Continued*

**Table 8.1**    Examples of Common Antihistamines, Leukotriene Inhibitors, and Mast Cell Stabilizers—cont'd

| DRUG/ADULT DOSAGE | NURSING IMPLICATIONS |
|---|---|
| **Mast Cell Stabilizers (Cromones)** | |
| cromolyn sodium (NasalCrom) 1 spray (5.2 mg/spray) in each nostril three to four times per day; may be increased to six times a day if needed *or* 20 mg oral inhalation by nebulizer every 6 hours nedocromil sodium (Tilade) 2 inhalations (1.75 mg each) four times a day | • Remind patients that there may be mild stinging or burning of the nasal lining with use, but this is an expected side effect, not an allergy.<br>• Teach patients to rinse the mouth and gargle after using the nebulizer to minimize dry mouth or throat, throat irritation, and hoarseness.<br>• Remind patients that these drugs must be used as prescribed daily to reduce symptoms because they are not rapid acting. |

*CNS*, central nervous system; *IM*, intramuscular; *IV*, intravenous; *WBCs*, white blood cells.

capillary leak, swelling, and bronchoconstriction. Blocking $H_2$ receptors decreases stomach acid production (discussed in Chapter 14). Antihistamines also limit the release of acetylcholine, which produces a drying effect (anticholinergic), particularly in the bronchioles and the GI system. Table 8.1 lists common antihistamines, their actions, and nursing implications.

## Uses

Antihistamine $H_1$-receptor blockers (antagonists) are used to treat almost any type of allergic reaction, including allergic rhinitis (nasal stuffiness and drainage). They are also used to treat asthma that is triggered by an allergic reaction. Histamine plays a central role in producing most of the typical eye and nasal signs and symptoms such as sneezing, nasal stuffiness, and postnasal drip.

Antihistamines are classed as first-generation drugs or second-generation drugs. First-generation drugs are available over the counter (OTC). Most of these products cross the blood–brain barrier and cause sedation (sleepiness) along with the antiallergy and anticholinergic effects. These drugs are effective in helping reduce symptoms of sneezing, itching, and rhinorrhea (runny nose) when used for a short time. According to the Beers Criteria, first-generation sedating antihistamines are considered potentially inappropriate medications in elderly patients. Use in the elderly should be avoided as they are highly anticholinergic, there is reduced clearance in advanced age, tolerance develops when used as hypnotics, and there is a greater risk of anticholinergic effects (e.g., confusion, dry mouth, constipation) and toxicity compared to use in younger adults.

Second-generation antihistamines are newer and usually have a more rapid onset of relief of sneezing, pruritus (itching), and rhinorrhea. These drugs do not cross the blood–brain barrier and therefore do not cause significant sedation. Some are available by prescription, and some are OTC. In general, they are less effective against nasal congestion than the first-generation antihistamines.

## Expected Side Effects

Drowsiness is an expected side effect for most antihistamines. In fact, many OTC sleep aids contain the antihistamine diphenhydramine. Patients should also expect dry mouth, increased heart rate, increased blood pressure, dilated pupils, and urinary retention to occur because of the anticholinergic effect of the antihistamines.

## Adverse Effects

Most adverse effects are related to severe anticholinergic symptoms, such as cardiac dysrhythmias or dangerously high blood pressure. A rising intraocular pressure (pressure inside the eye) in patients with glaucoma can worsen the disease and could cause blindness. Symptoms of overdosage include nervousness, anxiety, fear, agitation, restlessness, weakness, irritability, talkativeness, and insomnia. These symptoms may progress to dizziness, lightheadedness, tremor, and hyperreflexia, with progression to confusion, delirium, hallucinations, and euphoria. Antihistamines, especially first-generation drugs, should be used with great caution in children because responses can be unpredictable.

Problems with memory have been reported with continuous use of these agents, especially in older patients. Children and some older adults may have the opposite reaction (a *paradoxical* reaction) with hyperexcitability, agitation, or confusion.

 **Lifespan Considerations**

**Older Adults**

Older adults often have pronounced anticholinergic effects such as constipation, dry mouth, and urinary retention (especially men).

## Drug Interactions

The sedative effect often seen with antihistamines is increased when other CNS depressants (e.g., hypnotics, sedatives, tranquilizers, depressant analgesics, alcohol) are used along with the antihistamine. The sedative effect of antihistamines also adds to the effect of anticholinergic drugs, and they can strengthen the anticholinergic side effects of monoamine oxidase inhibitors (MAOIs) and tricyclic antidepressants.

When antihistamines are used along with *ototoxic drugs* (drugs that can damage hearing), such as large doses of aspirin or other salicylates or streptomycin, the antihistamine may relieve some of the symptoms of ototoxicity, such as dizziness; as a result, these important symptoms may be masked. They may also interfere with the effects of anticholinesterase drugs.

### ❖ Nursing Implications and Patient Teaching

◆ *Assessment.* Ask the patient about the presence of drug allergy, other drug use, and the presence of asthma, glaucoma, peptic ulcer disease, prostatic hypertrophy, bladder neck obstruction, respiratory or cardiac disease, and the possibility of pregnancy. A patient with thyroid disease or migraine headaches may be unable to take antihistamines because of the *tachycardia* (rapid heartbeat) produced. These conditions are contraindications or precautions for the use of antihistamines.

◆ *Planning and implementation.* Antihistamines for allergy should be taken only when needed. The type and dose should be chosen for the desired effect and the person being treated. For example, first-generation drugs make people very sleepy, and people who do tasks that require alertness probably should not use them. Sleepiness is also a concern in older patients who are prone to falls.

Giving oral doses with food or drink can limit GI side effects; however, some antihistamines must be taken on an empty stomach. Check a drug reference guide to determine whether the drug can be given with food or certain liquids or if it needs to be taken on an empty stomach.

When an intramuscular (IM) preparation such as diphenhydramine is used, inject it deep into the muscle to prevent tissue irritation. Intravenous (IV) injection of these agents is done slowly, with the patient lying down because of the risk of low blood pressure that can be caused by these drugs. Long-term use of topical nasal antihistamines increases the risk for sensitization, often causing a *rebound* effect (increase in the symptoms you are trying to stop).

◆ *Evaluation.* Assess the patient to determine whether allergy symptoms are reduced. Watch for any side effects.

Assess older adults for side effects such as dizziness, *syncope* (lightheadedness and fainting), and confusion. Problems with *dyskinesia* (difficulty in movements of the body), *bradykinesia* (slow movement), stiffness, and tremor are reactions that may also develop and must be reported to the prescriber.

◆ *Patient and family teaching.* Tell the patient and family:
- Unless you must restrict your fluid intake because of another health problem, drink extra fluids to help prevent the respiratory tract dryness that often occurs with antihistamine use.

- If any skin reactions occur, stop taking the drug at once and notify your healthcare provider. Do not increase the dose or drink alcohol while taking antihistamines because the CNS depressant effects of antihistamines may be increased.
- Avoid tasks such as driving or activities that require alertness until you know how antihistamines affect you, because they cause drowsiness in many patients.
- If the drug causes stomach upset, take it with meals or milk to decrease this problem.
- You may develop tolerance to an antihistamine. If one drug seems to stop working over time, your healthcare provider may suggest trying another antihistamine for better control of symptoms.

While taking an antihistamine, do *not* take any other drugs without the knowledge of your healthcare provider, especially sedative drugs.

## LEUKOTRIENE RECEPTOR ANTAGONISTS
### Action
A **leukotriene receptor antagonist (LTRA)**, also called a *leukotriene inhibitor*, is a drug that blocks the leukotriene response and lessens or prevents the symptoms of allergy and asthma. Different leukotriene inhibitors have different actions to reduce inflammation. Zileuton (Zyflo) blocks production of leukotriene within WBCs. Montelukast (Singulair) and zafirlukast (Accolate) block the leukotriene receptors on tissues. As a result of either action, the inflammatory response is reduced. Table 8.1 lists common leukotriene inhibitors, their actions, and nursing implications.

### Uses
Some leukotriene inhibitors are used for allergic rhinitis. Use of these inhibitors can relax respiratory smooth muscle and increase airflow through the bronchial tubes because leukotriene can also trigger bronchospasms. These drugs also are used for prevention and long-term treatment of asthma.

### Expected Side Effects, Adverse Reactions, and Drug Interactions
Leukotriene inhibitors are generally safe and well tolerated. Headache, nausea, and diarrhea are the most common side effects.

Although adverse reactions to the leukotriene inhibitors are rare, liver dysfunction is possible with long-term use. The leukotriene inhibitors interact with drugs that stimulate liver metabolism, such as phenytoin, phenobarbital, carbamazepine, and rifampin. Montelukast has the least number of drug interactions.

### ❖ Nursing Implications and Patient Teaching
◆ *Assessment.* Ask patients about the other drugs they take. Ask about the possibility of pregnancy, breastfeeding, or liver disease.

◆ *Planning and implementation.* Leukotriene inhibitors are not started if the patient is having an acute asthma attack. They are given as part of an asthma treatment regimen but will not relieve an acute attack of asthma. Watch for any adverse interactions with other drugs the patient is taking. Some of these drugs are to be given with food or on an empty stomach.

◆ *Evaluation.* Therapeutic effect is usually seen in 3 to 7 days with a reduction in the number and severity of allergic reactions or asthma attacks.

◆ *Patient and family teaching.* Tell the patient and family:
- Report to your healthcare provider any increase in asthma attacks or allergic symptoms.
- Consider not taking these drugs if you are pregnant or breast-feeding, although this is an individual decision to be made by you and your healthcare provider based on risk and benefit.
- These drugs are used to prevent (rather than stop) an asthma attack or allergic response; therefore do not suddenly stop taking the prescribed drug or decrease the dosage.

### MAST CELL STABILIZERS (CROMONES)

Another type of drug that reduces the amount of histamine and leukotriene release and can be helpful for allergy or asthma is the class of mast cell stabilizers (cromones). They work on the surface of mast cells and prevent them from opening to release the inflammatory mediators. For nasal allergies and asthma they are used as inhaled drugs. Common cromones and their nursing implications are listed in Table 8.1.

### DECONGESTANTS

#### Actions and Uses

Nasal congestion occurs because the nasal tissue is inflamed and swollen or because nasal secretions are thick and obstruct the nasal passage. A decongestant is a drug that reduces the swelling of nasal passages. There are two kinds of decongestants: sympathomimetics and corticosteroids.

Sympathomimetics are drugs that produce or mimic stimulation of the sympathetic (adrenergic) nervous system and have the same action as the body's own adrenaline. When blood vessels are stimulated by the sympathetic nervous system (alpha receptors), they shrink (*constrict*). After the blood vessels shrink, the secretions in the membranes of the nose can drain better, and stuffiness and pressure are thereby relieved. These drugs may also be used to decrease congestion around the eustachian tubes with middle ear infections. Most of these products are now available OTC. They can be taken orally or by nasal spray. Saline nasal spray and saline irrigations using a neti pot are an effective alternative to nasal sprays and can be used routinely to relieve nasal symptoms. There

are no side effects to the use of saline, and it can be used as often as necessary.

A corticosteroid is a drug built on the structure of cholesterol that is able to prevent or limit inflammation and allergy by slowing or stopping production of the mediators histamine and leukotriene. Corticosteroid nasal sprays are effective at controlling nasal inflammation. They stabilize the membranes of the WBCs, which produce the histamines and leukotrienes that cause inflammation. They work on the WBCs that help to fight infection; therefore their use is not recommended for people with sinus infections or for those who have immune diseases or are taking immune-suppressing drugs. If they are absorbed systemically, illness may result because of the lessened response of infection-fighting WBCs. It takes up to 2 weeks for corticosteroid nasal sprays to begin working. Oral, IV, and IM corticosteroids can also be used for allergic reactions but have many side and adverse effects. They may be used orally for allergies and asthma but are more commonly given as inhaled drugs. Table 8.2 lists common decongestants, their actions, and nursing implications. Chapter 13 discusses the actions and uses of corticosteroids and the nursing responsibilities.

#### Uses

Nasal decongestants are used to shrink nasal mucous membranes and relieve nasal congestion caused by allergies or cold symptoms.

#### Expected Side Effects

Topically applied nasal decongestants (sprays or drops) are well tolerated because the amount that enters the bloodstream is too small to cause side effects. Local effects include irritation and dryness of the mucous membranes. Sympathomimetic nasal sprays that are overused can enter the bloodstream and cause nervousness, insomnia, tremors, and heart palpitations. Expected side effects of oral decongestants include headache, nervousness, dizziness, insomnia, and tremors. A slight nosebleed is common with corticosteroid nasal sprays, but if it becomes severe, it would be considered an adverse effect.

#### Adverse Reactions

Oral sympathomimetic decongestants can have adverse side effects related to mimicking the sympathetic nervous system response. The sympathetic nervous system (beta$_1$ receptors) increases heart rate, increases the force of contraction of the heart muscle, increases the speed of electrical conduction in the heart, and constricts the blood vessels. The adverse effects that can be seen are cardiac dysrhythmias, hypertension, and palpitations, which could lead to a heart attack.

Sympathomimetic nasal decongestants can cause rebound congestion if overused or used for longer

## Table 8.2   Examples of Common Decongestants

*Nasal corticosteroids* decrease inflamed and swollen nasal membranes by preventing mast cells and white blood cells in the nasal mucosa from releasing histamine, leukotriene, and other mediators of inflammation.

*Sympathomimetic drugs* shrink swollen nasal membranes by activating the adrenergic receptors on blood vessels in the nasal mucosa, causing them to constrict. Swelling is reduced, and sinus drainage is improved.

| DRUG/ADULT DOSAGE | NURSING IMPLICATIONS |
|---|---|
| **Nasal Corticosteroids** | |
| fluticasone (Flonase Sensimist) two sprays of 110 mcg once daily<br>triamcinolone (Nasacort) two to four sprays of 55 mcg once daily | • Remind patients that relief is not immediate because these drugs take time to build up an effect.<br>• Caution patients not to swallow the spray to prevent absorbing the drug systemically and causing more side effects.<br>• Remind patients to clean and dry the applicator after each use (and never to share their inhaler with another person) to prevent infection because these drugs reduce the local immune response.<br>• Tell patients to watch for white patches in the nose or throat that may indicate a fungal infection because these drugs reduce the local immune response. |
| **Sympathomimetic Drugs** | |
| oxymetazoline, nasal spray (Afrin, many others), two to three sprays in each nostril as needed every 10–12 hours<br>phenylephrine, spray or drops (Neo-Synephrine, many others), 0.5%–1% solution sprayed or dropped into the nose every 6 hours<br>phenylephrine, oral tablets or liquids (Nasop, Sudafed, many others), 10–20 mg every 6 hours as needed<br>pseudoephedrine (Dimetapp, Sudafed, many others) 60 mg orally every 6 hours *or* 120 mg orally every 12 hours | • Tell patients that relief of nasal congestion is immediate because these sprays and drops work on contact with nasal membranes.<br>• Remind patients to use the nasal sprays for only a few days because tolerance and rebound stuffiness occur quickly.<br>• Caution patients not to swallow the spray to prevent absorbing the drug systemically and causing more side effects.<br>• Warn patients with high blood pressure, heart disease, glaucoma, or prostate enlargement to use these drugs with caution and not to exceed the prescribed dose because the drugs increase blood pressure, cause urinary retention, and increase intraocular pressure.<br>• Suggest that patients who are using the oral forms of any of these drugs take them at least 4 hours before going to bed because these drugs can cause insomnia. |

than 3 to 5 days. Rarely, a severe shocklike syndrome with hypotension and coma has been reported in children. Psychological dependence and toxic psychoses have been reported with long-term, high-dose therapy. The severity of overdosage varies, resulting in a variety of symptoms. The US Food and Drug Administration (FDA) stipulates that these products are not to be used in infants and toddlers because of problems with inadvertent overdosage in very young patients.

Corticosteroid nasal sprays can reduce the protective immune responses in the nose and throat. This action increases the risk of upper respiratory infections and overgrowth of oral fungus (yeast). As a result, redness, sores, or white patches may appear in the mouth or throat.

## Drug Interactions

Drugs that interact with sympathomimetics include caffeine, MAOIs, amphetamines, ergotamine, selegiline, and linezolid, which can cause hypertension and increasing heart rate with dysrhythmias. These drugs should not be taken with beta-blocking eye drops used for open-angle glaucoma. Corticosteroid nasal sprays should not be used with antibiotics or immunosuppressive drugs.

❖ **Nursing Implications and Patient Teaching**

◆ *Assessment.* Monitor heart rate and blood pressure in people taking sympathomimetic drugs, especially in those with a history of cardiac disease. Notify the prescriber if a rapid or irregular heart rate develops or if hypertension worsens. For patients using corticosteroid nasal sprays, assess the nasal and mouth area for white patches or redness that may indicate a fungal infection. For people who are susceptible to infection, take their temperature and monitor any signs and symptoms that might indicate an infectious process rather than an allergy (e.g., thick green nasal discharge, shortness of breath, wheezing).

◆ *Planning and implementation.* Oral sympathomimetic drugs can decrease the effectiveness of some drugs for high blood pressure and should not be used by people with uncontrolled hypertension or cardiac insufficiency. Patients taking antibiotics, antifungals, immunosuppressives, or HIV drugs and those who have sinus infections should not use corticosteroid nasal sprays.

◆ *Evaluation.* Nasal stuffiness and inflammation should be relieved instantly with use of a sympathomimetic nasal spray and within 1 hour with oral sympathomimetics. Nasal corticosteroids can take up to 2 weeks to reduce symptoms.

◆ *Patient and family teaching.* Tell the patient and family:
- Before using a decongestant, check with your prescriber if you have heart disease, high blood pressure, glaucoma, diabetes, an enlarged prostate, or thyroid disease because decongestants can make these problems worse.
- Avoid caffeine, alcohol, or other stimulant drugs while using oral sympathomimetic decongestants because heart rate and blood pressure problems will increase.
- Avoid taking sympathomimetic drugs within 4 hours of bedtime because these drugs may cause insomnia.
- If you develop extreme restlessness, insomnia, tremors, and heart palpitations, stop using the drug and notify your healthcare provider.
- Do not take sympathomimetic drugs if you are pregnant or breast-feeding.
- Do not overuse a sympathomimetic nasal spray or use it for longer than 3 days because rebound stuffiness and congestion are likely to occur.
- If you have high blood pressure or heart problems, check with the pharmacist before using OTC cold preparations that are advertised to relieve nasal congestion or stuffiness because OTC cold preparations often contain sympathomimetic drugs.
- If you have glaucoma or cataracts, check with your healthcare provider before using corticosteroid nasal sprays.
- Contact your healthcare provider if white patches develop in the nose or mouth, you have worsening nasal discharge, or flu-like symptoms and fever develop while taking corticosteroid nasal sprays.

## ASTHMA AND CHRONIC OBSTRUCTIVE PULMONARY DISEASE

### ASTHMA

Asthma is a long-term condition of the airways that causes smooth muscle constriction and inflammation of the airways and lungs. As a result of airway narrowing, airflow to lung tissue, where oxygen is picked up by the blood, can be greatly reduced. Although the actual symptoms of asthma may occur from time to time rather than continuously (known as an *intermittent problem*), the disorder is chronic and the person is always at risk for an asthma attack. However, the symptoms of asthma are reversible, and between attacks the patient usually has no signs or symptoms.

Two different problems can cause the airways to shrink and become obstructed (Fig. 8.2). Internal airway obstruction occurs when inflammation, often caused by an allergy, causes the mucous membrane lining to swell and secrete extra mucus. When the

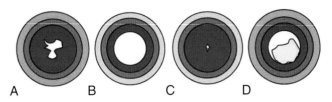

Fig. 8.2 Causes of narrowed airways: (A) Mucosal swelling. (B) Constriction of smooth muscle. (C) Mucosal swelling and constriction of smooth muscle. (D) Mucous plug. (From Workman, M. L., LaCharity, L. A., & Kruchko, S. L. (2011). *Understanding pharmacology* (1st ed.). Elsevier.)

smooth muscle surrounding the airway tightens (constricts), it narrows the outside structure of the airway through *bronchoconstriction*. Many patients with asthma have both types of airway obstruction because an allergy can irritate bronchiolar smooth muscle. Drug therapy for asthma usually requires more than one type of drug to manage the two causes of the disorder. Asthma can be triggered by dust mites, cockroaches, smoke, air pollution, pets, weather changes, exercise, and other irritants. Key recommendations from the 2021 Global Initiative for Asthma (GINA) for controlling asthma are to individualize and adjust asthma therapy in a continual cycle of assessment, treatment, and review. Treatment of modifiable risk factors and comorbidities are also incorporated to control asthma and exacerbations. This includes nonpharmacological strategies such as education and skills training, particularly for inhaler use and adherence.

 **Memory Jogger**

Inflammation narrows airways from the inside, and bronchoconstriction narrows airways from the outside.

Symptoms of an asthma attack are shortness of breath, wheezing (similar to the whistling sound a vacuum pipe makes when it becomes clogged), a dry, hacking cough, and a feeling of tightness in the chest. Asthma episodes can occur frequently every day, a few times per week, during the day or night, with exercise, or on a seasonal basis. Management depends on the severity and frequency of symptoms.

### CHRONIC OBSTRUCTIVE PULMONARY DISEASE

Chronic obstructive pulmonary disease (COPD) is a progressive disease that causes breathing difficulty. It obstructs airflow passages in the upper and lower airways, including the alveoli—where gas exchange takes place. The usual cause of COPD is cigarette smoking or exposure to secondhand smoke and air pollution that causes a constant inflammation of the upper airways known as *chronic bronchitis*. The inflammation causes large amounts of sticky mucus to be produced, which obstructs the upper airways, makes the work of breathing very difficult, and prevents air from flowing into the lungs and alveoli. Bronchitis affects only the airways, not the alveoli.

The same things that cause chronic bronchitis also cause the emphysema that is seen in COPD. Emphysema is damage to the lower airways involving the lung tissue and alveoli. When the alveoli become damaged, they can no longer stretch for oxygen to enter or shrink to force carbon dioxide out. The alveoli begin to collapse and die; the fewer alveoli that exist, the less oxygen is available to be moved into the bloodstream and the more carbon dioxide the body retains. COPD causes a chronic cough that produces clear, white, yellow, or green sticky mucus, wheezing, shortness of breath, chest tightness, and an enlarged chest.

In contrast to asthma, the person diagnosed with COPD always has symptoms. Symptoms become worse with increases in inflammation resulting from pulmonary infections and response to pollution and other triggers. The lung damage resulting from COPD, unlike that with asthma, is *not* reversible, although patients may have periods with less severe symptoms. Drug therapy for COPD involves most of the same drugs used for asthma because the symptoms are similar, although the actual causes differ.

## DRUG THERAPY FOR ASTHMA AND CHRONIC OBSTRUCTIVE PULMONARY DISEASE

Drug therapy for asthma and COPD includes bronchodilators and anti-inflammatory agents. Although both types of drugs are used, the dosage and delivery method used for COPD may be different (i.e., some drugs are more often delivered by nebulizer rather than as a sprayed inhalant). Drugs that help thin secretions (mucolytics) are used more often in COPD therapy than in asthma therapy (discussed later).

The goals of drug therapy for asthma are (1) to prevent acute asthma attacks and (2) to stop an asthma attack as quickly as possible after it has started. Some drugs are **asthma controller drugs** (asthma prevention drugs) that have the main purpose of preventing an asthma attack. Controller drugs must be taken daily to be effective, even when the person has no symptoms of asthma. Controller drugs usually include longer-acting bronchodilators and corticosteroids that prevent excessive inflammation (anti-inflammatories). Drugs that have the main purpose of stopping an asthma attack after it has started are **asthma reliever drugs** (asthma rescue drugs). They are usually short-acting bronchodilators that have no role in asthma prevention. The Global Initiative for Asthma has published guidelines for asthma diagnosis and drug management and recommends a stepwise plan for using asthma drugs that takes into account asthma severity (Fig. 8.3).

Approximately 60% of people have allergic asthma, making allergic asthma the most common type of asthma in both adults and children. The immune system responds to allergens by releasing immunoglobulin E (IgE), which causes inflammation of the

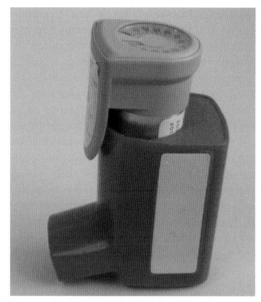

Fig. 8.3 Metered-dose inhaler with counter. (From Patel, M., Pilcher, J., Travers, J., et al. (2013). Use of metered-dose inhaler electronic monitoring in a real-world asthma randomized controlled trial. *Journal of Allergy and Clinical Immunology: In Practice, 1*(1), 83–91.)

airways. Blood tests for specific IgE and skin testing can be done so specific therapy can be ordered. Omalizumab (Xolair) is an add-on asthma medication that is administered according to the result of IgE units obtained from the blood tests. It is administered subcutaneously. Odactra is a sublingual immunotherapy (SLIT) tablet that is administered for those hypersensitive to dust mites. Both of these drugs should be administered for the first time in a healthcare provider's office with emergency medications available in case of anaphylaxis.

> 💡 **Memory Jogger**
> - Asthma controller drugs prevent asthma attacks and must be taken daily even when asthma symptoms are not present.
> - Asthma reliever drugs can rescue a person having an asthma attack. They are used only as needed and not on a schedule.

### BRONCHODILATORS

#### Action

A **bronchodilator** is a drug that relaxes the airway smooth muscles, allowing the lumens of the airways to widen. The respiratory and cardiac systems have special receptors (alpha- and beta-receptors) in the muscle cells that help in speeding up or slowing down the respiratory and cardiac processes. The main action of bronchodilators in asthma and other respiratory diseases when the airways are constricted is to act like the body's own adrenaline, which binds to and stimulates the beta$_2$-adrenergic receptors within bronchial tube smooth muscle and allows them to relax. The most common class of drugs with this action are the beta$_2$-adrenergic agonists. (Recall from Chapter 3 that an agonist drug binds to its receptor and activates it.) Another class of drugs that allows relaxation of bronchial smooth muscle is the **cholinergic** antagonists, also called *long-acting muscarinic antagonists.* (Recall from Chapter 3 that an antagonist drug blocks a receptor rather than activating it.) Cholinergic drugs and agents (e.g., acetylcholine) have exactly the opposite action of adrenaline. When a **long-acting muscarinic antagonist (LAMA)** is given, there is less acetylcholine present to interfere with the work of the body's adrenaline. This action allows natural adrenaline to bind to more beta$_2$-adrenergic receptors, causing relaxation of bronchial smooth muscle. Long-acting muscarinic antagonists are also useful in decreasing the excessive thick and sticky secretions seen in chronic bronchitis.

## Uses

The use of a bronchodilator in asthma and COPD depends on the drug's duration of action. A **short-acting beta$_2$-adrenergic agonist (SABA)** is an orally inhaled drug that binds rapidly to beta$_2$-adrenergic receptors and can start smooth muscle relaxation within seconds to minutes. As a result, SABAs are used during an actual asthma attack and when the person with COPD has symptoms of bronchospasm. SABAs may also be used during other respiratory infections when patients experience bronchospasm. SABAs are *reliever* drugs that act quickly. Their effects also wear off quickly, and a person may need more than one dose to stop a bronchospasm or asthma attack. SABAs are frequently prescribed to be given with inhaled corticosteroids. These drugs work together to prevent bronchospasm. While the SABA relaxes smooth muscle to open the airway, the corticosteroid prevents the release of inflammation mediators that caused the bronchospasm. When using SABA and an inhaled corticosteroid together, it is important to always use the SABA first to open the airway and allow the corticosteroid to reach the respiratory tract. Examples of common SABAs are listed in Table 8.3. Common corticosteroid inhalers can be found in Table 8.4.

 **Top Tip for Safety**

Teach patients with asthma to always have their SABA reliever drug with them at all times because an attack can occur anywhere and only a SABA can work fast enough to prevent a severe attack and death.

**Memory Jogger**

When using a SABA and an inhaled corticosteroid together, always use the SABA first.

Some beta$_2$-adrenergic agonists are long-acting drugs. Although they work in the same way as SABAs, they take time to build up an effect, and the effect lasts longer. A **long-acting beta$_2$-adrenergic agonist (LABA)** is an orally inhaled drug that binds over time to beta$_2$-adrenergic receptors and is used as an asthma controller drug. It must be taken on a daily schedule to prevent bronchospasms and asthma attacks even when symptoms are not present. LABAs are not helpful during an acute attack because they take time to work. Examples of common LABAs are shown in Table 8.3. Sometimes, so that patients have fewer drugs to take and remember, a LABA may be combined with an inhaled corticosteroid in one inhaler. An example is Breo Ellipta, which is the LABA vilanterol combined with the inhaled corticosteroid fluticasone.

 **Memory Jogger**

SABAs are reliever (rescue) drugs that are effective in stopping an asthma attack or bronchospasm. LABAs and cholinergic antagonists are controller (prevention) drugs and are not helpful during an asthma attack or bronchospasm.

 **Memory Jogger**

- Activated beta$_1$-adrenergic receptors and beta$_1$-agonist drugs increase heart rate, force of contraction, and speed of conduction. (Hint: You have only one heart.)
- Activated beta$_2$-adrenergic receptors and beta$_2$-agonist drugs cause bronchodilation. (Hint: You have two lungs.)
- Activated alpha-adrenergic receptors or alpha-agonists cause vasoconstriction.

*Cholinergic antagonists* are also used as orally inhaled controller drugs. Their response is slower, but they work by relaxing the muscles around the airways so the airway can open wider and breathing is improved. Like LABAs, cholinergic antagonists cannot stop an asthma attack or a bronchospasm after it has started. Examples of common cholinergic antagonists are shown in Table 8.3.

*Xanthine-based drugs* are older types of bronchodilators that are given systemically. They are rarely used because the dose that is effective is close to the dose that produces many dangerous side effects. This class of drugs includes theophylline and aminophylline. They are used only when other types of management are not effective. Patients must have blood levels measured frequently to ensure that the drug level is within the therapeutic range and not in the toxic range. The use of xanthines is not within the scope of this chapter.

## Expected Side Effects

Orally inhaled bronchodilators usually have few and only mild side effects because most of the drug goes into the airways. The action of all types of bronchodilators results in the stimulation of beta$_1$- and beta$_2$-adrenergic receptors throughout the body, especially in the heart and blood vessels. When bronchodilators are heavily used, common side effects include

## Table 8.3   Examples of Common Bronchodilators

*Short-acting beta$_2$-agonists (SABAs)* cause bronchodilation by rapidly binding to beta$_2$-adrenergic receptors in bronchial smooth muscle and stimulating muscle relaxation quickly, which widens the airways. These are *reliever/rescue* inhaled drugs used during an asthma attack or just before engaging in activity that usually triggers an attack.

*Long-acting beta$_2$-agonists (LABAs)* cause bronchodilation by binding to beta$_2$-adrenergic receptors in bronchial smooth muscle over time and eventually stimulating continued smooth muscle relaxation. LABAs are *controller/prevention* inhaled drugs used to prevent an asthma attack or bronchospasm and should not be used as rescue drugs.

*Long-acting muscarinic antagonists (LAMAs)* are inhaled controller drugs that cause bronchodilation by preventing the nervous system from releasing some acetylcholine, which then allows more of the body's own adrenaline to activate beta$_2$-receptors in bronchial smooth muscle.

| DRUG/ADULT DOSAGE | NURSING IMPLICATIONS |
|---|---|
| **Short-Acting Beta$_2$-Agonists** | |
| albuterol (Apo-Salvent ♣, ProAir HFA, PMS-Salbutamol ♣, Respirol, Ventolin HFA, VoSpire ER) one to two inhalations (90 mcg each) every 4–6 hours as needed<br>levalbuterol (Xopenex) one to two inhalations (45 mcg each) every 4–6 hours<br>pirbuterol (Maxair) two inhalations (0.4 mg each) every 4–6 hours | • Teach patients to carry the drug with them at all times because it can stop or reduce a life-threatening asthma attack or bronchoconstriction.<br>• Teach patients to monitor heart rate and other responses because excessive use causes rapid heart rate, nervousness, and tremors.<br>• When taking this drug with other inhaled drugs, teach patients to use this drug first and wait at least 5 minutes before taking the other inhaled drugs to allow the bronchodilating effect to increase the movement of the other drugs into the lungs.<br>• Teach patients to use the directions in Box 8.1 for correct technique to ensure that the drug reaches the airways.<br>• Instruct patients to use a spacer with the MDIs. If a spacer is not available, teach them to hold the mouthpiece 1–2 inches away from the mouth when the inhaler is activated and then to inhale the mist so that the drug reaches the airways and does not just stick to the back of the throat. |
| **Long-Acting Beta$_2$-Agonists** | |
| arformoterol (Brovana) 15 mcg every 12 hours (one vial) by nebulizer<br>formoterol (Foradil, Oxeze, Perforomist) 12 mcg (one capsule) every 12 hours by DPI<br>salmeterol (Serevent) 50 mcg (one inhalation) every 12 hours by DPI | • Remind patients to use LABAs daily as prescribed, even when symptoms are not present, to prevent an asthma attack or bronchospasm.<br>• Remind patients to *not* use LABAs as reliever/rescue drugs because their onset of action is too slow to help in an acute attack.<br>• Teach patients using a DPI and to follow the instructions in Box 8.2 and the directions on the inhaler to ensure the best effect of the drug. |
| **Long-Acting Muscarinic Antagonists** | |
| ipratropium (Atrovent) two to four inhalations (17 mcg each) over 6–8 hours<br>tiotropium (Spiriva HandiHaler) one inhalation (18 mcg) every day by DPI<br>tiotropium (Spiriva Respimat) two inhalations (2.5 mcg) daily by MDI | • Teach patients using an MDI to shake it well before using because the drug separates easily.<br>• Teach patients to drink plenty of liquids because the drugs cause mouth dryness.<br>• Teach patients about the expected side effects of stuffy nose, sore throat, and constipation because knowing the side effects helps relieve anxiety when they appear.<br>• Instruct patients to report urinary retention or consistently increased heart rate to their healthcare provider because these are serious adverse effects of the drugs. |

*DPI*, dry-powder inhaler; *MDI*, metered-dose inhaler.

hypertension, tachycardia, headache, and insomnia. Some people feel "nervous" and may have tremors with these drugs. Dry mouth and a bad taste are common side effects. Cardiovascular side effects are more noticeable with the SABAs because the onset of action is so rapid.

### Adverse Reactions

Some inhalers contain a preservative, and some patients may have an allergic reaction to it. If the bronchodilator is heavily used, it can be absorbed throughout the body and cause constriction of blood vessels in the heart muscle, leading to chest pain or even a myocardial infarction (heart attack).

### Drug Interactions

Drug interactions may occur between bronchodilators and MAOIs, tricyclic antidepressants, beta-blockers (beta-adrenergic antagonists), other antihypertensive agents, digoxin, potassium-losing diuretics, and caffeine-containing herbs. The combination of two or more of these agents may produce an additive effect.

Many general anesthetics may cause dysrhythmias when they are used with these drugs. Nonselective

### Table 8.4 Examples of Common Inhaled Corticosteroids

*Inhaled corticosteroids* decrease inflamed airways by preventing mast cells and WBCs in the respiratory mucosa from releasing histamine, leukotriene, and other mediators of inflammation. These drugs do *not* cause bronchodilation and should *not* be used as rescue drugs. An advantage is that the effects of inhaled corticosteroids are limited to the respiratory tract.

| DRUG/ADULT DOSAGE | NURSING IMPLICATIONS |
|---|---|
| beclomethasone (Qvar) one to two inhalations (40 mcg each) twice daily by MDI<br>budesonide (Pulmicort) two inhalations (180 mcg each) twice daily<br>flunisolide (Aerospan HFA) two inhalations (80 mcg each) twice daily<br>fluticasone (Flovent HFA, Flovent Diskus) two inhalations (80 mcg each) twice daily<br>mometasone (Asmanex) one inhalation (220 mcg) once or twice daily | • Do not use in patients who have sputum that contains *Candida* or who have systemic fungal infections because these drugs reduce the immune responses to those infections.<br>• Suggest that patients rinse their mouths after each use to minimize fungal infection of the mouth from immunosuppressive effects.<br>• Warn patients that inhaled corticosteroids are not to be used to treat an acute asthma attack because they are not bronchodilators.<br>• Teach patients to use these drugs daily as prescribed, even when no symptoms are present, because they are long-term controller drugs.<br>• Advise patients to notify their healthcare professional if white patches in the mouth or throat or soreness and redness in the mouth or throat appear because these are indications of infection.<br>• Teach patients how to properly use the MDI and DPI devices (see Boxes 8.1 and 8.2) because improper use reduces drug effectiveness. |

*DPI,* dry-powder inhaler; *MDI,* metered-dose inhaler; *WBCs,* white blood cells.

beta-blockers and beta-adrenergic blocking agents such as propranolol (Inderal) may block the bronchodilating effects of these beta$_2$-receptor–stimulating drugs. Bronchodilators can interfere with the action of some antihypertensive drugs.

#### ❖ Nursing Implications and Patient Teaching

◆ *Assessment.* Ask whether the patient is pregnant, is breast-feeding, or has a history of hyperthyroidism, heart disease, hypertension, diabetes, glaucoma, seizures, or psychoneurotic disease. Ask whether the patient is taking other drugs that may interact with bronchodilators or has a history of allergy. Any of these conditions may present contraindications or precautions to the use of bronchodilators. Take a baseline set of vital signs to be able to assess for drug-related changes.

◆ *Planning and implementation.* Beta$_2$-adrenergic receptors in bronchial smooth muscle cells must be stimulated to relieve bronchial spasm. One of the drawbacks of bronchodilators is that they may also stimulate receptors in the heart (beta$_1$), increasing the rate and force of cardiac contraction. Therefore bronchodilators should be given with extreme caution to patients who already have cardiovascular, endocrine, or convulsive disorders that may be affected by these drugs.

The routes of administration of bronchodilators vary according to how ill the patient is (the diagnostic classification) and the preparation to be used. Drugs may be given parenterally, orally, or, most often, by oral inhalation (nebulizers or metered-dose inhalers [MDIs]). How well the orally inhaled drug works to control or relieve asthma and bronchospasm depends on correct use of the inhaler. Show a patient who is using an inhaler for the first time how to use the inhaler

and give written instructions to refer to later. Research shows that many patients do not use inhalers correctly. Every time the patient comes in for a healthcare visit, ask for a demonstration of how the MDI is being used. Fig. 8.3 shows an MDI. Box 8.1 describes how to use an MDI, and Fig. 8.4 shows a patient using the inhaler with a spacer. Fig. 8.5 shows a typical dry-powder inhaler, and Box 8.2 describes how to use it. Chapter 4 provides instructions for the use of a nebulizer to deliver orally inhaled drugs.

Irritation of the lung passages, mouth, and throat may occur with use of powdered drug forms or other inhaled agents. Rinsing the mouth with water after each treatment helps reduce this problem.

◆ *Evaluation.* Check the patient's pulse and blood pressure and compare them with the baseline findings to assess whether the heart is affected by the drug. Response to therapy varies among patients. Assess for rate, depth, and ease of respiration to determine whether breathing problems have improved.

◆ *Patient and family teaching.* Tell the patient and family:
• Take the drug as directed by the healthcare provider and do not change the dose.
• Overuse of these drugs may result in severe side effects.
• Contact your healthcare provider if the drug is not helping your breathing problems.
• Contact your healthcare provider if bronchial irritation, dizziness, chest pain, insomnia, or any changes in symptoms occur.
• Drinking lots of fluid, especially water, makes the mucus thinner and helps the drug work better.
• Do not take any OTC drugs without first checking with your healthcare provider.

| Box 8.1 | Teaching a Patient How to Correctly Use a Metered-Dose Inhaler |

**WITH A SPACER (PREFERRED TECHNIQUE)**

1. Before each use, remove the caps from the inhaler and the spacer.
2. Insert the mouthpiece of the inhaler into the nonmouthpiece end of the spacer.
3. Shake the whole unit vigorously three or four times.
4. Fully exhale, and then place the mouthpiece into your mouth, over your tongue, and seal your lips tightly around it.
5. Press down firmly on the canister of the inhaler to release one dose of the drug into the spacer.
6. Breathe in slowly and deeply. If the spacer makes a whistling sound, you are breathing in too rapidly.
7. Remove the mouthpiece from your mouth and, while keeping your lips closed, hold your breath for at least 10 seconds and then breathe out slowly.
8. Wait at least 1 minute between puffs.
9. Replace the caps on the inhaler and the spacer.
10. At least once a day, clean the plastic case and cap of the inhaler by thoroughly rinsing in warm, running tap water; at least once a week, clean the spacer in the same manner.

**WITHOUT A SPACER**

1. Before each use, remove the cap, and shake the inhaler according to the instructions in the package insert.
2. Tilt your head back slightly, and breathe out fully.
3. Open your mouth, and place the mouthpiece 1 to 2 inches away.
4. As you begin to breathe in deeply through your mouth, press down firmly on the canister of the inhaler to release one dose of the drug.
5. Continue to breathe in slowly and deeply (usually for 5 to 7 seconds).
6. Hold your breath for at least 10 seconds to allow the drug to reach deep into the lungs, and then breathe out slowly.
7. Wait at least 1 minute between puffs.
8. Replace the cap on the inhaler.
9. At least once a day, remove the canister and clean the plastic case and cap of the inhaler by thoroughly rinsing in warm, running tap water.
10. Avoid spraying in the direction of your eyes.

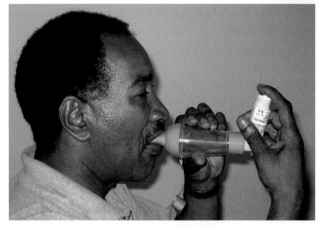

**Fig. 8.4** Patient using an aerosol (metered-dose inhaler) with a spacer. (From Ignatavicius, D., Workman, M. L., & Rebar, C. (2018). *Medical-surgical nursing* (9th ed.). Elsevier.)

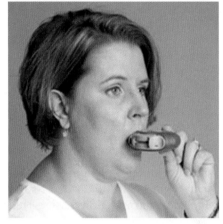

**Fig. 8.5** A dry-powder inhaler with a counter. (From Potter, P. A., Perry, A. G., Stockert, P., & Hall, A. (2019). *Essentials for nursing practice* (9th ed.). Elsevier.)

- A corticosteroid inhaler must be used after a SABA inhaler when you are using them both.

### ANTI-INFLAMMATORY DRUGS

Anti-inflammatory drugs have a major role as controller drugs for asthma therapy and the inflammation associated with COPD. Leukotrienes and cromones are some of the drugs used, and they have been discussed earlier in this chapter. Corticosteroids work to slow or stop the inflammatory mediators histamine and leukotriene, and they work like the corticosteroid nasal spray discussed earlier (see Decongestants). These are drugs that control asthma and COPD and, quite frequently, they are combined with a long-acting inhaler. Table 8.4 lists commonly inhaled anti-inflammatory drugs used for asthma and COPD.

## MUCOLYTICS AND ANTITUSSIVES

### MUCOLYTICS
**Action and Uses**

A **mucolytic**, sometimes called an *expectorant*, is a drug that decreases the thickness of respiratory secretions

- To prevent exercise-induced bronchospasm, use your reliever bronchodilator inhaler 15 to 30 minutes before starting to exercise.
- Shake the inhaler well before using it.
- Follow the instructions for correct use of your inhaler.
- After using your inhaler, rinse your mouth with water to decrease dry mouth and bad taste.
- Keep a count of the total number of sprays used and discard the inhaler after 200 sprays or check the inhaler's counter to know when it is time to get a new one.
- For an MDI, clean the mouthpiece and dry it at least once a week.

| Box 8.2 | Teaching a Patient How to Use a Dry-Powder Inhaler |

**FOR INHALERS THAT REQUIRE LOADING**
- Load the drug by:
  - Turning the device to the next dose of drug, *or*
  - Inserting the capsule into the device, *or*
  - Inserting the disk or compartment into the device.

**AFTER LOADING THE DRUG AND FOR INHALERS THAT DO NOT REQUIRE DRUG LOADING**
- Read your healthcare provider's instructions for how fast you should breathe for your particular inhaler.
- Exhale fully away from the inhaler.
- Place your lips over the mouthpiece, and breathe in forcefully. (There is no propellant in the inhaler; only your breath pulls the drug in.)
- Remove the inhaler from your mouth as soon as you have breathed in.
- Never exhale (breathe out) into your inhaler. Your breath moistens the powder, causing it to clump and not be delivered accurately.
- Never wash or place the inhaler in water.
- Never shake your inhaler.
- Keep your inhaler in a dry place at room temperature.
- If the inhaler is preloaded, discard it after it is empty.
- The drug is a dry powder, and there is no propellant. You may not feel, smell, or taste it as you inhale.

and aids in their removal. They are thought to work by increasing the amount of fluid in the respiratory tract and may help break down or dissolve mucus, making removal of the secretions easier. Thinning the secretions promotes ciliary action and makes coughing more effective by increasing the amount of sputum available to spit out. Guaifenesin is a mucolytic drug contained in many combination OTC cough and cold products. It is available as a single agent in OTC drugs (e.g., Mucinex, Robitussin, Organidin NR) and in prescription-only products (e.g., Humibid LA, Touro EX tablets). The drug is available in immediate-release (e.g., oral solutions), extended-release, and combination immediate/extended-release formulations.

Guaifenesin is used to treat symptoms of productive cough. These drugs are also useful in COPD disease when thick mucus is a complication, and they are indicated in patients with coughs associated with viral upper respiratory tract infections. Table 8.5 lists common mucolytic or expectorant drugs.

### Lifespan Considerations

**Pediatric Patients**

The FDA recommends that these products not be given to children younger than 2 years and some products not to children younger than 6 years because of cases of overdosage.

### Expected Side Effects and Adverse Reactions

GI upset is a common adverse reaction to mucolytics. Dizziness, headache, and rash may also occur.

### ❖ Nursing Implications and Patient Teaching

◆ *Assessment.* Ask the patient about a history of cough, the presence of other respiratory disease or allergy, and the use of other drugs that may cause drug interactions.

◆ *Planning and implementation.* Mucolytics are not to be used for persistent cough without the advice of a healthcare provider. Chronic or persistent cough may be the result of a serious condition and should not be ignored.

In addition to drug therapy, teach patients to drink more fluid each day and breathe humidified air to help thin secretions. Suggest that they take the mucolytic with a full glass of water.

◆ *Evaluation.* Monitor the patient to ensure that secretions become thinner and are decreased. If the patient uses more than the recommended dosage, adverse reactions may occur.

◆ *Patient and family teaching.* Tell the patient and family:
- The purpose of mucolytics is to make the sputum more liquid and easier to spit out when you cough. The mucolytic drug alone will not make you stop coughing.
- Use a humidifier and drink at least 2 quarts of water daily while taking a mucolytic unless there is a medical reason for fluid restriction. These actions will help get the mucus out.
- Notify your healthcare provider if the cough is present with a high fever, rash, or persistent headaches, or if the cough returns after it has been under control.
- Use the drug only in the dosage recommended to decrease the odds of side effects.
- Take the drug with at least one full glass of water.
- To cough effectively, sit upright and take several deep breaths before trying to cough.
- Avoid driving or other activities that require alertness until you know how you respond to the drug because it may cause dizziness.

### ANTITUSSIVES

#### Action and Uses

An **antitussive** is a drug that is used to relieve or suppress coughing. These drugs may act (1) centrally on the cough center in the brain; (2) peripherally by anesthetizing stretch receptors in the respiratory tract; or (3) locally, primarily by soothing irritated areas in the throat. Products vary in their effectiveness. Antitussives are commonly combined with other drugs and are usually sold OTC. Antitussives containing controlled substances usually require a prescription, although some states may allow codeine combination products to be sold OTC if the patient signs for them.

The main action of an antitussive depends on whether an opioid antagonist is included. Narcotic or

| Table 8.5 | Common Examples of Mucolytics and Antitussives |

*Mucolytics* are drugs that decrease the thickness and stickiness of respiratory secretions. They also enhance the action of respiratory cilia. Both actions improve movement of mucus out of the airways.

*Antitussives* suppress coughing by depressing the cough centers in the central nervous system (CNS) reducing the response of respiratory tract stretch receptors, or reducing throat irritation.

| DRUG/ADULT DOSAGE | NURSING IMPLICATIONS |
|---|---|
| **Mucolytics** | |
| guaifenesin (Mucinex), part of many over the counter (OTC) and prescription preparations for coughs and colds, 200–400 mg orally every 4 hours | • Ask patients with any side effects how much and how often they are taking this drug because when it is taken in recommended dosages, side effects are rare.<br>• Ask patients about back pain and difficulty passing urine because high dosages are associated with the formation of kidney stones.<br>• Instruct patients to notify the healthcare provider if symptoms have not improved within a few days or have worsened, because this may indicate more serious respiratory problems.<br>• Make sure the patient is drinking plenty of fluids to assist in liquifying the secretions to assist with expectoration. |
| **Antitussives** | |
| benzonatate (Tessalon Perles, Zonatuss) 100 mg orally every 8 hours | • Tell patients to avoid driving or performing tasks that require concentration because this drug may cause sedation and dizziness.<br>• Warn patients to swallow capsules whole because chewing them may result in an anesthetized throat that can make breathing and swallowing difficult and cause choking.<br>• If using syrup, teach patients to avoid drinking water after swallowing because this action can dilute the drug and reduce its effectiveness.<br>• Instruct patients to notify the healthcare provider if symptoms have not improved within a few days or have worsened because this may indicate more serious respiratory problems. |
| dextromethorphan (Delsym, Robitussin, Triaminic, many others) 10–20 mg orally every 4 hours as needed *or* 30 mg orally every 6–8 hours as needed | • Tell patients to avoid driving or performing tasks that require concentration because this drug may cause sedation and dizziness.<br>• Warn parents not to give their child a higher or more frequent dose than prescribed because overdoses can cause dangerous CNS responses, respiratory depression, and seizures.<br>• If using syrup, teach patients to avoid drinking water after swallowing because this action can dilute the drug and reduce its effectiveness.<br>• Instruct patients to notify the healthcare provider if symptoms have not improved within a few days or have worsened, because this may indicate more serious respiratory problems. |
| codeine-containing antitussives: promethazine and codeine (Pentazine with codeine, many others) 7.5 to 30 mg of codeine | • Warn patients that taking additional narcotics (opioids) drugs can result in additional drowsiness.<br>• Warn patients and families (especially with older adult patients) to check respiratory rate frequently because respiratory depression is possible.<br>• Tell patients to watch for nausea and constipation because these are the most common side effects.<br>• Tell patients to avoid driving or performing tasks that require concentration because this drug may cause sedation and dizziness.<br>• Tell patients that physical addiction is rare, but it is possible because codeine is an opioid.<br>• Instruct the patient to increase fluids, because codeine can cause constipation.<br>• Instruct patients to notify the healthcare provider if symptoms have not improved within a few days or have worsened because this may indicate more serious respiratory problems. |

antitussives that contain narcotics (opioids) suppress the cough reflex by acting directly on the cough center in the medulla of the brain. Nonopioid antitussives reduce the cough reflex at its source by anesthetizing stretch receptors in respiratory passages, lungs, and pleura, and by decreasing their activity.

## Expected Side Effects, Adverse Reactions, and Drug Interactions

Common side effects of antitussives include drowsiness, dry mouth, nausea, and *postural hypotension* (low blood pressure resulting in dizziness when a person suddenly stands up). Some cough preparations contain a decongestant as well. Pseudoephedrine has been diverted for use as a substrate for the illegal synthesis of amphetamine and methamphetamine, and the sale and purchase of all OTC products containing pseudoephedrine or ephedrine are controlled and must be signed for at the pharmacy counter. Those antitussives that contain codeine are also likely to cause constipation.

Opioid antitussives have an additive effect with other CNS depressants, and the dosage should be reduced.

### ❖ Nursing Implications and Patient Teaching

◆ *Assessment.* Ask the patient about allergy to antitussives, presence of COPD that may influence the patient's response to an opioid, possibility of pregnancy, and use of other drugs or alcohol that may cause drug interactions. These conditions may be contraindications or precautions to the use of antitussives.

Ask about a history of a nonproductive cough or a prolonged and productive cough that may keep the patient awake at night or cause muscular pain.

◆ *Planning and implementation.* Patients with allergy to these drugs and patients with COPD who have problems with breathing are not usually given opioid antitussives. Opioid antitussives may cause drug dependence. Some of the antitussives are Schedule II controlled substances and will require a prescription written for no refills because the drugs may become abused.

These preparations may cause drowsiness. Teach the patient to avoid tasks that require alertness after taking the drug.

Antitussives are oral drugs that should be used only for short periods. Short therapy decreases the risk of rebound symptoms from prolonged use or the possibility of abuse.

◆ *Evaluation.* Check for therapeutic effects, including stopping of the cough, decreased frequency and duration of coughing spells, and ability to sleep better at night. Monitor the patient for adverse reactions and drug tolerance.

◆ *Patient and family teaching.* Tell the patient and family:
* Take the drug as prescribed and do not change the dose or frequency.
* Use caution when doing tasks that require alertness while taking an opioid antitussive because these drugs cause drowsiness.
* Overuse of codeine-containing antitussives may cause severe constipation.
* Do not take opioid antitussives with alcohol or any other drugs that slow the central nervous system (CNS) because the side effects will be intensified.
* Change positions slowly when getting up from a lying or sitting position because many antitussives occasionally cause lightheadedness, dizziness, or fainting when you get up quickly.

## Get Ready for the Next-Generation NCLEX® Examination!

### Key Points

* Allergies can be caused by any substance (allergen) that is inhaled, swallowed, or touched. Allergens are viewed as antigens by the immune system.
* IgE is the antibody that the immune system makes to counteract the antigens; it prompts the release of histamine and leukotrienes to combat the antigens.
* The release of histamine and leukotrienes causes the respiratory symptoms of runny nose; watery, itchy eyes; rashes; sneezing; and wheezing caused by bronchoconstriction.
* Antihistamines, leukotriene inhibitors, and decongestants can ease the symptoms of allergies.
* Nasal decongestants (sympathomimetics) can cause rebound congestion and should not be used for longer than 3 days.
* Asthma causes bronchoconstriction and difficulty breathing.
* Leukotriene inhibitors, bronchodilators, and anti-inflammatory drugs can help control asthma.
* COPD is a chronic disease involving upper and lower airways (bronchitis and emphysema).

* Short-acting bronchodilator agents (SABAs) are used as rescue drugs only because they work immediately to relieve a bronchospasm or asthma attack.
* Patients with asthma should always carry a SABA.
* Long-acting bronchodilator agents (LABAs) are used to control asthma and must be used every day as directed to prevent an asthma attack.
* Bronchodilators should be used first when multiple inhalers are prescribed. The patient should wait 5 minutes before using other inhalers.
* Teach patients the proper use of measured-dose inhalers (MDIs) and dry-powder inhalers (DPIs), as described in Boxes 8.1 and 8.2.
* Cortisone inhalers and nasal decongestants can cause fungal infections because they reduce the local immune responses.
* Cortisone inhalers are *not* rescue drugs and should be taken as prescribed every day to prevent asthma attacks and bronchospasms.
* Mucolytic drugs thin secretions and must be taken with water and increased fluids.
* Teach patients to use cough suppressants only as needed to prevent secretions from building up.
* Cough suppressants can cause CNS depression.

## Clinical Judgment and Next-Generation NCLEX® Examination-Style Questions

### Case Study

Mr. Clarke is a 75-year-old overweight retired coal miner with a 10-year history of COPD and asthma. He lives with his wife and two dogs in a low-income neighborhood that was flooded after a recent hurricane. He currently is smoking one pack of cigarettes a day and has done that for the last 25 years, despite a left cerebrovascular accident with right-sided weakness.

Medications: fluticasone/salmeterol two puffs twice a day
Albuterol inhaler two puffs every 8 hours and PRN

He is complaining of shortness of breath, chest discomfort, and cough and cold symptoms that started 3 days ago. Bilateral wheezes are heard in both lower bases of the lungs.

Vital signs:
Temperature:102°F (38.9°C)
Heart Rate: 112
Respirations: 30 breaths/minute
Blood Pressure: 160/94 mm Hg
Oxygen Saturation: 84% on 1 liter of oxygen per nasal cannula

1. **What is the priority action of the nurse?**

   1. Increase the oxygen to maintain an $O_2$ sat of 90%.
   2. Place the patient on a cardiac monitor.
   3. Apply personal protective equipment (PPE).
   4. Call the rapid rescue team.

2. **Which prescriptions/orders will the nurse expect the healthcare professional to write? Select all or any that apply.**

   1. Complete blood count (CBC)
   2. COVID-19 antigen test
   3. Venturi mask at 30%
   4. Nicotine patch
   5. Diphenhydramine 25 mg as needed for sleep
   6. Formoterol 15 mcg nebulizer every 12 hours
   7. Peak flow
   8. Chest x-ray
   9. Azithromycin 250 mg orally for 3 days

3. **Which of Mr. Clarke's modifiable risk factors should be assessed and or adjusted to improve symptom control? Select all or any that apply.**

   1. Pets
   2. Age
   3. Mold
   4. Cigarette smoking
   5. Right-sided weakness
   6. Weight

4. **Which additional drug would the nurse anticipate the healthcare provider will order to further improve direct relaxation of bronchial smooth muscle?**

   1. pseudoephedrine
   2. fexofenadine
   3. tiotropium
   4. montelukast

5. **Which statements made by the patient exhibits the correct use of using a metered dose SABA inhaler? Select all or any that apply.**

   1. I will wait 3 minutes between puffs.
   2. I will clean the plastic case once a day.
   3. I will inhale slowly for 3 to 5 seconds.
   4. I will hold my breath for 10 seconds after inhaling.
   5. I will hold the mouthpiece 1 to 2 inches away from my mouth.
   6. I will use a spacer when I can.
   7. I will shake the inhaler before I use it.
   8. If I start to shake when using, I will call the healthcare provider.
   9. I will rinse the spacer with running water once a week.

6. **Instructions: Match the number or name of each drug listed in the left column with the correct nursing implication in the right column.**

   | DRUG | NURSING IMPLICATION |
   | --- | --- |
   | 1. levalbuterol | ___ Should not be used in elderly patients |
   | 2. benzonatate | ___ Drug takes 2 weeks to control symptoms |
   | 3. guaifenesin | ___ Is used as a rescue drug |
   | 4. mometasone | ___ Is used as a controller drug |
   | 5. codeine | ___ Can cause oral candida |
   | 6. diphenhydramine | ___ Causes choking if not swallowed whole |
   | 7. formoterol | ___ Causes constipation |
   | 8. levocetirizine | ___ Administered with a full glass of water |
   | 9. fluticasone | ___Should be taken at night |

7. **A patient on fexofenadine every morning tells the nurse that it is no longer working, and her nasal congestion is getting worse again. What is the correct response of the nurse?**

   1. "You can only use this drug for 5 days or your symptoms will worsen."
   2. "You should take an additional antihistamine if using this drug no longer works."
   3. "Eating grapefruit or drinking grapefruit juice will decrease the drug effectiveness."
   4. "You should not use this drug because you are over 65 years of age."

8. **Which is the correct order when administering asthma medications?**

   1. Long-acting beta agonist (LABA), inhaled corticosteroid (IC), short-acting beta agonist (SABA)
   2. IC, SABA, LABA
   3. SABA, LABA, IC
   4. IC, LABA, SABA

9. **A patient is receiving a drug for the first time in the healthcare provider's office when he starts feeling lightheaded with fast, shallow breathing and tachycardia. What is the first action of the nurse?**

   1. Apply 100% oxygen via nonrebreather mask.
   2. Call 911.
   3. Administer epinephrine 0.3 mg intramuscular.
   4. Administer diphenhydramine 50 mg by mouth.

10. Which instruction will the nurse include in a teaching plan for a patient with asthma?

1. Keep a diary to give to the healthcare provider that identifies triggers that caused wheezing.
2. Wash clothes and bedding in cold water.
3. Stay inside during days of high air pollution.
4. Use an air cleaner inside the house.
5. Remove mold from showers and damp areas.
6. Avoid milk products.

## Next-Generation NCLEX® (NGN) Examination–Style Question

**History and Physical**
**1000**

CC: "I'm short of breath."

HPI: An 8-year-old client presents to the emergency department with complaints of shortness of breath since this morning. According to the child's parents, the child woke up this morning and immediately asked for their inhaler. The parents state, "The inhaler hasn't really helped, and they aren't feeling better."

PMH: asthma

Home medications: albuterol HFA

Physical Exam:

General: anxious

HEENT: pallor to lips, mucous membranes moist, nasal flaring

Respiratory: tachypnea, diffuse bilateral wheezing, labored breathing with prolonged expiration, coughing

Cardiovascular: S1, S2, no murmur or rub

Neuro: minimal tremor, no confusion

**Nurse's Notes**
**1015**

Provider at the bedside assessing the client. Orders received and implemented.

**1100**

The nurse returns to the client's room to reassess the client.

**Flow Sheet**
**1000**

Blood Pressure: 108/71 mm Hg

Heart Rate: 104/min
Respiratory Rate: 28/min
Oxygen Saturation: 90% on room air
Weight: 52 pounds (23.6 kg)

**1015**

albuterol nebulizer 1.25 mg STAT
budesonide nebulizer 0.25 mg immediately following albuterol nebulizer

The nurse is performing a reassessment of the client at **1100**.

**For each assessment finding, click to indicate whether the assessment finding would be expected to have increased, decreased, or no change based on the medications administered per the provider's orders.**

**Each row must have only one response option selected.**

| ASSESSMENT FINDING | INCREASE | DECREASE | NO CHANGE ANTICIPATED |
|---|---|---|---|
| Oxygen Saturation | | | |
| Blood Pressure | | | |
| Heart Rate | | | |
| Respiratory Rate | | | |
| Expiratory Phase | | | |
| Tremor | | | |
| Weight | | | |

See answer on Evolve at http://evolve.elsevier.com/Visovsky/LPNpharmacology/.

# Drugs Affecting the Renal/Urinary and Cardiovascular Systems

## Learning Outcomes

1. List the names, actions, possible side effects, and adverse effects of diuretic drugs.
2. Explain what to teach patients and families about diuretic drugs.
3. List the names, actions, possible side effects, and adverse effects of drugs for benign prostatic hyperplasia and overactive bladder.
4. Explain what to teach patients and families about drugs for benign prostatic hyperplasia and overactive bladder.
5. List the names, actions, possible side effects, and adverse effects of drugs for high blood cholesterol and drugs for high blood pressure.

6. Explain what to teach patients and families about drugs for high blood lipid levels and high blood pressure.
7. List the names, actions, possible side effects, and adverse effects of drugs for angina and heart failure.
8. Explain what to teach patients and families about drugs for angina and heart failure.
9. List the names, actions, possible side effects, and adverse effects of drugs for dysrhythmias.
10. Explain what to teach patients and families about drugs for dysrhythmias.

## Key Terms

**adrenergics** A category of drugs that affect nervous system control of various organs and tissues by activating or blocking receptors that respond to the body's natural adrenergic substances, epinephrine and norepinephrine.

**alpha$_1$-adrenergic antagonist** A type of adrenergic drug that lowers blood pressure by blocking the adrenergic receptor sites in blood vessel smooth muscle that, when activated, cause vasoconstriction and raise blood pressure.

**alpha$_2$-adrenergic agonist** A type of adrenergic drug that works centrally (in the brain) to turn on special alpha$_2$-receptors that, when normally activated, cause vasodilation and decrease blood pressure.

**angiotensin-converting enzyme inhibitor (ACE-I)** A type of renin-angiotensin-aldosterone system drug that reduces high blood pressure by stopping the conversion of angiotensin I to angiotensin II (the hormone that causes the vasoconstriction and increased aldosterone).

**angiotensin II receptor blocker (ARB)** A type of renin-angiotensin-aldosterone system drug that blocks the vasoconstrictor and aldosterone-secreting effects of angiotensin II. It lowers blood pressure by selectively blocking the binding of angiotensin II at receptor sites found in many tissues.

**antidysrhythmic** A drug that makes heart rhythm more regular and reduces serious dysrhythmias.

**antihyperlipidemic** A drug that treats hyperlipidemia, particularly by targeting blood cholesterol levels.

**antihypertensive** A drug that has the main purpose of lowering blood pressure.

**beta-blocker** An antagonist drug that blocks the activity of beta-adrenergic receptors, which lowers blood pressure and slows heart rate.

**calcium channel blockers** A class of antihypertensive drugs that lower blood pressure by reducing the effect of calcium in the heart muscle and in the smooth muscles of arteries.

**diuretic** A drug that decreases fluid volume by increasing urine output.

**hydroxymethylglutaryl-coenzyme A (HMG-CoA) reductase inhibitors (statins)** Antihyperlipidemic drugs that lower blood low-density lipoprotein levels by slowing cholesterol production in the liver.

**inotropic drug** A drug that affects contractility of the myocardium. A positive inotropic drug increases contractility; a negative inotropic drug decreases contractility of the myocardium.

**loop diuretic** A drug that increases urine output by blocking active transport of chloride, sodium, and potassium in the thick ascending loop of Henle.

**nitrates** A class of drugs that dilate blood vessels by relaxing vascular smooth muscle in the peripheral venous system and reducing resistance to blood flow in the arterial system.

**potassium-sparing diuretic** A drug that increases the excretion of water and sodium, leading to increased urine output without the loss of potassium in the urine.

**renin-angiotensin-aldosterone system (RAAS) drugs** Drugs that interfere with the actions of angiotensin II and aldosterone to decrease blood pressure by decreasing vasoconstriction and fluid volume; include angiotensin-converting enzyme inhibitors and angiotensin II receptor blockers.

**thiazides and thiazide-like diuretics** Drugs that increase urine output by preventing water, sodium, potassium, and chloride from being reabsorbed into the blood through the walls of the nephron.

**urinary antispasmodics** Drugs that improve symptoms of overactive bladder and reduce incontinence by relaxing the bladder muscle.

**vasodilators** A class of drugs that prevent contraction of smooth muscle cells in the blood vessel walls and act in other ways to cause them to dilate (widen or relax).

---

Interactions between the renal/urinary system and the cardiovascular system help to maintain fluid balance, delivery of nutrients, and removal of waste products from cells, tissues, and organs. Many of the drugs that affect one system also affect the functioning of the other.

## DRUGS THAT AFFECT THE RENAL/ URINARY SYSTEM

The renal/urinary system consists of two kidneys, two ureters, the bladder, and the urethra (Fig. 9.1). This system controls blood volume in the body and the content of the fluid portion of the blood because of its close connection with the cardiovascular system. Although the kidneys do not regulate what comes into the body, they balance all body fluids and the blood by carefully controlling which substances remain in the body and which leave the body. The kidneys act like a filter for the blood, removing wastes, excess substances, and extra fluid. Most drugs that affect the renal/urinary system change how much water and other substances are retained by the body or excreted in urine.

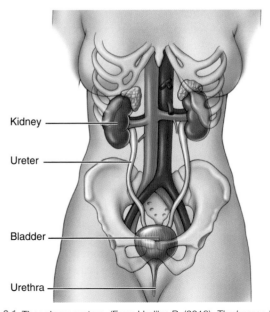

Fig. 9.1 The urinary system. (From Herlihy, B. (2018). *The human body in health and illness* (6th ed.). Elsevier.)

Labels: Kidney, Ureter, Bladder, Urethra

## DIURETICS

A **diuretic** is a drug that decreases fluid volume by increasing urine output. Although their site of action is the kidney, diuretics are chiefly used for cardiovascular problems, such as high blood pressure (HBP; hypertension) and heart failure, rather than for kidney problems. Diuretics typically work well, are safe, are well tolerated by the patient, and are cost effective.

Diuretics are usually classified into three groups: (1) thiazides (e.g., chlorothiazide, hydrochlorothiazide) and thiazide-like diuretics (e.g., metolazone, indapamide), (2) loop diuretics (e.g., furosemide, bumetanide), and (3) potassium-sparing diuretics (e.g., amiloride, triamterene, spironolactone). The most effective diuretics are those that work at the ascending loop of Henle in the nephron (Fig. 9.2).

>  **Memory Jogger**
>
> The three main categories of diuretics are:
> - Thiazide and thiazide-like diuretics
> - Loop diuretics
> - Potassium-sparing diuretics

## ACTIONS

**Thiazides and thiazide-like diuretics** work at the end of the ascending loop of Henle and the beginning of the distal convoluted tubule in the nephron (see Fig. 9.2). These drugs increase urine output by preventing water, sodium, potassium, and chloride from being reabsorbed into the blood through the walls of the nephron. As a result, the water and electrolytes stay within the tubules, making their way through the renal system into the bladder, and then are excreted from the body. Thiazide and thiazide-like drugs are the most commonly used type of diuretic and often are first-line agents in the management of HBP.

Over the long term, thiazides also dilate the smooth muscles in the smallest vessels in the arterial system, the arterioles. The heart does not have to work as hard to pump blood into the vascular system because the arterioles are dilated. Table 9.1 gives the dosages and nursing implications of selected thiazide diuretics.

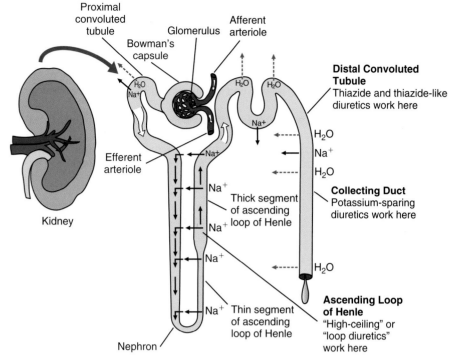

**Fig. 9.2** Sites of diuretic actions on the kidney and nephron. (From Workman, M. L., & LaCharity, L. A. (2016). *Understanding pharmacology* (2nd ed.). Elsevier.)

## Lifespan Considerations

### Pregnancy and Breast-Feeding

Thiazide diuretics are approved for use during pregnancy and may be used in low doses for breast-feeding mothers without adverse effects on the infant. More powerful diuretics are usually not recommended during pregnancy unless they are essential for the mother's health. High doses of diuretics in breast-feeding women may suppress lactation.

A **loop diuretic** is a drug that increases urine output by blocking active transport of chloride, sodium, and potassium in the thick ascending loop of Henle (see Fig. 9.2). Loop diuretics (also known as *high-ceiling diuretics*) are widely considered the most powerful of the diuretics. Use can result in significant decrease in fluid volume and increase in urine output. Loop diuretics are used in a variety of conditions, including heart failure, pulmonary edema, and cirrhosis of the liver with ascites.

Potassium is one of the major electrolytes that can be lost after loop diuretic administration. Monitor potassium levels carefully because significant changes in potassium can result in cardiac dysrhythmias. Table 9.1 provides the dosages and nursing implications of selected loop diuretics.

## Memory Jogger

Water always follows sodium. Diuretics that work by increasing sodium excretion in the urine always increase the water in urine output.

A **potassium-sparing diuretic** is a drug that increases the excretion of water and sodium, leading to increased urine output without the loss of potassium in the urine. They are called *potassium-sparing drugs* because they do not "waste" potassium, which often occurs with thiazide and loop diuretics. Potassium-sparing diuretics act by slowing the sodium pump in the collecting duct of the nephron so that more sodium and water are excreted as urine (see Fig. 9.2). Table 9.1 gives the dosages and nursing implications of selected potassium-sparing diuretics.

## Lifespan Considerations

### Older Adults

Older adult patients taking diuretics are more likely to develop postural hypotension, confusion, low potassium levels (hypokalemia) (except with potassium-sparing diuretics), and increased serum glucose levels. Lower dosages may be required based on patient responses. Monitor older adults who are taking diuretics more frequently for dehydration and symptoms of hypokalemia such as muscle weakness and irregular heartbeat.

### Uses

Healthcare providers prescribe diuretics for a variety of conditions, including HBP, heart failure, and cirrhosis of the liver. They are typically used in conditions that require a decrease in edema (i.e., decreased fluid volume). Diuretics can sometimes increase the excretion of other drugs (e.g., aspirin) in cases of overdose.

### Expected Side Effects

Common side effects of diuretics include urinary urgency and frequency. Other expected side effects include

**Table 9.1** Common Diuretics

*Thiazides* lower blood pressure through increasing urine output by preventing water, sodium, potassium, and chloride from going through the walls of the nephron to be reabsorbed into the blood. They also dilate arterioles by relaxing the smooth muscle in these blood vessel walls.

As with thiazide diuretics, *thiazide-like diuretics* lower blood pressure by preventing water, sodium, potassium, and chloride from going through the walls of the nephron to be reabsorbed into the blood. They also dilate arterioles by relaxing the smooth muscle in these blood vessel walls.

*Loop diuretics* increase urine output by blocking active transport of chloride, sodium, and potassium in the thick ascending loop of Henle.

*Potassium-sparing diuretics* increase excretion of water and sodium, which increases urine output without loss of potassium. They slow the sodium pump in the distal tubule of the nephron so that more sodium and water are excreted in urine.

| DRUGS/ADULT DOSAGE | NURSING IMPLICATIONS |
|---|---|
| **Thiazides** | |
| chlorothiazide (Diuril) 500–1000 mg orally given in one to two divided doses<br>hydrochlorothiazide 12.5–50 mg orally daily in one to two divided doses | • Weigh the patient daily while he or she is taking diuretics to monitor trends and prevent dehydration.<br>• In the acute care setting, monitor intake and output to make sure that the patient achieves fluid balance.<br>• Monitor potassium levels to assess that they are within normal levels because these drugs reduce blood potassium levels.<br>• Monitor the patient's basic metabolic panel to check for abnormal electrolytes, blood urea nitrogen, and/or creatinine. These laboratory tests can indicate fluid and electrolyte imbalance or kidney problems.<br>• Report below-normal potassium levels to the healthcare provider because low potassium levels can have serious effects on muscles and breathing.<br>• Inform the healthcare provider if your patient has a history of gout because thiazide diuretics can cause a flare-up.<br>• If the patient has diabetes, monitor his or her glucose level carefully because diuretics can cause elevated blood sugar.<br>• Hold diuretics if the patient has a blood pressure lower than 90/60 mm Hg because this can be a symptom of dehydration or other adverse effects. |
| **Thiazide-Like Diuretics** | |
| indapamide (Lozol) 1.25–2.5 mg orally daily<br>metolazone (Zaroxolyn) 2.5–5 mg orally daily<br>chlorthalidone (generic form) 12.5–25 mg orally daily. Some patients may have doses up to 50–100 mg daily<br>chlortalidone (Thalitone) 15–25 mg once daily | • Weigh the patient daily while he or she is taking diuretics to monitor trends and prevent dehydration.<br>• Monitor potassium levels to assess that they are within normal levels because these drugs reduce blood potassium levels.<br>• Report potassium levels lower than 3.5 mEq/L (3.5 mmol/L) to the healthcare provider because low potassium levels can have serious effects on heart rhythm. |
| **Loop Diuretics** | |
| bumetanide (Bumex) 0.5–2 mg orally once daily; 0.5–1.0 mg intramuscular (IM) to maximum of 10 mg per day in divided doses<br>furosemide 40–240 mg orally daily as a single dose or in two divided doses; in certain situations, may be given as IM or intravenous dose 20 to 40 mg, may be increased by 20 mg every 2 hours until desired effect is achieved | • Side effects are more severe with loop diuretics than with other diuretics because drugs in this class are the most powerful diuretics.<br>• Watch for symptoms of low potassium, including dry mouth, increased thirst, muscle cramps, fatigue, weakness, and mood changes because low potassium levels can have serious effects on muscles and breathing.<br>• Report potassium levels lower than 3.5 mEq/L (3.5 mmol/L) to the healthcare provider because low potassium levels can have serious effects on heart rhythm.<br>• Remind patients to stand up slowly to avoid orthostatic hypotension.<br>• Notify the healthcare provider if the patient reports decreased hearing or a ringing in the ears because loop diuretics can be ototoxic (damage hearing). Discontinuing the drug typically reverses the changes in hearing.<br>• Monitor blood glucose in patients with diabetes because these drugs can cause hyperglycemia.<br>• Check and record urine output to make sure the drug is working properly. You may need to empty the Foley catheter more frequently.<br>• Urination typically occurs within 1 hour, so inform the patient that he or she will need to be close to a bathroom to avoid urinary urgency or incontinence. |

| Table 9.1   Common Diuretics—cont'd | |
|---|---|
| **DRUGS/ADULT DOSAGE** | **NURSING IMPLICATIONS** |
| **Potassium-Sparing Diuretics** | |
| amiloride (Midamor) 5–20 mg orally daily<br>spironolactone (Aldactone) 25–100 mg orally daily as a single dose or in two divided doses.<br>spironolactone (CaroSpir suspension) 20–75 mg in single or divided doses<br>triamterene (Dyrenium) 100 mg orally twice daily | • Monitor potassium levels to assess whether they are within normal levels because higher-than-normal blood potassium levels can occur with these drugs.<br>• Report potassium levels greater than 5.0 mEq/L (5.0 mmol/L) to the healthcare provider because high potassium levels can cause dangerous cardiac problems.<br>• Teach patients the signs of a high potassium level, including confusion, irregular heartbeat, nervousness, numbness or tingling in the hands or feet, unusual fatigue, and a heavy feeling in the legs.<br>• Teach patients to stand up slowly to avoid orthostatic hypotension because these drugs decrease fluid volume and decrease blood pressure.<br>• Teach patients to avoid foods high in potassium (see Box 9.1) to prevent hyperkalemia.<br>• Remind patients to avoid salt substitutes because they are often high in potassium. |

dry mouth, increased thirst, and lightheadedness. Fluid and electrolyte imbalances are common side effects. Thiazide diuretics can cause an increase in uric acid, which can cause flare-ups of gout in certain patients. Table 9.1 provides specific dosages and nursing implications associated with specific classes of diuretics.

## Adverse Effects

Diuretics increase urine output and, as a result, dehydration is a major adverse effect. Signs and symptoms of dehydration include increased heart rate, low blood pressure, decreased urine output or dark yellow urine, dry mouth with a sticky coating on the tongue, and tenting of the chest or the forehead (if you pinch the skin, the skin remains elevated like a tent when you release it). Thiazides and loop diuretics can cause severe hypokalemia (low potassium level), whereas potassium-sparing diuretics can cause hyperkalemia (high potassium level). Signs of hypokalemia include muscle cramping, abnormal heart rhythm, and changes in reflexes. Signs of hyperkalemia include confusion, irregular heartbeat, numbness of the hands or feet, and a feeling of heaviness in the legs.

Loss of sodium can cause confusion, irritability, fatigue, and even seizures in some patients. A major adverse effect of all diuretics is severe low blood pressure that can result in falls, particularly in high-risk and older patients.

## Drug Interactions

Increased loss of potassium can result from use of thiazide or loop diuretics if the patient is taking corticosteroids or certain antibiotics. For patients with bipolar illness using lithium, the loss of sodium caused by diuretics can increase the risk for lithium toxicity. Potassium-sparing diuretics with angiotensin-converting enzyme inhibitors (ACE-Is) or angiotensin receptor blockers (ARBs) can lead to hyperkalemia. Patients taking potassium-sparing diuretics should avoid salt substitutes to decrease the risk of hyperkalemia.

### Top Tip for Safety

Potassium levels that are too high or too low can cause life-threatening dysrhythmias.

### ❖ Nursing Implications and Patient Teaching

◆ *Assessment.* Assess the patient for changes in vital signs (particularly a decrease in blood pressure). Carefully assess the patient for any signs of dehydration before giving any diuretic. Monitor daily weight for changes from a baseline weight (patient's normal weight). If the patient's weight is below his or her normal weight, contact the healthcare provider before giving the diuretic. Check the patient's most recent potassium level. If the level is below the normal range (which can be caused by thiazide or loop diuretics) or above the normal range (which can be caused by potassium-sparing diuretics), contact the healthcare provider before you give the drug.

◆ *Planning and implementation.* Give diuretics in the morning to avoid disturbing the patient's sleep at night. Tell patients that they will most likely experience urinary frequency and urgency and therefore should be near a bathroom or have access to a urinal or bedside commode after taking the drug. Make sure patients know to ask for help when getting up if needed. Tell patients to notify you if they have any weakness, muscle cramping, numbness or tingling in the extremities, or sensation of irregular heartbeat because these may be symptoms of a decreased potassium level.

Continue to monitor trends in daily weight, peripheral edema, and blood pressure while the patient is taking diuretics. For thiazides and loop diuretics, teach patients *to eat* foods that are high in potassium (Box 9.1). For potassium-sparing diuretics, teach patients to *avoid* foods that are high in potassium (see Box 9.1).

◆ *Patient and family teaching.* Tell the patient and family:
- Take the drug exactly as prescribed. Do not skip or double doses.
- Doses are best taken early in the day to avoid affecting sleep at night.
- If you are taking a thiazide or loop diuretic, include several high-potassium foods in your diet every day.
- If you are taking a potassium-sparing diuretic, avoid foods high in potassium and salt substitutes, which may be high in potassium.
- Use sunscreen and protective clothing to avoid skin irritation and sunburn because of photosensitivity.
- Report to your healthcare provider any signs of abnormal potassium levels such as muscle cramping, weakness, numbness or tingling in the extremities, or sensation of irregular heartbeat.
- It will be helpful to monitor daily weight to observe any change in fluid levels above or below your normal weight. Notify your healthcare provider if you experience any unintentional weight loss or weight gain.
- If you are taking a diuretic for your blood pressure, remember that HBP is not cured by drugs, and you should not stop taking the drug without consulting a healthcare provider.
- Avoid taking any over-the-counter (OTC) drugs without discussing this with your healthcare provider to avoid a drug interaction.

## DRUGS FOR BENIGN PROSTATIC HYPERPLASIA

Benign prostatic hyperplasia (BPH) is a noncancerous growth of the prostate gland that is frequently seen as men age. When the prostate gland becomes large enough, the patient can have problems urinating because the prostate puts pressure on the bladder and urethra (Fig. 9.3). Drugs used in the management of BPH are alpha$_1$-adrenergic receptor blockers, which relax the smooth muscle of the prostate and bladder outlet, and the testosterone inhibitors, which shrink the prostate. Both types of drug can help the patient pass urine more easily. Table 9.2 lists the dosages and nursing implications of selected drugs to treat BPH.

## BLADDER ANESTHETICS

Bladder anesthetics are drugs that, when taken orally, are excreted into the urine and act as a local anesthetic on the mucous membranes of the urinary tract. The only drug in this class is phenazopyridine. It can control symptoms of urinary irritation, including burning, pain, and urinary frequency, that often result from an acute urinary tract infection. Phenazopyridine is said to work like an "aspirin for the bladder." The usual adult dosage is 200 mg orally three times daily after meals for 2 days. Warn patients that this drug turns the urine an orange-red color that can stain the toilet and clothing. Phenazopyridine does not treat the cause of irritation to the bladder. It is not an antibiotic and cannot cure a urinary tract infection when used alone.

 **Top Tip for Safety**

Phenazopyridine can be used a maximum of 2 days. If the patient is still having symptoms of bladder irritation after 2 days, notify the healthcare provider.

### DRUGS FOR OVERACTIVE BLADDER

In people with overactive bladder (OAB), the detrusor muscle (bladder wall muscle) contracts before the

| Box 9.1 | Foods with High or Very High Potassium Levels | |
|---|---|---|
| **CATEGORY** | **HIGH (200–300 mg/serving)** | **VERY HIGH (> 300 mg/serving)** |
| Fruits | Apricots (canned)<br>Oranges (1 medium)<br>Orange juice<br>Peaches, fresh (1 medium) | Bananas (1 small)<br>Mango (1 medium)<br>Dried fruits (¼ cup)<br>Prune juice |
| Vegetables | Asparagus (4 spears)<br>Beets, fresh or cooked<br>Brussels sprouts<br>Okra | Beet greens (¼ cup)<br>Black beans, cooked (½ cup)<br>Potatoes with skin; baked potato (½ medium)<br>Baby carrots (10 pieces)<br>Sweet potatoes, yams |
| Miscellaneous | Peanut butter (2 tablespoons)<br>Nuts and seeds (1 ounce)<br>Chocolate (1.5-ounce bar)<br>Salmon, canned (3 ounces) | Bouillon, low sodium (1 cup)<br>Milk, chocolate (1 cup)<br>Pizza (2 slices)<br>Salt substitute (¼ teaspoon)<br>Yogurt (6 ounces)<br>Milkshake (1 cup)<br>Cappuccino (1 cup) |

Modified from Mahan, L. K., & Raymond, J. (2017). *Krause's food & the nutrition care process* (14th ed.). Elsevier; USDA Agricultural Research Service, FoodData Central. (2019). https://fdc.nal.usda.gov.

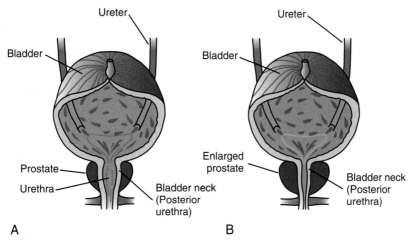

Fig. 9.3 (A) Normal prostate gland. (B) Enlarged prostate gland showing the narrowing of the urethra, decreasing urine flow. (From Workman, M. L., & LaCharity, L. A. (2016). *Understanding pharmacology* (2nd ed.). Elsevier.)

## Table 9.2   Common Drugs for Benign Prostatic Hyperplasia

*Dihydrotestosterone (DHT) inhibitors* shrink the prostate by working as a counterfeit drug that mimics testosterone and binds to the enzyme that normally converts testosterone to DHT, its most powerful form. With less DHT in the prostate, the cells do not receive the signal to grow, and the gland shrinks and exerts less pressure on the urethra, allowing better urine flow.

*Selective alpha$_1$ blockers* relax smooth muscle tissue in the prostate gland, the neck of the bladder, and the urethra by binding to the alpha$_1$-adrenergic receptors in these tissues. When the receptors are activated, the smooth muscle constricts, tightening the prostate, which increases the pressure and squeezes the urethra. When the receptors are bound to selective alpha$_1$ blockers, smooth muscle relaxes, placing less pressure on the urethra and improving urine flow.

| DRUGS/ADULT DOSAGE | NURSING IMPLICATIONS |
|---|---|
| **Dihydrotestosterone (DHT) Inhibitors** | |
| dutasteride (Avodart) 0.5 mg orally once daily<br>finasteride (Proscar) 5 mg orally once daily | • Teach patients that the most common side effect of these drugs is a decreased interest in sexual activity because knowing about the side effects reduces anxiety when they occur.<br>• Instruct patients to report to their healthcare provider breast enlargement, nipple drainage, or pain in the testicles because these drugs may affect other hormones and sex tissues.<br>• Warn patients and family members that pregnant women should not handle or touch these drugs because they can cause birth defects when absorbed through the skin.<br>• Teach men who are having sex with a pregnant woman to wear a condom to prevent exposure of the fetus because this drug is present in seminal fluid. |
| **Selective Alpha1 Blockers** | |
| alfuzosin (Uroxatral) 10 mg orally once daily with food<br>silodosin (Rapaflo) 8 mg orally once daily with food<br>tamsulosin (Flomax) 0.4–0.8 mg orally once daily 30 minutes after a meal<br>terazosin 1–10 mg orally once daily at bedtime | • Ask patients who are taking tamsulosin whether they have an allergy to sulfa drugs because tamsulosin is made from a sulfonamide and may cause an allergic reaction in patients who are allergic to sulfa drugs.<br>• Teach patients that the most common side effect of these drugs is a decreased interest in sexual activity because knowing about the side effects reduces anxiety when they occur.<br>• Warn patients to change positions slowly because these drugs lower blood pressure and can cause dizziness. |

bladder is full (Fig. 9.4). The person with OAB feels a sudden, urgent need to urinate (urgency) and may lose bladder control before reaching a toilet (urinary incontinence). Although OAB can occur in men or women, the problem is more common in women. The prevalence increases with age, and it can significantly affect quality of life.

Drugs prescribed for OAB are **urinary antispasmodics**, which improve symptoms and reduce incontinence by relaxing the bladder muscle. Table 9.3 gives the dosages and nursing implications of selected urinary antispasmodics.

## DRUGS THAT AFFECT THE CARDIOVASCULAR SYSTEM

The primary purpose of the cardiovascular system is to supply oxygenated blood that includes water (plasma), nutrients, and hormones to tissues and organs while removing carbon dioxide and waste products for elimination. Any breakdown in cardiovascular functioning can lead to uncomfortable symptoms, decreased quality of life, and even death if not managed carefully.

The cardiovascular system consists of the heart and blood vessels working together to move blood throughout the body. Using specialized cardiac muscle and nerve cells, electrical impulses cause the heart muscle to contract, pumping blood from the heart into the aorta and to the arteries (Fig. 9.5). The oxygenated blood moves through the arteries to the arterioles and then to capillaries, where oxygen exchanges with carbon dioxide. The deoxygenated blood moves from the capillaries to the venules and then to the larger veins and back into the vena cava, where it returns to the heart.

Healthcare providers use a variety of approaches to prevent or manage symptoms and to treat abnormalities in the cardiovascular system. Some drugs work by helping to prevent high cholesterol levels that narrow arteries, others by reducing HBP, and still others by managing symptoms associated with diseases of the heart itself.

This chapter addresses some of the most common cardiovascular drugs that you may see in practice to give you an overview of how these drugs can help provide the best health and quality of life possible for your patients. The discussion proceeds from drugs typically used to reduce the risk of cardiovascular disease to those that treat cardiovascular disease.

Two major risk factors for cardiovascular disease are high levels of blood lipids (hyperlipidemia) and HBP (hypertension). Effective drug therapy can modify both of these risk factors. High levels of blood lipids, including cholesterol, can lead to thickening of the lining of arteries with fatty plaque, a condition called *atherosclerosis* (Fig. 9.6). Eventually, atherosclerosis blocks some blood flow through the arteries. When HBP coexists with atherosclerosis, greater amounts of plaque occur with further blood vessel narrowing, and the heart has to work harder to pump blood through them.

Decreased blood flow through the coronary arteries that supply the heart muscle with oxygen can result in ischemia (lack of oxygen to the tissue) and pain called *angina*. To treat angina, selected cardiovascular drugs can dilate (widen) the coronary arteries, which delivers more blood and oxygen to the heart muscle. If the blood flow is severely impaired through the coronary arteries or a clot forms in a coronary artery, the patient can experience a myocardial infarction (heart attack) that results from a severe lack of oxygen to the heart muscle.

Over time, the ability of the heart to pump decreases in patients with prolonged HBP and/or changes in heart muscle resulting from a myocardial infarction. The decreased ability of the heart to pump effectively is called *heart failure*. Heart failure is managed by using a variety of cardiovascular drugs to improve the ability of the heart to pump and reduce the associated symptoms.

Damage to the heart muscle from HBP and atherosclerosis causes changes in the electrical conduction system

**Normal Bladder**
Detrusor muscle
contracts when
bladder is full

Urine

Urethra

**Overactive Bladder**
Detrusor muscle
contracts before
bladder is full

Urine

Urethra

**Fig. 9.4** Pathophysiology of overactive bladder. (From Workman, M. L., & LaCharity, L. A. (2016). *Understanding pharmacology* (2nd ed.). St. Louis: Elsevier.)

of the heart (see Fig. 9.5A). These changes can result in dysrhythmias (abnormal heart rhythms). The dysrhythmias can cause significant decreases in cardiac output and even death if not managed effectively. Several cardiovascular drugs are used to restore normal heart rhythms.

The cardiovascular drug groups discussed in this chapter include cholesterol-lowering drugs, blood pressure–lowering drugs, blood vessel dilators (antianginals), drugs to improve heart muscle contraction (positive inotropic drugs), and drugs to make electrical conduction through the heart more regular (antidysrhythmics). A patient may be taking drugs from a variety of cardiovascular drug categories.

 **Memory Jogger**

The five most common types of cardiovascular drugs are:
- Antihyperlipidemics
- Antihypertensives
- Drugs for angina
- Drugs for heart failure
- Antidysrhythmics

## ANTIHYPERLIPIDEMICS

Hyperlipidemia is the condition of having high levels of lipids (primarily cholesterol) and other fatty acids in the blood. **Antihyperlipidemics** are drugs that treat

| Table 9.3 | Common Drugs for Overactive Bladder |
|---|---|

*Urinary antispasmodics* inhibit involuntary nerve-induced contractions of the detrusor muscle in the bladder wall, allowing the bladder to relax and hold more urine without the strong urge to urinate.

| DRUGS/ADULT DOSAGE | NURSING IMPLICATIONS |
|---|---|
| **Urinary Antispasmodics** | |
| oxybutynin (Ditropan) 2.5–5 mg orally two to three times daily<br>oxybutynin (Ditropan XL) 5–10 mg orally once daily<br>oxybutynin transdermal patch (Oxytrol) 3.9 mg/day applied transdermally every 3–4 days<br>oxybutynin chloride 10% topical gel (Gelnique) one sachet or actuation topically once daily<br>tolterodine (Detrol) 1–2 mg orally twice daily<br>tolterodine (Detrol LA) 2–4 mg orally once daily<br>solifenacin (Vesicare) 5–10 mg orally once daily<br>darifenacin (Enablex) 7.5–15 mg orally once daily<br>trospium chloride (Sanctura) 20 mg orally twice daily 1 hour before meals or on an empty stomach<br>trospium chloride extended release (Sanctura XR) 60 mg once daily 1 hour before breakfast | • Tell patients that common side effects include dry mouth, dry eyes, headache, and constipation because knowing the expected side effects reduces anxiety.<br>• Teach patients to check their heart rate at least once daily and report irregularities or chest pain because these are symptoms of an adverse reaction.<br>• Remind patients to avoid taking antihistamines with these drugs because the combination can cause urinary retention and/or constipation.<br>• Teach patients to weigh themselves and report to the prescriber weight gain (more than 2 lb/day) or increased swelling because these drugs can cause urinary retention and heart failure.<br>• Remind patients to avoid becoming overheated or dehydrated during exercise or hot weather because these drugs decrease sweating and increase the risk for heatstroke.<br>• Teach patients to avoid consuming alcohol within 2 hours of taking these drugs because side effects such as drowsiness are increased.<br>• Teach patients to avoid driving or any other activities that require clear vision until they know how the drug will affect them because this class of drugs can cause blurred vision.<br>• Teach patients using the transdermal patch system to remove the old patch before applying a new one to prevent drug overdose.<br>• Teach patients using the transdermal patch system to rotate sites (abdomen, hip, or buttock) with every application.<br>• Teach patients using the topical gel to squeeze the entire contents of one packet sachet or one actuation of the metered-dose pump into the palm of the hand or directly onto the skin then gently rub the gel into the skin until it is dried. Wash hands with soap and water right away after applying. Do not exercise, bathe, or swim for at least 1 hour after applying to avoid washing away the drug. |

hyperlipidemia, particularly by targeting blood cholesterol levels. The body needs a certain amount of cholesterol for making healthy cell membranes, hormones, vitamin D, and bile acids, and it is a normal and vital part of blood plasma. The liver produces much of the body's cholesterol. Cholesterol levels in blood are a combination of the cholesterol ingested in the diet and the cholesterol produced by the liver. The liver contributes much more cholesterol to blood cholesterol levels than does the food you eat.

Blood lipids (cholesterol and other fatty acids) move through the body attached to protein carriers called *lipoproteins*. When considering cardiovascular disease and atherosclerosis, the most important lipoproteins are the high-density lipoproteins (HDLs), which are protective, and low-density lipoproteins (LDLs), which are harmful.

As you think about drugs for reducing cholesterol, you can consider the effect of the drug on the levels of "good" cholesterol (protective HDLs) and "bad" cholesterol (harmful LDLs). HDLs remove cholesterol from the blood and transport it to the liver. If you have ever seen a catfish in action, you can see that it acts as a scavenger for food and cleans the bottom of the fish tank. HDLs scavenge harmful lipids from the blood so that they do not stick to blood vessels and contribute to plaque. LDL cholesterols, on the other hand, are major contributors to the onset and progression of heart disease and stroke.

For some patients, lipid levels can be improved through diet, exercise, and lifestyle changes. Others may require lipid-lowering drugs (antihyperlipidemics). Most lipid-lowering drugs tend to reduce LDLs and other fatty acids. Some drugs can increase the scavenger HDLs.

### Memory Jogger

LDLs are the "bad" cholesterol; HDLs are the "good" cholesterol.

Four classes of drugs are used to treat hyperlipidemia: HMG-CoA reductase inhibitors (statins), selective cholesterol absorption inhibitors, fibric acid derivatives, and bile acid sequestrants. Niacin or nicotinic acid was once commonly prescribed for hyperlipidemia but is rarely used today because of its side effects and because it is no longer considered to be effective.

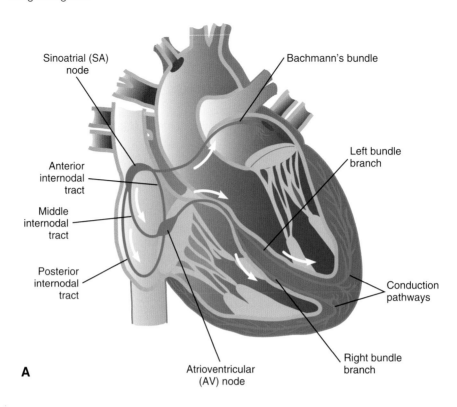

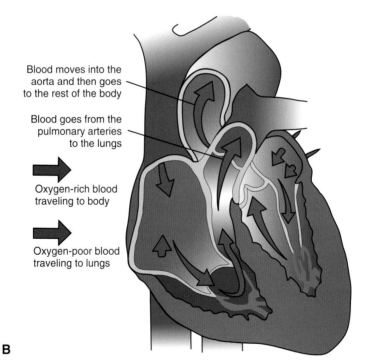

Fig. 9.5  (A) Using specialized cardiac muscle and nerve systems, electrical impulses cause the heart muscle to contract. (B) The contraction pumps blood from the heart into the aorta and to the arteries. (From Workman, M. L., & LaCharity, L. A. (2016). *Understanding pharmacology* (2nd ed.). Elsevier.)

 **Memory Jogger**

The four classes of antihyperlipidemics are:
- HMG-CoA reductase inhibitors (most common)
- Cholesterol absorption inhibitors
- Fibric acid derivatives (fibrates)
- Bile sequestrants

## HMG-CoA REDUCTASE INHIBITORS (STATINS)

### Actions

**Hydroxymethylglutaryl-coenzyme A (HMG-CoA) reductase inhibitors (statins)** are antihyperlipidemic drugs that lower blood LDL levels by slowing cholesterol production in the liver. They do not remove dietary cholesterol from the blood. The statins are the most

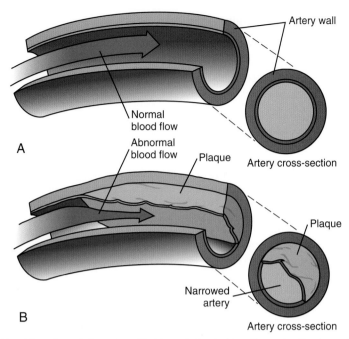

Fig. 9.6 (A) Normal blood flow through the artery. (B) Artery obstructed by atherosclerotic plaque. Notice the restricted blood flow through the artery. (From Workman, M. L., & LaCharity, L. A. (2016). *Understanding pharmacology* (2nd ed.). Elsevier.)

effective drugs for lowering LDL levels and raising HDL levels. Table 9.4 provides the dosages and nursing implications of commonly prescribed HMG-CoA reductase inhibitors. Consult a drug reference source or handbook for information on other statin drugs.

## Uses

The main use of statins is to lower blood LDL levels to reduce the risk for atherosclerosis, hypertension, heart attack, peripheral arterial disease, and stroke. Although other benefits have been described for statins, they are approved only to lower blood cholesterol levels.

## Expected Side Effects

The most common side effects of statins are abdominal pain, headache, diarrhea, muscle pain (myalgia), and joint discomfort. Other side effects are sore throat and heartburn. Patients with diabetes may experience elevated blood glucose levels.

## Adverse Effects

The action of statins is in the liver, and liver function is therefore affected to some degree. Liver failure has been reported rarely. With higher doses of statins, patients may experience rhabdomyolysis (muscle breakdown). This is a very serious condition that can be life-threatening. Signs and symptoms of rhabdomyolysis include general muscle soreness, muscle pain, muscle weakness, stomach pain, and brown (tea-colored) urine. The brown urine results from the kidneys trying to filter the products of muscle breakdown. Ultimately, patients experience kidney failure.

Statins are dangerous if used during pregnancy. Although cholesterol is important for normal brain

development, if taken during pregnancy statins can lower the cholesterol levels in the fetus, which results in brain deformities. For the same reason, statins are contraindicated in women who are breast-feeding.

> ### 🍂 Lifespan Considerations
> #### Pregnancy and Breast-Feeding
> Statins are contraindicated during pregnancy and breast-feeding because of the effects of lower cholesterol levels on the developing brain.

## Drug Interactions

Alcohol and acetaminophen increase the liver toxicity effects of statins. Aspirin and antacids decrease the effectiveness of statins. Grapefruit juice can increase the concentration of statins in the blood and should be avoided to reduce the risk for toxic side effects.

### ❖ Nursing Implications and Patient Teaching

◆ *Assessment.* Carefully assess the patient's dietary patterns. Even though the patient is taking a drug to decrease cholesterol, it is not a good reason to continue eating foods high in saturated fats, such as fatty meats, fried foods, and baked goods made with trans fats (e.g., donuts, cookies).

Review liver function test results in the medical record before giving statins. If you see any abnormalities or have questions, contact the registered nurse (RN) or the healthcare provider. If you are working in a community setting, it will be important to know whether your female patients are pregnant or planning pregnancy because statins are very dangerous to the fetus. Women must avoid statins while breast-feeding. In

Table 9.4    Common HMG-CoA Reductase Inhibitors (Statins)

*HMG-CoA reductase inhibitors (statins)* lower blood low-density lipoprotein levels by slowing liver production of cholesterol. They do not remove dietary cholesterol from the blood.

| DRUGS/ADULT DOSAGE | NURSING IMPLICATIONS |
|---|---|
| **Hmg-CoA Reductase Inhibitors (Statins)** | |
| atorvastatin (Lipitor) 10–80 mg orally once daily<br>fluvastatin (Lescol) 20–40 mg orally once or twice daily<br>fluvastatin extended release (Lescol XL) 80 mg orally once daily<br>lovastatin 10–80 mg orally once daily with evening meal; the 80 mg dose may be given in divided dose<br>lovastatin extended release (Altoprev) 20–60 mg orally once daily with evening meal<br>pravastatin (Pravachol) 40–80 mg orally once daily<br>rosuvastatin (Crestor) 5–40 mg orally once daily<br>simvastatin (Zocor, FloLipid) 5–40 mg orally once daily in the evening | • Remind patients to remain on a low-cholesterol diet while taking statins because drugs do not reverse a high-cholesterol diet.<br>• Check drug references for individual statins because some have best effects when taken in the evening and others can be taken without regard to meals for best effect.<br>• Teach patients to avoid alcohol because drinking alcohol puts stress on the liver.<br>• Tell patients to report severe muscle aches, changes in urine color, or decreased urine output because statins can cause rhabdomyolysis, a disorder resulting from broken muscle cells that damage the kidneys.<br>• Teach patients that they should avoid grapefruit juice because it interacts with statins and can cause drug toxicity.<br>• Remind patients to follow up with their healthcare provider for regular laboratory work because statins can cause liver problems.<br>• Monitor patients for signs of liver problems, such as nausea, yellowing of the eyes or roof of the mouth, darkened urine, or light-colored stools, because these symptoms suggest damage to the liver.<br>• Side effects are rare, but some patients experience GI symptoms, including upset stomach, gas, constipation, and stomach cramps. Some patients experience mild muscle or joint ache. If patients experience these symptoms, remind them to contact their healthcare provider rather than stopping the drug. |

other adults, assess for any symptoms of impaired liver function. Ask patients about their use of alcohol before starting statin therapy. Heavy use of alcohol contributes to liver problems while taking statins, and patients need to understand this before beginning therapy.

◆ *Planning and implementation.* While on statin therapy, patients may have scheduled blood lipid levels drawn as ordered by the prescriber. Levels are typically measured 4 to 12 weeks after beginning statin therapy and after dosage changes to evaluate the response to treatment. Patients need to fast at least 12 hours before having blood samples drawn for measurement of cholesterol, HDL, LDL, and triglycerides.

The timing of statin administration may impact patient response. Consulting a pharmacist or drug reference is helpful in determining the best time to give a specific statin. Some statins work best when given in the evening, many can be taken once a day without regard to meals, and some may need to be taken twice a day. Do not give a statin with grapefruit juice because it inhibits drug breakdown, allowing higher drug blood levels that can cause toxic side effects.

◆ *Evaluation.* Monitor for expected side effects, including headache, upset stomach, sore throat, and diarrhea. These side effects are typically short term and get better over time. Check the patient for jaundice (yellowing of the skin and mucous membranes, including whites of the eyes) and for darkening of the urine or clay-colored stools, which are indications of liver toxicity (hepatotoxicity). Patients who exhibit these symptoms should

be given liver function tests. Report any severe muscle aches or signs of liver problems to the RN or healthcare provider immediately.

### Top Tip for Safety

Immediately report to the healthcare provider any severe muscle ache or signs of liver problems that the patient has noticed, such as jaundice or dark urine, because those symptoms can be signs of serious adverse effects of statins.

◆ *Patient and family teaching.* Tell the patient and family:
• Lifestyle changes such as exercise, a low-cholesterol diet, and good weight management are just as important as taking the statins to help prevent cardiovascular disease.
• Make note of the recommended best time of day to take your statin, and take it at the same time each day.
• Inform your healthcare provider if you may be pregnant or plan to become pregnant because statins can cause birth defects.
• Avoid grapefruit juice when you are taking statins because it can cause the drug to accumulate in the blood and increase the risk of toxic effects.
• If you have any signs of liver problems, such as light-colored stools, yellowish tinge to the skin or eyes, or dark urine, notify your healthcare provider immediately because these are indications of adverse drug effects.
• If you have severe muscle aches, notify your healthcare provider because this is an indication of a possible adverse drug effect.

- Expected side effects include headache, upset stomach, and mild achiness. These usually get better within a few weeks after starting the statin.
- Web sites such as that of the American Heart Association (https://www.heart.org) have resources to help you learn about cholesterol and low-cholesterol diets.

## NONSTATIN ANTIHYPERLIPIDEMIC DRUGS

Nonstatin antihyperlipidemic drugs use a variety of actions to reduce the levels of blood cholesterol derived from ingested food. These drugs are used less often because they are not as effective as statins. They would most likely be prescribed if the person is not responsive to or unable to tolerate statins.

### Selective Cholesterol Absorption Inhibitors

Selective cholesterol absorption inhibitors are the next most commonly prescribed drugs for lowering cholesterol. Ezetimibe was the first agent introduced in this category. The drug stays in the intestinal wall and acts on the intestinal epithelial cells to limit the absorption of cholesterol from food and from other sources in the body. Selective cholesterol absorption inhibitors are often combined with statins in pill form to give the patient the best chance of lowering LDL cholesterol and raising HDL cholesterol.

### Fibric Acid Derivatives (Fibrates)

Gemfibrozil and fenofibrate are the preferred drugs among fibric acid derivatives because they are more effective and have fewer adverse effects than some other drugs. Both are highly effective at lowering triglyceride levels and increasing HDL levels, but they have little effect on lowering LDL levels. Gemfibrozil and fenofibrate are generally well tolerated but can cause liver toxicity and cholelithiasis (gallstones). These drugs are not recommended for patients with a history of gallbladder disease.

### Bile Acid Sequestrants

Bile acid sequestrants, such as cholestyramine and colestipol, increase excretion of cholesterol and reduce LDL levels. They do this by forming a solid compound with bile salts, which increases bile loss through the feces (stool). Normal fat digestion is disturbed, and many patients do not tolerate these drugs because of uncomfortable GI side effects (e.g., constipation, bloating, nausea). Bile acid sequestrants are not absorbed and do not have some of the severe systemic adverse effects that other antihyperlipidemics have.

Other drugs taken with bile acid sequestrants may not get absorbed because they act by binding to substances in the intestinal tract. In particular, bile acid sequestrants reduce absorption of fat-soluble vitamins (i.e., vitamins A, D, E, and K), and the patient may show symptoms of vitamin deficiency, especially if taking the drugs in high doses or for a long time. Watch for bleeding problems that may result from vitamin K deficiency, which affects the clotting cycle.

## NIACIN OR NICOTINIC ACID

You may have heard of niacin as one of the B-complex vitamins found in animal proteins, green vegetables, and whole wheat. Although recent guidelines suggest that niacin is not recommended for reducing cardiovascular risk, you may see patients in your clinical practice who are taking niacin. The main problem with niacin use is the expected side effect of flushing (sensation of warmth or "prickly heat" with redness that usually occurs on the face, neck, or trunk). Flushing occurs shortly after taking the drug and is very uncomfortable. Taking aspirin 30 minutes before niacin and increasing the niacin dosage from 500 to 1000 mg three times daily very slowly over 3 to 4 weeks may reduce the flushing. Flushing may decrease over time while taking the drug. Other side effects include indigestion, gas, hot flashes, rapid heart rate, and sweating.

❖ **Nursing Implications and Patient Teaching**
◆ *Assessment.* As with statins, it is important to assess the patient's diet history, including his or her ability to adhere to lifestyle recommendations. These factors are just as important as the drug therapy because no cholesterol-reducing drug cures hyperlipidemia. Assess the patient's liver function tests; if there are any abnormal results, notify the RN or the healthcare provider. Assess the patient's use of alcohol because alcohol can increase the risk of damage to the liver.

◆ *Planning and implementation.* For patients taking the nonstatin antihyperlipidemic drugs that affect absorption of cholesterol from the GI tract, you will likely be giving supplemental doses of vitamins A, D, and K. As for statins, carefully review the proper timing of these drugs in relation to meals. By themselves, selective cholesterol absorption inhibitors can be given without regard to meals. However, they are often combined with statins, and their timing would be similar to that of statin drugs.

For best results, fibric acid derivatives such as gemfibrozil should be given 30 minutes before the morning and evening meals. Bile acid sequestrants are usually taken one or two times a day before meals. The drugs come in powder form and must be mixed with water, milk, or juice. Monitor how well the patient is tolerating the drug. If there are any signs of severe GI symptoms such as abdominal pain, severe bloating, or severe constipation, notify the RN or the healthcare provider. If the patient is taking niacin, make sure to notify the healthcare provider in case they want the patient to discontinue the drug.

◆ *Evaluation.* The healthcare provider will order follow-up blood tests to determine the patient's responses to cholesterol-lowering therapy. Compare these results with those obtained before the drug was started to evaluate drug effectiveness and any changes in liver function.

◆ *Patient and family teaching.* Tell the patient and family:
- Take the drug at the time prescribed because timing is important for cholesterol-lowering drugs.
- Notify your healthcare provider and your pharmacist that you are taking a cholesterol-lowering drug so that they will carefully review drug interactions with other drugs you are taking.
- If you have any significant side effects, notify your healthcare provider before you consider stopping the drug. Dosages may be adjusted by your healthcare provider, or you may be switched to a different drug.
- The drugs do not by themselves cure your high cholesterol problem. Continue making healthy lifestyle choices.

 **Bookmark This!**

The American Heart Association has great information for you and your patients about heart health and heart disease: https://www.heart.org.

## ANTIHYPERTENSIVE DRUGS

Blood pressure is the pressure of circulating blood on the walls of arteries and veins as the blood moves through the body with each contraction and relaxation of the heart. A healthy blood pressure maintains circulation to major organs and all parts of the body during rest and during activity. Blood pressure that is too high or too low can cause critical problems that affect blood vessels, organs, and tissues. Many things can affect the blood pressure, including heart rate, how well the heart contracts, certain hormones, blood volume, physical activity, and stress.

Hypertension (HBP) is a disorder in which the patient's blood pressure is consistently elevated above normal values. If left untreated, hypertension damages major organs, including the heart, brain, and kidneys. Managing hypertension dramatically reduces the odds of heart attack, stroke, and kidney failure.

There are two kinds of hypertension. In primary hypertension, the specific cause is unknown. In secondary hypertension, the blood pressure changes result from a specific cause. If the cause is treated or managed, the blood pressure naturally returns to normal. About 90% of cases are primary hypertension, which cannot be cured but can be well managed with good drug therapy. This section focuses on managing primary hypertension.

Although *hypertension* is the technical term, we use the phrase *high blood pressure (HBP)* to discuss drugs and nursing management. In the past, use of the term *hypertension* created the impression that a person would be feeling "hyper" if his or her blood pressure was too high, even though HBP is often without symptoms. When patients felt calm, they believed their blood pressure was normal and did not think they needed drugs. This led to much confusion between patients and their healthcare providers. *HBP* is a simpler term, and patients understand it better than hypertension.

According to the American Heart Association, HBP affects as many as one in three adults 20 years of age or older. Although the exact cause of HBP is unknown, risk factors include a family history of HBP, black race, overweight or obesity, physical inactivity, current cigarette smoking or exposure to secondhand smoke, and too much alcohol consumption. People with diabetes, elevated blood lipid levels, or kidney disease also are at higher risk for HBP. Risk increases with age, and it is not surprising that as the population ages, there will be a need for a good understanding of HBP management. Whatever the cause, when HBP is untreated or poorly treated, serious health problems and even death can develop.

Severity of HBP is classified according to the stages listed in Table 9.5. The term *prehypertension* has been eliminated in favor of the more accurate term *elevated blood pressure*. Accurate diagnosis is essential to determine the best treatments for patients. LPNs have an important role in using the proper technique for blood pressure screening, and you will work with the healthcare team to reinforce recommended lifestyle changes (Box 9.2).

If lifestyle changes alone are not effective in reducing the patient's blood pressure, healthcare providers will begin drug therapy. Choices of prescribed drugs may depend on the patient's age and race and whether the patient has diabetes or chronic kidney disease, which can complicate treatment. Do not hesitate to communicate with the healthcare provider if you are not clear about your patient's blood pressure goals.

An **antihypertensive** is a drug that has the main purpose of lowering blood pressure. A variety of drugs can lower blood pressure by different mechanisms. Not all patients respond to any one class of blood pressure–lowering drugs in the same way.

| Table **9.5** | Categories of Blood Pressure | | |
|---|---|---|---|
| **CLASSIFICATION** | **SYSTOLIC BLOOD PRESSURE** | | **DIASTOLIC BLOOD PRESSURE** |
| Normal | < 120 mm Hg | and | < 80 mm Hg |
| Elevated | 120–129 mm Hg | and | < 80 mm Hg |
| Stage 1 hypertension | 130–139 mm Hg | or | 80–89 mm Hg |
| Stage 2 hypertension | ≥ 140 mm Hg | or | ≥ 90 mm Hg |

From Whelton, P. K., Carey, R. M., Aronow, W. S., et al. (2018). 2017 ACC/AHA/AAPA/ABC/ACPM/AGS/APhA/ASH/ASPC/NMA/PCNA Guideline for the prevention, detection, evaluation, and management of high blood pressure in adults: A report of the American College of Cardiology/American Heart Association task force on clinical practice guidelines. *Journal of the American College of Cardiology, 71*(6), 127–248.

Drug therapy for HBP often requires trial periods to establish the right drug or drug combinations to help a patient achieve his or her blood pressure goal. For the general population, non-black patients typically begin with thiazide diuretics. These drugs may be prescribed alone or in combination with angiotensin-converting enzyme inhibitors (ACE-Is) or angiotensin II receptor blockers (ARBs). For black patients, thiazide diuretics and calcium channel blockers are used alone or in combination for best management. For patients with diabetes and/or chronic kidney disease, ACE-Is and ARBs are used. Additional classes of drugs commonly used in the management of HBP include beta-blockers, alpha blockers, alpha$_2$-agonists, combined alpha and beta-blockers, and vasodilators.

Although the antihypertensive drugs have different actions, some nursing implications are the same for all of them. Box 9.3 describes the common nursing considerations for giving antihypertensive drugs. Nursing considerations and patient teaching issues specific to any single antihypertensive drug type are listed within the individual drug categories.

Many types of drugs are available to treat HBP. The drug selected for use depends on the severity of the disease. The drugs act at many sites in the body and in several different ways (Fig. 9.7). Patients may need several types of drugs to achieve the best management of their blood pressure. Antihypertensive drugs are grouped in five main categories:

1. Diuretics indirectly reduce blood pressure by producing sodium and water loss, thereby reducing fluid volume. (See Drugs That Affect the Renal/Urinary System for the actions and nursing implications of diuretics.)
2. Renin-angiotensin-aldosterone system (RAAS) drugs, which work by decreasing vasoconstriction and decreasing fluid volume to decrease blood pressure, include these drugs:
   a. Angiotensin-converting enzyme inhibitors (ACE-Is)
   b. Angiotensin II receptor blockers (ARBs)

---

**Box 9.2  Recommended Lifestyle Changes for Patients with High Blood Pressure**

- Stop smoking.
- Eat a well-balanced diet.
- Decrease sodium (salt) intake.
- Explore ways to reduce stressors in your life.
- Maintain a healthy weight.
- Try to get 40 minutes of moderate-intensity exercise three to four times each week.
- Limit alcohol to no more than two drinks per day for men or one drink per day for women.
- Avoid all over-the-counter drugs that can raise blood pressure.

---

**Box 9.3  General Nursing Implications for Antihypertensive Drug Therapy**

**ASSESSMENT**

- Gather baseline vital signs before giving any drug for high blood pressure (HBP).
- Get a complete list of all drugs that the patient is currently taking, including prescription, over-the-counter, and herbal drugs.
- Assess the patient's use of alcohol and/or illegal drugs that may interfere with the drug therapy or increase the risk of adverse effects.
- Review the patient's laboratory work, particularly that related to kidney tests (blood urea nitrogen and creatinine levels) and serum sodium and potassium concentrations.
- Assess for fluid balance, including the presence of edema or symptoms of dehydration.

**PLANNING AND IMPLEMENTATION**

- Teach the patient to report all over-the-counter drugs and check with the healthcare provider to avoid dangerous drug interactions.
- Remind the patient to avoid sudden changes in position because most antihypertensive drugs cause orthostatic hypotension.
- Withhold blood pressure drugs if the patient has a blood pressure measurement lower than 90/60 mm Hg, and notify the healthcare provider.
- Monitor blood pressure every 4 to 8 hours and as needed at the beginning of therapy in case the patient has a significant drop in blood pressure.
- Monitor potassium levels to assess whether they are within the normal range. Report abnormal levels to the healthcare provider.
- Teach the patient to avoid alcohol because it can cause hypotension in patients who are taking blood pressure drugs.
- Give the patient the drug at the same time every day. It is important to avoid missing doses because missed doses can cause rebound HBP.
- Teach the patient to keep taking the drugs as prescribed because they do not cure HBP.
- Initiate fall risk precautions for older adult patients who are taking HBP drugs.

**EVALUATION**

- Monitor the patient's blood pressure regularly to determine how well the patient is responding to the drug.
- Report any side effects or adverse effects to the healthcare provider.
- Track the patient's response to the drugs to determine whether they are effective.
- Continue to reinforce healthy lifestyle changes (see Box 9.2).

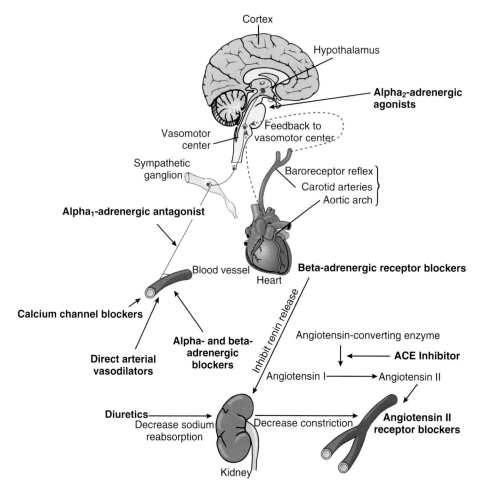

Fig. 9.7 Common sites of action of antihypertensive drugs. (From Lilley, L., Collins, S., & Snyder, J. (2019). *Pharmacology and the nursing process* (9th ed.). Elsevier.)

3. Calcium channel blockers decrease blood pressure by relaxing vascular smooth muscle in the coronary and systemic arteries, leading to decreased peripheral resistance.

4. Adrenergic agents used for the treatment of HBP affect epinephrine and norepinephrine (neurotransmitters) in the nervous system. Depending on the receptor, these drugs can decrease vasoconstriction and decrease contractility of the heart, thereby decreasing blood pressure. Adrenergic agents include these:
   a. Beta-blockers
      i. Nonselective
      ii. Selective
   b. Alpha$_1$-antagonists
   c. Alpha$_2$-agonists
   d. Combined alpha- and beta-antagonists

5. Vasodilators directly affect the arterial and/or venous system to decrease peripheral resistance.

Diuretics were discussed earlier in this chapter, and the remaining four categories are discussed here. Each class works a bit differently, and we discuss them separately so that you can better understand how to care for patients taking one or more HBP drugs at the same time. In addition, several of the drug categories work well for patients with other cardiovascular illnesses.

## ANTIHYPERTENSIVE DRUG ACTIONS

### Renin-Angiotensin-Aldosterone System Drugs

**Renin-angiotensin-aldosterone system (RAAS) drugs,** including ACE-Is and ARBs, interfere with the actions of angiotensin II and aldosterone to decrease blood pressure by decreasing vasoconstriction and fluid volume. When a person's blood pressure drops, cells in the kidney release a hormone called *renin* into the blood. Renin helps produce angiotensin I. Angiotensin I is converted to angiotensin II by an enzyme called the *angiotensin-converting enzyme (ACE).* Angiotensin II is a hormone that causes vasoconstriction and stimulates the adrenal cortex to increase aldosterone secretion; aldosterone then can increase water and sodium reabsorption. This works very well in helping to raise blood pressure back to normal. A good grasp of this process is helpful in understanding how ACE-Is and ARBs act to reduce HBP.

An **angiotensin-converting enzyme inhibitor (ACE-I)** is a type of RAAS drug that reduces HBP by stopping the conversion of angiotensin I to angiotensin II (the hormone that causes the vasoconstriction and increased aldosterone). An **angiotensin II receptor blocker (ARB)** is a type of RAAS drug that blocks the vasoconstrictor and aldosterone-secreting effects of angiotensin II. It lowers blood pressure by selectively blocking the binding of angiotensin II at receptor sites found in many tissues. Both ACE-Is and ARBs decrease vasoconstriction and decrease the release of aldosterone, decreasing fluid volume and lowering blood pressure. Table 9.6 lists the dosages and nursing implications of selected ACE-Is and ARBs.

 **Memory Jogger**

ACE-I drug names typically use the suffix -pril (e.g., captopril, enalapril, prinivil). ARBs typically end with the suffix -sartan (e.g., valsartan, losartan).

 **Top Tip for Safety**

Advise patients that garlic supplements can increase antihypertensive effects and that black licorice can decrease antihypertensive effects.

## Calcium Channel Blockers

Calcium ions are very important in the contraction of the heart and vascular smooth muscle. Calcium flows into muscle cells through tiny channels in their membranes and works as a switch that allows muscle fibers to slide past each other and shorten to contract. At the end of each contraction, calcium flows out of the channels, which allows the muscles to relax and lengthen again.

Calcium channel blockers are a class of antihypertensive drugs that lower blood pressure by reducing the effect of calcium in the heart muscle and in the smooth muscles of arteries. They work in two main ways. Calcium channel blockers help slow the flow of calcium ions across cell membranes, reducing the amount of calcium available for arterial smooth muscle contraction and producing relaxation of coronary and systemic arteries. With relaxation of the smooth muscle, blood flow improves, and blood pressure decreases. The oxygen can then get into the heart muscle, where it is needed. Some calcium channel blockers slow the flow of electricity through the cardiac conduction system, slowing the heart rate, and can be used to treat abnormal heart rhythms. You may see them used in patients with HBP, patients with angina, and patients with abnormal heart rhythms (dysrhythmias). Table 9.6 gives the dosages and nursing implications of selected calcium channel blockers.

 **Memory Jogger**

Fluid retention is a common side effect of calcium channel blockers, and these drugs should be avoided in patients with heart failure.

## Adrenergic Drugs

Adrenergics are a category of drugs that affect nervous system control of various organs and tissues by activating or blocking receptors that respond to the body's natural adrenergic substances, epinephrine and norepinephrine. To better comprehend how adrenergic drugs work,

you need to understand the role of the sympathetic nervous system in blood pressure control. The sympathetic nervous system relies on two main neurotransmitters, epinephrine and norepinephrine; these neurotransmitters are also called *catecholamines*. The neurotransmitters carry impulses to receptors on the surfaces of the heart, lungs, and blood vessel smooth muscle; after these receptors are turned on, a response is created.

There are two main types of adrenergic receptors: alpha-receptors and beta-receptors. Drugs that stimulate these receptors (called *agonists*) turn on the response; drugs that block the receptors (called blockers or antagonists) prevent the expected response. (Recall the discussion of receptors, agonists, and antagonists from Chapter 3.)

*Beta-blockers.* There are two main types of beta-receptors: beta$_1$-receptors located primarily in the heart and beta$_2$-receptors located primarily in the lungs. An easy way to remember which type of receptor is affected by the drug is this: *beta$_1$, one heart; beta$_2$, two lungs.* Stimulation of beta$_1$-receptors leads to increased heart rate and increased contractility of the heart. This is very helpful when you are healthy and need the fight-or-flight mechanism to work for you. In patients with HBP, however, these responses can be harmful, and drugs are used to block the response.

A beta-blocker is an antagonist drug that blocks the activity of beta-adrenergic receptors. These drugs are classified in two groups: nonselective and selective beta-antagonists. The nonselective agents block both beta$_1$ and beta$_2$ sites—that is, they affect both beta$_1$ (heart) receptors and beta$_2$ (lung) receptors. Blocking beta$_1$ receptors decreases heart contractility and heart rate (which can decrease blood pressure). On the other hand, blocking beta$_2$-adrenergic receptors causes bronchoconstriction, which can be a problem, especially in patients with asthma. For that reason, the newer selective beta$_1$ blockers are better for patients with HBP or other heart problems (Fig. 9.8). They do not have an effect on the lungs at normal doses.

Names of beta-blockers typically end with the suffix -olol; examples include metoprolol, propranolol, and sotalol. The -olol ending gives you the hint that the drug is a beta-blocker. Table 9.6 lists the dosages and nursing implications of selected beta-blockers.

 **Memory Jogger**

You can use the terms *antagonist* and *blocker* interchangeably to describe a drug that turns off a receptor. For example, you can refer to metoprolol as a beta-blocker or a beta-antagonist.

*Alpha$_1$-adrenergic antagonists.* Stimulation of alpha$_1$-adrenergic receptors causes arterial vascular smooth muscle constriction (Fig. 9.9). For example, if the

| Table 9.6 | **Common Antihypertensive Drugs** |

*Diuretics* reduce blood pressure by producing sodium and water loss, thereby decreasing fluid volume.
*Renin-angiotensin-aldosterone system (RAAS) drugs* decrease vasoconstriction and fluid volume, which lowers blood pressure.
*Calcium channel blocking agents* decrease blood pressure by relaxing vascular smooth muscle in the coronary and systemic arteries, which decreases peripheral resistance.
*Adrenergic agents* affect nervous system control of various organs and tissues by activating or blocking receptors that respond to the body's natural adrenergic substances, epinephrine and norepinephrine.
*Vasodilators* directly affect the arterial and/or venous system to decrease peripheral resistance.

| DRUGS/ADULT DOSAGE | NURSING IMPLICATIONS |
|---|---|
| **Diuretics** | |
| See Table 9.1 for dosages. | • See Table 9.1 for nursing implications. |
| **Renin-Angiotensin-Aldosterone System (Raas) Drugs** | |
| ACE-Is<br>captopril 6.25–50 mg orally two to three times daily<br>enalapril (Vasotec, Epaned) 2.5–40 mg orally daily as a single dose or in two divided doses<br>lisinopril (Prinivil, Zestril, Qbrelis) 2.5–40 mg orally once daily<br>quinapril (Accupril) 10–80 mg orally daily as a single dose or in two divided doses<br>ARBs<br>losartan (Cozaar) 50–100 mg orally daily as a single dose or in two divided doses<br>valsartan (Diovan) 40–320 mg orally once daily or in two divided doses<br>irbesartan (Avapro) 75–300 mg orally once daily<br>candesartan (Atacand) 4–32 mg orally daily as a single dose or in two divided doses<br>olmesartan (Benicar) 20–40 mg orally once daily | • Avoid sudden changes in position because most antihypertensive drugs cause orthostatic hypotension.<br>• Teach patients that these drugs can have a first-dose effect, which increases the risk of falls and dizziness.<br>• Remind patients to keep taking the drugs as prescribed because they do not cure HBP.<br>• ACE-Is and ARBs can cause hyperkalemia (high potassium levels); remind patients to avoid high-potassium foods (see Box 9.1), including salt substitutes.<br>• Monitor patients' blood pressure levels regularly to determine how well they are responding to the drug.<br>• Some patients may experience a dry cough while taking ACE-Is. If so, report this to the healthcare provider who may switch the patient to an ARB because they do not cause a cough.<br>• If the patient experiences swelling of the eyes, mouth, face, or tongue, contact the healthcare provider immediately because this could be a sign of angioedema (Fig. 9.10), a potentially life-threatening condition.<br>• These drugs can cause severe birth defects if taken during pregnancy, and they should not be taken by patients who are or may become pregnant.<br>• Teach patients taking these drugs to avoid alcohol because it can cause hypotension.<br>• Remind patients to avoid all OTC drugs until checking with their healthcare provider to avoid dangerous drug interactions. |
| **Calcium Channel Blocking Agents** | |
| amlodipine (Norvasc) 2.5–10 mg orally once daily<br>diltiazem (Cardizem) 30–120 mg orally three to four times daily, up to 480 mg daily<br>diltiazem extended release (Cardizem CD, Dilacor XR) 120–360 mg orally once daily<br>felodipine (Plendil) 2.5–10 mg orally daily<br>nicardipine (Cardene) 20–40 mg orally three times daily<br>nicardipine sustained release (Cardene SR) 30–60 mg twice daily<br>nifedipine (Adalat, Procardia) 10–30 mg orally three times daily, not to exceed 180 mg daily<br>nifedipine extended release (Adalat CC, Procardia XL) initially 30–60 mg orally once daily, not to exceed 120 mg daily<br>verapamil (Calan, Isoptin) 40–120 mg orally every 8 hours<br>verapamil extended release (Calan SR, Isoptin SR) 180–480 mg once daily at bedtime<br>verapamil extended release (Verelan PM extended-release capsules, controlled onset) 200–400 mg once daily at bedtime | • Avoid sudden changes in position because most antihypertensive drugs cause orthostatic hypotension.<br>• Remind patients to keep taking the drugs as prescribed because they do not cure HBP.<br>• Monitor patients' blood pressure levels regularly to determine how well they are responding to the drug.<br>• Patients should avoid alcohol because it can cause hypotension in patients taking drugs for HBP.<br>• Remind patients to avoid all OTC drugs until checking with the healthcare provider to avoid dangerous drug interactions.<br>• Notify the provider if the patient experiences swelling in the legs because this can be a sign of fluid retention caused by calcium channel blockers.<br>• Calcium channel blockers are avoided in patients with heart failure because of the potential for fluid retention.<br>• Teach patients to avoid grapefruit and grapefruit juice while taking calcium channel blockers, as it may increase the risk of toxicity.<br>• Be alert for signs of Stevens-Johnson syndrome (erythema multiforme), a life-threating skin condition that can be an adverse effect of calcium channel blockers. The condition is associated with skin lesions, fever, and aching joints.<br>• Before giving the drug and in order to avoid significant hypotension, report to the healthcare provider heart rates slower than 60 beats/min and blood pressure levels lower than 90 mm Hg systolic.<br>• If you are caring for a patient who is receiving IV calcium channel blockers, check with the RN or the healthcare provider regarding the need for a bed with a cardiac monitor. |

**Table 9.6** Common Antihypertensive Drugs—cont'd

| DRUGS/ADULT DOSAGE | NURSING IMPLICATIONS |
|---|---|
| **Adrenergic Agents** | |
| **Beta-Blockers**<br>acebutolol (Sectral) 400–1200 mg orally once a day or in divided doses<br>atenolol (Tenormin) 25–200 mg orally once daily or in divided doses<br>betaxolol (Kerlone) 5–20 mg orally once daily<br>metoprolol (Lopressor, Toprol) 50–100 mg one to two times daily, up to 450 mg per day in two divided doses<br>metoprolol (Toprol XL) 12.5–100 mg orally once daily, up to 400 mg once daily<br>nadolol (Corgard) 40–320 mg orally once daily<br>propranolol (Inderal) 10–40 mg orally two to four times daily, up to 160–640 mg daily in two to four divided doses<br>propranolol extended release (Inderal LA, Inderal XL) 80 mg orally once daily, up to 160–320 mg once daily | **All Adrenergic Agents**<br>• Avoid sudden changes in position because most antihypertensive drugs cause orthostatic hypotension.<br>• Remind patients to keep taking the drugs as prescribed because they do not cure HBP.<br>• Monitor patients' blood pressure regularly to determine how well they are responding to the drug.<br>• Patients should avoid alcohol because it can cause hypotension in patients who are taking drugs for HBP.<br>• Remind patients to avoid all OTC drugs until checking with the healthcare provider to avoid dangerous drug interactions.<br><br>**Beta-Blockers**<br>• To prevent adverse effects, withhold the drug if the heart rate is slower than 60 beats/minute or systolic blood pressure is less than 90 mm Hg.<br>• Teach patients that common side effects include decreased sexual ability, dizziness, drowsiness, difficulty sleeping, or weakness. Some patients may experience cold hands or feet.<br>• Tell patients to report symptoms of depression to their healthcare provider.<br>• Teach diabetic patients that beta-blockers can mask signs of hypoglycemia (except for sweating). Remind them to check blood sugar levels regularly and to treat low blood sugar.<br>• To avoid rebound HBP, do not stop beta-blockers suddenly. |
| **Alpha Blockers**<br>doxazosin (Cardura) 1–16 mg orally once daily<br>prazosin (Minipress) 1–5 mg orally two to three times daily; usual dose 2–20 mg daily<br>terazosin (Hytrin) 1–5 mg orally daily as a single dose at bedtime or in two divided doses; usual dose range is 1–20 mg daily. | **Alpha Blockers**<br>• A side effect of doxazosin, prazosin, and terazosin is hypotension caused by a first-dose effect. These drugs may be given at night to prevent severe orthostatic hypotension, and the effects diminish over time.<br>• Monitor patients carefully for side effects, including dizziness, nervousness, fatigue, headache, and stuffy or runny nose, which can occur with alpha blockers.<br>• Weigh patients at least two times a week because alpha blockers can cause fluid retention.<br>• Tell patients to avoid driving or using heavy machinery until at least 24 hours after the first dose because alpha blockers can cause a sudden drop in blood pressure. |
| **Alpha/Beta-Blockers**<br>carvedilol (Coreg) 3.125–25 mg orally twice daily<br>carvedilol extended release (Coreg CR) 10 mg orally once daily, up to 80 mg once daily<br>labetalol HCl (Normodyne, Trandate) 100 mg twice daily (usual dosage range is 200–400 mg twice daily), up to 2400 mg orally in two or three divided doses | **Alpha/Beta-Blockers**<br>• Alpha/beta-blockers have the same side effects and adverse effects that occur with either type of drug. |
| **Alpha$_2$-Agonists**<br>clonidine (Catapres, Duraclon, Kapvay) 0.1 mg orally twice daily; usual maintenance dosage range is 0.1–0.8 mg daily<br>clonidine transdermal patch (Catapres TTS-1, TTS-2, TTS-3 [0.1, 0.2, 0.3 mg, respectively]) patch applied to a hairless site on the body every 7 days<br>methyldopa (Aldomet) 250 mg orally two to three times daily; may increase up to 3 g daily in divided doses | **Alpha$_2$-Agonists (Centrally Acting Adrenergic Agents)**<br>• These drugs affect the CNS, causing decreased vasoconstriction and dilation of blood vessels, and they have a higher risk of side effects than other blood pressure drugs. They are used only in cases of difficult-to-manage HBP.<br>• Teach patients the common side effects, including dizziness, fatigue, dry mouth, and nasal congestion.<br>• Oral rinses, good oral care, and sugarless gum may help decrease dry mouth in patients who are taking alpha$_2$-agonists.<br>• Read the directions for applying the clonidine patch very carefully to ensure that you are using the system correctly, and then write the time and date on the patch before placing it on the patient.<br>• To prevent rebound HBP, do not stop alpha$_2$-agonists suddenly. |
| **Vasodilators** | |
| hydralazine (Apresoline) 10 mg orally four times daily; usual dose 100–200 mg daily in two to four divided doses | • Monitor blood pressure carefully at the beginning of therapy in case the patient has a significant drop in blood pressure.<br>• Teach patients to weigh themselves every day and to report swelling of the hands or feet to their healthcare provider.<br>• Remind patients to take the drug at the same time every day. It is important to avoid missing doses because missed doses can cause rebound HBP.<br>• Teach patients to change position slowly to avoid orthostatic hypotension. |

ACE-I, angiotensin-converting enzyme inhibitor; ARB, angiotensin II receptor blocker; CNS, central nervous system; HBP, high blood pressure; OTC, over-the-counter.

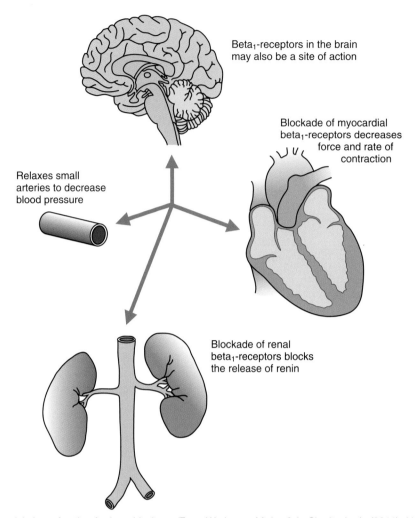

Beta₁-receptors in the brain may also be a site of action

Blockade of myocardial beta₁-receptors decreases force and rate of contraction

Relaxes small arteries to decrease blood pressure

Blockade of renal beta₁-receptors blocks the release of renin

Fig. 9.8 Potential sites of action for beta-blockers. (From Workman, M. L., & LaCharity, L. A. (2011). *Understanding pharmacology.* Elsevier.)

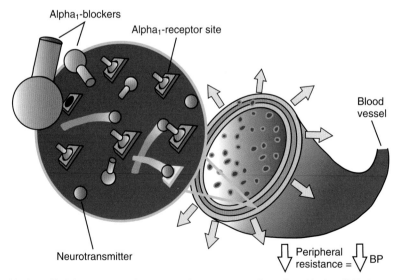

Alpha₁-blockers

Alpha₁-receptor site

Blood vessel

Neurotransmitter

Peripheral resistance = ⇩ BP

Fig. 9.9 Alpha₁-blockers fill alpha₁-receptor sites, preventing neurotransmitters from binding. With fewer receptors being stimulated, vasoconstriction is prevented or reversed, and blood pressure *(BP)* is lowered. (From Workman, M. L., & LaCharity, L. A. (2011). *Understanding pharmacology.* Elsevier.)

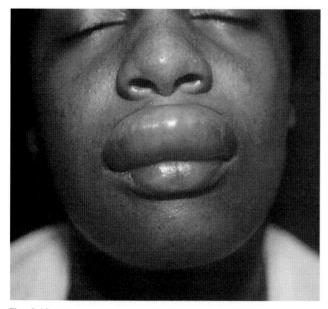

Fig. 9.10 Angioedema. (From Workman, M. L., & LaCharity, L. A. (2011). *Understanding pharmacology.* Elsevier.)

blood pressure is very low, certain drugs increase blood pressure by targeting the alpha$_1$-adrenergic receptors. For patients with HBP, the alpha$_1$-adrenergic inhibitor drugs work through selective blocking of alpha$_1$-adrenergic receptor sites, leading to decreased peripheral vascular resistance and decreased blood pressure. An **alpha1-adrenergic antagonist** is a drug that lowers blood pressure by blocking the adrenergic receptor sites in blood vessel smooth muscle that, when activated, cause vasoconstriction and raise blood pressure.

*Centrally acting alpha$_2$-adrenergic agonists.* The **alpha2-adrenergic agonists** work centrally (in the brain) to turn on special alpha$_2$-adrenergic receptors that, when normally activated, cause vasodilation and decrease blood pressure. These drugs can be very helpful in reducing blood pressure but have significant side effects, and they need to be used very carefully and with regular blood pressure monitoring.

*Combination alpha/beta-blockers.* Combination alpha/beta-blockers have the benefit of affecting the responses of both types of adrenergic receptors. They relax the blood vessels like the alpha$_1$ blockers do, and they slow the heart rate and contractility of the heart like the beta$_1$ blockers do.

*Vasodilators.* **Vasodilators** are a class of drugs that dilate (widen or relax) blood vessels in several ways. Some dilate arteries and veins by preventing contraction of smooth muscle cells. Others cause vasodilation by affecting the CNS. Some drugs work primarily on the arterial system, some more on the venous system, and some work on both arteries and veins. Dilation of the blood vessels decreases blood pressure, improves

blood flow to the major organs, and decreases the workload of the heart.

## USES OF ANTIHYPERTENSIVE DRUGS

Antihypertensives and diuretics are used alone or in combination to decrease elevated blood pressure to a desired level according to accepted guidelines. By maintaining normal blood pressure, these drugs help prevent complications of acute and chronic HBP. As you work with patients, you may see that several trials of different prescriptions are often needed before the right combination of drugs is achieved for the best control. Careful monitoring is essential.

## EXPECTED SIDE EFFECTS OF ANTIHYPERTENSIVE DRUGS

All blood pressure drugs can cause hypotension, which is blood pressure that is too low to maintain adequate circulation. Most can cause orthostatic hypotension, which is dizziness that occurs when changing positions. Symptoms associated with blood pressure that is too low include dizziness, weakness, and confusion (particularly in older adults). These symptoms can lead to an increased risk of falling. As you study each class of drugs, remember that you need to be able to recognize the difference between expected side effects and adverse reactions. When the blood pressure drops below 90/60 mm Hg or the patient is experiencing severe side effects, you should notify the healthcare provider to determine whether an alternative drug would work with fewer side effects.

## ADVERSE REACTIONS OF ANTIHYPERTENSIVE DRUGS

Each class and each drug has many potential serious adverse reactions. The specific adverse effects are discussed in Table 9.6.

 **Lifespan Considerations**

**Older Adults**

Older adults are particularly at risk for dizziness when taking antihypertensive drugs. The orthostatic hypotension they experience places them at risk for falling when they rapidly change positions, such as getting up quickly from a chair or bed.

 **Top Tip for Safety**

**ANTIHYPERTENSIVES**
Teach patients who are taking antihypertensive drugs to stand up slowly to avoid dizziness and prevent falls.

## DRUG INTERACTIONS WITH ANTIHYPERTENSIVES

Frequently a patient with HBP has to take many different drugs because he or she has other medical problems. All antihypertensive drugs can have drug interactions. Check each drug the patient is taking; interactive effects that lower the blood pressure too much or make the blood pressure go even higher can occur. Consult a drug reference book or a pharmacist for more information about interactions between the patient's prescribed antihypertensive drug and any other drug he or she is taking.

### ❖ Nursing Implications and Patient Teaching

◆ *Assessment.* In assessing your patient with HBP, remember to consider all modifiable and nonmodifiable risk factors. For example, knowing that black patients have a higher risk of HBP than whites will remind you to carefully screen for HBP as black patients may require drug therapy at a younger age than whites. Assessing patients for smoking, levels of physical activity, and high-sodium/high-fat diets is also important. Lifestyle changes are critical whether the patient is taking drugs for HBP or has elevated blood pressure.

For all patients with HBP, it is critical to gather a thorough drug history. Certain prescription drugs, OTC drugs, herbal preparations, and even illegal drugs can cause HBP. Common prescription drugs such as glucocorticoids, oral contraceptives, nonsteroidal anti-inflammatory drugs (NSAIDs), and OTC drugs for cough and cold symptoms may cause the patient to have elevated blood pressure. Patients who use illegal drugs such as cocaine, anabolic steroids, and amphetamines often are diagnosed with HBP when they are seen for any reason by healthcare providers. This can occur even in teenagers and young adults. As an LPN/VN, you may have the most contact of any healthcare professional with patients in your care settings, and building a trusting relationship can help you screen for these and other risk factors for HBP.

Before giving any drug that affects blood pressure, baseline blood pressure and heart rate checks are essential. Knowing the patient's blood pressure and heart rate before you give a drug helps you to evaluate the patient's response to the drug. Drugs such as beta-blockers affect the blood pressure and the heart rate. If the heart rate is lower than 60 beats/min, withhold the drug, and contact the healthcare provider. For several categories of drugs, you need to monitor electrolyte levels (e.g., potassium). If you are giving an ACE-I and the potassium level is greater than 5.0 mEq/L (5.0 mmol/L), withhold the drug, and contact the healthcare provider because ACE-Is can cause hyperkalemia. If you are giving a diuretic such as furosemide, you should watch for hypokalemia (potassium levels lower than normal).

◆ *Planning and implementation.* HBP has no cure, but it can be well managed. It is important to involve your patient in planning care as much as possible so that he or she will better understand why taking a prescribed antihypertensive drug is important. For best results, patients need both drug therapy and lifestyle changes. HBP usually does not have symptoms, and patients may not feel sick. It is important for you to reinforce with the patient why treating HBP is important for maintaining good health even if no symptoms are present.

---

### 🔊 Top Tip for Safety

Ask patients about any herbal or OTC drugs they are taking because some may cause HBP and some may increase the side effects of drugs used to treat HBP.

---

◆ *Evaluation.* It is important to evaluate the patient's response to the drug. Compare his or her current blood pressure with the baseline values. Is the blood pressure improving? Is the patient tolerating the blood pressure drug without side effects? Evaluate how the patient is doing with lifestyle changes. Some patients are able to stop smoking but have difficulty with the dietary changes. Others may have made changes to their diet but have not been physically active.

The healthcare provider may order laboratory work, including a complete blood count, electrolytes, and blood urea nitrogen/creatinine to monitor renal function. This laboratory work helps identify adverse effects from the drug, and it checks for evidence of organ damage caused by chronic HBP.

Ask the patient about side effects the antihypertensive drug may be producing. Some of these drugs can cause impotence in men. If this occurs, men may want to discuss possible changes in their drug therapy with their healthcare providers. Always refer patients to their healthcare provider if they have stopped taking their HBP drugs because of side effects (see Box 9.3).

◆ *Patient and family teaching.* Tell the patient and family:
- Take this drug exactly as ordered. If a dose is missed, it should be taken as soon as it is remembered; if the next scheduled dose is close, skip the missed dose and return to the regular dosing schedule.
- Teach proper techniques for home monitoring of blood pressure and heart rate. If the blood pressure is lower than 90/60 mm Hg or the heart rate is less than 60 beats/min, contact your healthcare provider.
- Keep a daily record of your blood pressure to bring to your appointments. This helps the healthcare provider make sure you are taking the most effective drugs.
- Remember to get up slowly from a lying or sitting position to avoid dizziness from getting up too fast.
- Notify your healthcare provider of any new or uncomfortable symptoms that develop. These symptoms may indicate an adverse effect or may be relieved by simply changing to a new drug.

- Avoid alcoholic beverages while taking drugs for HBP.
- Keep a list of the drugs that you take and share it with all healthcare providers so they will be aware of the doses and types of drugs you are taking.

 **Bookmark This!**

The National Institutes of Health has a wide variety of health information available to everyone in English (https://www.nih.gov/health-information) and in Spanish (https://salud.nih.gov).

## DRUGS USED FOR ANGINA AND MYOCARDIAL INFARCTION

### ANTIANGINALS

Coronary arteries supply blood, oxygen, and nutrients to heart muscle. For patients with atherosclerosis, plaque within the blood vessel leads to lack of blood flow and oxygen to the heart and potentially other areas of the body. Partial blood flow to the heart muscle can cause a lack of oxygen and chest pain called *angina*. If the blood flow is significantly reduced, the heart muscle can die and the patient has a heart attack (myocardial infarction).

Major classes of drugs used to manage angina are nitrates, beta-blockers, and calcium channel blockers. All of these drugs can improve circulation and reduce cardiac workload, thereby reducing myocardial oxygen demand (how much oxygen the heart needs).

### NITRATES

#### Action

Nitrates are a class of drugs that dilate blood vessels by relaxing vascular smooth muscle in the peripheral venous system and reducing resistance to blood flow in the arterial system. Relaxing the smooth muscle in the veins helps increase pooling of venous blood, thereby decreasing the amount of blood returned to the heart (preload). Relaxing the arterial system decreases the pressures the heart has to pump against (afterload). These effects work together to help the heart receive more oxygen and pump more easily.

#### Uses

Rapid-acting nitrates such as sublingual nitroglycerin (NTG) and intravenous NTG are used to relieve pain in acute angina. The long-acting oral nitrates, topical NTG paste, and transdermal patches can prevent angina and reduce the severity and frequency of angina attacks. Nitrates reduce the work of the heart after a myocardial infarction or in patients with heart failure.

#### Expected Side Effects

Throbbing headaches, caused by rapid blood vessel dilation in the head and face, occur in more than 50% of patients who take nitrates. The headaches usually occur very quickly after taking the drug and usually go away quickly if the patient is taking low doses. For patients who are taking high doses, acetaminophen or other analgesics may be needed to help reduce the pain. For patients who require long-term use of nitrates, headaches typically become less severe over time. It is common for patients to experience a slight drop in blood pressure after taking the drug because of venous dilation.

#### Adverse Effects

Some patients may have strong reactions to nitrates depending on the route of administration. Severe postural hypotension (low blood pressure when a person suddenly stands up), reflex tachycardia (rapid heartbeat) or paradoxical bradycardia (heart rate < 60 bpm), vertigo (feeling of dizziness or spinning), or severe weakness may occur.

#### Drug Interactions

Alcohol, antihypertensive drugs, opioids, and diuretics can increase the effect of nitrate drugs, causing tachycardia and severe hypotension. Caffeine, pseudoephedrine, methylphenidate, and certain antidiabetic drugs can decrease the effectiveness of nitrates. Drugs given for erectile dysfunction (e.g., sildenafil) can cause severe hypotension if given while the patient is taking nitrates.

❖ **Nursing Implications and Patient Teaching**

◆ *Assessment.* A good patient history, including all OTC and prescription drugs, is important to avoid drug interactions. It is important to get a baseline assessment of heart rate and blood pressure before giving a nitrate drug. For patients with acute angina, get a good description of the patient's symptoms, including onset, duration, and characteristics of the pain. Ask patients if they have ever had pain like this before and, if so, what they did to relieve the pain. This will be very important as you monitor the effectiveness of the nitrate. Box 9.4 gives the current recommendation for giving sublingual NTG to patients with acute angina.

◆ *Planning and implementation.* An advantage of NTG and other nitrates is that they come in a variety of forms. NTG tablets are easily absorbed under the tongue and are recommended in an emergency for quick action. However, swallowing the same tablets would destroy the NTG. Other forms, such as isosorbide, are given orally for longer action. NTG also is available as a paste or a transdermal patch, which allows the NTG to be absorbed into the bloodstream through the skin. Carefully titrating intravenous NTG relieves pain in severe angina.

Whatever the route, you need to follow proper administration guidelines. Place sublingual NTG under the tongue for absorption into the bloodstream.

| Box 9.4 | Patient Education for Taking Nitroglycerin Sublingual or Spray for Sudden Onset of Chest Pain |
| --- | --- |

Step 1: Make sure to sit or lie down, and then take one dose of NTG (sublingual or spray) immediately after the chest pain starts. If the symptoms do not improve or get worse, call 911.

Step 2: If the symptoms improve after the first dose but do not go away completely, you can take a second dose after 5 minutes. If the symptoms do not improve or get worse, call 911.

Step 3: If the symptoms continue to improve but do not go away completely, you can take a third dose 5 minutes after the second dose. If the symptoms do not improve or get worse, call 911. Do not take more than three doses in 15 minutes.

Step 4: Call 911 if:
- Symptoms do not get better within 5 minutes or they get worse after the first dose.
- Symptoms do not continue to get better after the second dose.
- Chest pain does not go away completely within 5 minutes after taking the third dose.
- You feel that you have taken more than the required dose.

Remind the patient that the drug is absorbed under the tongue and is not to be chewed or swallowed. If the patient is prescribed NTG paste, measure the dose carefully, using the directions and the proper measuring paper. Remove all old NTG paste before applying the new paste to prevent dosage accumulation. Wear gloves when applying NTG paste because it is absorbed through the skin (on patients and on nurses!).

 **Top Tip for Safety**

Teach patients not to chew or swallow sublingual NTG tablets because the drug is destroyed in the GI system and will not help the angina.

 **Top Tip for Safety**

Wear gloves to apply NTG paste to avoid absorbing it through the skin into your bloodstream.

Carefully monitor the patient's response to NTG. Almost all patients who are taking NTG experience a drop in blood pressure because it is a vasodilator. Do not give NTG if the patient's blood pressure is lower than 90/60 mm Hg. Patients often experience a headache after taking NTG. Administration of acetaminophen or another pain reliever can help reduce the headache. These headaches typically go away within a few weeks as the patient begins to get used to the drug.

Patients develop a tolerance to NTG, and they must have time off of the drug so that it does not lose effectiveness. For example, an NTG patch may be placed in the morning and then removed at bedtime as directed.

If the patch were left on the body for 24 hours, the next dose would be less effective, and the patient would no longer receive the benefit of the nitrate. Time off during the night ensures that the drug will continue to work. Table 9.7 provides additional information about NTG and nursing implications.

◆ *Evaluation.* It is important to evaluate the patient for effectiveness of the drug. Sublingual NTG is given to patients with sudden onset of angina. It is fast and can be effective. For evaluation, ask whether the NTG relieves or reduces the patient's angina; if it does not, call 911. In any emergency situation, failure of the drug to relieve pain is an indicator that the patient may be having a heart attack and is likely to have heart muscle damage unless emergency care is received.

Evaluate the patient's blood pressure carefully after giving any nitrates until you are clear about the patient's usual response. For sublingual NTG, you may monitor blood pressure every 5 minutes until the pain is relieved or until emergency care providers have arrived to transport the patient to the acute care setting.

 **Top Tip for Safety**

**ANGINA ATTACKS**

For acute angina, teach the patient to put one NTG tablet under the tongue as soon as the pain begins and not to chew or swallow the drug. Tell the patient to let the drug dissolve under the tongue while he or she lies down and rests. If the pain is not relieved or reduced within 5 minutes, the patient should call 911 or report to the emergency room. The patient should not drive if he or she is having chest pain! While waiting for the ambulance, the patient may take a second pill. If the pain is not relieved within another 5 minutes, the patient may take a third pill. The patient should not take more than three sublingual tablets.

◆ *Patient and family teaching.* Tell the patient and family:
- Keep the NTG tablets in a dark glass container to prevent breakdown of the drug.
- Carefully check the expiration dates of NTG tablets. Tablets that have expired are not effective for treating chest pain.
- Do not drink alcoholic beverages while taking nitrate products. If you have a special occasion, notify your healthcare provider before you decide to drink alcohol.
- If you are using NTG spray, do not smoke or use the spray near an open flame because the drug is flammable.
- For transdermal patch application, select a hairless spot (or clip your skin hair) and apply the patch to the skin. Do not cut the patch because it will affect the dose of the drug. If the patch comes off, discard and replace it with a new one at a different site. Rotate the sites each day to prevent skin irritation.

| Table **9.7** | **Common Antianginal Drugs** |
|---|---|

*Nitrates* vasodilate by relaxing vascular smooth muscle in the peripheral venous system and reducing resistance to blood flow in the arterial system. These effects help the heart get more oxygen and pump more easily.

*Beta-blockers* reduce sympathetic stimulation to the heart, decreasing heart rate and contractility of the heart muscle, which lowers myocardial oxygen demand.

*Calcium channel blocking agents* decrease blood pressure by relaxing vascular smooth muscle in the coronary and systemic arteries, which decreases peripheral resistance and myocardial oxygen demand.

| DRUGS/ADULT DOSAGE | NURSING IMPLICATIONS |
|---|---|
| **Nitrates** | |
| isosorbide mononitrate (Ismo, Monoket) 5–20 mg orally twice daily 7 hours apart<br>isosorbide mononitrate extended release (Imdur) 30–60 mg orally once daily (up to 240 mg/day)<br>isosorbide dinitrate 5–20 mg orally two to three times daily (up to maximum 480 mg/day)<br>isosorbide dinitrate extended-release (Isochron, IsoDitrate) 40 mg orally once daily (up to maximum of 160 mg/day)<br>nitroglycerin (NTG) (many brand names)<br>Sublingual or buccal 0.3–0.6 mg; may repeat every 5 minutes up to three doses<br>Sublingual or lingual spray one to two sprays; may repeat every 5 minutes up to three doses<br>Oral (sustained-release capsules) 2.5–6.5 mg three to four times daily<br>Topical 2% ointment 0.5 inches (7.5 mg) twice daily; may have up to 1 inch (15 mg) twice daily; include a nitrate-free interval of up to 12 hours<br>Transdermal patch 0.1–0.8 mg/hour, is worn 12–14 hours/day; include a nitrate-free interval of 10–12 hours | • Monitor blood pressure carefully while the patient is taking nitrates because a decrease in blood pressure is a common side effect of this drug.<br>• For immediate-release isosorbide mononitrate, giving drugs 7 hours apart helps to prevent tolerance to nitroglycerin.<br>• Teach patients that they may experience a headache with NTG drugs because blood vessel dilation in the head and face causes pain. Mild headaches may be treated with a mild pain reliever such as acetaminophen (Tylenol).<br>• Wear gloves when applying NTG ointment or paste to avoid absorption into your skin.<br>• Make sure to remove used patches according to directions (most often at bedtime) because patients need a drug-free period to avoid tolerance to the drug.<br>• Rotate sites when using paste or patches as directed to prevent skin breakdown.<br>• If using paste or patch, choose a hairless area on the upper arm, back, or chest for best drug absorption. Apply paste as directed in thin layer. Do not rub paste into skin.<br>• For acute episodes of chest pain, give sublingual NTG or lingual spray (spray onto or under the tongue) for best drug absorption into the blood vessels of this area.<br>• Store NTG tablets in a dark glass container to prevent breakdown of the drug.<br>• Make sure to check the expiration dates of NTG tablets because they deteriorate quickly and then are not effective in treating chest pain.<br>• Teach male patients that drugs for erectile dysfunction, if taken with nitrates, can cause a severe drop in blood pressure. |
| **Beta-Blockers** | |
| See Table 9.6 for dosage ranges. | • See Table 9.6 for nursing implications. |
| **Calcium Channel Blocking Agents** | |
| See Table 9.6 for dosage ranges. | • See Table 9.6 for nursing implications. |

- Avoid drugs for erectile dysfunction such as sildenafil (Viagra) because they can cause a severe drop in blood pressure.
- Keep a record of every angina attack. If you are having an increase in the frequency of attacks or change in symptoms, notify your healthcare provider.

## ANTIDYSRHYTHMICS

The heart has its own electrical conduction system made of specialized cells that can automatically create, conduct, and respond to electrical impulses. Electrical impulses travel through the heart muscle, causing the heart to contract and pump blood. The primary pacemaker of the heart is the sinoatrial node (see Fig. 9.5). When working properly, the heart's pacemaker automatically creates impulses that cause an orderly contraction of the atria and ventricles, which can be felt as a smooth and regular pulse. The heart muscle contracts, and blood flows through the heart chambers into the lungs and the rest of the body.

The pacemaker can respond to the needs of the body for increased oxygen. For example, heart rate increases during exercise so that the muscles receive enough oxygen. If the patient has a drop in blood pressure, the heart usually responds by increasing the rate to restore blood pressure. If there are threats to the functioning of the pacemaker of the heart, the patient can experience an abnormal rhythm, and cardiac output is reduced.

When the cells in the conduction system do not have enough oxygen or are damaged through disease or when electrolytes are out of balance, irregular heart rhythm results. The abnormal heart rhythm (whether too slow or too fast) can have a significant impact on cardiac output. These abnormal rhythms may be benign (not requiring drugs), or they may be life-threatening. You may hear nurses in the clinical area using the term *arrhythmia* to describe abnormal heart rhythm. We use the term *dysrhythmia* (irregular rhythm) rather than *arrhythmia* (without rhythm) to describe abnormal heart rhythm.

Dysrhythmias may be fast or slow, with an irregular or a regular pattern. Common causes of dysrhythmias include hypoxia (e.g., caused by blockage of a coronary artery), fluid and electrolyte imbalances (e.g., high or low potassium levels), adverse effects of certain drugs, and interventions for the heart (e.g., cardiac catheterization, open heart surgery).

Dysrhythmias are usually classified according to the site of origin and type of rhythm abnormality produced. For example, atrial dysrhythmias start in the atria, supraventricular dysrhythmias start above the ventricles, and ventricular dysrhythmias start in the ventricles. One type of atrial dysthymia is atrial fibrillation; the rhythm starts in the atria, and the rate is irregular. Ventricular tachycardia is a rapid heart rate that starts in the ventricles. The primary nursing issue is whether the rhythm affects how well the patient's heart can pump. The goal of any treatment plan or therapeutic regimen is for the patient's heart to regain a normal rate and rhythm so that normal circulation is restored. Most acute care settings offer specific courses to help nurses identify specific dysrhythmias.

### Action

An **antidysrhythmic** drug works to make heart rhythm more regular and reduces serious dysrhythmias. Even though many dysrhythmias require nonpharmacologic treatments (ranging from pacemaker insertion to giving the heart an electric shock), drugs play an important role in treating abnormal heart rhythms to help the heart achieve a more normal rhythm. Antidysrhythmic drugs affect the cells that are beating irregularly during different phases of electrical conduction. Some of the drugs used to help regulate heart rhythm are also used to treat HBP and other cardiovascular problems.

Antidysrhythmic drugs are classified using the Vaughan-Williams classification system. It organizes the drugs according to where they act in the conduction cycle:
1. Class I drugs are sodium channel blockers (e.g., quinidine, procainamide, disopyramide).
   a. They lengthen the period during which the cells cannot release or discharge their electrical activity.
   b. They make the heart less excitable, slowing the impulse conduction through the heart.
2. Class II drugs are beta-blockers (e.g., propranolol, esmolol, acebutolol).
   a. They reduce sympathetic stimulation to the heart, decreasing the heart rate.
   b. They decrease contractility of the heart muscle.
3. Class III drugs are potassium channel blockers (e.g., amiodarone).
   a. They make the cells less excitable.
   b. They can slow the heart rate.
4. Class IV drugs are calcium channel blockers (e.g., diltiazem, verapamil).
   a. They selectively block the ability of calcium to enter the heart muscle cells.
   b. They slow conduction through the sinoatrial and/or atrioventricular node.
5. Other drugs (e.g., digoxin, magnesium sulfate)

### Uses

The cause of the dysrhythmia determines which drug class will be most effective for treatment. Whatever the abnormal rhythm, the goal is to restore the rhythm to normal and maintain adequate cardiac output.

Digoxin is used primarily to treat heart failure, but it also plays a role in treating fast dysrhythmias, such as atrial fibrillation or supraventricular tachycardia. It reduces the heart rate by slowing how fast the sinoatrial node fires and slowing conduction through the atrioventricular node. It also strengthens the contraction of the heart. Toxic levels of this drug can also cause dysrhythmias.

Other drugs that affect heart activity are the beta-adrenergic blockers such as sotalol or acebutolol. Drugs in this class act very much like quinidine on the heart, but they also decrease the response of the heart muscle to epinephrine and norepinephrine (other chemical neurotransmitters) by blocking the stimulation of the heart's beta-receptors.

 **Memory Jogger**

Learning the common suffixes can help you recognize the specific class of drugs:
1. Beta-blockers often end with -olol.
2. ACE-Is often end with -pril.
3. ARBs often end with -sartan.

Many antidysrhythmic drugs are so powerful that they are given only in critical care units, where the patients are closely monitored. As the patient's condition becomes more stable, oral versions of the drug or another antidysrhythmic may be used for long-term therapy. Table 9.8 lists drugs that are commonly used in the treatment of acute and chronic dysrhythmias.

### Adverse Reactions

Drugs that are given to control dysrhythmias may cause other dysrhythmias. All patients who are receiving these drugs should have their hearts carefully monitored by electrocardiogram (ECG) for any change.

| Table **9.8** | **Common Antidysrhythmic Drugs** |
|---|---|

*Sodium channel blockers* increase the length of time during which the cells cannot discharge their electrical activity, slowing conduction of impulses through the heart and making it less excitable. They are used to treat supraventricular and ventricular dysrhythmias and life-threatening dysrhythmias such as atrial or fibrillation and ventricular fibrillation.

*Beta-blockers* reduce sympathetic stimulation of the heart, decreasing the heart rate and heart muscle contractility. They are often used to treat rapid dysrhythmias that originate above the ventricle, such as supraventricular tachycardia.

*Potassium channel blockers* make cardiac cells less excitable and reduce the heart rate. They are often used to help convert atrial fibrillation and/or atrial flutter to a normal sinus rhythm and can be used to treat dangerous ventricular dysrhythmias.

*Calcium channel blockers* impede the ability of calcium to enter heart muscle cells, which slows conduction of electrical impulses through the sinoatrial and atrioventricular nodes. These drugs are primarily used to treat supraventricular tachycardia.

*Cardiac glycosides* decrease the speed of conduction through the atrioventricular node, decreasing the number of atrial polarizations, and they slow the ventricular rate.

| DRUGS/ADULT DOSAGE | NURSING IMPLICATIONS |
|---|---|
| **Sodium Channel Blockers** | |
| quinidine<br>As quinidine sulfate 200–300 mg orally every 6–8 hours<br>As quinidine sulfate extended release 300–600 mg every 8–12 hours<br>As quinidine gluconate extended release 324–648 mg orally every 8–12 hours<br>disopyramide (Norpace) 100–200 mg every 6 hours (range 400–800 mg in four divided doses); some cases may require a loading dose of 200–300 mg orally one time only<br>disopyramide (Norpace XL) 200–300 mg every 12 hours; maximum is 800 mg/day<br>propafenone (Rythmol) 150–300 mg orally every 8 hours<br>propafenone sustained release (Rythmol SR) 225–425 mg every 12 hours | • Carefully monitor the heart rate and blood pressure of the patient because these drugs can cause hypotension and dysrhythmias.<br>• Teach patients to avoid all OTC drugs to prevent dangerous interactions.<br>• Quinidine can cause significant GI side effects. Remind patients to take the drug with food to ease these symptoms.<br>• Give the drug exactly as scheduled to avoid irregular blood levels. Patients may need to use timers to remember to take the drug on schedule.<br>• Monitor patient weight and intake and output because some of these drugs can cause urinary retention.<br>• Older adult patients are more likely to experience dizziness and confusion and therefore are at greater risk for falls.<br>• Teach family members to assess the patients for any confusion and report to the healthcare provider.<br>• Carefully review your drug reference or manual before giving any sodium channel blocker to see additional side effects and adverse effects specific to each drug. |
| **Beta-Blockers** | |
| acebutolol (Monitan, Sectral) 200 mg orally twice daily (usual therapeutic range 600–1200 mg daily)<br>propranolol (Inderal) 10–30 mg orally three to four times daily; may increase to 160–320 mg daily in three or four divided doses<br>sotalol (Betapace, Sorine) 80 mg orally every 12 hours; average dosage 160–240 mg daily | • Monitor the patient's heart rate and blood pressure. Hold the drug if the heart rate is less than 60 beats/min or systolic blood pressure is less than 90 mm Hg.<br>• Teach patients that stopping beta-blockers can cause serious complications, including rapid heart rate, hypertensive crisis, and heart attack.<br>• Monitor blood sugar regularly in patients with diabetes because beta-blockers can increase or decrease blood sugar levels. They can also mask the signs of hypoglycemia (e.g., increased heart rate).<br>• Teach patients that depression can be a side effect of taking beta-blockers. If they experience symptoms of depression, contact their healthcare provider. |
| **Potassium Channel Blockers** | |
| amiodarone (Cordarone) usual dose 200–800 mg orally daily in one dose or in divided doses | • Monitor for common side effects such as photosensitivity, nausea, vomiting, dizziness, fatigue, and hypotension.<br>• Be sure to monitor the respiratory status of patients who are taking amiodarone because this drug may cause pulmonary complications.<br>• Teach patients who are taking amiodarone that the drug causes sensitivity to light and that they may need to wear dark glasses when going outside. They also should wear protective clothing and a sunscreen barrier.<br>• Remind patients that they may not have side effects until they have taken the drug for several days or weeks.<br>• Tell patients that long-term use of amiodarone may cause a bluish discoloration of the face, neck, or arms. Reassure them that this side effect is reversible and will fade away over several months.<br>• Patients need to schedule eye examinations every 6–12 months because amiodarone can cause corneal microdeposits or other eye changes.<br>• Remind male patients to report pain or swelling in the scrotum to the healthcare provider. The patient may need a decrease in drug dosage. |

Table **9.8** Common Antidysrhythmic Drugs—cont'd

| DRUGS/ADULT DOSAGE | NURSING IMPLICATIONS |
|---|---|
| **Calcium Channel Blockers** | |
| diltiazem extended-release capsules (Cardizem CD, Cardizem, LA, Dilacor XR) 120–360 mg orally once daily<br>verapamil (Calan, Isoptin) 240–480 mg orally in 3–4 divided doses<br>verapamil extended release (Calan SR, Isoptin SR, Covera-HS) 180–480 mg orally once daily or in two divided doses; some forms may be given at bedtime | • Avoid sudden changes in position because these drugs cause orthostatic hypotension.<br>• Remind patients to keep taking the drugs as prescribed because they do not cure HBP or irregular heart rate.<br>• Monitor patients' blood pressure and heart rate regularly to determine how well they are responding to the drug.<br>• Teach patients to avoid alcohol because it can cause hypotension in patients taking calcium channel blockers.<br>• Teach patients to avoid grapefruit and grapefruit juice while taking calcium-channel blockers, as they may increase the risk of toxicity.<br>• Avoid all OTC drugs until checking with the healthcare provider to avoid dangerous drug interactions.<br>• Notify the healthcare provider if the patient experiences swelling in the legs because this can be a sign of fluid retention caused by calcium channel blockers.<br>• Calcium channel blockers are avoided in patients with heart failure because of the potential for fluid retention.<br>• Be alert for signs of Stevens-Johnson syndrome (erythema multiforme), a life-threating skin condition that can be an adverse effect of calcium channel blockers. This condition is associated with skin lesions, fever, and aching joints.<br>• Report heart rates of less than 60 beats/min and blood pressure levels lower than 90 mm Hg systolic to the healthcare provider before giving the drug to avoid significant hypotension.<br>• If you are caring for a patient who is receiving intravenous calcium channel blockers, check with the registered nurse or healthcare provider regarding the need for a bed with a cardiac monitor. |
| **Cardiac Glycosides** | |
| digoxin (Digitek, Lanoxicaps, Lanoxin) 0.125–0.5 mg daily orally (dose varies depending on patient weight, drug form, and patient response); in older adults, maximum dose of 0.125 mg daily | • Calcium channel blockers such as verapamil and diltiazem are replacing digoxin for treatment of atrial dysrhythmias. If you have a patient who is taking digoxin, monitor very carefully for symptoms of digoxin toxicity, such as lack of appetite, nausea, vomiting, and vision changes.<br>• Monitor potassium levels carefully because a low potassium level can cause dangerous dysrhythmias.<br>• In rare cases, patients may be given a loading dose to begin therapy and then switched to a normal dose after 24 hours. This is becoming a much less common practice.<br>• If the patient experiences any symptoms of digoxin toxicity, contact the healthcare provider. Optimal blood levels are 0.5–0.8 ng/mL.<br>• Take the apical pulse before giving digoxin. Do not give the drug if the pulse is less than 60 beats/min.<br>• Give digoxin at the same time every day to prevent irregular drug blood levels.<br>• Teach patients that a missed dose may be taken within 12 hours of the scheduled time and to never take double doses because of the high risk of drug toxicity. |

*GI,* gastrointestinal; *HBP,* high blood pressure; *OTC,* over the counter.

 **Top Tip for Safety**

Drugs given to control dysrhythmias may cause other dysrhythmias. Monitor the patient for symptoms of irregular heartbeats.

❖ **Nursing Implications and Patient Teaching**
◆ *Assessment.* Ask about the patient's health history, including any drug allergies, other drugs taken that may

cause drug interactions, and other medical problems. It is best practice to assess the apical heart rate using your stethoscope before giving the drug. Some irregular heart rates are very weak and are difficult to palpate using a radial pulse.

◆ *Planning and implementation.* The healthcare provider typically obtains an ECG before giving the drugs. This test helps the provider determine how well the drugs work. In addition, take the baseline and follow-up vital signs when you are giving antidysrhythmic drugs. In some settings, you may have the responsibility of monitoring changes in blood pressure or pulse as the patient begins taking the drug. Any significant changes must be reported to the RN or healthcare provider. Hospitalized patients often continue their antidysrhythmic drugs when they go home, and you should take advantage of every opportunity to teach patients about these drugs.

◆ *Evaluation.* In some settings, the patient is monitored using telemetry (24-hour-a-day cardiac monitoring). Specially trained staff (e.g., monitor technicians, nurses, LPN/VNs with training) monitor for changes in the ECG patterns. Monitor for changes in vital signs because improvement in rhythm often leads to improvement in vital signs.

◆ *Patient and family teaching.* Tell the patient and family:
- Take this drug exactly as ordered, and do not skip doses or double the dose.
- Report any new or distressing symptoms to the nurse or other healthcare provider, especially any sudden weight gain, trouble breathing, or increased coughing.
- Return regularly for checkup visits to the healthcare provider to see how the drug is affecting your heart function.
- Do not take any other drugs before consulting with the healthcare provider to make sure the combination is safe. This includes aspirin, laxatives, cold and sinus products, and other OTC drugs.

## INOTROPIC DRUGS

The term *inotrope* is used to describe contractility of the heart. An **inotropic drug** affects contractility of the myocardium (heart muscle). A positive inotropic drug increases contractility; a negative inotropic drug decreases contractility of the myocardium. In heart failure, positive inotropic drugs increase contractility and therefore increase the ability of the heart to pump blood.

 **Memory Jogger**
- A positive inotropic drug increases contractility and the ability of the heart to pump.
- A negative inotropic drug decreases contractility and the ability of the heart to pump.

Examples of positive inotropes include cardiac glycosides such as digoxin, phosphodiesterase inhibitors such as milrinone, and dobutamine. The major cardiac glycoside is digoxin. Between the 1960s and the early 2000s, digoxin was one of the main drugs used in heart failure to increase the contractility of the heart. As researchers learned more about the pathophysiology of

heart failure, other drugs have replaced digoxin as a drug of choice. Digoxin is still used as an antidysrhythmic and as an adjuvant agent in heart failure. Names, dosages, and nursing implications for common antidysrhythmics are listed in Table 9.8. For more information about specific antidysrhythmics, consult a drug reference book or a pharmacist.

### Action
As a positive inotrope, digoxin activates contractile proteins in the heart muscle, increasing their ability to contract. This increase in contractility continues even if the patient is taking a beta-blocker (a negative inotrope; recall that beta-blockers can decrease contractility to decrease how hard the heart works). In patients with heart failure, an increased force of contraction may lead to an improvement in cardiac output.

Digoxin affects the conduction system of the heart, decreasing the heart rate. As a result, digoxin can effectively treat atrial fibrillation in some cases. Other inotropic agents that are used in patients with heart failure include milrinone and dobutamine. These agents are used in seriously ill, symptomatic patients. Both require extensive monitoring, and they are typically used in acute care or palliative care settings to reduce symptoms of heart failure.

Patients with heart failure are more likely to receive ACE-Is or ARBs, beta-blockers, and/or diuretics to manage symptoms and decrease progression of the illness. Nevertheless, digoxin is still used in some cases and has significant implications for monitoring a patient who is taking it.

### Uses
Positive inotropic drugs are primarily used for symptom management in patients with advanced heart failure and in critical care areas to increase contractility of the heart muscle and improve cardiac output.

### Adverse Reactions
Inotropic drugs are very powerful and can be toxic. Symptoms of digoxin toxicity include anorexia, nausea, vomiting, diarrhea, visual disturbances such as blurred or yellow vision, and irregular heart rate (at times with palpitations). Patients may experience anxiety, depression, or confusion. Older adult patients are at particular risk for the adverse effects of inotropic drugs, including digoxin.

A blood test that tells the level of digoxin (often called *dig level*) is a tool that determines the correct dose and protects the patient from toxicity. Patients are more likely to develop high digoxin blood levels if they are older, have renal insufficiency, or have electrolyte imbalances caused by dehydration or drugs taken for other types of heart conditions. Treatment of digoxin toxicity begins by stopping the drug and treating the associated symptoms, as needed.

Adverse reactions in patients taking dobutamine include chest pain, palpitations, shortness of breath, bronchospasm, severe allergic reaction, and dysrhythmias. Adverse reactions associated with milrinone are similar and include chest pain, bronchospasm, severe allergic reaction, and dysrhythmias.

 **Lifespan Considerations**

**Older Adults**

Digoxin has a very narrow therapeutic range, which means that the effective dose is close to the dose that can cause toxicity. Older adults are particularly at risk for digoxin toxicity. Symptoms of toxicity may begin slowly and are often easy to overlook. These symptoms include loss of appetite, nausea, vomiting, and changes in vision (blurred or with a yellow-green tint).

### Drug Interactions

Beta-adrenergic blocking agents, calcium gluconate, calcium chloride, succinylcholine, and verapamil increase the therapeutic and the toxic effects of inotropic drugs. Any drug that changes the electrolyte balance may also lead to digoxin toxicity. Patients who take drugs that reduce potassium levels, such as diuretics, are particularly susceptible to digoxin toxicity.

### ❖ Nursing Implications and Patient Teaching

◆ *Assessment.* Take vital signs before giving digoxin or any inotropic agents. While improving contractility of the heart, they can also affect the heart rate. For digoxin, make sure that the patient's heart rate is 60 beats/min or higher. If you have a patient in an acute care setting who is taking digoxin for atrial fibrillation, it is important to have a skilled monitor technician available to monitor for any changes in the ECG. You also need to assess whether the patient's potassium level is within normal limits because a low potassium level can increase the risk of digoxin toxicity. Should you have any questions about your assessment, notify the RN or the healthcare provider before giving these drugs. Assess for any potential adverse effects each time you give the drug.

If you are caring for a patient who is receiving intravenous milrinone or dobutamine, carefully monitor for a rapid heart rate and negative changes in the patient's condition (e.g., increased shortness of breath, chest pain) that may indicate adverse effects.

◆ *Planning and implementation.* Know about two types of doses for patients taking digoxin: the initial loading dose and the maintenance (regular daily) dose. The healthcare provider may prescribe a higher and/or more frequent dose when a patient begins taking digoxin to reach a target blood level for a specific response. When the target blood level is reached, a smaller dose is given once daily to maintain the blood level.

 **Top Tip for Safety**

Digoxin lowers the patient's heart rate. Always measure the patient's apical heart rate for 60 seconds with a stethoscope before giving these drugs. This safety measure is essential to avoid an overdose. If the patient's pulse is irregular, you may not feel an accurate heart rate using the radial pulse alone.

**Top Tip for Safety**

**DIGOXIN**

Remember the rules for leading and trailing zeroes when giving digoxin. The usual dosage for digoxin in adults is very small compared with other drugs, ranging from 0.125 to 0.25 mg.

◆ *Evaluation.* Monitoring for drug toxicity is important for any patient who is taking a positive inotropic drug. If you notice any significant change in vital signs, notify the RN or the healthcare provider in charge of the patient. You may be caring for patients with multiple chronic illnesses, and it is important to monitor for any adverse effects. The healthcare provider will order blood tests to measure the serum digoxin level. The therapeutic level of digoxin is 0.5–2 ng/mL (nanograms per milliliter). If the level is 2 ng/mL or above, hold the drug, and notify the healthcare provider for best action.

Should a patient become severely digoxin toxic, the healthcare provider may prescribe digoxin immune fab (Digibind). This drug requires careful monitoring of the patient's vital signs and potassium levels and special plans for slowly reducing the amount of drug that is given to avoid causing other life-threatening events.

◆ *Patient and family teaching.* Teach the family and patient:
- Let your healthcare provider know if you have any loss of appetite, nausea, vomiting, diarrhea, or vision changes that can be an indication of digoxin toxicity.
- Do not skip a dose or stop taking the drug without discussing this with your healthcare provider.
- Keep appointments with your healthcare provider to make sure that the drug is still effective. Blood levels of the drug may be ordered.
- Do not take any other prescription or OTC drugs without the approval of your healthcare provider.
- Notify your healthcare provider of any chest pain, shortness of breath, or peripheral edema that may indicate worsening heart failure.
- Include foods rich in potassium in your diet (unless contraindicated by your healthcare provider). Good sources of potassium include bananas, orange juice, green leafy vegetables, and baked potatoes.

# Get Ready for the Next-Generation NCLEX® Examination!

## Key Points

- Thiazide and thiazide-like drugs are the most commonly used type of diuretic and often are the first line in the management of HBP.
- Loop diuretics are widely considered the most powerful of the diuretics. Use can result in significant decreases in fluid volume and increase in urine output.
- Potassium is one of the major electrolytes lost after loop diuretic administration. Monitor potassium levels carefully because significant changes in potassium can result in cardiac dysrhythmias.
- Potassium-sparing diuretics increase the excretion of water and sodium, leading to increased urine output without the loss of potassium.
- Monitor older adults taking diuretics more frequently for dehydration and symptoms of low potassium levels, such as muscle weakness and irregular heartbeats.
- Common side effects of diuretics include urinary urgency and urinary frequency.
- Diuretics can cause low blood pressure that can result in falls, particularly by high-risk patients.
- Patients who are taking potassium-sparing diuretics should avoid salt substitutes to decrease the risk for hyperkalemia.
- Potassium levels that are too high or too low can cause life-threatening dysrhythmias.
- Assess the patient carefully for any signs of dehydration before giving any diuretic.
- Warn patients and family members that pregnant women should not handle or touch dihydrotestosterone (DHT) inhibitors used for BPH because these drugs can cause birth defects if absorbed through the skin.
- Warn patients who are taking selective alpha₁ blockers for BPH to change positions slowly because these drugs lower blood pressure and can cause dizziness.
- Remind patients who are taking urinary antispasmodics to avoid becoming overheated or dehydrated during exercise or hot weather because these drugs decrease sweating and increase the risk for heatstroke.
- LDLs are the "bad" cholesterol; HDLs are the "good" cholesterol.
- All patients who are taking statins should have liver function studies shortly after starting the drug and then yearly or if they experience any symptoms of liver problems.
- Statins are contraindicated during pregnancy and breast-feeding because of the effects of lower cholesterol levels on the developing brain.
- For patients who are taking statins, immediately report to the healthcare provider any severe muscle ache or signs of liver problems, such as jaundice or dark urine, because those symptoms can be signs of serious adverse effects.
- One of the main problems for patients taking niacin is the expected side effect of flushing (red color in the face and neck).
- No cholesterol-reducing drug cures hyperlipidemia.
- Drug therapy for HBP often requires trial periods to establish the right drug or drug combinations to help the patient achieve his or her blood pressure goal.
- You can use the terms *antagonist* and *blocker* interchangeably to describe a drug that turns off a receptor.

- ACE-Is and ARBs can cause hyperkalemia (high potassium levels); remind patients taking them to avoid high-potassium foods.
- Fluid retention is a common side effect of calcium channel blockers and should be avoided in patients with heart failure.
- Beta-blockers typically end with the suffix -olol—for example, metoprolol, propranolol, and sotalol.
- A side effect of prazosin and terazosin is first-dose hypotension. As a result, they may be given at night to prevent orthostatic hypotension. The effects diminish over time.
- To prevent rebound HBP, do not stop alpha₂-agonists suddenly.
- Antihypertensives and diuretics are used alone or in combination to decrease elevated blood pressure to a desired level according to accepted guidelines and to prevent complications of acute and chronic HBP.
- All blood pressure drugs can cause hypotension (blood pressure too low to maintain adequate circulation). Most can cause orthostatic hypotension (dizziness that occurs when changing positions).
- Older adults are particularly likely to experience dizziness when taking blood pressure drugs. The orthostatic hypotension they experience places them at risk for falling when they rapidly change positions, such as getting up quickly from a chair or bed.
- Teach your patient to stand up slowly when taking drugs for HBP to avoid dizziness and prevent falls.
- For all patients with HBP, it is critical to gather a thorough drug history. Certain prescription drugs, OTC drugs, herbal preparations, and illegal drugs can cause HBP.
- Baseline blood pressure checks are essential before giving any drug that affects blood pressure,.
- HBP has no cure; it can, however, be well managed.
- Notify the healthcare provider of any new or uncomfortable symptoms that develop. They may indicate an adverse effect, or they may be relieved simply by changing to a new drug.
- Teach patients to avoid alcoholic beverages while taking drugs for HBP.
- Rapid-acting nitrates (e.g., sublingual NTG, intravenous NTG) are used to relieve pain in acute angina. The long-acting oral nitrates, topical NTG paste, and transdermal patches can prevent angina and reduce the severity and frequency of angina attacks.
- Throbbing headaches occur in more than 50% of patients who take nitrates.
- Remember that all antidysrhythmic drugs can cause dysrhythmias.
- Positive inotropic drugs are primarily used for symptom management in patients with advanced heart failure and in critical care areas to increase contractility of the heart muscle and improve cardiac output.
- Digoxin has a very narrow therapeutic range, which means the dose that is effective is close to the dose that causes toxic reactions. Older adults are particularly at risk for digoxin toxicity. Symptoms of toxicity may begin slowly and are often easy to overlook. They include loss of appetite, nausea and vomiting, and changes in vision.
- Digoxin lowers the patient's heart rate; always measure the patient's apical heart rate for 60 seconds with a stethoscope before giving these drugs. If the patient's

pulse is irregular, you may not feel an accurate heart rate using the radial pulse alone.

- Remember the rules for the "leading" and "trailing" zeroes when giving digoxin. For example, a patient may be receiving a dose of 0.125 or 0.25 mg/day.

## Clinical Judgment and Next-Generation NCLEX® Examination-Style Questions

1. A patient with benign prostatic hypertrophy is receiving tamsulosin, a selective alpha$_1$ blocker, to help improve urine flow. Which of the following health factors would the LPN/VN report to the healthcare provider before giving the drug? **Select all or any that apply.**

   1. The patient reports a history of allergy to sulfa antibiotics.
   2. The patient has a history of smoking 15 years ago.
   3. The patient is exercising three times a week.
   4. The patient's potassium level is 4.0 mEq/mL.
   5. The patient has a history of orthostatic hypotension.

2. A patient with a history of overactive bladder is prescribed oxybutynin 5 mg orally twice a day. Which of the following statements by the patient indicates a need for more teaching?

   1. "I need to avoid drinking alcohol at least 2 hours within taking my oxybutynin."
   2. "I will weigh myself every day and notify my healthcare provider if I have more than a 2-pound weight gain."
   3. "Antihistamines can cause me to retain urine."
   4. "I really like to take a sauna after swimming."

3. The patient has a history of acute angina. Which of the following should the LPN/VN teach the patient regarding taking NTG tablets for chest pain? **Select all or any that apply.**

   1. Take one dose of NTG immediately at the onset of the pain. If the symptoms get a little better but do not go away, take the second dose 5 minutes later. You can even take a third dose 5 minutes after the second dose.
   2. Take no more than three doses in 15 minutes.
   3. Call emergency services if your symptoms do not improve or if they worsen after the first dose.
   4. You may feel a slight burning under the tongue when you take the NTG.
   5. Common side effects include lightheadedness, muscle aches, and seizures.
   6. The NTG will work better if you also dissolve an aspirin under your tongue at the same time.

4. The patient is taking digoxin 0.25 mg every morning with breakfast for atrial fibrillation. The LPN/VN checks the apical pulse and determines the rate to be 68 beats/min. Which of the following actions is appropriate by the LPN/VN?

   1. Ask the patient to drink a cup of coffee and return to the room in 1 hour so you can give the drug.
   2. Hold the drug and notify the healthcare provider.
   3. Give the drug and document it in the medical record.
   4. Give the drug and notify the healthcare provider.

5. Which of the following laboratory tests must be carefully monitored in a patient taking triamterene?

   1. Potassium level
   2. Liver function studies
   3. Arterial blood gases
   4. Cholesterol level

6. Which of the following symptoms are associated with digoxin toxicity? **Select all or any that apply.**

   1. Nausea
   2. Anorexia
   3. Blurred vision
   4. Constipation
   5. Enlarged liver

7. A patient is receiving a new statin drug for an elevated cholesterol level. Which of the following statements by the patient indicates a need for additional teaching?

   1. "I can add cholesterol back in my diet now that I have started this drug."
   2. "I will notify my healthcare provider if I have any severe muscle aches or changes in my urine."
   3. "I will work with my healthcare provider to have my cholesterol checked in 4 to 12 weeks to see how the drug is working."
   4. "I have to monitor my blood sugar daily because the drug can increase my blood sugar."

8. Match the following drugs with their classification.

| | |
|---|---|
| 1. chlorothiazide (Diuril) | A. loop diuretic |
| 2. furosemide (Lasix) | B. potassium-sparing diuretic |
| 3. metolazone (Zaroxolyn) | C. thiazide diuretic |
| 4. spironolactone (Aldactone) | D. thiazide-like diuretic |
| 5. bumetanide (Bumex) | |
| 6. amiloride (Midamor) | |

9. Which of the following types of food should be avoided in patients taking angiotensin-converting enzyme inhibitors?

   1. Foods high in folic acid, such as lentils and avocado
   2. Foods high in vitamin K, such as green leafy vegetables
   3. Foods high in iron, such as red meat and salmon
   4. Foods high in potassium, such as bananas and orange juice

10. Match the drug action with the drug class.

| DRUG ACTION | DRUG CLASS |
|---|---|
| 1. Slows the sodium pump in the distal tubule of the nephron | a. __ Angiotensin-converting enzyme inhibitor |
| 2. Decreases heart rate and decreases contractility of the heart | b. __ Loop diuretic |
| | c. __ Beta-blocker |
| 3. Blocks active transport of sodium, chloride, and potassium in the loop of Henle | d. __ Alpha$_2$-adrenergic agonist |
| 4. Blocks the formation of angiotensin II | e. __ Potassium-sparing diuretic |
| 5. Causes vasodilation centrally by affecting receptors in the brain | |

## Case Study

A patient with a history of chronic HBP is on a prescription of losartan 100 mg daily. The healthcare provider added a dose of hydrochlorothiazide 25 mg/day.

1. Losartan is available in 50 mg tablets. How many tablets of losartan will the nurse administer?

2. Based on the patient's complaint, what nursing action should be initiated?

## Drug Calculation Review

A patient is receiving 10 mg of simvastatin at bedtime. The patient prefers the oral suspension of simvastatin available as 20 mg/5 mL How many mL will you prepare to give the patient?

## Case Study

### Question 1

Mr. Johnson is a 58-year-old black male with primary hypertension diagnosed 15 years ago by his primary care physician. According to his family history, his father had HBP and his grandfather died of a stroke at the age of 62. Mr. Johnson is currently 5 feet 10 inches tall and weighs 242 pounds (BMI 34.7) . During his visit, he tells you that his daughter was recently killed in a car accident and that this has been devastating for his family. He is currently prescribed a combination of a thiazide-like diuretic (chlorthalidone) and a calcium channel blocker (amlodipine) to manage his blood pressure. Which risk factors contribute to Mr. Johnson's hypertension?
**Select all or any that apply.**
__ A. Psychosocial stress
__ B. Black race
__ C. Family history
__ D. Calcium channel blockers
__ E. Smoking history
__ F. Retired from job
__ G. Obesity

### Question 2

Mr. Johnson's blood pressure is found to be 156/90 mg Hg, heart rate 92 beats/min, and respirations 16 breaths/min. He has 2+ pitting edema in both feet and reports that he sometimes gets short of breath when he does even a small amount of physical activity. His lab work is normal except for a potassium level of 3.3 mmol/L Choose the **most likely** options for the information missing from the statements below by selecting from the list of options provided.

The nurse recognizes that _____, a drug from the _____ category, is the most likely cause of the increase in peripheral edema. Evaluation of his lab work reveals a(n) _____ potassium level that is commonly associated with _____. Besides his HBP, Mr. Johnson is showing symptoms associated with _____.

| OPTIONS |
| --- |
| Amlodipine |
| Chlorthalidone |
| Thiazide-like diuretics |
|    Myocardial infarction |
|    Increased |
|    Decreased |
|    Calcium channel blockers |
|    Potassium-sparing diuretic |
|    Heart failure |
|    Gout |

## Learning Outcomes

1. List the names, actions, possible side effects, and adverse effects of drugs for Parkinson's disease.
2. Explain what to teach patients and families about drugs for Parkinson's disease.
3. List the names, actions, possible side effects, and adverse effects of drugs for Alzheimer's disease.
4. Explain what to teach patients and families about drugs for Alzheimer's disease.
5. List the names, actions, possible side effects, and adverse effects of drugs for epilepsy and other seizure problems.
6. Explain what to teach patients and families about drugs for epilepsy and other seizure problems.
7. List the names, actions, possible side effects, and adverse effects of drugs for multiple sclerosis.
8. Explain what to teach patients and families about drugs for multiple sclerosis.
9. List the names, actions, possible side effects, and adverse effects of drugs for amyotrophic lateral sclerosis and myasthenia gravis.
10. Explain what to teach patients and families about the drugs for amyotrophic lateral sclerosis and myasthenia gravis.

## Key Terms

**antiepileptic drug (AED)** Drug that reduces or prevents seizures.

**biological response modifier (BRM)** Drug that modifies the patient's immune response to abnormal triggers of immunity and inflammation.

**10 catechol-*O*-methyltransferase (COMT) inhibitor** Drug that suppresses the activity of the COMT enzyme so that naturally occurring dopamine and dopamine agonist drugs remain active in the body longer, helping to restore the acetylcholine–dopamine balance in the brain.

**cholinesterase inhibitor** Drug that delays memory loss by binding to the enzyme acetylcholinesterase and slowing its action, which allows any acetylcholine produced to remain functional longer; also used to treat myasthenia gravis.

**delirium** A distressed state of mind that causes irrational beliefs characterized by illusions and paranoia.

**dopamine agonist** Drug that has the same chemical structure as natural dopamine and is used to increase the levels of dopamine in the brain and restore balance between the actions of acetylcholine and dopamine.

**dyskinesia** An abnormality and distortion in performing voluntary movements. It results in jerky motions and looks much like uncoordinated dance movements.

**dystonia** Abnormal involuntary movements such as chewing, grinding of the teeth, protrusion of the tongue, opening and closing the mouth, head bobbing, or jerky, constant movements of the feet or hands.

**monoamine oxidase type B (MAO-B) inhibitor** Drug that suppresses the action of MAO-B, allowing dopamine levels to increase and reducing the symptoms of Parkinson's disease.

**neurotransmitter** Chemical that is released from the end of one nerve, crosses a synaptic cleft, and then binds to receptors on the beginning of the next nerve in the line (or on a skeletal muscle) to transmit the electrical signal.

***N*-methyl-D-aspartate (NMDA) blocker** Drug that slows the progression of Alzheimer's disease by blocking the entrance of calcium into neurons, which reduces or slows neuronal damage.

**10 phenytoin** An antiepileptic drug that reduces or prevents seizures by binding to sodium channels on nerve membranes in the brain and making them less active, which prevents the spread of neuron excitation.

## CENTRAL NERVOUS SYSTEM FUNCTIONS

The central nervous system (CNS) consists of the brain and the spinal cord (Fig. 10.1). The nerves coming from the spinal cord are part of the peripheral nervous system (PNS) and are controlled by the brain. The PNS nerves serve to relay signals between the brain and the body by connecting the CNS to organs, limbs, muscles, blood vessels, and glands.

The CNS has many critical structures and actions that work together to ensure continuous and normal whole-body functioning. The brain monitors and regulates the coordination of body systems and activities, including movement, endocrine secretions, and intellectual functions such as thinking and decision making. It monitors body conditions by receiving sensory information from elsewhere in the body and from the environment through vision, hearing, smell, taste, spatial awareness, and touch. The brain interprets this information and determines how the body should respond. For example, we actually see with our brain, not our eyes. The nerve endings of specialized photoreceptor cells (rods and cones) in the retina detect and convert light into signals that are then sent through the optic nerve to the brain. The brain translates the light signals into what we "see" (perceive). Altered perception is how optical illusions work. Magicians create illusions by taking advantage of how our brains interpret stimuli.

Many problems that occur inside or outside the CNS can affect brain function. This chapter focuses on drug therapy for CNS problems that mainly affect physical function, including Parkinson's disease (PD), Alzheimer's disease (AD), epilepsy, and multiple sclerosis (MS). Drug therapy for problems that primarily affect behavior and mental health is described in Chapter 11.

Movement is an important motor function that involves the brain, spinal cord, nerves, muscles, and bones. For example, your decision to deliberately move your arm starts when you think about it, which excites nerve cells *(neurons)* in a particular part of the brain. Initial excitation is turned into an electrical signal that causes your muscles to move the arm in the direction you planned. Getting the signal from your brain to your arm muscles involves a relay of signals (conduction) through a specific line of connected nerves. At each connection, signals are conducted across an intervening space called a *synapse* (Fig. 10.2). Transmission of electrical impulses between neurons depends on the release of neurotransmitters.

A **neurotransmitter** is a chemical that is released from the end of one nerve, crosses a synaptic cleft, and then binds to receptors on the next nerve in the line. This action transmits the electrical signal that started in your brain through the line of connected nerves. When the last nerve in the line gets to your arm muscles, the neurotransmitter binds to receptors on the muscle and triggers the muscle contractions needed to make your arm move.

Neurotransmitters can be excitatory or inhibitory. *Excitatory neurotransmitters* include acetylcholine (ACh), epinephrine, and norepinephrine. When the excitatory neurotransmitter ACh is released from the end of a nerve in response to thinking about moving your arm, it ensures that this action signal gets transmitted to the next nerve in the line. At the point where the last nerve in the line is stimulated, the ACh it releases binds to receptors on the arm's skeletal muscles, and they contract and move your arm as you intended.

*Inhibitory neurotransmitters* include dopamine, some types of serotonin, and gamma-aminobutyric acid (GABA). Smooth movement requires input from an excitatory neurotransmitter (ACh) and an inhibitory neurotransmitter (dopamine). These inputs are balanced in such a way that when you decide to move your arm, you can control the direction, degree, and strength of the movement. You do not need the same strength to rub your eye gently as you do to throw a baseball 60 feet. Without dopamine to modify arm muscle contractions, your arm movement would be fast, jerky, and wild. Think of how much hot coffee you would spill moving a cup to your mouth if dopamine were not modifying this arm movement.

Some problems that occur in the CNS, such as PD, result from an imbalance of excitatory and inhibitory

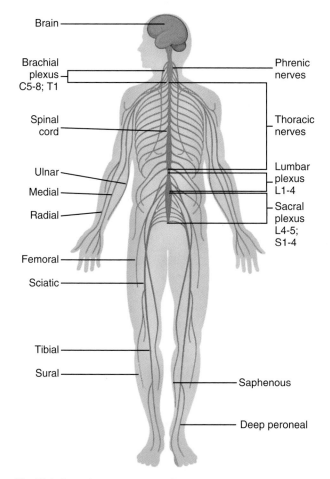

Fig. 10.1 Central nervous system. *C*, cervical; *L*, lumbar; *T*, thoracic.

Brain

Brachial plexus C5-8; T1

Spinal cord

Ulnar

Medial

Radial

Femoral

Sciatic

Tibial

Sural

Phrenic nerves

Thoracic nerves

Lumbar plexus L1-4

Sacral plexus L4-5; S1-4

Saphenous

Deep peroneal

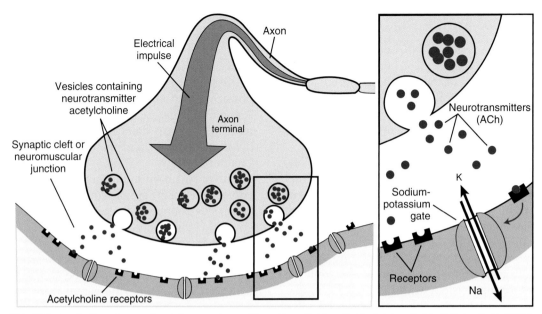

FIG. 10.2 Conduction of nerve signals by neurotransmitters. (From Fulcher, E. M., Fulcher, R. M., & Soto, C. D. (2012). Pharmacology (3rd ed.). St. Louis: Saunders.)

neurotransmitters. Others problems, such as epilepsy, are caused by conditions in the brain that allow neurons to become excited when the excitation is not needed. Still others, such as AD and MS, result from degenerative changes that occur in nerves or the support cells of the brain.

## DRUGS FOR PARKINSON'S DISEASE

Second only to AD, PD is the most common neurodegenerative disease. The exact cause of PD is unknown, but it is thought to be caused by a combination of genetic, protective, and environmental factors. The incidence of PD increases with age, but it can occur before age 50. The disease strikes more men than women.

The diagnosis of PD takes quite a while because there is no specific test for the disease. Diagnosis is made after all other neurologic disease processes have been ruled out. The disease manifests as movement disorders and is associated with the presence of Lewy bodies in the brain. Lewy bodies are protein deposits in the brain cells associated with thinking, movement, and memory, and they cause dementia. If cognitive problems occur a year or more after the movement difficulties begin, the patient is said to have Parkinson's disease dementia.

PD is a CNS disorder in which not enough dopamine is available to modify excitatory signals to skeletal muscles. Dopamine is an inhibitory neurotransmitter that is mostly produced deep in the midbrain area known as the *substantia nigra*, which is part of the basal ganglia. When this brain area slows or stops production of dopamine, the balance between excitatory motor nerve signals and inhibitory motor nerve signals is reduced, causing mostly excitatory input (Fig. 10.3). Movements become hard to control and jerky, and some muscles are rigid because they fail to relax sufficiently. When the arms and legs move, they "catch" at certain points in a stop-and-go

fashion known as *cogwheel rigidity*. The neurologic problems also cause facial features to become masklike (Fig. 10.4). The gait becomes slow and shuffling with short steps. The risk of falls greatly increases. Other common symptoms of PD include tremors, stooped posture, difficulty stopping motion after it has started, difficulty chewing and swallowing, and drooling.

Depression, hallucinations, anxiety, and delusions are frequent complications of PD. Delusions and hallucinations can result from the changes in the brain that PD causes, or they can occur from the adverse effects of PD drugs themselves. The PD drugs increase the dopamine levels to improve the motor symptoms, but unfortunately, increasing the dopamine supply can also cause hallucinations and delusions. Symptoms of PD worsen over time until the patient eventually requires total care. Box 10.1 lists the motor and nonmotor symptoms of PD.

 **Bookmark This!**

Ongoing clinical trials and research are changing the understanding of PD. Check out the Michael J. Fox Web site: https://www.michaeljfox.org.

Although drug therapy does not cure PD, it can delay worsening of symptoms and allow patients to remain independent longer. Drug therapy for PD includes dopamine and dopamine agonists, catechol-*O*-methyltransferase (COMT) inhibitors, and monoamine oxidase type B (MAO-B) inhibitors. The common drugs in these classes are listed in Table 10.1.

At one time, anticholinergic drugs were the main therapy for PD. These drugs were used to balance decreased dopamine levels because they reduced ACh levels. However, this action did not address the main problem of PD (i.e., lack of dopamine), and they caused many side effects and adverse reactions. As a result,

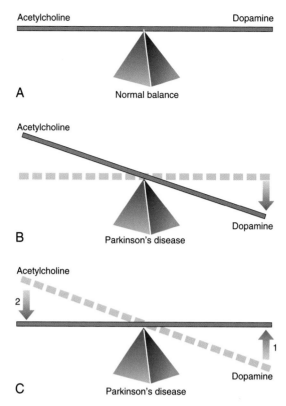

A, Normal balance of acetylcholine and dopamine in the CNS.
B, In Parkinson's disease, a decrease in dopamine results in an imbalance.
C, Drug therapy in Parkinson's disease is aimed at correcting the imbalance between acetylcholine and dopamine. This can be accomplished by:
  1. increasing the supply of dopamine
  2. blocking or lowering acetylcholine levels

Fig. 10.3 The neurotransmitter abnormality in Parkinson's disease. *CNS,* central nervous system. (From Lilley, L. L., Rainforth Collins S., & Snyder, J. (2019). *Pharmacology and the nursing process* (9th ed.). Elsevier.)

anticholinergic drugs are no longer the most common therapy for PD. Amantadine (Symmetrel) comes in an immediate-release form and is a drug that is used in early and advanced PD to lessen tremors. Amantadine is an antiviral agent used as a prophylactic for influenza A. It has dopamine agonist properties that have been found helpful in reducing extrapyramidal reactions and motor symptoms that occur with dopamine drug.

Pimavanserin (Nuplazid) is an atypical antipsychotic that is the only drug specifically approved only for Parkinson's disease psychosis.

**Black Box Warning: Pimavanserin**

Pimavanserin carries a black box warning, however, of increased stroke risk and death in elderly patients with dementia. It is considered a potentially inappropriate drug for use in older adults according to the Beers Criteria.

**Memory Jogger**

There are three classes of drugs for managing PD:
- Dopamine agonists
- COMT inhibitors
- MAO-B inhibitors

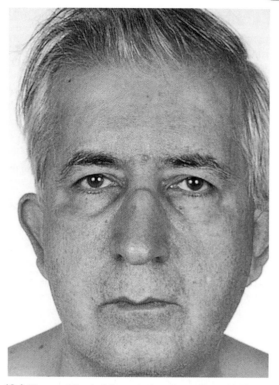

Fig. 10.4 The masklike facial expression of a patient with Parkinson's disease. (From Perkin, D. (1998). *Mosby's color atlas and test of neurology.* Mosby-Wolfe.)

**Box 10.1  Symptoms of Parkinson's Disease**

| MOTOR SYMPTOMS | NONMOTOR SYMPTOMS |
|---|---|
| • Slow movements (bradykinesia)<br>• Decreased arm swing when walking<br>• Difficulty rising from a chair or turning in bed<br>• Absence of facial expressions<br>• Instability when standing up<br>• Freezing in place and having a rigid stance<br>• Stooped, shuffling gait<br>• Tremors | • Constipation<br>• Diminished sense of smell<br>• Depression, anxiety, and irritability<br>• Problems with focused attention and planning<br>• Slowing of thought; language and memory difficulties<br>• Personality changes; dementia<br>• Hallucinations and delusions<br>• Sleep disturbances<br>• Urinary frequency<br>• Orthostatic hypotension |

**DOPAMINE AGONISTS**

**Action and Uses**

A dopamine agonist is a drug that has the same chemical structure as natural dopamine and is used to increase the levels of dopamine in the brain to restore balance between the actions of acetylcholine and dopamine. The therapeutic effect of these drugs helps reduce muscle tremors and rigidity and improves mobility, muscular coordination, and performance. Dopamine agonists can be used alone, or as symptoms progress, they can be used in combination. The National Parkinson

| Table **10.1** | Examples of Common Drugs Used to Manage Parkinson's Disease |

*Dopamine and dopamine agonists* have the same chemical structure as natural dopamine and improve symptoms of Parkinson's disease by increasing the levels of dopamine in the brain to restore balance between acetylcholine and dopamine action.

*COMT inhibitors* reduce the symptoms of Parkinson's disease by suppressing the activity of the COMT enzyme so that naturally occurring dopamine and dopamine agonist drugs remain active in the body longer, helping to restore the acetylcholine–dopamine balance in the brain.

*Selective MAO-B inhibitors* allow existing dopamine to remain active in the brain longer by inhibiting MAO-B, which breaks down dopamine in the brain and elsewhere in the body.

| DRUG/ADULT DOSAGE | NURSING IMPLICATIONS |
|---|---|
| **Dopamine and Dopamine Agonists** | |
| carbidopa/levodopa (Rytary, Sinemet) levodopa (Inbrija) 42 mg inhalation powder capsule with an inhaler device Rytary (23.75 mg carbidopa/95 mg levodopa) orally three times per day initially, increasing to a maximum daily dose of 612.5 mg/2450 mg Sinemet (25 mg carbidopa/100 mg levodopa) orally three times a day, increasing to a total of 200 mg/2000 mg/day pramipexole (Mirapex, Mirapex ER) 0.125 mg orally three times per day initially, increasing by 0.125–0.25 mg/dose every 5–7 days to a maximum dosage of 1.5 mg orally three times per day (4.5 mg/day) ropinirole (Requip, Requip XL) 0.25 mg orally three times per day for the first week; gradually titrate at weekly intervals to a maximum of 24 mg/day rotigotine (Neupro) transdermal patch at an initial dose of 2 mg/24 hours, increasing to a maximum of 8 mg/24 hours | • Carbidopa/levodopa tablets come in different dosages and are increased frequently from three times daily up to five times daily based on improvement of symptoms. For levodopa (Inbrija), inhale the contents of two capsules via oral inhalation with the provided inhaler as needed for wearing off symptoms up to five times daily. The dose should be taken when symptoms of a wearing-off period start to return.<br>• Tablets also come in extended-release form. Extended-release tablets are scored.<br>• Do not crush or chew whole or half tablets; they must be swallowed intact.<br>• Extended-release forms of tablets that are not scored should not be halved, crushed, or chewed to retain the slow-release effect.<br>• Give with 6–8 ounces of water at least 30–60 minutes before eating to maximize absorption.<br>• Give with a nonprotein snack to avoid nausea.<br>• Do not give with high-protein foods because they decrease absorption.<br>• Instruct patients to get up slowly to avoid postural hypotension with all dopamine agonists.<br>• Monitor blood glucose levels closely in diabetic patients to avoid hypoglycemia caused by increased sympathetic tone.<br>• Closely monitor patients with a history of cardiac disease for hypotension and increasing dysrhythmias.<br>• Monitor liver function studies because these drugs are metabolized in the liver, and monitor complete blood counts because these drugs can increase the risk of gastrointestinal bleeding.<br>• Notify the healthcare provider about any behavioral changes, hallucinations, or delusions.<br>• Monitor for worsening dyskinesia and/or dystonia reactions and notify the healthcare provider if they occur because this can indicate a need for dosage change.<br>• Skin reactions are common with the use of the rotigotine (Neupro) patch. Do not apply the patch in the same place more than once every 14 days, and after removing the patch, gently clean the skin with mild soap and water. |
| **COMT Inhibitors** | |
| entacapone (Comtan) 200 mg orally with each levodopa/carbidopa dose up to a maximum of 1600 mg/day tolcapone (Tasmar) initially, 100 mg orally three times daily with the first dose given with carbidopa/ levodopa; maximum dose 600 mg/ day opicapone (Ongentys) 50 mg at bedtime on an empty stomach | • Give entacapone with every dose of carbidopa/levodopa to enhance drug effect.<br>• Give the first dose of tolcapone with the first dose of carbidopa/levodopa and subsequent doses 6–12 hours later.<br>• Review liver function studies and monitor for liver failure in patients who are taking tolcapone.<br>• Report signs of liver failure, such as abdominal pain, jaundice, and dark urine with nausea and vomiting, to the healthcare provider.<br>• Remind patients that these drugs may cause a nondangerous side effect of turning the urine a brownish-orange color.<br>• These drugs enhance the effect of dopamine, and symptoms of worsening dyskinesia or psychosis may occur. Notify the healthcare provider if these changes occur.<br>• These drugs cannot be given with nonselective MAO inhibitors (i.e., those that inhibit both type A and type B MAOs) because of the increased cardiovascular risk.<br>• Anticipate that the carbidopa/levodopa dose may be decreased as these drugs take effect.<br>• Opicapone causes drowsiness and can cause orthostatic hypotension.<br>• Concomitant use of opioid agonists (codeine, hydrocodone, oxycodone) with COMT inhibitors may cause excessive sedation and somnolence. |

| Table 10.1   Examples of Common Drugs Used to Manage Parkinson's Disease—cont'd | |
| --- | --- |
| **DRUG/ADULT DOSAGE** | **NURSING IMPLICATIONS** |
| **Selective MAO-B Inhibitors** | |
| rasagiline (Azilect) 0.5–1 g orally once daily<br>safinamide (Xadago) 50–100 mg orally once daily<br>selegiline (Eldepryl, Emsam, Zelapar) 5 mg tablet orally twice daily | • Give these drugs at the same time every day. Once-a-day doses can be taken at nighttime because they can cause drowsiness.<br>• Teach patients to avoid foods and beverages that contain large amounts of tyramine (see Box 10.2) when using any of these drugs and for 2 weeks after therapy is stopped.<br>• Monitor vital signs, particularly blood pressure.<br>• Teach patients and families to report severe headache, palpitations, nausea, and vomiting to the healthcare provider immediately because these are signs of a hypertensive crisis.<br>• These drugs enhance the effect of dopamine, so symptoms of worsening dyskinesia or psychosis may occur. Teach patients and families to notify the healthcare provider if these changes occur.<br>• Anticipate that the healthcare provider may decrease the dosage of carbidopa/levodopa as these drugs take effect. |

*COMT*, catechol-O-methyltransferase; *MAO-B*, monoamine oxidase type B.

Foundation recommends that carbidopa/levodopa (Sinemet, Rytary) be used as a first-line treatment for patients with PD who are older than 70 years of age and that the newer dopamine agonists, such as pramipexole (Mirapex, Mirapex ER), ropinirole (Requip, Requip XL), and rotigotine (Neupro), be used as first-line treatment in patients between the ages 50 and 70.

All patients will eventually require levodopa because dopamine becomes deficient in PD. Levodopa is synthesized in the brain and converted to natural dopamine. For this reason, levodopa is the most important drug used to manage the symptoms of PD. Carbidopa is usually given in combination with levodopa because it allows more levodopa to get into brain cells; this means that lower doses of levodopa can be used, preventing the nausea and vomiting that accompany the continually increasing levodopa doses needed to control disease symptoms. Levodopa (Larodopa) is rarely given alone for this reason.

*Wearing off* is an issue of a drug losing its effectiveness; it can occur after levodopa has been used for several years. The action of levodopa peaks in about 1 hour after administration and wears off in 4 or 5 hours. The wearing-off effect causes rapid swings of symptoms. Symptoms improve when adequate levels of dopamine are present and worsen as the amount of dopamine decreases and its therapeutic effect wears off. This is also called an *on/off effect*. The extended-release form of carbidopa/levodopa and the longer half-lives of dopamine agonists help to prevent this effect. Carbidopa/levodopa is also available as an intestinal infusion pump (Duopa). The pump is inserted directly into the small intestine through a small feeding tube and can deliver 16 continuous hours of carbidopa and levodopa therapy to reduce motor symptoms. Levodopa comes in an inhaled form as well (Inbrija). It can be inhaled up to five times a day to counteract wearing off.

## Expected Side Effects and Adverse Reactions

The most common side effects of carbidopa/levodopa and all dopamine agonists include postural and general hypotension, headache, GI disturbances, insomnia, dream abnormalities, decreased impulse control, and confusion. The most common adverse reaction to carbidopa/levodopa is dyskinesia, which results in involuntary muscle movements that look like uncoordinated dance movements. Dyskinesia is common in patients on long-term carbidopa/levodopa therapy (longer than 3 years). The effect of dyskinesia is minimized with the use of pramipexole, ropinirole, rotigotine, and other dopamine agonists. Dopamine agonists can also cause delirium (a distressed state of mind that causes irrational beliefs characterized by illusions and paranoia), psychosis, and hallucinations. If these problems occur, the healthcare provider needs to determine whether the symptoms are related to the advancing disease process, depression, or the PD drug.

> **⮂ Do Not Confuse**
> • *Risperidone* is an antipsychotic drug that is sometimes used to combat psychosis in PD.
> • *Ropinirole* is used to treat symptoms of PD, including stiffness, tremors, muscle spasms, and poor muscle control.

Carbidopa/levodopa dosages may be decreased as COMT inhibitors and MAO-B inhibitors are added to the drug regimen. This can precipitate *neuroleptic malignant syndrome*, with symptoms of agitation, coma, muscle rigidity, tremors, high fever, and an unstable blood pressure. Remember that as COMT inhibitors and MAO-B inhibitors are added to the regimen of dopamine agonists, the amount of available dopamine rises; this can increase the adverse effects of dopamine agonists until their dosages are adjusted by the healthcare provider.

When dopamine agonists are taken with protein as a meal or a snack, the effectiveness of the drug is reduced. These drugs are best absorbed on an empty stomach.

## Drug Interactions

Use of antihypertensive agents with dopamine agonists can cause severe hypotension. Use of older, nonselective MAO inhibitors such as phenelzine (Nardil) along with dopamine agonists can precipitate a hypertensive crisis. Phenytoin (Dilantin) reduces the effectiveness of dopamine agonists. Multivitamins that contain iron decrease the effects of carbidopa/levodopa. Vitamin $B_6$ (pyridoxine) increases the metabolism of levodopa taken without carbidopa. Metoclopramide (Reglan) can reduce the effectiveness of the dopamine agonists because metoclopramide is a dopamine antagonist that prevents dopamine from combining with dopamine receptors. Use of dopamine agonists with sedatives worsens drowsiness and increases the risk of confusion, hallucinations, and delusions, especially in those persons already suffering from mental illnesses.

### ❖ Nursing Implications and Patient Teaching

◆ *Assessment.* Dopamine agonists frequently cause postural hypotension, and you should take a full set of vital signs, including orthostatic blood pressure readings (supine, sitting, and standing). Assessment of the patient's motor skills and functional ability for walking and eating is important to establish a baseline and to ensure safety from falls and aspiration. Ask whether patients have had melanoma or closed-angle glaucoma; these conditions are contraindications for dopamine agonist therapy because the drugs can worsen them. Closely monitor blood glucose levels because the sympathetic effects of levodopa can cause hypoglycemia. Observe for symptoms such as headache, anxiety, shakiness, weakness, and irritability that can indicate low blood glucose. Check blood urea nitrogen (BUN) and creatinine levels before starting pramipexole to rule out renal impairment because 90% of the drug is excreted by the kidneys. Monitor liver enzymes before and at intervals during treatment because other drugs used in the treatment of PD are metabolized by the liver.

◆ *Planning and implementation.* Dopamine agonists are recommended to be given 30 to 60 minutes before meals for better absorption and for maximum effect so that the patient has less difficulty chewing and swallowing, which lessens the risk of aspiration. Never crush the extended-release tablets. When using rotigotine transdermal patches, apply them at the same time every day, and rotate application sites. Do not apply to the same site more than once every 14 days to avoid a skin reaction.

Dopamine agonists should be withdrawn slowly because these drugs have a long half-life. When withdrawing one preparation and beginning a new preparation, the new drug is started in small doses and the old drug is withdrawn gradually. These agents are usually started at the lowest dose possible, and the dose is increased gradually until the maximum therapeutic effect has been obtained.

Dopamine agonists are available in patches, tablets, sustained-release capsules, syrups, and elixirs. They are generally well absorbed from the GI tract. Peak blood levels of carbidopa/levodopa, one of the main treatment drugs, is achieved in 1 to 6 hours, depending on the route of administration and the formulation of the drug given. Sustained-release capsules reach peak plasma levels in 8 to 12 hours. Sustained-release capsules are not recommended for initial therapy because they do not allow enough flexibility in dosage regulation.

◆ *Evaluation.* Long-term use of dopamine agonists may lead to *akinesia* (loss of movement), *tardive dyskinesia* (abnormal and involuntary movements, especially of the lower face), and *dystonia* (impairment of muscle tone). The dosage is likely to be reduced to the minimum effective level to reverse these effects, and very slow and careful changes in dosages are made as necessary to avoid overdrug. Monitor all patients closely for behavior changes because these drugs can exacerbate depression and psychosis. Report abnormal involuntary movements such as chewing, grinding of the teeth, protrusion of the tongue, repeated opening and closing of the mouth, head bobbing, or jerky, constant movements of the feet or hands because these can indicate **dystonia**, which can be related to progression of the disease itself or wearing off of dopamine. If these symptoms appear, alert the healthcare provider because the drug dosage may need to be adjusted.

◆ *Patient and family teaching.* Tell the patient and family:
- Clinical improvements are cumulative (get better over time) and may take 2 to 3 weeks to reach full effect. Continue to take the drug even if you see no changes at first.
- If possible, take the drug on an empty stomach 30 to 60 minutes before a meal or snack so that the drug is absorbed well and can help you chew and swallow better.
- If the drug causes nausea, you can take it with some crackers or other carbohydrates. Do not take the drug with food containing protein because this can reduce the drug's effectiveness.
- Avoid taking levodopa with vitamin $B_6$ (pyridoxine) because the vitamin accelerates inactivation of the drug. This is not a problem if you are taking levodopa/carbidopa.
- Contact your healthcare provider immediately if symptoms suddenly become worse, if you have intermittent winking or muscle twitching, or if abdominal pain, constipation, distention, or urinary problems occur.
- Take care when using drugs—along with your drugs for PD—for sleep, for pain, to relax muscles, or to control bladder function because the combination can lead to confusion, hallucinations, and other symptoms.
- Change positions slowly from lying down to standing up because low blood pressure can occur and cause you to fall.

- Contact your healthcare provider as soon as possible if you develop hallucinations or delusions.

## CATECHOL-*O*-METHYLTRANSFERASE INHIBITORS

### Action and Uses

Catechol-*O*-methyltransferase (COMT) is an enzyme that breaks down (metabolizes) naturally occurring catecholamine-based neurotransmitters, including dopamine and dopamine agonist drugs. A catechol-*O*-methyltransferase (COMT) inhibitor is a drug that suppresses the activity of the COMT enzyme so that naturally occurring dopamine and dopamine agonists remain active in the body longer, helping to restore the ACh–dopamine balance in the brain. Levodopa is the main dopamine agonist drug used in PD. A COMT inhibitor is given with levodopa to allow blood levels of levodopa to stay high enough to enter the brain, where it is converted to dopamine. Entacapone (Comtan) and tolcapone (Tasmar) are COMT inhibitors that are used for PD.

### Expected Side Effects and Adverse Reactions

Entacapone and tolcapone can potentiate the dopaminergic adverse effects of levodopa and cause dyskinesia and hypotension. The most common expected effects are GI upset and discoloration (brownish-orange color) of the urine. Both drugs are metabolized by the liver, but tolcapone leads to a higher risk of severe liver failure, and it is not used unless other measures have failed. Tolcapone is not used in persons with existing hepatic disease. Liver function must be closely monitored every 6 months if tolcapone is used.

### Drug Interactions

Neither entacapone nor tolcapone should be taken with other MAO inhibitors, such as phenelzine (Nardil), because they reduce catecholamine metabolism and can cause cardiovascular problems such as severe hypertension, tachycardia, and dysrhythmias. Likewise, any direct catecholamine drugs, such as epinephrine or methyldopa, may increase heart rates, cause dysrhythmias, and lead to severely high blood pressure levels. The MAO-B inhibitors selegiline (Eldepryl, Zelapar) and rasagiline (Azilect) are used in PD and considered safe to take with COMT inhibitor drugs because they are selective in blocking the breakdown of dopamine but not other catecholamines, and the adverse cardiac effects are avoided.

### ❖ Nursing Implications and Patient Teaching

◆ *Assessment.* The patient may experience orthostatic hypotension because COMT inhibitors potentiate the action of carbidopa/levodopa. Take a full set of vital signs and orthostatic blood pressure levels, and remind patients to rise slowly to avoid falls. Monitor for indications of dyskinesia and hyperkinesia, and notify the healthcare provider if they occur.

◆ *Planning and implementation.* Entacapone is given with every dose of carbidopa/levodopa; tolcapone is given with the first dose of carbidopa/levodopa, and subsequent doses are given 6 to 12 hours later. If tolcapone is used, monitor patients for liver failure and review liver function studies.

◆ *Evaluation.* Evaluate patients for akinesia, dystonia, and tardive dyskinesia (discussed earlier) because these drugs are given with carbidopa/levodopa and increase the response of dopamine agonists. Monitor patients for depression and psychosis.

◆ *Patient and family teaching.* Tell the patient and family:

- Take entacapone with each levodopa/carbidopa dose for best effect.
- The first dose of tolcapone is given with levodopa/carbidopa, and subsequent doses are given about 6 and 12 hours later.
- Notify your healthcare provider if you develop jaundice, abdominal pain, or swelling because these symptoms may indicate liver failure. This is especially important if taking tolcapone.
- Notify your healthcare provider if you have worsening depression, delirium, or hallucinations.
- Do not suddenly stop taking either of these drugs because they must be tapered off slowly to avoid a worsening condition.
- Your urine may have a brownish-orange discoloration; this is an expected side effect and is not dangerous.
- Rise slowly from a sitting or lying position to prevent faintness, dizziness, and falls caused by an unexpected drop in blood pressure.

## MONOAMINE OXIDASE TYPE B INHIBITORS

### Action and Uses

MAO is made in the mitochondrial membranes in most cells of the body. The enzyme breaks down (metabolizes) many substances. MAO type A (MAO-A) breaks down many neurotransmitters, including epinephrine, norepinephrine, serotonin, and dopamine. MAO type B (MAO-B) is more specific for metabolizing dopamine and serotonin. A monoamine oxidase type B (MAO-B) inhibitor suppresses the action of MAO-B, which allows dopamine levels to increase and reduces the symptoms of PD. MAO-B inhibitors are sometimes used to treat depression because this drug category also reduces the breakdown of serotonin. These drugs have fewer side effects than MAO-A inhibitors, which are nonselective.

Three MAO-B inhibitor drugs—selegiline, rasagiline, and safinamide (Xadago)—are used in combination with carbidopa/levodopa. They typically are used early in the disease course as monotherapy or in addition to dopamine agonist drugs. Adding MAO-B inhibitors to the drug regimen allows the dose of levodopa to be decreased, which lessens the side effects of higher levodopa levels.

## Expected Side Effects and Adverse Reactions

The usual side effects of MAO-B inhibitors are dry mouth, nausea, constipation, and lightheadedness. Confusion and hallucinations can occur, especially in older adults. The adverse effect of severe hypertension can occur if MAO-B inhibitors are used in high doses, but this is unlikely to occur at lower doses. Tyramine-rich foods should be avoided when taking any MAO inhibitor because they can cause a severe hypertensive crisis. Box 10.2 is a partial list of foods to avoid when taking MAO inhibitors. Photosensitivity also can occur and increase the risk of sunburn. These drugs cause drowsiness.

## Drug Interactions

MAO-B inhibitors interact with some opiate drugs used for pain, such as meperidine, tramadol, and methadone, and can cause a hypertensive crisis. They should not be used with droperidol or cyclobenzaprine. Taking MAO-B inhibitors with tricyclic antidepressants, such as amitriptyline; with selective serotonin reuptake inhibitors, such as fluoxetine; or with other MAO inhibitors can cause serotonin syndrome, which cause muscle spasms, agitation, hyperthermia, tremors, seizures, or delirium. Drugs that stimulate the sympathetic (fight-or-flight) nervous system, such as amphetamines, phenylephrine (decongestant), and dextromethorphan (cough medicine), can cause a hypertensive crisis. Ginseng, ephedra, ma huang, and St. John's wort can also cause a hypertensive crisis and should be avoided with MOA inhibitors.

### ❖ Nursing Implications and Patient Teaching

◆ *Assessment.* Monitor vital signs, especially during dose increases. Alert the healthcare provider for any changes, especially in blood pressure and pulse because orthostatic hypotension, hypertension, or tachycardia with new dysrhythmias may indicate adverse reactions to these drugs. Monitor all patients closely for behavior changes because these drugs can cause hallucinations, delusions, depression, or confusion.

---

| Box **10.2** | Foods That Contain Tyramine |
| --- | --- |

- Cured or smoked meats, fish, and cheeses (e.g., salami, anchovies)
- Avocados, bananas, figs, and raisins
- Beer and red wine
- Sauerkraut
- Sour cream
- Soy sauce or soy-containing foods such as miso soup
- Yeast extract found in some breads, canned foods, and snacks
- Yogurt
- Pickled herring

---

◆ *Patient and family teaching.* Tell the patient and family:
- These drugs can take several weeks to begin working.
- Do not exceed the prescribed drug dose because doing so can cause dangerously high blood pressure levels.
- Avoid foods that contain tyramine, such as beer, red wine, aged cheese, smoked meat, cheese, fish, soy products, and pickled herring.
- Report symptoms of very high blood pressure, such as a severe headache, irregular pulse, or nausea and vomiting, to your healthcare provider immediately.
- Very low blood pressure, dizziness, lightheadedness, and fainting are possible, so move slowly when arising from a sitting or lying position.
- Do not take over-the-counter (OTC) drugs or herbs without checking with the pharmacist or your healthcare provider.
- These drugs cause drowsiness. Avoid driving or using dangerous machinery until you know how the drug affects you.
- Wear sunscreen, sunglasses, and protective clothing when outside because this drug increases the risk of serious sunburn, even if you have dark skin.

## DRUGS FOR ALZHEIMER'S DISEASE

Alzheimer's disease (AD) is a common form of dementia. *Dementia* is the progressive loss of brain function. There are many causes and types of dementia, and AD is one that can be helped initially with drug therapy. In AD, there is a familial tendency or genetic predisposition to develop problems in and around brain neurons that affect their function. The protein beta-amyloid builds up and forms deposits in the brain. The microtubules in the neurons also become tangled and form nonfunctional meshes in the brain. Levels of the excitatory neurotransmitter ACh are decreased in the brain, which results in more difficulty with memory and learning. Blood flow throughout the brain decreases, and over time these changes reduce the size of the brain and all aspects of brain function (Fig. 10.5).

The symptoms of early AD involve memory issues and can be mistaken for normal aging. The disease is progressive, and memory problems become increasingly more challenging, such as getting confused regarding times and places or forgetting how to get home. Changes in mood, judgment, and personality eventually occur. Box 10.3 lists 10 warning signs of AD.

More than 5 million persons suffer from AD. Risk factors include older age (greater than 65 years), a family history of AD, and having the *APOE-e4 gene.* Unfortunately, no single test can be used to diagnose AD. Instead, the diagnosis is made based on symptoms, family interviews, physical examination, and neurologic and cognitive examinations.

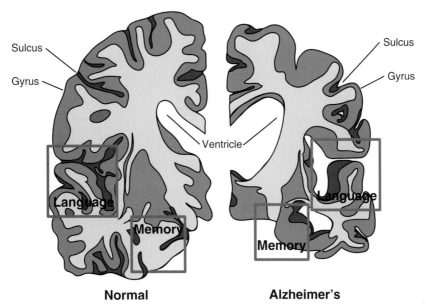

Sulcus
Gyrus
Ventricle
Sulcus
Gyrus
Language
Memory
Language
Memory

**Normal**          **Alzheimer's**

**Fig. 10.5** Cross-sections of a normal brain and a brain affected by Alzheimer's disease. Neurons die in areas of the brain that are important for memory and language. (From Workman, M. L., & LaCharity, L. A. (2016). *Understanding pharmacology* (2nd ed.). Elsevier.)

| Box 10.3 | Ten Warning Signs of Alzheimer's Disease |
|---|---|

1. Memory loss that disrupts daily life
2. Challenges in planning or solving problems
3. Difficulty completing familiar tasks at home, at work, or at leisure
4. Confusion about time or place
5. Trouble understanding visual images and spatial relationships
6. New problems with words in speaking or writing
7. Misplacing things and losing the ability to retrace steps
8. Decreased or poor judgment
9. Withdrawal from work or social activities
10. Changes in mood and personality

Drug therapy does not cure AD. Drugs used for AD, which provide only temporary improvement in symptoms, include cholinesterase inhibitors and *N*-methyl-D-aspartate (NMDA) blockers. Effectiveness of the drugs varies from person to person, and the length of time for which a drug is therapeutic is limited. Table 10.2 lists the names, adult dosages, and nursing implications for these drugs. Research in the area of AD is ongoing, and help for family and professional caregivers is available.

Aducanumab (Aduhelm) is a monoclonal antibody that was approved in June 2021 under the Accelerated Approval Program of the US Food and Drug Administration (FDA). It is an intravenously administered beta-amyloid beta-directed antibody that has shown to reduce beta-amyloid plaque in people with mild cognitive impairment who had evidence of build-up of amyloid plaques in the brain. Aduhelm does not improve cognitive abilities or reverse cognitive impairment and dementia. This drug is designed to slow the progression of the disease. Beta-amyloid pathology must be confirmed prior to initiating treatment. After an initial titration schedule, the maintenance dosage of aducanumab is 10 mg/kg intravenous (IV) infusion over 60 minutes given every 4 weeks (at least 21 days apart). The most common side effects listed are a headache and falls. No adverse drug interactions have been reported. However, the drug is under scrutiny because the current evidence available would suggest that a yearly cost of aducanumab ($56,000) is not reasonable considering drug safety, effectiveness, and clinical benefits. Medicare will cover the drug only for recipients enrolled in a clinical trial approved by CMS or supported by the National Institutes of Health (NIH).

 Bookmark This!

The Alzheimer's Foundation of America provides care and services to individuals living with AD and to their families and caregivers: https://alz.org.

## CHOLINESTERASE INHIBITORS

### Action and Uses

Drug therapy attempts to increase ACh levels because this excitatory neurotransmitter is reduced in the brains of patients with AD. Acetylcholinesterase is an enzyme that specifically breaks down ACh. A **cholinesterase inhibitor** is a drug that binds to acetylcholinesterase and slows its action, which allows any ACh produced to remain functional longer. This action appears to delay memory loss and improve the patient's ability to perform his or her activities of daily living. Unfortunately, the drug is useful only temporarily. As the disease progresses, fewer intact neurons are available to make ACh. When this occurs, the drug is no longer effective.

| Table 10.2 | Examples of Common Drugs for Management of Alzheimer's Disease |

*Cholinesterase inhibitors* delay memory loss in Alzheimer's disease by binding to the enzyme acetylcholinesterase and slowing its action, which allows any acetylcholine produced to remain functional for a longer period.

*NMDA blockers* slow the progression of Alzheimer's disease by blocking the entrance of calcium into neurons, which reduces or slows neuronal damage.

| DRUG/ADULT DOSAGE | NURSING IMPLICATIONS |
| --- | --- |
| **Cholinesterase Inhibitors** | |
| donepezil (Aricept) 5–10 mg orally once daily<br>rivastigmine (Exelon) 1.5–3 mg orally twice daily; 4.6 mg/24 hours to 9.5 mg/24 hours transdermal patch<br>galantamine (Razadyne) 4–8 mg orally twice daily; extended-release tablets 8–16 mg orally once daily | • Give donepezil once a day in the evening.<br>• If using the disintegrating tablet, place the tablet on the tongue before swallowing.<br>• Teach patients and families to measure and give the oral solution with a syringe.<br>• Rivastigmine must be given with food.<br>• If using the transdermal rivastigmine patch:<br>  • Apply once daily to clean, dry, hairless, intact healthy skin on the upper or lower back to prevent removal by the patient.<br>  • Do not use on areas with recent application of lotions, creams, or powder.<br>  • Rotate application sites daily. Do not apply to the same site more than once every 14 days.<br>  • May be used while bathing or showering.<br>  • Apply patch at about the same time every day.<br>  • Always remove the old patch before applying a new patch.<br>• Give galantamine twice-a-day oral dosage with food, or give the once-a-day oral dosage in the morning with food.<br>• If using the liquid oral form of galantamine, measure the ordered dose with the enclosed pipette into 3–4 ounces of a nonalcoholic drink.<br>• Monitor weekly weights because these drugs may cause weight loss.<br>• Monitor laboratory work as ordered to ensure safety from adverse effects.<br>• Donepezil is the only cholinesterase inhibitor approved for severe Alzheimer's. |
| **NMDA Blockers** | |
| memantine (Namenda, Namenda XR) 5–10 mg orally twice daily; extended-release capsules 7–28 mg orally once daily | • Extended-release capsules can be opened and the contents sprinkled on applesauce before swallowing. Do not divide the contents of the capsule because this will result in unequal dosing.<br>• If the oral solution of the drug is used, do not mix it with other liquids. Use a syringe or dropper to measure, and give it directly into the mouth.<br>• Monitor the patient's neurologic function, serum creatinine levels, blood urea nitrogen, and liver function studies, and notify the healthcare provider of any changes from baseline.<br>• Weigh the patient weekly because this drug can cause weight loss. |

Three cholinesterase inhibitors are used in the treatment of AD: donepezil (Aricept), rivastigmine (Exelon), and galantamine (Razadyne). Table 10.2 lists the common names, adult dosages, and nursing implications for these drugs.

### Expected Side Effects and Adverse Reactions

Expected side effects of cholinesterase inhibitors include mild diarrhea, especially when starting treatment. Drowsiness, headache, loss of appetite, GI discomfort, joint pain, and muscle cramping can occur. Adverse effects include hallucinations, dysrhythmias, GI bleeding, infection, and difficulty urinating or incontinence. These drugs increase ACh concentration. They are considered to be cholinergic agonists and can have adverse effects on other body systems, causing symptoms of overstimulation of the parasympathetic (rest-and-digest) nervous system. Box 10.4 lists these adverse effects.

| Box 10.4 | Common Adverse Effects of Cholinergic Agonists and Cholinesterase Inhibitors |

• Cardiac: slow heart rate, low blood pressure, heart blocks, fainting
• Central Nervous System: convulsions, headaches, seizures, sweating
• Gastrointestinal: increased secretions, increased salivation, abdominal cramps, vomiting, diarrhea
• Respiratory: increased secretions and bronchospasm
• Urinary: urinary incontinence

### Drug Interactions

Cholinesterase inhibitors should not be given with other drugs that can prolong the QT interval on the ECG because this can cause a fatal dysrhythmia known as *torsade de pointes*, a form of ventricular tachycardia. Dextromethorphan (found in OTC cough drugs), quinidine, and fluconazole are three such drugs. Consult a drug reference or pharmacist to determine whether these drugs interact with any other drugs the patient is taking. Anticholinergic drugs decrease the effectiveness of cholinesterase inhibitors, and taking the drug with other cholinesterase inhibitors, such as edrophonium (Tensilon), increases the risk of adverse effects.

### ❖ Nursing Implications and Patient Teaching

◆ *Assessment.* Obtain a baseline weight measurement and reassess at weekly intervals because these drugs can cause a loss of appetite. Observe for signs and symptoms that may indicate a GI bleed, such as dark, tarry stools and decreasing hemoglobin and hematocrit levels. Monitor blood test levels and report abnormal baseline liver function studies and BUN/creatinine levels to the healthcare provider because abnormalities can affect metabolism of the drugs. Assess the urinary patterns, and reassess for changes that indicate side effects of the drugs.

Before a patient starts a cholinesterase inhibitor, assess the patient using an Alzheimer's Disease Assessment Scale (ADAS) so that an objective evaluation can be made when evaluating for symptom improvement. The assessment tools of the ADAS evaluate cognition, functional capacity, behavior, general health, and quality of life. By using these tools, you can better gauge how and whether the drug is helping the patient. Also assess for swallowing difficulties so that the proper drug formulation can be given (e.g., liquid, sublingual tablets).

◆ *Planning and implementation.* Carefully monitor patients who have asthma for worsening of symptoms. Check vital signs, especially heart rate, and look for adverse signs and symptoms indicating parasympathetic stimulation, as indicated in Box 10.4.

◆ *Evaluation.* Monitor for improvement using an Alzheimer's Disease Assessment Scale. Monitor for any changes in vital signs and for adverse reactions.

◆ *Patient and family teaching.* Tell the patient and family:
- It may take several weeks for the drugs to have a therapeutic effect.
- These drugs do not cure AD.
- If difficulty breathing, fainting, or GI bleeding occurs, notify your healthcare provider immediately.
- Notify your healthcare provider if expected side effects are causing increased discomfort or new symptoms develop.
- Use the bathroom every 2 hours to avoid urinary incontinence because these drugs increase urination.
- Take donepezil at bedtime.
- Take galantamine and rivastigmine at the same time twice a day with food to avoid GI upset.
- Your risk for falls is increased because these drugs can cause dizziness and weakness.
- Keep all follow-up appointments so that the effects of these drugs can be evaluated.

 **Bookmark This!**

A list of cognitive assessment and family informational tools can be found on the Alzheimer's Association Web site: https://www.alz.org/health-care-professionals/cognitive-tests-patient-assessment.asp.

## *N*-METHYL-D-ASPARTATE BLOCKERS

### Action and Uses

There are NMDA receptors in the brain. When activated, these receptors allow more calcium into brain neurons, which appears to be important in memory and learning. However, too much calcium damages neurons. It is thought that excess calcium is one mechanism that causes neurofibrillary tangles to form in the brains of patients with AD. *N*-methyl-D-aspartate (NMDA) blockers are drugs that prevent the entrance of calcium into neurons, which reduces or slows the neuronal damage in AD. Memantine (Namenda, Ebixa) is used with the drugs donepezil, rivastigmine, and galantamine to increase the effects of these cholinergic agonists.

### Expected Side Effects and Adverse Reactions

The expected side effects of memantine are headaches, dizziness, and constipation. Adverse side effects include hallucinations, worsening confusion, depression, somnolence, shortness of breath, incontinence, and weight loss. This drug can also cause hypertension in certain individuals.

### Drug Interactions

Drugs that increase the urine pH (alkaline) or are excreted by the kidneys can interfere with the renal excretion of memantine and increase the expected and adverse side effects. Carbonic anhydrase inhibitors such as acetazolamide (which are used for treating glaucoma and high-altitude sickness), quinidine, and dextromethorphan are examples of such drugs.

### ❖ Nursing Implications and Patient Teaching

◆ *Assessment.* Memantine is eliminated primarily by the kidney and should be used with caution in patients with kidney disease, people at risk for renal impairment due to age, and people taking other drugs that also have a risk of renal impairment. Baseline measurements of creatinine, BUN, and liver enzymes should be obtained. Urinary tract infections can increase the levels of memantine by increasing the pH. If the patient has symptoms of a urinary tract infection, obtain a urinalysis, and consult with the healthcare provider before starting drug therapy. Monitor the respiratory rate and vital signs, especially the blood pressure in patients with heart disease. Report symptoms such as ataxia, dizziness, and other adverse reactions to the healthcare provider.

◆ *Patient and family teaching.* Tell the patient and family:
- Take or give memantine at the same time every day.

- The extended-release capsule can be opened, and all of the contents can be sprinkled on applesauce if swallowing is difficult.
- If using the liquid form of the drug, do not mix it with other liquids to avoid interactions.
- Report problems with vision, rash, shortness of breath, agitation or restlessness, confusion, dizziness, incontinence, and weight loss to your healthcare provider.
- Avoid driving or engaging in hazardous activities until you know how the drug affects you.
- Report symptoms of a urinary tract infection (e.g., acute changes in mental status, frequency of urination, pain or discomfort during urination, concentrated and bad-smelling urine) to your healthcare provider.

## DRUGS FOR EPILEPSY

*Epilepsy* is a common type of chronic seizure disorder in which neurons of the brain become hyperexcitable and trigger electrical signals when they are not needed. The unnecessary signals cause rapid and repeated refiring of nerves in the brain, leading to seizures. *Seizures* are the body's total responses to those inappropriate brain signals. When the signals reach the skeletal muscles, a *convulsion* may occur, which is a sudden contraction of many muscle groups without the person's conscious control. A convulsion is the part of a seizure that is seen as the motor response to these brain signals. Other parts of seizure activity include changes in or loss of consciousness; a variety of sensory changes in vision, hearing, touch, smell, and taste; and autonomic symptoms such as facial flushing, incontinence, nausea, and drooling. Symptoms of seizures vary with the area of the brain affected and the type of seizure experienced.

Seizures are classified as partial or generalized. Each classification has subtypes based on symptoms, how long an episode lasts, whether convulsions occur, how widespread the response is, and the degree of change in consciousness. Box 10.5 lists the classifications of seizures.

A variety of problems can produce seizures. For example, high temperatures in infants and children, strokes, head trauma, brain tumor, meningitis, and poisoning (especially from excessive alcohol intake or drugs) may induce seizures. Epilepsy is one cause of chronic and recurring seizures.

Although other types of epilepsy management exist, most often drug therapy is used. An **antiepileptic drug (AED)** is a drug that reduces or prevents seizures. AEDs are divided into traditional and newer categories. Some drugs categorized as AEDs have additional uses for other problems and disorders.

### TRADITIONAL ANTIEPILEPTIC DRUGS

The traditional AEDs include phenytoin, carbamazepine, ethosuximide, phenobarbital, and valproic acid. Although these drugs have different actions, side effects, adverse effects, and drug interactions, some nursing implications are the same for all of them. Many of the points to teach patients and families about these drugs are also the same. Box 10.6 describes the common nursing considerations for AEDs, and

## Box 10.5 Classification of Major Seizure Types

| SEIZURE TYPE | SYMPTOMS |
| --- | --- |
| **PARTIAL SEIZURES** | |
| Simple | No loss of consciousness, isolated or discrete motor symptoms (e.g., twitching of one toe or foot), changes in one or more senses, one or more autonomic symptoms (e.g., drooling, facial flushing); usually lasts 20–60 seconds |
| Complex | Consciousness altered or impaired and person does not respond to environmental stimulation, may have a fixed gaze stare and be motionless, automatism (performance of repetitive motions such as head-turning from side to side, foot-pedaling motions); usually lasts 45–90 seconds |
| Partial with secondary generalization | Begins as a partial seizure with the patient retaining consciousness and then progresses to loss of consciousness |
| **GENERALIZED SEIZURES (ALL FEATURE LOSS OF CONSCIOUSNESS)** | |
| Absence (petit mal) | Consciousness loss is brief (10–30 seconds) without loss of posture; minimal or no change in motor activity |
| Tonic-clonic (grand mal) | Often preceded by an aura or a cry, whole-body convulsions starting with muscle rigidity followed by powerful contractions, loss of posture, urinary incontinence, confusion after muscle responses are over; usually lasts less than 90 seconds |
| Atonic | Muscle tone loss in one or more muscle groups; usually lasts 10–60 seconds |
| Myoclonic | Brief (1–2 seconds) contraction of one (focal) or more muscle groups (can involve the whole body) |
| Status epilepticus | Single seizure lasting 15–30 continuous minutes or a series of recurring seizures between which the patient does not regain consciousness; may be convulsive, absence, myoclonic, or generalized convulsive (life-threatening) |
| Febrile | Tonic-clonic seizures induced by temperature elevation (usually in children); last 15–30 seconds |

Box 10.7 describes general patient teaching points. Nursing considerations and patient teaching issues specific to single drugs are listed with the individual

drug categories in Table 10.3. Although the older AED drugs have more side effects and other issues than do some newer ones, they are still used effectively today for most patients, often in combination with newer AEDs.

| Box 10.6 | General Nursing Considerations for Antiepileptic Drugs |

**ASSESSMENT**

- Before giving an antiepileptic drug (AED), obtain a complete list of drugs that the patient is taking, including over-the-counter and herbal preparations, because these drugs interact with numerous other drugs, herbals, and supplements.
- Always consult a drug reference or pharmacist to determine possible interactions between AEDs and any other drug a patient is prescribed.
- Check baseline vital signs, level of consciousness, and gait, all of which can change as a result of AEDs.
- Assess adolescents for recent changes in height and weight because these changes affect the dosage needed to prevent seizures.
- Ask female patients of childbearing age if they are pregnant, planning to become pregnant, or breast-feeding because many AEDs increase the risk of birth defects and/or enter breast milk and affect the infant.
- Ask patients whether an aura occurs before any seizure.
- Tell the patient to put on his or her call light if he or she feels that a seizure is about to occur.

### Memory Jogger

There are five traditional antiepilepsy drugs:
- phenytoin
- carbamazepine
- ethosuximide
- phenobarbital
- valproic acid

### Actions and Uses

**Phenytoin** is an AED that reduces or prevents seizures by binding to sodium channels on nerve membranes and making them less active, which prevents the spread of neuron excitation. This and similar anticonvulsants are among the oldest drugs used in the management of epilepsy and are available as tablets, capsules, liquid suspensions, and solutions for injection. A prodrug of phenytoin is fosphenytoin (Cerebyx), which is available only intravenously and is used on a short-term basis; it is converted to phenytoin in the body. Phenytoin anticonvulsants are approved only for treatment of seizure disorders.

| Box 10.7 | General Patient and Family Teaching Points for Antiepileptic Drugs |

- Teach patients about the importance of keeping follow-up appointments with the healthcare provider to monitor drug effectiveness and drug blood levels.
- Instruct patients to take the drug exactly as prescribed and not to suddenly stop taking it because seizures may occur.
- Teach patients to take a missed dose as soon as it is remembered but not to take a double dose. Teach patients to immediately report to the healthcare provider any new, worsening, or unusual symptoms.
- Remind patients to avoid adding any over-the-counter drugs or supplements without checking with their healthcare provider to prevent possible interactions.
- Instruct patients to avoid alcoholic beverages or other drugs known to depress the central nervous system (CNS) because severe CNS depression may occur. For some patients, alcohol triggers seizure activity.
- Remind patients to avoid driving, operating dangerous equipment, or doing anything that requires mental alertness until they know how the antiepileptic drug (AED) affects their level of consciousness and reflexes.
- Tell patients and families to notify the healthcare provider immediately if signs of increasing depression are seen because many of these drugs increase depression and suicidal ideation.

**PLANNING AND IMPLEMENTATION**

- Place the patient's bed in the lowest position, and raise the side rails to prevent injury.
- Remind the patient to call for help when getting out of bed, and make sure that the call light is within easy reach because many AEDs cause dizziness.
- Make sure that oxygen and suction equipment are in the patient's room and in good working order in case a seizure does occur.
- Monitor the patient for seizure activity and be prepared to protect the patient from injury if one occurs.
- Monitor regularly scheduled blood drug measurements to determine whether levels are in the effective range or could cause adverse reactions.
- Many AEDs increase suicidal ideation. Report to the healthcare provider immediately any patient statements or actions that indicate he or she may be considering self-harm.
- AEDs work in the CNS and depress its activity to some degree. They should not be taken with alcohol or any other type of CNS depressant.
- Suddenly stopping AED therapy can result in seizures. When changing drugs or discontinuing drugs, taper doses slowly to reduce the risk for seizures.

**Table 10.3    Examples of Common Traditional Antiepileptic Drugs**

| DRUG/ADULT DOSAGE | NURSING IMPLICATIONS |
|---|---|
| phenytoin (Dilantin, Phenytek)<br>Loading dose: 15–20 mg/kg orally or intravenous (IV) given in divided doses throughout the day<br>Maintenance dose: 4–7 mg/kg per day orally divided into 2–3 doses | • Dosages for different forms of phenytoin are not interchangeable because the drug concentrations vary by type.<br>• Warn patients that gum hyperplasia is a side effect of this drug and that good oral hygiene is needed to prevent tooth loss from gum disease.<br>• Remind patients who take warfarin that closer monitoring is needed and the warfarin dose may need to be adjusted because phenytoin has mixed interactions with warfarin's effect.<br>• Ask patients about all other drugs they take because phenytoin interacts with many other drugs. Check with a pharmacist and the patient's healthcare provider about the need for dosage adjustments with any drug.<br>• Avoid giving this drug by the intramuscular (IM) route because it is a severe tissue irritant.<br>• Phenytoin causes birth defects and is not used during pregnancy.<br>• Teach patients to measure their pulse rate daily and to report changes and irregularities to their healthcare provider because these drugs can cause bradycardia and other heart rhythm problems.<br>• Monitor the patient's blood pressure and heart rate and rhythm before giving the drug IV, every 15 minutes during the infusion, and after the infusion is complete to identify severe hypotension or heart rhythm problems. |
| carbamazepine (Epitol, Tegretol, Tegretol XR)<br>Initial dose: 200 mg orally daily; over time, increase to 100–400 mg orally every 6–8 hours<br>Sustained-release forms: 200–800 mg orally every 12 hours | • This drug causes birth defects and is not used during pregnancy.<br>• Teach patients to measure their pulse rate daily and to report changes and irregularities to their healthcare provider because these drugs can cause tachycardia, atrial fibrillation, and other heart rhythm problems.<br>• Instruct patients to walk slowly and carefully, especially on stairs, because this drug may cause ataxia and increase the risk of falls.<br>• Remind patients who take warfarin that closer monitoring is needed and that the warfarin dose may need to be increased because carbamazepine reduces the effect of warfarin.<br>• Ask patients about all other drugs they take because carbamazepine interacts with many other drugs. Check with a pharmacist and the patient's healthcare provider about the need for dosage adjustments with any drug.<br>• Suggest that patients take the drug with meals or a substantial snack to decrease gastrointestinal (GI) problems.<br>• Carbamazepine is autoinducer: half life variable for first 3–5 weeks. Slower titration during this time to avoid toxicity. |
| ethosuximide (Zarontin)<br>Initial dose: 250 mg orally every 12 hours<br>Maintenance dose: 20–40 mg/kg per day orally in two divided doses | • Ask patients about all other drugs they take because ethosuximide interacts with many other drugs. Check with a pharmacist and the patient's healthcare provider about the need for dosage adjustments with any drug.<br>• If the patient has GI side effects, suggest that he or she take the drug with meals or a substantial snack to decrease these problems.<br>• This drug may be used during pregnancy because it has a lower risk of birth defects than do other traditional antiepileptic drugs. |
| phenobarbital 1–3 mg/kg per day orally or IV or IM, once or twice daily<br>primidone (Mysoline) initially 125–250 mg orally once daily at bedtime; gradually increase to 250–500 mg orally every 8 hours to a maximum of 2 g/day | • This drug causes birth defects and is not used during pregnancy.<br>• Observe mental status and respiratory effectiveness carefully and often because this drug can cause profound CNS depression, respiratory depression, and cognitive impairment.<br>• Check with a pharmacist before giving phenobarbital with any other drug because it has many incompatibilities.<br>• Warn patients and families that there is an increased risk of falls, especially when first starting the drug, because of CNS depression and ataxia. |
| valproic acid (Depakote, Depakene, Depacon [injectable form]) 10–15 mg/ kg per day orally or IV, in divided doses if the total is more than 250 mg; may be increased up to 60 mg/kg per day in divided doses | • Remind patients who take warfarin that closer monitoring is needed and that the warfarin dose may need to be decreased because valproic acid increases blood levels of warfarin.<br>• Remind parents of young children who are taking this drug to check the child weekly for yellowing of the skin or whites of the eyes, darkening of the urine, or light-colored stools because severe liver toxicity can occur. If any of these changes are present, notify the healthcare provider.<br>• Give IV infusions slowly over 60 minutes to avoid injection-site pain and severe dizziness.<br>• This drug causes birth defects and is not used during pregnancy. |

Carbamazepine is an AED that limits the spread of neuron excitation by altering the sodium channels of nerve membranes to prevent or slow the refiring of neurons. Its structure is similar to that of the tricyclic antidepressants. This drug is often used to control epilepsy in children. It is also used as a mood stabilizer and to reduce skeletal muscle spasms.

Ethosuximide is an AED that raises the seizure threshold by altering calcium channels on neuron membranes. The number of seizures is reduced because stronger excitation is needed to stimulate them. Although this drug can help reduce all types of seizures, it is most effective for absence seizures. Ethosuximide is used to reduce seizures during pregnancy because it is less likely to cause birth defects than phenytoin, fosphenytoin, or carbamazepine.

Phenobarbital is a drug from the barbiturate class that raises the seizure threshold by enhancing the action of the inhibitory neurotransmitter GABA, resulting in widespread CNS depression. It is the oldest drug used to control seizures, and it is also used as a sedating agent. Phenobarbital has the longest duration of action of the traditional AEDs. It is used for all types of seizures except absence seizures and is used on a short-term basis for insomnia and anxiety. This drug is available in tablet form, oral solutions, and solutions for injection.

Primidone is a prodrug that is converted to phenobarbital in the body. It has the same actions, side effects, interactions, and precautions as phenobarbital.

Valproic acid is an AED that raises the seizure threshold by possibly increasing the activity of one of the inhibitory neurotransmitters, GABA. Not all of its actions are known. It is often combined with divalproex sodium to increase its duration of action and to reduce the frequency of dosing. In addition to treatment of most seizure types, valproic acid is used to help manage manic types of bipolar disorders.

### Expected Side Effects

The most common side effect of phenytoin is gum hyperplasia, especially with long-term use. Other common side effects include abdominal discomfort. Unlike many other AEDs, phenytoin does *not* cause drowsiness.

The most common side effects of carbamazepine are constipation, nausea and vomiting, and *ataxia* (unsteadiness when walking). Other side effects include itching, rash, muscle weakness, and an increased risk of sunburn.

Ethosuximide has fewer side effects than other traditional AEDs. The most common side effects of this drug are heartburn (*dyspepsia*), nausea and vomiting, dizziness, drowsiness, and fatigue. Adverse effects of this drug are rare.

Phenobarbital and primidone have many CNS side effects, especially drowsiness and ataxia. Additional side effects include blurred vision, dizziness, and mental status changes. These problems are most apparent when therapy first begins and become less severe over time.

The most common side effects of valproic acid are drowsiness, muscle weakness, nausea, diarrhea, and menstrual irregularities. Additional side effects include anorexia, double vision, and blurred vision. Instead of drowsiness, some patients have insomnia.

### Adverse Reactions

Phenytoin is a known *teratogen* that causes birth defects. It should be avoided during pregnancy. Other adverse effects of phenytoin include the red blood cell problem of anemia, reduced white blood cell counts with increased risk of infection, and reduced platelet counts with increased risk of bleeding. Although they are not common, heart rhythm problems, especially *bradycardia* (slow heart rate), can occur. Rashes caused by phenytoin can progress to a widespread and serious problem known as *Stevens-Johnson syndrome*, which can result in skin sloughing and other complications that require immediate medical attention.

### Top Tip for Safety

Development of a rash in a patient who is taking phenytoin, carbamazepine, and/or lamotrigine may signify the onset of a severe adverse reaction. Notify the healthcare provider immediately.

Carbamazepine, like phenytoin, affects the bone marrow, leading to anemia, reduced white blood cell counts with increased risk of infection, and reduced platelet counts with increased risk of bleeding. Heart rhythm problems may lead to *tachycardia* (rapid heart rate), atrial fibrillation, and severe hypertension.

Phenobarbital (and primidone) can cause severe CNS depression, especially when given parenterally. It can cause respiratory depression and should not be given to patients who have chronic obstructive pulmonary disease or any other severe respiratory impairment. Phenobarbital has an increased risk of physical and psychological dependency, especially with long-term use, and is classified as a Schedule IV controlled substance. The many other possible adverse effects include bone marrow depression, cognitive impairment, exfoliative dermatitis, liver impairment, bradycardia, and coma. In cases of acute overdose, the patient may show exaggerated CNS depression, slow and shallow respirations, small pupil size (*miosis*), tachycardia, absence of reflexes (*areflexia*), shock, or coma. Death may occur as a result of cardiorespiratory failure. Consult a drug reference for a more complete list of adverse reactions associated with phenobarbital.

Valproic acid has been known to cause amnesia and heart rhythm irregularities, especially tachycardia. Hearing loss and GI bleeding are also possible.

**Lifespan Considerations**

**Pediatric Patients**

Serious liver toxicity may be seen in some children who are taking valproic acid, especially those younger than 2 years and those receiving multiple AEDs. The risk of liver toxicity decreases as the child ages.

 **Lifespan Considerations**

**Pregnancy**

Phenytoin, carbamazepine, phenobarbital, primidone, and valproic acid are known teratogens that commonly cause birth defects. These drugs are not to be used during pregnancy unless epilepsy cannot be controlled any other way.

## Drug Interactions

The list of drugs that interact with all of the traditional AEDs is very long and includes very common drugs such as aspirin, acetaminophen, oral contraceptives, proton pump inhibitors, and drugs for diabetes. Of particular note are the drugs used to manage psychiatric problems and warfarin. To prevent severe complications and adverse reactions, avoid other prescription drugs unless the benefit outweighs interaction risks. Instruct patients to avoid OTC drugs and supplements unless prescribed by their healthcare provider. Always consult a drug reference or pharmacist to determine possible interactions between AEDs and any other drug a patient is prescribed.

 **Top Tip for Safety**

Always consult a drug reference or pharmacist to determine possible interactions between AEDs and any other drug a patient is prescribed.

## NEWER ANTIEPILEPTIC DRUGS

More than a dozen drugs are considered to be newer AEDs. Some are drugs that have been used for many years for other conditions and have been found to help control some types of seizures. However, most must be used along with or added to a regimen that includes traditional AEDs. This type of add-on therapy is known as *adjuvant therapy.*

Five drugs have been approved for use as single-drug therapy *(monotherapy)* for epilepsy in place of a traditional AED. These drugs may also be used along with traditional AEDs. Table 10.4 lists the names, dosages, and nursing implications of the five AEDs approved as monotherapy for epilepsy: oxcarbazepine, lamotrigine, lacosamide, levetiracetam, and topiramate. Table 10.5 lists the newer AEDs that are approved only for use as adjuvant therapy along with one or more traditional AEDs. For more information about the newer AEDs used as adjuvant therapy, consult a drug reference.

 **Memory Jogger**

Five newer AEDs are approved for use as monotherapy:
- oxcarbazepine
- lamotrigine
- lacosamide
- Topiramate
- levetiracetam

## Oxcarbazepine

*Action and uses.* Oxcarbazepine is an AED derived from carbamazepine (see Traditional Antiepileptic Drugs) that reduces seizures by blocking sodium channels on neuron membranes, requiring greater stimulation for them to depolarize (fire). It raises the seizure threshold. Although the structure is similar to that of carbamazepine, it has fewer CNS side effects. It is approved for use to control partial seizures.

*Expected side effects and adverse reactions.* The most common side effects of oxcarbazepine are drowsiness, dizziness, headache, and nausea. Visual side effects of double vision and blurred vision may also occur.

The most common adverse effects are amnesia and low sodium levels *(hyponatremia)*. Rare problems include bone marrow suppression and confusion. As with traditional AEDs, depression and suicidal ideation are possible. Although oxcarbazepine is less likely than traditional AEDs to cause birth defects, it is still not recommended during pregnancy.

*Drug interactions.* Oxcarbazepine lowers blood sodium levels; this effect is intensified when the patient also takes sodium-excreting diuretics. Oxcarbazepine interacts with many drugs, especially aspirin, acetaminophen, oral contraceptives, proton pump inhibitors, drugs for psychiatric problems, drugs for HIV disease, and drugs for diabetes. To prevent severe complications and adverse reactions, avoid other prescription drugs unless the benefit outweighs interaction risks. Consult a drug reference or pharmacist for possible interactions with other drugs the patient is prescribed.

❖ **Nursing Implications and Patient Teaching**

◆ *Planning and implementation.* In addition to the general nursing implications for patients who are taking AEDs that are listed in Box 10.6, the following issues and actions are important for patients who are taking oxcarbazepine. Ask the patient about changes in vision such as blurred vision or double vision, which are common side effects of therapy with oxcarbazepine. If these visual changes are present, instruct the patient not to drive or operate dangerous machinery to avoid an accident or injury.

This drug can cause blood levels of sodium to be low. Check laboratory values for sodium levels whenever they are measured. Report levels lower than

## Table 10.4   Epileptic Drugs Approved as Monotherapy

| DRUG/ADULT DOSAGE | NURSING IMPLICATIONS |
|---|---|
| oxcarbazepine (Trileptal): initially, 300 mg orally every 12 hours; gradually increase to 1200 mg orally every 12 hours<br><br>oxcarbazepine (Oxtellar XR): initially, 600 mg orally once daily; gradually increase to 2400 mg orally once daily | • Monitor blood sodium levels because this drug can cause hyponatremia.<br>• Assess patients for symptoms associated with low sodium levels, such as headache, increased muscle weakness, and decreased deep tendon reflexes, and report these to the healthcare provider.<br>• To avoid falls, caution patients to walk carefully and use hand rails on stairs whenever they feel some muscle weakness.<br>• Instruct patients not to drive or operate dangerous equipment when their vision is blurry or doubled to prevent an accident or injury. |
| lamotrigine (Lamictal): initially, 50 mg orally once daily for 2 weeks, then 50 mg orally twice daily for 2 weeks, gradually increasing to maintenance at 250 mg orally twice daily<br><br>lamotrigine extended release (Lamictal XR): start at 50 mg orally once daily for 2 weeks, then 100 mg orally once daily for 2 weeks, then increase by 100 mg per week until maintenance dose of 400–600 mg once daily is reached | • Use the correct starter kit when drug therapy begins to avoid complications and interactions.<br>• Assess the patient daily for a rash, which can signal the beginning of life-threatening skin reactions. If a rash is detected, withhold the dose and notify the healthcare provider immediately.<br>• Teach patients to check themselves daily for rashes, and tell them to notify their healthcare provider immediately if a rash is found.<br>• Check with the healthcare provider to determine whether folic acid supplements are needed because this drug interferes with the production of folic acid in the body and some patients may become folic acid deficient.<br>• Carefully check the dosages prescribed for black patients because clearance rates are lower, and lower dosages are often needed for these patients to prevent drug overdose.<br>• To prevent an accident or injury, instruct patients not to drive or operate dangerous equipment when their vision is blurry or doubled. |
| lacosamide (Vimpat): initially, 100 mg orally twice daily or 100 mg intravenous (IV) infusion twice daily; maintenance, 150–200 mg/day orally twice daily | • Monitor patients for orthostatic hypotension and take steps to prevent falls, such as accompanying the patient during ambulation.<br>• Instruct patients to change positions slowly, especially when moving from a lying or sitting position to a standing position, because this drug can cause orthostatic hypotension and syncope.<br>• Remind patients that even if they like the mood produced by the drug not to increase the dosage or how often they take the drug in order to avoid psychological dependence.<br>• Instruct patients not to drive or operate dangerous equipment when their vision is blurry or doubled to prevent an accident or injury.<br>• Give IV infusions slowly, over 30–60 minutes, to avoid injection-site pain and heart rhythm problems.<br>• Monitor the patient's blood pressure and heart rate and rhythm before giving the drug IV, every 15 minutes during the infusion, and after the infusion is complete to identify severe hypotension or heart rhythm problems. |
| topiramate (Qudexy, Topamax, Trokendi XR)<br>Quick-release forms: initially, 25 mg orally twice daily; gradually increase over 6–7 weeks to 200 mg orally twice daily<br>XR forms: initially, 50 mg orally once daily; gradually increase over 6–7 weeks to 400 mg orally once daily<br>Levetiracetam (Keppra, Spritam) 1500 mg orally twice daily | • Monitor laboratory values, especially blood pH, electrolytes, and ammonia levels because this drug can cause metabolic acidosis, elevated ammonia levels, and encephalopathy.<br>• Assess patients for symptoms of encephalopathy, such as the development of lethargy, vomiting, changes in mental status, or hypothermia, and report these immediately to the healthcare provider so that prompt encephalopathy treatment can begin.<br>• The risk of metabolic acidosis is greater if the patient is also taking metformin for diabetes control.<br>• Assess patients for symptoms of metabolic acidosis (slow heart rate, hypotension, muscle weakness, and warm, flushed skin) and, if present, report these symptoms to the healthcare provider immediately.<br>• Follow dose-increasing schedules exactly to avoid adverse reactions.<br>**All patients beginning treatment with levetiracetam should be closely monitored for emerging or worsening depression or suicidal thoughts/behavior.**<br>**Blood urea nitrogen and creatinine clearance should be monitored during therapy and dosage reduced in those people with renal insufficiency. A complete blood count should be drawn for baseline values as blood abnormalities can occur.**<br>**This drug should be taken at the same time each day. The tablet or the extended-release tablet should be swallowed whole. Do not break, crush, or chew it.** |

| Table **10.5** | Examples of Newer Antiepileptic Drugs Approved as Adjuvant Therapy | | |
|---|---|---|
| **DRUG** | **ADULT MAINTENANCE DOSAGE** | **TYPE OF SEIZURE ACTIVITY TREATED** |
| ezogabine (Potiga) | 200–400 mg orally three times daily | Partial |
| felbamate (Felbatol) | 400–800 mg orally three times daily | Lennox-Gastaut syndrome and severe seizures that cannot be controlled with any other drugs |
| gabapentin (Horizant, Gralise, Neurontin) | 300–800 mg orally three times daily | Partial |
| pregabalin (Lyrica) | 200 mg orally three times daily | Partial |
| rufinamide (Banzel) | 1600 mg orally twice daily | Lennox-Gastaut syndrome |
| tiagabine (Gabitril) | 8–14 mg orally four times daily or 16–28 mg orally twice daily | Partial |
| vigabatrin (Sabril) | 1500 mg orally twice daily | Complex partial |
| Zonisamide (Zonegran | 100–600 mg orally once a day | Partial |

135 mEq/L (135 mmol/L) to the healthcare provider. Assess for symptoms associated with low sodium levels, such as headache, increased muscle weakness, and decreased deep tendon reflexes. If these symptoms are present, document them, and report them to the healthcare provider.

◆ *Patient and family teaching.* In addition to the teaching points listed in Box 10.7, tell the patient who is taking oxcarbazepine and his or her family:

- Keep all appointments for laboratory testing because this drug can cause electrolyte problems and decrease blood counts.
- Do not drive or operate dangerous equipment if you are experiencing blurred vision or double vision.
- If you notice increased muscle weakness and persistent headache, notify your healthcare provider because these may indicate low sodium levels.
- If you are taking oral contraceptives, use an additional form of contraception to prevent an unplanned pregnancy because this drug reduces the effectiveness of hormonal contraceptives.

### Lamotrigine

*Action and uses.* Lamotrigine is a newer AED with an unknown mechanism of action that is thought to reduce seizures by blocking sodium channels on neuron membranes. It is approved for use as monotherapy for partial seizures, tonic-clonic seizures, and seizures associated with Lennox-Gastaut syndrome. It is approved for some types of bipolar disorders. Table 10.4 lists the names, dosages, and nursing implications for lamotrigine.

*Expected side effects.* The most common side effects of lamotrigine are drowsiness, abdominal pain, and visual disturbances (e.g., double vision, blurred vision). Other side effects include ataxia, dry mouth, and dizziness. An unusual issue with lamotrigine is that its clearance rate is lower among black patients, which can lead to symptoms of overdose even with the usual recommended dosages.

*Adverse reactions.* Lamotrigine can cause life-threatening rashes, including Stevens-Johnson syndrome and toxic epidermal necrolysis. It has a black box warning that instructs immediate discontinuation of the drug if a rash appears during treatment. Although this problem can occur in patients of any age, it is more likely to occur in children. The drug interferes with the formation of folic acid, an important vitamin, and some patients may become folic acid deficient. Although lamotrigine is less likely than traditional AEDs to cause birth defects, it is still not recommended during pregnancy. Just as with traditional AEDs, depression and suicidal ideation are possible.

> **Top Tip for Safety**
>
> If any rash appears during therapy with lamotrigine, stop the drug and notify the healthcare provider immediately because this could signal the beginning of a life-threatening skin problem.

*Drug interactions.* Lamotrigine interacts with many drugs, especially aspirin, acetaminophen, oral contraceptives, proton pump inhibitors, cardiac drugs, drugs for psychiatric problems, drugs for HIV disease, drugs for tuberculosis, and drugs for diabetes. To prevent severe complications and adverse reactions, avoid other prescription drugs unless the benefit outweighs interaction risks. Consult a drug reference or pharmacist for possible interactions with other drugs the patient is prescribed.

❖ *Nursing Implications and Patient Teaching.* In addition to the general nursing implications for patients who are taking AEDs (see Box 10.6), the following issues and actions are important for patients who are taking lamotrigine.

◆ **Planning and implementation.** When drug therapy with lamotrigine is begun, three starter kits are available for prescription, depending on whether the patient will be taking lamotrigine as monotherapy or with other specific AEDs. Be sure to use the correct starter kit to avoid complications and interactions.

Assess the patient daily for rash, which can signal the beginning of life-threatening skin reactions. If a rash is present, withhold the dose, and notify the healthcare provider immediately. Assess black patients very carefully for side effects and adverse reactions because the drug clearance rate is about 25% lower than for patients of other races.

◆ **Patient and family teaching.** In addition to the teaching points listed in Box 10.7, tell the patient who is taking lamotrigine and his or her family:

- Check yourself every day for rashes. If a rash appears, notify your healthcare provider immediately because this response may be the start of a life-threatening reaction.
- If you are taking the extended-release form of the drug, swallow it whole, and do not crush, open, or chew it to keep the drug release even throughout the day.
- If your mouth becomes uncomfortably dry, chewing gum, sucking hard candy, and drinking more water may help the problem.
- Do not drive or operate dangerous equipment if your vision is blurred or you have double vision.

## Lacosamide

*Action and uses.* Lacosamide is a modified amino acid with an unknown mechanism of action that appears to control seizures by acting at sodium channels to stabilize neuron membranes and prevent repetitive excitation and firing. It is approved for use as monotherapy to control partial seizures and can be used as adjuvant therapy with some other AEDs. Table 10.4 lists the names, dosages, and nursing implications for lacosamide.

*Expected side effects.* The most common side effects of lacosamide are headache, dizziness, blurred vision, and double vision. Other side effects include fatigue, nausea, and ataxia.

*Adverse reactions.* Many people who are taking lacosamide experience *euphoria*, a feeling of intense well-being and happiness. This is considered an adverse reaction because it can lead to psychological dependence (but not addiction). Orthostatic hypotension (low blood pressure on moving to a standing position) with brief *syncope* (loss of consciousness) has been reported, leading to an increased risk of falls and injury.

Unlike other newer AEDs, lacosamide does not reduce the effectiveness of oral contraceptives. Intravenous infusions of lacosamide can cause pain at the injection site, rapid lowering of blood pressure, and heart rhythm problems, especially bradycardia. Although lacosamide is less likely than traditional AEDs to cause birth defects, it is still not recommended during pregnancy. As with traditional AEDs, depression and suicidal ideation are possible.

*Drug interactions.* Lacosamide interacts with many drugs, especially cardiac drugs, antihypertensives, drugs for psychiatric problems, drugs for HIV disease, antifungal drugs, and drugs for tuberculosis. To prevent severe complications and adverse reactions, avoid other prescription drugs unless the benefit outweighs interaction risks. Consult a drug reference or pharmacist for possible interactions with other drugs the patient is prescribed.

❖ *Nursing implications and patient teaching.* In addition to the general nursing implications for patients who are taking AEDs (see Box 10.6), the following issues and actions are important for patients who are taking lacosamide.

◆ **Planning and implementation.** Assess the patient's blood pressure before and after giving this drug because it can cause severe hypotension. This problem is worse in patients whose blood pressure is normally low. If the blood pressure is lower than normal, walk with the patient during ambulation, and instruct him or her not to walk alone.

Ask the patient about changes in vision such as blurred vision or double vision, which are common side effects of therapy with lacosamide. If these visual changes are present or the drug makes the patient dizzy, instruct him or her not to drive or operate dangerous machinery to avoid an accident or injury.

When giving this drug intravenously, infuse it slowly over 30 to 60 minutes. Faster rates increase the risk of pain at the injection site, severe hypotension, and heart rhythm problems. Monitor the patient's blood pressure and heart rate and rhythm before giving the drug, every 15 minutes during the infusion, and after the infusion is complete.

Observe the patient for mood changes after taking this drug. Some people feel euphoric, which can increase the risk of psychological dependency.

◆ **Patient and family teaching.** In addition to the teaching points listed in Box 10.7, tell the patient who is taking lacosamide and his or her family:

- Change positions slowly, especially when moving from a lying or sitting position to a standing position, because you may experience a sudden drop in blood pressure.
- Report any unexpected loss of consciousness to your healthcare provider because this is a possible adverse reaction to the drug.
- Do not drive or operate dangerous equipment if your vision is blurred, if you have double vision, or if you are dizzy, to prevent an accident or injury.
- Some people feel especially happy or even "high" when they take this drug and may be tempted to take it more often (i.e., become dependent on this

feeling). Regardless of this mood change, do not take the drug more often than prescribed.

## Topiramate

*Actions and uses.* Although the exact mechanisms are not clear, topiramate appears to reduce seizures by preventing the spread of excitation in the brain rather than raising the seizure threshold. It seems to have three actions that produce this response. Topiramate acts at sodium channels to stabilize neuron membranes and prevent repetitive excitation and firing, enhances the inhibitory neurotransmitter GABA, and blocks some excitatory receptors. It is approved for use as monotherapy for partial seizures, tonic-clonic seizures, and seizures associated with Lennox-Gastaut syndrome. It is also approved as adjuvant therapy for control of epilepsy. The drug has been used to treat migraines but is not approved for this use. Table 10.4 lists the names, dosages, and nursing implications for topiramate.

*Expected side effects.* Common side effects of topiramate are abdominal pain, nausea, dizziness, drowsiness, and fatigue. Additional side effects include taste changes, anorexia, and *paresthesias* (sensations of numbness, tingling, or "pins and needles").

*Adverse reactions.* Topiramate can cause memory impairment and electrolyte imbalances, especially low levels of phosphorus and calcium. At higher doses, topiramate can cause metabolic problems, particularly acidosis and elevated ammonia concentrations. When ammonia levels become too high, they can cause encephalopathy, which leads to brain damage and death. Symptoms of elevated ammonia levels and encephalopathy are unexplained lethargy, vomiting, changes in mental status, and low core body temperature (hypothermia).

Topiramate is a known teratogen that causes birth defects. It is not to be used during pregnancy unless epilepsy cannot be controlled any other way. As with other AEDs, depression and suicidal ideation are possible.

> ### 👁 Top Tip for Safety
>
> If blood ammonia levels are high or if symptoms of encephalopathy are present, the drug is immediately discontinued and treatment for encephalopathy is started.

*Drug interactions.* Topiramate interacts with many drugs, especially aspirin, acetaminophen, oral contraceptives, cardiac drugs, diuretics, antihypertensives, antifungals, drugs for psychiatric problems, drugs for HIV disease, drugs for tuberculosis, drugs that affect blood clotting, and drugs for diabetes. To prevent severe complications and adverse reactions, avoid other prescription drugs unless the benefit outweighs interaction risks. Consult a drug reference or pharmacist for possible interactions with other drugs the patient is prescribed.

❖ *Nursing implications and patient teaching.* In addition to the general nursing implications for patients taking AEDs (see Box 10.6), the following issues and actions are important for patients who are taking topiramate.

◆ **Planning and implementation.** Assess patients who are taking topiramate for the development of lethargy, vomiting, changes in mental status, or hypothermia (lower than normal core body temperature) because these may be signs of encephalopathy caused by high blood ammonia levels. Report any symptoms to the healthcare provider immediately. Be prepared to draw blood for measurement of ammonia level (normal ammonia levels are 10–80 mcg/dL [6–47 mmol/L]).

Monitor laboratory values, especially pH and electrolytes, because this drug increases the risk of metabolic acidosis. The risk is greater if the patient is also taking metformin for diabetes control. Symptoms of acidosis include slow heart rate, hypotension, muscle weakness, and warm, flushed skin. If the patient has several of these symptoms, notify the healthcare provider immediately.

◆ **Patient and family teaching.** In addition to the teaching points listed in Box 10.7, tell the patient who is taking topiramate and his or her family:

* If you suddenly become lethargic and confused and have vomiting or if your temperature falls below 95°F (35°C), call your healthcare provider immediately because these are symptoms of a life-threatening complication.
* Do not chew or crush capsules because this ruins the slow-release feature, and the drug may be absorbed so quickly that the risk of side effects and adverse reactions is increased.
* Do not chew or break the tablet form of the drug because it is very bitter tasting.

## Levetiracetam

*Actions and uses.* The exact mechanism of how levetiracetam prevents partial onset, primary generalized tonic-clonic, and myoclonic seizures is unknown, but what is known is that it connects with a protein that is involved with the release of inhibitory and excitatory neurotransmitters in the brain. It is being used as monotherapy for adults and children older than 16 years with focal seizures.

*Expected side effects and adverse reactions.* Headache, dizziness, and drowsiness as well as other CNS side effects were frequently reported. This drug may increase agitation, anger, anxiety, apathy, depersonalization, depression, hyperkinesis, nervousness, neurosis, and personality disorders.

It is listed under Beers Criteria as being potentially inappropriate drug use in older adults due to drug-disease or drug-syndrome interactions that may exacerbate the disease or syndrome.

*Drug interactions.* There are over 200 drugs that cause moderate interactions when given with levetiracetam, so precaution is warranted. Alcohol should be avoided when taking all anti-epileptics

❖ *Nursing implications and patient teaching*
◆ **Planning and implications.** BUN and creatinine clearance should be monitored during therapy and dosage reduced in those people with renal insufficiency. A CBC should be drawn for baseline values as blood abnormalities can occur.
◆ **Patient and family teaching.** All patients beginning treatment with levetiracetam should be closely monitored for emerging or worsening depression or suicidal thoughts/behavior.

This drug should be taken at the same time each day. The tablet or the extended-release tablet should be swallowed whole. Do not break, crush, or chew it.

### Epidiolex (Cannabidiol)

There are two syndromes that cause seizures in childhood that benefit from the FDA approval in 2018 of Epidiolex (Cannabidiol). Traditionally, seizures in both these syndromes have been extremely difficult to treat. Dravet syndrome is a genetic condition that causes frequent febrile seizures that later turn into myoclonic seizures and status epilepticus. Lennox-Gastaut syndrome presents between the ages of 3 and 5 and causes multiple types of seizures. Both conditions have a profound impact on the quality of life of the patients and their families because of the uncontrolled seizures.

Epidiolex's mechanism of action is not entirely understood, but it may decrease/prevent seizures by modification of the endocannabinoid system. Cannabidiol prevents the degradation of anandamide, which is an endocannabinoid that may have a role in seizure inhibition. It is orally administered to children and adults using a titration schedule either with or without food. Obtaining serum transaminases (alanine transaminase [ALT] and aspartate transaminase [AST]) and total bilirubin concentrations before treatment is recommended in all patients. Abrupt discontinuation of cannabidiol should be avoided to minimize the risk of increased seizure and status epilepticus

Anorexia, diarrhea, vomiting, nausea, and drowsiness were the most common side effects.

### DRUGS FOR MULTIPLE SCLEROSIS

Multiple sclerosis (MS) is an autoimmune disease that affects the fatty tissue *(myelin)* in the brain and spinal cord. Myelin surrounds and protects neurons and is important in providing support for neuron function in the CNS. Immune system cells and their products

attack myelin and destroy patches of it in the CNS, creating plaques, which reduce nerve function (Fig. 10.6). Although the nerves are not directly attacked, nerve transmission is interrupted, which causes the symptoms of MS. Specific early symptoms depend on where in the brain and spinal cord the myelin is destroyed. Box 10.8 lists common symptoms of MS. The disorder develops in women twice as often as in men.

MS manifests in a variety of types, the most common being relapsing-remitting MS (RRMS). A patient with RRMS has periods of worsening symptoms *(relapsing)* followed by periods in which symptoms are not present or are very mild *(remitting* or *remission periods)*. The disorder is progressive with worsening symptoms, longer duration of symptoms, and fewer remission periods over time. Eventually, symptoms are always present, and most motor functions decline. Some patients with RRMS have lived more than 30

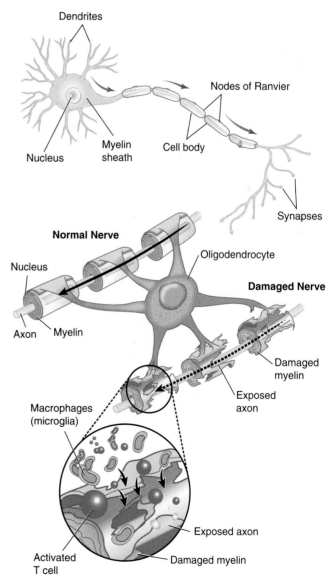

**Fig. 10.6** Pathogenesis of multiple sclerosis. (From McCance, K., & Huether, S. (2019). *Pathophysiology: The biologic basis for disease in adults and children* (8th ed.). Elsevier.)

| Box 10.8 | **Common Early Symptoms of Multiple Sclerosis** |
|---|---|

- Fatigue
- Double vision/blurry vision
- Muscle weakness
- Numbness of arms and legs
- Difficulty walking
- Urinary tract infections
- Bowel and bladder dysfunction
- Depression
- Difficulty with concentration

years with the disease; however, life expectancy is always decreased. MS cannot be cured, but drug therapy can slow progression and allow patients to remain functionally independent longer.

Management of MS is performed by neurologic healthcare providers and specialized clinics. Initial drug therapy is started with these specialists. However, patients with MS can develop other acute problems and be hospitalized, where some drug therapy must continue. As motor function decreases, many patients with MS are placed in long-term care facilities. The drugs discussed in this chapter are primarily used for RRMS.

### NONSPECIFIC ANTI-INFLAMMATORY DRUGS

For many years, treatment for MS consisted of generalized reduction of inflammation and immunity with powerful anti-inflammatory agents, such as corticosteroids. These drugs may relieve some symptoms but do not alter the course of the disease and have significant side effects. Corticosteroids may be used occasionally at lower dosages in addition to more specific drug therapies for MS. Chapter 13 discusses corticosteroids in detail.

### SPECIFIC DRUGS FOR MULTIPLE SCLEROSIS

More therapeutic options are now available for MS. The three broad categories of drugs to reduce MS symptoms, slow progression, and increase the duration of remissions (for RRMS) are the biological response modifiers (BRMs), monoclonal antibodies, and neurologic drugs. The names, dosages, side effects, and adverse reactions to check for in patients who are receiving these drugs are listed in Table 10.6.

#### Biological Response Modifiers

A biological response modifier is a drug that alters the patient's immune response to abnormal triggers of immunity and inflammation. This drug class contains two drugs given by subcutaneous injection and two oral preparations. Both types of drugs are taken regularly. The two injectable BRMs are beta-interferon (Avonex, Betaseron, Extavia, Plegridy, Rebif) and glatiramer (Copaxone, Glatopa). The oral drugs are fingolimod (Gilenya) and teriflunomide (Aubagio). The BRMs are

prescribed by healthcare providers who are specialists in the care of patients with MS. These specialists and specialty nurses are responsible for patient teaching and for managing side effects and adverse reactions. The names, dosages, side effects, and adverse reactions to check for in patients who are receiving BRMs are listed in Table 10.6.

### Monoclonal Antibodies for Multiple Sclerosis

Monoclonal antibodies for MS attack and inactivate or destroy lymphocytes that are involved in direct destruction of myelin or produce chemicals (cytokines) that trigger the immune system to destroy myelin. The lymphocyte population in the periphery of the body is reduced along with lymphocytes in the CNS. All of these drugs increase the risk of infection by reducing general immunity and can trigger severe allergic reactions.

These drugs are all given as intravenous infusions on a specific schedule that ranges from once monthly to once every 6 months to once yearly. They are given only in specialized centers or in offices of healthcare providers who are specialists in the care of patients with MS. These specialists and specialty nurses are responsible for monitoring patients during and after infusion, patient teaching, and managing side effects and adverse reactions. The names, dosages, side effects, and adverse reactions to check for in patients who are receiving these drugs are listed in Table 10.6.

### Specific Neurologic Drugs for Multiple Sclerosis

Neurologic drugs approved specifically for MS are dimethyl fumarate (Tecfidera) and dalfampridine (Ampyra). Both are oral drugs that must be taken daily to help improve some symptoms of MS. They are likely to be part of the prescribed drug regimen for patients with MS when they are admitted to the hospital or another care facility. The benefits of the drugs are achieved only if therapy continues in all care settings.

Dimethyl fumarate reduces inflammation in the CNS, which helps protect neurons and myelin from damage. Dalfampridine blocks potassium channels in unmyelinated nerves, helping them to continue to function. It is used to help improve the walking ability of patients with MS. The names, dosages, side effects, and adverse reactions to check for in patients who are receiving these drugs are listed in Table 10.6.

## DRUGS FOR AMYOTROPHIC LATERAL SCLEROSIS

Amyotrophic lateral sclerosis (ALS) is a progressive, fatal neurodegenerative disease that affects the motor nerves of the brain and spinal cord. It can strike anyone at any time; however, it usually affects persons between 40 and 70 years of age. The cause of ALS is unknown, and there is no cure. There are no diagnostic tools available that detect the disease. Diagnosis is made when other neurodegenerative diseases have been ruled out.

## Table 10.6  Examples of Drugs for Relapsing-Remitting Multiple Sclerosis

*Biological response modifiers* alter the immune response of MS patients to abnormal triggers of immunity and inflammation, which slows progression of the disease, improves symptoms, and increases the duration of remission periods.

*Monoclonal antibodies* slow the progression of MS by attacking and inactivating or destroying lymphocytes that are involved in direct destruction of myelin or that produce chemicals (cytokines) that trigger the immune system to damage myelin.

*Neurologic drugs* slow progression and reduce the symptoms of MS using several mechanisms to protect nerves and myelin from destruction or improve impulse transmission of demyelinated nerves.

| DRUG/ADULT DOSAGE | EXPECTED SIDE EFFECTS AND ADVERSE REACTIONS |
|---|---|
| **Biological Response Modifiers** | |
| beta-interferon (Avonex, Betaseron, Extavia, Plegridy, Rebif): maintenance, depends on strength and formulation of the drug; given subcutaneously three times weekly, every other day, or once every 14 days for long-duration formulas<br>fingolimod (Gilenya) 0.5 mg orally once daily<br>glatiramer (Copaxone, Glatopa) 20 mg subcutaneously daily of the 20 mg/mL solution *or* 40 mg subcutaneously three times per week of the 40 mg/mL solution<br>teriflunomide (Aubagio) 7 *or* 14 mg orally once daily | • Flulike symptoms<br>• Headache<br>• Injection-site reactions<br>• Peripheral neuropathy<br>• Elevated levels of liver enzymes<br>• Slow heart rate<br>• Thinning scalp hair |
| **Monoclonal Antibodies** | |
| alemtuzumab (Lemtrada) 12 mg IV daily for 3 consecutive days (total dose of 36 mg) for maintenance<br>daclizumab (Zinbryta) 150 mg injected subcutaneously once monthly for maintenance<br>natalizumab (Tysabri) 300 mg IV infusion given over 1 hour every 4 weeks<br>ocrelizumab (Ocrevus) 600 mg IV infusion every 6 months for maintenance | • Increased risk of infection<br>• Higher risk of severe allergic reactions<br>• Infusion-site reactions<br>• Flulike symptoms<br>• Back pain<br>• Hypotension<br>• Edema<br>• Patient should not be taking more than one monoclonal antibody at a time. |
| **Neurologic Drugs** | |
| dalfampridine (Ampyra) 10 mg orally every 12 hours<br>dimethyl fumarate (Tecfidera) 240 mg orally twice daily | • Increased risk of infection<br>• Headache, dizziness, muscle weakness<br>• Gastrointestinal problems, heartburn, constipation<br>• Confusion, seizure activity<br>• Nausea, diarrhea, abdominal pain<br>• Flushing, itching, rashes |

*IV*, Intravenous; *MS*, multiple sclerosis.

Most patients die within 3 to 5 years of diagnosis. Loss of coordination is usually the first symptom of the disease. As the voluntary muscles begin to be affected, the patient progressively loses the ability to move, speak, eat, and breathe. The involuntary muscles become atrophied and die, and the patient becomes paralyzed. Because it is a motor neuron disease, cognitive functioning and the sensory neurons of sight, hearing, smell, taste, and touch usually are not affected.

ALS patients have excess glutamate in their brain and spinal cord. Glutamate is an amino acid that can be toxic to nerve cells, and drug therapy is designed to moderate and inhibit the action of glutamate.

## GLUTAMINE ANTAGONISTS

Riluzole reduces the actions of glutamate by inhibiting or blocking the action and/or release of glutamate. Riluzole has a neuroprotective effect and is thought to delay injury to and death of the neurons. This action helps to prolong the life of an ALS patient by 3 months. A thickened form of riluzole is manufactured as a liquid suspension for easier administration as

swallowing becomes difficult. Table 10.7 lists the nursing implications of riluzole

### Expected Side Effects and Adverse Reactions
Weakness, lack of energy, diarrhea, anorexia, nausea, and vomiting are the most frequently reported side effects. Hepatic enzyme elevation and hepatotoxicity can occur. Neutropenia, anemia, and kidney dysfunction are rare adverse reactions of the drug.

### Drug Interactions
Riluzole should be used with caution with dextromethorphan. Signs and symptoms of hepatic injury during coadministration of riluzole and quinidine should be monitored because hepatotoxicity can occur.

❖ *Nursing implications and patient teaching*
◆   **Assessment.** Liver function enzymes should be monitored before and during the course of therapy every month for the first 3 months, every 3 months for the remainder of the first year, and periodically as needed after that. If a febrile illness develops, the WBC count should be monitored because neutropenia can occur with this drug.

Several cases of interstitial lung disease have been reported with riluzole, and you should check with the healthcare provider if the patient has pulmonary disease. Withhold the drug and notify the healthcare provider if liver enzyme levels are elevated.

◆ **Planning and implementation.** Riluzole should be given at least 1 hour before or 2 hours after a meal. Liver function tests, serum bilirubin, and neurologic functioning should be monitored before and during use. As swallowing becomes difficult, the liquid suspension of riluzole can be used. This drug should not be given to patients who are pregnant or breast-feeding.

◆ **Evaluation.** Differentiating adverse side effects from the actions of riluzole is difficult because the manifestations of ALS (weakness and lack of energy) are often associated with side effects. Care should be taken when evaluating for side effects.

◆ **Patient and family teaching.** Tell the patient and family:
- The dose should not be increased. There is no added benefit with daily doses greater than 50 mg every 12 hours, and increased side effects can occur.
- Report any febrile illness to the healthcare provider.
- Driving or engaging in potentially hazardous activities before the response to the drug is known is dangerous and should not be undertaken.
- Do not breast-feed while taking this drug.
- Do not drink alcohol while taking this drug because of potential adverse effects.

### ANTIOXIDANT

Radicava (Edaravone) is an antioxidant which slows the decline of functional abilities that occur with ALS by scavenging free radicals and serving as an antioxidant that is neuroprotective against the oxidative stress that contributes to neurodegeneration and the development of ALS. Edaravone can decrease the decline of physical function significantly after 6 months of use. It comes in both oral and intravenous forms. There are few side effects and no adverse reactions other than hypersensitivity to the drug. There are no interactions reported.

## DRUGS FOR MYASTHENIA GRAVIS

Myasthenia gravis is an autoimmune disease that attacks the neuromuscular junction (connection between the nerve and muscle). It can affect anyone regardless of age but is more prevalent among women younger than 40 years and men older than 60 years.

The disease is characterized by weakness and fatigue of the voluntary muscles. Eye drooping and double vision are often the first signs of disease because the eye muscles are some of the first to be affected. Other symptoms include arm and leg weakness, dysphasia, and difficulty with chewing, swallowing, and breathing. The muscles become weaker as they are exercised; consequently, muscle weakness and fatigue are worse in the afternoon and evening. Chewing and swallowing become more difficult during and after meals.

### ACETYLCHOLINESTERASE INHIBITORS

#### Action and Uses

Acetylcholinesterase (AChE), or cholinesterase, is an enzyme that breaks down acetylcholine (ACh) in the brain. ACh is a neurotransmitter released by nerve cells that causes muscles to contract. In myasthenia gravis, ACh levels are deficient, which explains the muscle weakness and fatigue that are experienced by patients

| Table 10.7 Example of Drugs Used for Amyotrophic Lateral Sclerosis | |
|---|---|
| *Glutamine antagonists* inhibit or block the action or release of glutamate. | |
| **DRUG/ADULT DOSAGE** | **NURSING IMPLICATIONS** |
| riluzole (Rilutek) 50 mg tablets to be given twice daily for a total of 100 mg/day at least 1 hour before or 2 hours after a meal riluzole (Tiglutik), 50 mg/10 mL suspension to be given twice daily for a total of 100 mg/day at least 1 hour before or 2 hours after a meal<br>Edavarone (Radicava) 105 mg orally once daily in the morning after overnight fasting for 14 days followed by a 14-day drug-free period for an initial treatment cycle. For subsequent treatment cycles, administer for 10 days out of 14-day periods followed by 14-day drug-free periods | • As the disease progresses, the liquid suspension may be given for easier swallowing.<br>• Liver function enzymes should be monitored before and during the course of treatment every month for the first 3 months, every 3 months for the remainder of the first year, and periodically as needed after that.<br>• If liver enzymes are elevated, withhold the drug and notify the healthcare provider.<br>• Report signs of jaundice and yellowing of the sclerae to the healthcare provider because liver toxicity can occur.<br>• Call the healthcare provider if the patient has a febrile illness so the white blood cell count can be monitored.<br>• Administration by via of nasogastric tube feedings or orally is relative to type of food consumption:<br>• High fat meal (800 to 1,000 calories, 50% fat): Fast 8 hours before and 1 hour after administration.<br>• Low fat meal (400 to 500 calories, 25% fat): Fast 4 hours before and 1 hour after administration.<br>• Calorie supplement (250 calories, e.g., protein drink): Fast 2 hours before and 1 hour after administration.<br>• Only water may be consumed in the 1 hour after administration. |

| Table 10.8   Examples of Common Drugs Used for Myasthenia Gravis | |
| --- | --- |
| **DRUG/ADULT DOSAGE** | **NURSING IMPLICATIONS** |
| pyridostigmine bromide (Mestinon) 30 mg tablet: given every 6 hours for a daily dose of 600 mg but not to exceed 1500 mg/day; pyridostigmine bromide 60 mg tablet: given every 6 hours for a daily dose of 600 mg but not to exceed 1500 mg/day<br>pyridostigmine bromide 60 mg/5 mL solution: given every 6 hours for a daily dose of 600 mg but not to exceed 1500 mg/day<br>pyridostigmine bromide 180 mg extended-release tablet: 180 mg to 540 mg once or twice daily | • Dosage varies according to patient response.<br>• Monitor patients for clinical improvement. If improvement does not occur, it may be due to underdosage or overdosage.<br>• Monitor for increasing muscle weakness, which may indicate overdosage (cholinergic crisis).<br>• Monitor for increasing muscle weakness, which may indicate myasthenic crises (worsening of the disease).<br>• Notify the healthcare professional if there are signs of increasing muscle weakness.<br>• Monitor vital signs and notify the healthcare provider about any changes in heart rate, blood pressure, or breathing.<br>• Administer at intervals when the muscles are strongest or before activity (e.g., early in the morning, before meals) to assist swallowing and prevent aspiration. |

with the disease. Inhibiting the enzyme AChE makes more ACh available, producing stronger muscles.

AChE inhibitors (also called *cholinesterase inhibitors*) are the basic treatment for myasthenia gravis. Edrophonium has a short half-life of about 12 minutes, and it is used only as a diagnostic tool. Patients test positive for myasthenia gravis if their muscles get stronger after being injected with edrophonium. This is also known as the *Tensilon (edrophonium) test*.

Pyridostigmine (a cholinesterase inhibitor) has a half-life of 3 to 4 hours and is used for long-term maintenance therapy for the disease. Table 10.8 lists the nursing implications for pyridostigmine.

## Expected Side Effects and Adverse Reactions

The most common side effects for the use of edrophonium and pyridostigmine are related to the cholinergic activity of the GI system. Nausea, vomiting, diarrhea, stomach cramps, abdominal pain, difficult swallowing, and increased salivation are the most common side effects. Bradycardia and other dysrhythmias can occur. Hypotension due to a fall in cardiac output (from bradycardia) may also occur. This happens because ACh is the neurotransmitter for the parasympathetic nervous system that increases gastric activity and decreases heart rate.

Severe adverse reactions include respiratory depression and respiratory arrest. Cardiac arrest can occur during a cholinergic crisis (overstimulation of the parasympathetic nervous system). Increased bronchial secretions, laryngospasm, and bronchial constriction can also occur. Pyridostigmine is combined in tablet and syrup form with bromide, and if the serum bromide level becomes too high, it can cause abnormalities in electrolyte levels.

## Drug Interactions

Other cholinesterase inhibitors can produce additive effects and increase the chance for a cholinergic crisis. Amifampridine, a potassium channel blocker approved for use in other rare neuromuscular diseases, can precipitate severe adverse reactions. Tricyclic antidepressants such as amoxapine, amitriptyline, and chlordiazepoxide may antagonize some of the effects of drugs that mimic or enhance the parasympathetic nervous system. Other drugs that interact with pyridostigmine are atropine, bethanechol, disopyramide, and medicines that block muscle or nerve pain.

❖ *Nursing implications and patient teaching*

◆ **Assessment.** Pyridostigmine should be used with caution in patients with bronchial asthma, chronic obstructive pulmonary disease (COPD), bradycardia, or cardiac arrhythmias. Patients being treated for hypertension or glaucoma with beta-adrenergic receptor blockers may be at risk for unopposed cholinergic activity because of the indirect cholinergic activity of pyridostigmine.

◆ **Planning and implementation.** Space doses at least 6 hours apart. Giving the extended-release product at bedtime to treat weakness that occurs at night and on awakening may enhance patient safety from falls. Extended-release products should be swallowed whole and not crushed or chewed. A syrup is available for use and may be given over ice chips. Atropine should be readily available in the event of a symptomatic bradycardia such as hypotension.

◆ **Evaluation.** Evaluate and report muscular weakness, cramps, or muscular fasciculations. If the patient does not show improvement in symptoms, underdosage or overdosage may be responsible. Monitor vital signs frequently, especially respiratory rate, because increasing muscle weakness can lead to respiratory arrest.

◆ *Patient and family teaching.* Tell the patient and family:
• If you miss a dose, take it as soon as you can. If it is almost time for your next dose, take only that dose. Do not take double or extra doses.
• The duration of the drug action can vary with physical and emotional stress and disease severity.
• Report onset of rash to the healthcare provider.
• Sustained-release tablets can become spotted in appearance, but this does not affect the potency of the drug.

- Do not breast-feed while taking this drug without consulting the healthcare provider.

Efgartigimod alfa (Vygart) is a human immunoglobulin that can be used in about 80% of patients with myasthenia gravis. The drug reduces the antibodies that interfere with communication between nerves and muscles and improves the weakness and fatigue of voluntary muscles. It is an IV infusion that is administered once a week for 4 weeks. It may increase the risk of infection and immunosuppression. Live vaccines should not be given to a patient on this drug.

# Get Ready for the Next-Generation NCLEX® Examination!

## Key Points

- The symptoms of Parkinson's disease (PD) are caused by an imbalance in neurotransmitters in which the amount of ACh (an excitatory chemical) is normal but there is too little dopamine (inhibitory chemical) in the brain. Motor and sensory symptoms are progressive and debilitating.
- Dopamine agonists are best absorbed on an empty stomach. When taken 30 to 60 minutes before a meal or snack, they help the patient to be better able to chew and swallow.
- Taking dopamine agonists with food that is high in protein reduces the drug's effectiveness.
- Levodopa peaks in about 1 hour and wears off in 4 or 5 hours. As it wears off, there are rapid swings of symptoms. This is also called an *on-off effect*.
- Long-term use of dopamine agonists may lead to *akinesia* (loss of movement), *tardive dyskinesia* (abnormal and involuntary movements, especially of the lower face), and *dystonia* (impairment of muscle tone).
- Dopamine agonists can exacerbate depression and psychosis.
- Monitor blood glucose levels closely when using dopamine agonists because the sympathetic effects can cause hypoglycemia.
- Teach people who are taking MAO-B inhibitors to avoid tyramine-containing foods such as beer, wine, and aged meats and cheeses.
- In Alzheimer's disease (AD), microtubules within neurons become tangled and form nonfunctional meshes in the brain, and the level of the excitatory neurotransmitter ACh is decreased in brain tissue. These changes result in progressive difficulty with memory and learning.
- Cholinesterase inhibitors are drugs that bind to acetylcholinesterase and slow its action, allowing ACh to remain functional longer, possibly delaying memory loss and improving functional ability.
- Cholinesterase inhibitors are parasympathetic agonists, and they can cause adverse side effects throughout the body, including bradycardia, hypotension in the cardiac system, and seizures in the neurologic system.
- Memantine (Namenda) is an NMDA blocker that can allow more calcium into brain neurons, possibly improving memory. It is given with cholinesterase inhibitors to boost their effect.
- Patients with AD should be weighed weekly to monitor for weight loss that can be caused by all the drugs used to improve memory.
- Donepezil (Aricept) should be given at night.
- Phenobarbital is a Schedule IV controlled substance with an increased risk of physical and psychological dependency.
- Stopping AEDs suddenly can trigger seizure activity. The drugs are tapered slowly to reduce this possibility.
- With any AED, depression and suicidal ideation are possible.
- Phenytoin, carbamazepine, phenobarbital, primidone, and valproic acid are known teratogens that commonly cause birth defects. These drugs are not to be used during pregnancy unless epilepsy cannot be controlled any other way.
- Epidiolex is a cannabidiol (CBD) that treats seizures associated with two rare and severe forms of epilepsy in children.
- Always consult a drug reference or pharmacist to determine possible interactions between AEDs and any other drug that a patient is prescribed.
- Serious liver toxicity may be seen in some children who are taking valproic acid, especially those younger than 2 years of age and those receiving multiple AEDs.
- If any rash appears during therapy with lamotrigine, stop the drug and notify the healthcare provider immediately because this could signal the beginning of life-threatening skin problems.
- Topiramate can increase blood levels of ammonia and cause encephalopathy with brain damage.
- There is no cure for MS.
- Monoclonal antibodies for MS have a high risk of severe allergic reactions.
- The monoclonal antibodies for MS all increase the risk of infection.

## Clinical Judgment and Next-Generation NCLEX® Examination-Style Questions

### Case Study

The nurse is caring for Mr. Smith an 82-year-old male patient with a 5-year history of Parkinson's disease and dementia. His observed symptoms of Parkinson's are a slow, shuffling gait, cogwheel rigidity, and a masklike facial expression. He has a history of arthritis and frequently complains of joint pain. He also complains of chronic nasal stuffiness and headaches. Vital signs are stable, and he has no known drug allergies.

1. Instructions: For each potential prescription listed below, place an X in the box to indicate whether the prescription is anticipated, nonessential or contraindicated.

| POTENTIAL PRESCRIPTION | ANTICIPATED | NON-ESSENTIAL | CONTRA-INDICATED |
|---|---|---|---|
| Carbidopa/ levodopa | | | |
| Tolcapone | | | |
| Nuplazid | | | |
| Pramipexole | | | |
| Tramadol | | | |
| Selegiline | | | |
| Phenylephrine | | | |
| Amantadine | | | |

2. The nurse has asked the nursing assistant to help Mr. Smith fill out the next day's menu. The nurse then reviews the patient's menu choices. Which menu choice will prompt the nurse to reinforce dietary teaching to the patient?

   1. Grapefruit juice, poached egg, and toast with jelly
   2. Oatmeal, orange juice, and toast with butter
   3. Granola with blueberries and raisins with oat milk
   4. Hamburger, french fries, and chocolate milkshake
   5. Linguini with white sauce, salad, and iced tea
   6. Bean burrito with cola

3. As Mr. Smith's Parkinson's disease advances, which symptom/symptoms present the greatest risk for safety?

   1. Shuffling gait
   2. Depression
   3. Cogwheel rigidity
   4. Difficulty chewing

4. The nurse administers Mr. Smith's drugs at 0600 (6 a.m.), 1400 (2 p.m.), 2200 (10 p.m.). What time will the nurse expect to see worsening motor symptoms?

   1. 1600 (4:00 p.m.)
   2. 1100 (11:00 a.m.)
   3. 0500 (5:00 a.m.)
   4. 0700 (7:00 a.m.)

5. A 32-year-old female patient with new onset seizures is prescribed phenytoin 100 mg orally twice a day. Which information given by the nurse is correct?

   1. "A slight rash is normal when taking this medication."
   2. "Feeling drowsy is a side effect of this medication."
   3. "Floss your teeth at least once a day when taking this medication."
   4. "The dizziness you experience will go away in time"

6. Scenario: The healthcare provider (HCP) has written a prescription for a rivastigmine transdermal patch for an asthmatic patient with Alzheimer's disease. Before administering the patch, the nurse will first _____1_____. The patch must _____2_____. It is most important for the nurse to monitor the patient for _____3_____.

| OPTIONS FOR 1 | OPTIONS FOR 2 | OPTIONS FOR 3 |
|---|---|---|
| Utilize the Alzheimer's Disease Assessment Scale | Be placed on the back every day | Urinary retention |
| Obtain a 12-lead EKG | Be covered with plastic wrap when showering | Headaches |
| Obtain a chest x-ray | Be changed at the same time every 48 hours | Cough |
| Assess for swallowing problems | Be rotated to different sites on the arms and legs | BUN/creatinine levels |

7. Which are the best times for a patient with myasthenia gravis to take pyridostigmine bromide?

   1. Every 6 hours while awake
   2. 1 hour before meals
   3. With each meal
   4. 2 hours after each meal

8. Which signs and symptoms will the nurse monitor for in a patient who is taking a monoclonal antibody to slow the progression of MS? Select all or any that apply.

   1. Sore throat
   2. Nasal congestion
   3. Shortness of breath
   4. Fever
   5. Peripheral neuropathy
   6. Constipation
   7. Urinary incontinence
   8. Back pain
   9. Yellow skin and sclera

9. The nurse is caring for a patient diagnosed with Lennox-Gastaut syndrome. Which adjuvant antiepileptics would the nurse expect the HCP to prescribe? Select all or any that apply.

   1. tiagabine
   2. gabapentin
   3. phenytoin
   4. cannabidiol
   5. rufinamide
   6. felbamate
   7. levetiracetam
   8. zonisamide
   9. carbamazepine

10. Which antiepileptics carry an increased risk of psychological dependency?

   1. carbamazepine
   2. cannabidiol
   3. ethosuximide
   4. phenytoin
   5. phenobarbital
   6. valproic acid
   7. lacosamide

## Learning Outcomes

1. List the names, actions, possible side effects, and adverse effects of drugs for anxiety and sleep.
2. Explain what to teach patients and families about drugs for anxiety and sleep.
3. List the names, actions, possible side effects, and adverse effects of antidepressant drugs and mood stabilizers.
4. Explain what to teach patients and families about antidepressant drugs and mood stabilizers.
5. List the names, actions, possible side effects, and adverse effects of typical and atypical antipsychotic drugs.
6. Explain what to teach patients and families about typical and atypical antipsychotic drugs.
7. List the names, actions, possible side effects, and adverse effects of drugs that treat tardive dyskinesia.
8. Explain what to teach patients and families about drugs that treat tardive dyskinesia.

## Key Terms

**anxiolytic** A description for any drug that can reduce anxiety.

**atypical antidepressants** Drugs that affect the neurotransmitters dopamine, norepinephrine, and/or serotonin to help reduce depression.

**atypical antipsychotics** Drugs that are usually a combination of dopamine and serotonin blockers and are used to reduce positive symptoms and improve negative symptoms of some types of psychosis without causing severe extrapyramidal effects. Also called *second-generation antipsychotics*.

**benzodiazepines (BNZs)** A class of sedative-hypnotic drugs that depress the central nervous system by binding to benzodiazepine receptors, which then act with gamma-aminobutyric acid (GABA) receptors to enhance GABA effects. Depending on the drug dose and concentration, they can reduce anxiety, induce sleep, and relax skeletal muscles.

**benzodiazepine agonist** Drug that has a different chemical structure from the benzodiazepines (BNZs) but still binds strongly to BNZ receptors and acts in the same ways as BNZs to initiate sleep and promote longer sleep with less risk for dependence.

**dopamine system stabilizers (DSSs)** Drugs that affect dopamine and serotonin receptors slightly differently from other atypical antipsychotics. As a result, they have fewer motor side effects and adverse effects.

**drug-induced movement disorders (DIMDs)** Umbrella term for adverse effects associated with use of antipsychotics. These include extrapyramidal symptoms (EPS) of pseudoparkinsonism, acute dystonia, and akathisia, as well as tardive dyskinesia.

**hypnotics** Drugs in the sedative-hypnotic class that are used mainly to cause sleep; they promote sleep by changing signals in the central nervous system and reducing responses to stimulation. See *sedatives*.

**monoamine oxidase inhibitor (MAOI)** Drug that inhibits monoamine oxidases, enzymes that break down neurotransmitters, including dopamine, norepinephrine, and serotonin. Blocking these enzymes increases the amount of available neurotransmitters and reduces depressive symptoms.

**mood stabilizers** Drugs used primarily to treat patients with bipolar illness. They help manage or reduce the symptoms associated with mania and improve the symptoms of depression. Several drugs in this category are also used as antiseizure drugs.

**nonphenothiazines** Drugs that are chemically different from the phenothiazines but have similar actions, side effects, and adverse effects.

**phenothiazines** Drugs that block binding of dopamine to dopamine receptors and other neurotransmitters to acetylcholine and alpha-adrenergic receptors. These drugs reduce positive symptoms but have significant side and adverse effects.

**sedatives** Drugs in the sedative-hypnotic class that have a calming, relaxing effect at lower doses and cause sleep at higher doses; they promote sleep by changing signals in the central nervous system and reducing responses to stimulation. See *hypnotics*.

**selective serotonin reuptake inhibitor (SSRI)** Drug that blocks reabsorption of the neurotransmitter serotonin, increasing the concentration of serotonin that is available for binding postsynaptic receptors to improve a patient's sense of well-being and reduce depression.

**serotonin-norepinephrine reuptake inhibitor (SNRI)** Drug that prevents reabsorption of serotonin and norepinephrine, increasing the concentrations of both neurotransmitters available to postsynaptic receptors. These actions can improve a patient's sense of well-being and reduce depression.

**11 tricyclic antidepressants (TCAs)** An older class of drugs used to reduce depression. The precise action is unknown, but the drugs are thought to interfere with the reuptake of norepinephrine and serotonin.

**typical antipsychotics** Drugs that block dopamine receptors in the brain, which helps treat the positive symptoms of psychosis such as hallucinations and delusions. They do not affect the negative symptoms.

Blocking dopamine can result in a variety of side effects and adverse reactions, including pseudoparkinsonism, tardive dyskinesia, and other drug-induced movement disorders.

**vesicular monoamine transporter 2 inhibitors** Drugs that reduce persistent symptoms of tardive dyskinesia in patients who require long-term antipsychotic drug therapy to treat their mental illness.

## DRUG THERAPY AND MENTAL ILLNESS

More than half of Americans will be diagnosed with a mental illness at some time during their lifetime; about 4% will be diagnosed with a serious mental illness such as bipolar disorder, schizophrenia, or major depression. Fortunately, as we learn more about the brain, newer drug therapies can reduce some of the suffering associated with living with mental illness. As an LPN/VN, you will care for patients receiving treatment for mental illnesses in all care settings. Therefore it is really important to understand the role of drug therapy in treating mental illness as well as the potential for side and adverse effects in drug use.

Before we talk about drug therapy for mental illness, it is important to understand the basic concepts of mental health and mental illness. According to the World Health Organization (WHO), mental health is a state of well-being that includes the ability to cope with normal life stresses, work productively, acknowledge personal abilities, and contribute to the community. A person's mental health is influenced by biological and other factors, including environment, culture, and economic status.

Nevertheless, rather than categorizing any individual as having mental health or mental illness, it is important to consider the mental health–mental illness continuum (Fig. 11.1). At any time, a person may be coping very well with normal stressors, but at a later time a significant life event could trigger emotional problems or concerns. In contrast, some people experience far greater emotional problems related to common normal stressors and have marked distress or impairment. More severe impairment is consistent with mental illness. People with mental illness may experience changes in behaviors and emotions and significant changes in their ability to think. They often have difficulty coping with normal stressors, interacting with others, and otherwise functioning within their own cultural norms.

### Bookmark This!

The National Alliance on Mental Illness (NAMI) is a wonderful resource for caregivers, patients, and families: https://nami.org/Home. You can access information that is helpful to you and your agency. You may even find a local group that provides support for your patients and their families.

As described in Chapter 10, chemical neurotransmitters have important roles in transmitting messages between the brain and other areas of the nervous system. Neurotransmitters are involved in memory (storage and recall of information), mood (emotional state), and affect (response to a specific stimulus or event), and learning how drugs work will help you understand their impact on your patients. The main neurotransmitters

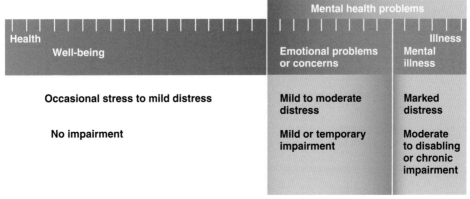

Fig. 11.1 The mental health–mental illness continuum. (University of Michigan. (2009). *Understanding U: A guide to help you manage the ups and downs of life. What is mental health?* https://hr.umich.edu/sites/default/files/resource_guide_final.pdf)

affected by psychiatric drugs are serotonin, dopamine, norepinephrine, gamma-aminobutyric acid (GABA), acetylcholine, and histamine. Table 11.1 describes these neurotransmitters and how they typically affect mental health and mental illness. This chapter focuses on drugs that are used for sleep difficulties, anxiety, depression, other mood disorders, and psychosis.

## DRUGS FOR SLEEP AND ANXIETY

### SEDATIVE-HYPNOTICS

Sleep is a state of rest for the mind and body in which conscious awareness is reduced partially or completely. Sufficient amounts of sleep are needed daily to restore energy levels and promote optimal mental and physical functioning. Adults vary in how much sleep they need daily and whether it must occur over 6 to 8 hours or can occur over multiple shorter periods throughout the day.

Most adults have experienced occasions when they could not get to sleep or did not remain asleep during an expected period. This problem is known as *insomnia*. Many people have occasional insomnia, but others struggle with this problem almost daily. When sleep is insufficient for adequate rest, all aspects of functioning are affected. Areas of obvious impairment include learning, remembering, concentration, judgment, reaction time, coordination, and general social interactions. You probably have been around someone who is sleep deprived or have had this problem yourself. People who suffer from sleep deprivation may feel irritable, impatient, and unable to concentrate.

People who have chronic insomnia usually require a more complex behavioral and pharmacologic approach to help the problem. For those who have intermittent problems with insomnia, drug therapy can be helpful. A sedative is a drug that promotes sleep by changing signals in the central nervous system (CNS) and reducing responses to stimulation. At lower doses, sedatives have a calming, relaxing effect, and at higher doses, they cause sleep. Drugs in this class that are used mainly to cause sleep are called hypnotics. Sometimes, people may use or be prescribed a drug that has a side effect of sedation, such as an antihistamine or muscle relaxant, but this discussion focuses only on sedatives.

### Action and Uses

The two main categories of drugs prescribed for sleep are the benzodiazepines (BNZs) and benzodiazepine agonists (also called *non-benzodiazepines*). BNZs are a class of sedative-hypnotic drugs that depress the CNS by binding to benzodiazepine receptors, which then act with GABA receptors to enhance GABA effects. Depending on the drug dose and concentration they reduce anxiety, induce sleep, and relax skeletal muscles. Thus sleep begins sooner after going to bed and total sleep time is increased.

Recall from Chapter 10 that GABA is an inhibitory neurotransmitter, and when GABA receptors are stimulated, CNS activity is reduced. Depending on which type of BNZ receptor a specific BNZ binds to, other responses can include reduced seizure activity and reduced anxiety. Depending on dose, drug concentration, and added chemicals, some BNZs are approved for use as sedatives but not to relieve anxiety; others are approved to reduce anxiety but are not approved for sedation.

A benzodiazepine agonist has a different chemical structure from the BNZs but still binds strongly to BNZ receptors; it acts in the same ways as BNZs to initiate sleep and promote longer sleep with less risk for drug dependence. These drugs are used more specifically for sedative effects and have less muscle-relaxing or antiseizure action than BNZs. Table 11.2 lists the names, adult dosages, and nursing implications for the most common BNZs and BNZ agonists prescribed to induce sleep. Table 11.2 also lists the BNZs most commonly used to reduce anxiety. Check with a drug

## Table 11.1 Examples of Neurotransmitters and Their Functions in Mental Health

| NEUROTRANSMITTER | FUNCTIONS | POSSIBLE CHANGES IN MENTAL HEALTH AND ILLNESS |
|---|---|---|
| norepinephrine | Sympathetic nervous system (fight-or-flight response) Alertness and arousal | Decreased in depression |
| Serotonin | Sleep, appetite, pain, mood | Decreased in depression |
| Dopamine | Learning, movement, motivation and drive, attention, pleasure and reward | Increased in schizophrenia |
| gamma-aminobutyric acid (GABA) | Inhibitory neurotransmitter Sleep, muscle tension, sedation | Decreased in anxiety and mood disorders Decreased in schizophrenia Decreased in autism spectrum disorders |
| Acetylcholine | Parasympathetic nervous system (rest or repose) | Decreased in Alzheimer's disease |
| Histamine | Sleep–wake cycle, memory, learning, pain, reward | Increased during stress |

## Table 11.2  Examples of Common Drugs for Sleep and Anxiety

*Benzodiazepines* induce and prolong sleep or reduce anxiety by binding to BNZ receptors to enhance the inhibitory effects of GABA and make the CNS less responsive to stimuli.

*Benzodiazepine agonists*, which have a chemical structure different from BNZs, act as agonists at the BNZ receptors to induce and prolong sleep or reduce anxiety by enhancing the inhibitory effects of GABA and making the CNS less responsive to stimuli. Newer drugs reduce anxiety through a variety of actions that affect the serotonin and dopamine neurotransmitters.

| DRUG/ADULT DOSAGE | NURSING IMPLICATIONS |
|---|---|
| **Drugs for Sleep** | |
| **Benzodiazepines**<br>estazolam 0.5–2 mg orally at bedtime<br>flurazepam 15–30 mg orally at bedtime<br>temazepam (Restoril) 7.5–15 mg orally at bedtime; maximum dose 30 mg<br>lorazepam (Ativan) 2–4 mg orally at bedtime | • Teach patients not to take sedatives with alcohol or any other CNS depressant to avoid severe CNS depression, coma, or death.<br>• Ask women if they are pregnant, because these drugs have a high risk of causing birth defects.<br>• Tell patients not to drive, operate dangerous equipment, or make serious decisions while under the influence of these drugs, because impaired judgment and memory are possible.<br>• Tell patients to take the drug only if they have sufficient sleep time available to prevent confusion and other effects while awake. |
| **Benzodiazepine Agonists**<br>eszopiclone (Lunesta) 1–3 mg orally at bedtime<br>zaleplon (Sonata) 5–20 mg orally at bedtime<br>zolpidem (Ambien; Edluar) 5–10 mg orally at bedtime; also available in sublingual form, 5–10 mg at bedtime | • Teach patients that these drugs should be taken immediately before going to bed and with at least 7–8 hours of planned time to sleep.<br>• Suggest that patients have a family member or close friend with them when they first start taking the drug because incidences of sleep-walking, sleep-eating, and sleep-driving have occurred.<br>• Tell patients not to drive, operate dangerous equipment, or make serious decisions while under the influence of these drugs because impaired judgment and memory are possible.<br>• Teach patients that eszopiclone may cause a metallic taste in the mouth.<br>• Teach patients not to take sedatives with alcohol or any other CNS depressant to avoid severe CNS depression, coma, or death.<br>• Tell patients to take the drug only if they have sufficient sleep time available to prevent confusion and other effects while awake.<br>• Report agitation to the healthcare provider because this may be a side effect of eszopiclone.<br>• Monitor the patient's level of consciousness carefully because higher doses can lead to greater risk of daytime memory impairment and decreased alertness. |
| **Drugs for Anxiety** | |
| **Benzodiazepines**<br>alprazolam (Xanax) 0.25–0.5 mg orally two to three times per day; maximum of 4 mg/day in divided doses; often used PRN<br>alprazolam extended release (Xanax XR) 0.5–10 mg orally once daily, preferably in the morning<br>diazepam (Valium) 2–10 mg orally two to four times per day<br>diazepam IM (Valium): 2–5 mg for moderate anxiety; for severe anxiety, 5–10 mg, may repeat in 3–4 hours if necessary<br>lorazepam (Ativan) initially 1–3 mg/day orally given in two or three divided doses; usual dose 2–6 mg daily in divided doses; maximum dose 10 mg/day<br>**Benzodiazepine Agonists**<br>buspirone (BuSpar) usual dose is 15–30 mg/day given in 2–3 divided doses; maximum dose is 60 mg/day | • These drugs may cause drowsiness; advise patients to avoid driving, operating heavy machinery, or making any important decisions while taking these drugs.<br>• Provide patients with a call light and remind them to ask for help if getting out of bed, because these drugs can cause dizziness and drowsiness.<br>• Patients who are taking these drugs should be assessed using your agency's fall-risk protocols because these drugs increase the risk of falls.<br>• These drugs are intended for short-term use because they can cause physical dependence. Notify the healthcare provider if you have a patient admitted to your facility who has been using these drugs for more than 2–4 weeks.<br>• Teach patients who have been taking BNZs for more than 2–3 weeks not to stop them suddenly to avoid physical withdrawal symptoms. If they need to discontinue, they may require gradual and individualized tapering.<br>• BNZs should not be used in older adults because they increase the risk of falls and mortality rates.<br>• Assess your patients for a history of alcohol or other substance use disorder because they are at increased risk for BNZ dependence.<br>• Teach patients to avoid using nicotine products (e.g., cigarettes, chewing tobacco) or drinking caffeinated beverages (e.g., coffee, tea, cola) because they can decrease the effect of anxiolytic drugs. Teach patients to avoid driving or operating machinery until they are certain that buspirone does not cause them to feel sleepy or dizzy.<br>• Tell patients that the drug may be taken with or without food but should be taken the same way each time to avoid inconsistency in the dosage.<br>• Remind patients to avoid eating grapefruit or drinking grapefruit juice while taking buspirone because it can increase the effect of the drug. Buspirone typically takes about 1–2 weeks for the patient to experience a decrease in symptoms. |

*BNZ*, benzodiazepine; *GABA*, gamma-aminobutyric acid.

reference guide or a pharmacist for information about other sedative-hypnotic drugs.

## Expected Side Effects and Adverse Reactions

Both classes of sedatives can cause mild daytime drowsiness and some memory loss. Both are metabolized by the liver and should not be used by anyone who has a liver disorder or impairment. The BNZs have a higher risk of addiction and dependency than do BNZ agonists. They also carry a black box warning for CNS depression. Overdoses are possible and serious. These drugs have a high risk of birth defects.

BNZ agonists might induce physical activity during sleep for some people. These activities have included sleep-walking, sleep-eating, and even sleep-driving— all without the person's awareness or remembrance of the action!

### Lifespan Considerations

**Pregnancy**

Pregnancy is an absolute contraindication to BNZs because these drugs have a high risk of birth defects. Although the chemical structure of BNZ agonists is different, they bind to the same receptors as BNZs and have similar actions. As a result, they are not recommended during pregnancy.

## Drug Interactions

Caffeine reduces the effectiveness of sedative drugs from both classes. The BNZs interact with any drug that causes CNS depression such as alcohol, anticonvulsants, sedating antidepressants, opioids and many others. Grapefruit juice may increase drug concentrations. Always consult a drug reference or a pharmacist to avoid possible drug interactions.

### Top Tip for Safety

The drug flumazenil is a BNZ receptor antagonist and is used as an antidote to reverse an overdose of a BNZ sedative or a BNZ agonist sedative. It is given intravenously for rapid reversal of sedation.

### ❖ Nursing Implications and Patient Teaching

◆ *Assessment.* Ask the patient about all other drugs he or she takes, including over-the-counter (OTC) drugs, to determine whether there are other drugs that depress the CNS. Assess the patient's level of consciousness and ask whether he or she has a history of depression, confusion, falls, or pain. Ask about the patient's use of alcohol because these drugs should not be taken with any type of alcoholic beverage.

Ask women of child-bearing age whether they may be pregnant. These drugs should not be used during pregnancy.

◆ *Evaluation.* Usually, sedatives begin to take effect in 15 to 30 minutes. Check the patient (without waking him or her) at that time for drug effectiveness and for changes in respiratory rate and depth. If this is the patient's first time taking a sedative, recheck at least hourly for about 4 hours, and assess for any unusual reactions or activity.

◆ *Patient and family teaching.* Tell the patient and family:
- Take these drugs for no longer than 2 to 3 weeks and only when needed, to avoid physical or psychological dependency.
- Take a drug for sleep only if you have at least 5 to 6 hours immediately available to sleep to avoid excessive drowsiness when you are supposed to be awake.
- Do not drive, operate dangerous equipment, or make important decisions while under the influence of these drugs because they may alter your ability to reason clearly.
- Do not take a sedative with alcohol or any other drug that depresses the CNS to prevent severe side effects, coma, and death.
- To avoid dangerous interactions, do not take any other drug without the approval of your healthcare provider.
- When taking a BNZ agonist, be aware that drugs from this class can cause you to be physically active at night, even leaving the house and driving a car, without your knowledge or memory of the event. It is best to have a family member or friend watch for these effects when you first start taking the drug.
- Report any new or unusual side effects to your healthcare provider.
- Drinking excessive amounts of caffeinated beverages can reduce the effectiveness of the sedative.
- Buspirone does not lead to long-term dependence with long-term administration.
- Avoid drinking grapefruit juice if taking buspirone.

## ANTIANXIETY DRUGS

We can all identify with feelings of anxiety at certain times in our lives. We may describe it in terms of feelings of unease, worry, or apprehension. When we are anxious, we may experience physical and behavioral symptoms. Perhaps our heart rate increases, and we may have a mild headache or breathe a little more rapidly. In some cases, we may find ourselves being a little more irritable, pacing, or experiencing muscle tension. These are all symptoms of anxiety.

Anxiety is very common, particularly in times of increased stress. Anxiety can be mild, moderate, or severe, depending on the situation. A person who has chronic or disabling anxiety may be experiencing an anxiety disorder. Advanced practice nurses or healthcare providers may diagnose, for example, general anxiety disorder, social anxiety disorder, panic disorder, obsessive-compulsive disorder, or posttraumatic stress disorder. Although a detailed discussion of each of these disorders is beyond the scope of this textbook, many can be well managed with a combination of nonpharmacologic strategies (including counseling) and pharmacologic therapy.

Any drug that can reduce anxiety may be described as an **anxiolytic**. Major categories of antianxiety agents are BNZs, BNZ agonists, and certain antidepressants (i.e., selective serotonin reuptake inhibitors [SSRIs] and serotonin-norepinephrine reuptake inhibitors [SNRIs]). In general, the choice of drug varies according to the needs of the patient, including whether the anxiety is an acute or a chronic condition.

## Action and Uses

The BNZ and BNZ agonist classes of drugs for sedation (discussed earlier) can also be used as anxiolytics. These drugs act with GABA receptors to enhance GABA effects, which reduces anxiety and decreases muscle tension. BNZs are recommended primarily for short-term use, such as during a panic attack, during alcohol withdrawal, or before surgery. They generally should not be prescribed on a PRN basis because irregular use can increase anxiety due to variations in blood drug levels. Long-term use of BNZs can result in physical dependence and withdrawal symptoms if the drug is stopped suddenly.

A newer drug from the BNZ agonist class, buspirone, reduces anxiety through a variety of actions that affect the serotonin and dopamine neurotransmitters. Onset of the anxiolytic effect is slower than with the BNZs and may take 1 to 2 weeks. Maximal effects of buspirone may take up to 3 to 6 weeks. This drug can reduce anxiety without the risk of physical dependence and the sedation that is often associated with BNZ drugs.

Certain drugs that are often considered antidepressants, such as SSRIs and SNRIs, are commonly used to relieve symptoms of anxiety. These drugs are discussed in the next section.

## Expected Side Effects and Adverse Reactions

The expected side effects and adverse reactions of anxiolytics are very similar to those presented in the section on drugs used for sleep. BNZs and BNZ agonists may cause some drowsiness and memory loss when used for anxiety. Other side effects can include dizziness, headache, and hypotension. Adverse effects include confusion, apnea, and seizures. In addition, it is important to remember that BNZs have a higher risk of addiction and dependency than the BNZ agonists.

## Drug Interactions

Do not give BNZs to patients who are taking sodium oxybate (drug prescribed for narcolepsy, a sleep–wake disorder). This combination can result in serious respiratory depression, even coma. Avoid giving BNZs to patients who are taking opioids or any other drug that can result in CNS depression.

Do not give buspirone with monoamine oxidase inhibitors (MAOIs), opioids, or drugs for tuberculosis. Drinking grapefruit juice can significantly increase the blood levels of buspirone, which increases the risk of adverse reactions.

### ❖ Nursing Implications and Patient Teaching

◆ *Assessment.* Check the patient's vital signs, including blood pressure, heart rate, and respiratory rate, before giving the drug. Patients with a history of lung, liver, or kidney problems may be more sensitive to the effects of the drug.

Assess the mental status of the patient before giving the drug. Is he or she oriented to time, place, and person? If not, contact the healthcare provider before giving the drug.

Assess the patient for a history of alcohol or other chemical dependency because there is an increased risk of BNZ dependence. This is less likely with the BNZ agonists. Ask patients to describe their feelings of anxiety to determine effectiveness after you have given the drug.

> ### Lifespan Considerations
> #### Older Adults
> BNZs are not recommended to treat insomnia, agitation, or delirium in patients 65 years of age or older, and they are avoided in all patients with cognitive impairment, dementia, or a history of falls or fractures.

◆ *Planning and implementation.* Many BNZs have a rapid onset and short duration of action, requiring multiple doses per day. They can be used very effectively for patients with acute anxiety or panic attacks. Buspirone, a BNZ agonist, and other antidepressants used for anxiety have a much longer onset of action, and it may take several weeks for the patient to notice an effect.

Monitor the patient for side effects of drowsiness or dizziness because these can cause an increased risk of falls. Report changes in mental status, such as confusion or agitation, to the registered nurse (RN) or healthcare provider. If patients have respiratory depression after BNZ use, flumazenil, a BNZ receptor antagonist, can quickly reverse the effects.

For long-term mental health, nonpharmacologic therapies such as counseling, mindfulness training, yoga, or other interventions are essential. Provide the patient and family with information about local resources, including crisis lines, support groups, and Web sites (e.g., www.nami.org/Home).

◆ *Evaluation.* Ask the patient whether he or she has experienced any relief from anxiety. Explore how the drug affects the patient's ability to focus, make decisions, and function. If the patient is still having symptoms, contact the healthcare provider for the next steps. If the patient has been using BNZs for longer than 2 to 4 weeks, suddenly stopping the drug will result in severe withdrawal symptoms, including panic, vomiting, sweating, abdominal and muscle cramps, and seizures. The risk of seizures is greatest during the first 24 to 72 hours after starting to withdraw the drug. Slow tapering of the drug dosage can decrease the risk of withdrawal symptoms.

◆ *Patient and family teaching.* Tell the patient and family:
  • Take this drug exactly as prescribed. Withdrawal symptoms can occur if the drug has been used for longer than 2 to 4 weeks; in that case, contact your healthcare provider because you will need to taper the dosage.
  • Do not use this drug if you are pregnant or breastfeeding because the effects can be passed to the fetus or infant.
  • Avoid drinking grapefruit juice while taking these drugs because doing so could cause an increase in effect.
  • Avoid driving, operating hazardous machinery, or performing activities that require alertness until your response to the drug has been determined.
  • Change positions slowly to minimize dizziness that may occur.
  • Avoid drinking alcohol with these drugs to reduce the risk of severe sedation and respiratory depression.
  • Do not use nicotine products (e.g., cigarettes, chewing tobacco) or drink caffeinated beverages (e.g., coffee, tea, cola) because they can decrease the effect of anxiolytic drugs.

## ANTIDEPRESSANTS AND MOOD STABILIZERS

### ANTIDEPRESSANTS

Depression, whether mild or severe enough to interfere with activities of daily living (ADLs), has been recognized for centuries. Most people have days when they feel "down" or "blue." Sometimes, depressive symptoms are triggered by difficult situations such as the loss of a loved one or by experiencing a sudden illness, and they are normal responses to these life-changing events. However, intense and prolonged inability to interact with others, go to work, or keep up with ADLs and loss of interest in pleasurable activities represent more significant depression.

Box 11.1 lists common depressive symptoms, which can go on for weeks or months. Risk factors for depression include a family history of depression, substance abuse, history of abuse, certain drugs, or chronic illnesses. Fig. 11.2 shows some examples of people with depression.

---

| Box 11.1 | Symptoms of Depression |

  • Abrupt changes in eating habits
  • Chronic fatigue; feeling slowed down
  • Decreased ability to perform normal daily tasks
  • Decreased appetite and/or weight loss or overeating and weight gain
  • Difficulty concentrating, remembering, or making decisions
  • Feelings of hopelessness or pessimism
  • Inability to experience pleasure in hobbies and activities that were once enjoyed
  • Insomnia, early morning awakening, or oversleeping
  • Irritability
  • Numb or empty feeling, or absence of any feelings at all
  • Persistent feelings of worthlessness, guilt, helplessness, or sadness
  • Persistent physical symptoms that do not respond to treatment (e.g., headaches, digestive disorders, chronic pain)
  • Recurrent thoughts of death or suicide
  • Restlessness

From Workman, M., & LaCharity, L. (2016). *Understanding pharmacology: Essentials for medication safety* (2nd ed.). Saunders.

There are several categories of depression, including dysthymic disorder (mild to moderate form of depression that lasts up to 2 years), major depressive disorder, and bipolar disorder (including bipolar I and bipolar II). They are often referred to as mood disorders. Many types of therapy have been explored, but only in the past 50 years have drugs been discovered that significantly reduce depressive symptoms.

Most patients require several trials of different drugs or drug combinations to determine which is most effective to manage their symptoms. This can be a time-consuming process for patients because most antidepressants take several weeks to take effect. Good communication between the patient and the healthcare provider is important during the process of finding the right drug with the fewest side effects.

---

### Top Tip for Safety

**988 SUICIDE AND CRISIS LIFELINE**
All patients with a history of depression or at risk for depression and their loved ones should be aware of the new three-digit dialing code (988) that will route callers to the National Suicide Prevention Lifeline. This is available to everyone in the United States.

---

MAOIs were the first drugs successfully used to treat depression. The tricyclic antidepressants (TCAs) became available in the 1960s. SSRIs were introduced in the 1970s, followed by SNRIs. One other category, described as atypical antidepressants, work slightly differently from the other antidepressants but do affect the neurotransmitters dopamine, norepinephrine, and/or serotonin to help reduce depression.

Screen all patients who are taking antidepressants for thoughts of suicide or self-harm (i.e., suicidal ideation). Observe your patients for any worsening of symptoms, suicidal thoughts, or unusual changes in behavior, particularly within the first few months of starting therapy or when dosage changes.

 **Bookmark This!**

The Centers for Disease Control and Prevention Web site contains extensive resources for healthcare professionals on suicide: https://www.cdc.gov/violenceprevention/suicide/index.html. You can find risk factors, prevention strategies, and links to other helpful Web sites. This is a great resource for all nurses.

Antidepressants should not be stopped suddenly, because this may cause withdrawal symptoms or a relapse of depressive symptoms. These drugs should be tapered or discontinued under the direction of the healthcare provider.

## SELECTIVE SEROTONIN REUPTAKE INHIBITORS
### Action and Uses

A **selective serotonin reuptake inhibitor (SSRI)** blocks reabsorption of the neurotransmitter serotonin, increasing the concentration of serotonin that is available for binding postsynaptic receptors to improve a patient's sense of well-being and reduce depression (Fig. 11.3). These drugs are similar to TCAs but are prescribed more frequently because they are much safer and better tolerated. They can be used in a variety of conditions, including depression, premenstrual dysphoric disorder, posttraumatic stress disorder, obsessive-compulsive disorder, and general anxiety disorder. Table 11.3 lists the names, adult dosages, and nursing implications of the most common SSRIs. Check a drug reference or with a pharmacist for information about other drugs in this category.

 **Memory Jogger**

The main categories of antidepressants are:
- Selective serotonin reuptake inhibitors (SSRIs)
- Serotonin-norepinephrine reuptake inhibitors (SNRIs)
- Tricyclic antidepressants (TCAs)
- Monoamine oxidase inhibitors (MAOIs)
- Atypical antidepressants

### Expected Side Effects and Adverse Reactions

Expected side effects of SSRIs include nausea (especially during the first 2 weeks), drowsiness, insomnia, dry mouth, decreased appetite, increased sweating, and constipation. Sexual side effects are common in men and women. They range from decreased sex drive to decreased ability to orgasm and erectile dysfunction.

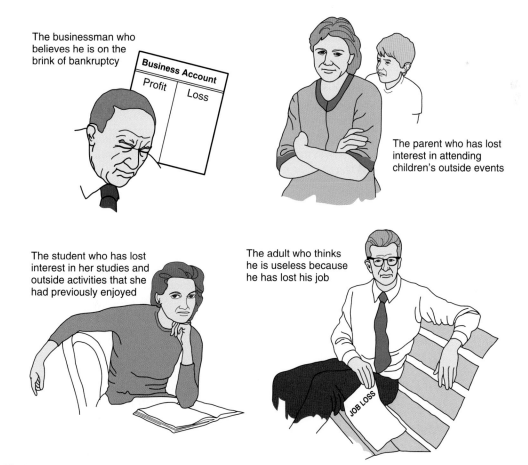

Fig. 11.2 Examples of depression. (From Workman, M. L., & LaCharity, L. (2017). *Understanding pharmacology: Essentials for medication safety* (2nd ed.). Elsevier.)

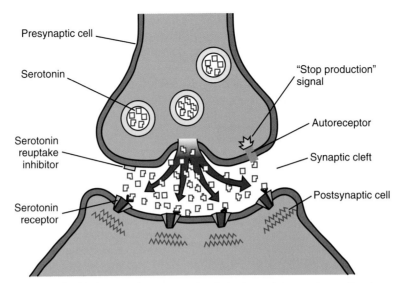

Fig. 11.3 Serotonin synthesized in the central nervous system helps to regulate mood, appetite, sleep, and other functions. The neurotransmitter is stored in granules in the presynaptic cell. An electrical impulse is transmitted when the chemical is secreted from the presynaptic nerve ending, diffuses across the synaptic cleft, and reversibly binds to postsynaptic serotonin receptors. Normally, the neurotransmitter is recycled (reabsorbed). When autoreceptors on the presynaptic membrane become bound by serotonin molecules in the synapse, they signal the cell to reduce its firing rate and therefore the release of the neurotransmitter (stop production). For depression resulting from low levels of serotonin, selective serotonin reuptake inhibitors can increase the amount of available serotonin by limiting its reabsorption (reuptake) into the presynaptic cell. (From Workman, M. L., & LaCharity, L. (2017). *Understanding pharmacology: Essentials for medication safety* (2nd ed.). Elsevier.)

### Table 11.3  Examples of Antidepressant Drugs

*Atypical antidepressants* work slightly differently from other antidepressants but do affect the neurotransmitters dopamine, norepinephrine, and/or serotonin.

*Selective serotonin reuptake inhibitors* prevent reabsorption of serotonin, increasing the amount of serotonin that is available for binding to postsynaptic receptors.

*Serotonin-norepinephrine reuptake inhibitors* prevent reabsorption of serotonin and norepinephrine, increasing the amount of both neurotransmitters available for binding to postsynaptic receptors.

*Tricyclic antidepressants* block the reuptake of norepinephrine and serotonin, which increases the availability of these neurotransmitters for activation of the postsynaptic receptors.

*Monoamine oxidase inhibitors* block the enzyme monoamine oxidase, which is responsible for breaking down neurotransmitters such as dopamine, norepinephrine, and serotonin in the brain. Blocking the MAO enzyme increases the concentrations of these neurotransmitters and results in reduction of depression and anxiety.

| DRUG/ADULT DOSAGE | NURSING IMPLICATIONS |
|---|---|
| **Atypical Antidepressants** | |
| bupropion 100–150 mg orally two to three times daily<br>bupropion sustained-release form (Wellbutrin SR) 150–200 mg one to two times daily<br>bupropion extended-release form (Wellbutrin XL) 150 mg orally one to two times daily; may gradually increase to 450 mg/day | • Work with the RN or other healthcare provider to screen all patients who are taking antidepressants for thoughts of suicide because they are at increased risk, particularly when starting to take antidepressants.<br>• Onset of antidepressant effect may take 1 to 3 weeks, with maximum effect up to 4 weeks.<br>• Notify the healthcare provider if you assess that the patient has a history of an eating disorder because it may increase the risk of seizures.<br>• Do not discontinue these drugs suddenly because the patient may experience withdrawal symptoms.<br>• Report any signs of agitation, irritability, or unusual behaviors to the RN or other healthcare provider because these drugs can trigger mania in some patients.<br>• These drugs may be used in some cases to help patients to stop smoking.<br>• Give the doses with food to decrease GI side effects.<br>• Give the drugs in the morning to decrease the risk of insomnia. Do not give at bedtime. |

| Table **11.3** | Examples of Antidepressant Drugs—cont'd |
|---|---|

### Selective Serotonin Reuptake Inhibitors

| | |
|---|---|
| escitalopram (Lexapro) start with 10 mg orally once daily; may be increased to a maximum of 20 mg/day<br>fluoxetine (Prozac, Sarafem) start with 10–20 mg/day orally; may be increased to a maximum of 80 mg/day<br>fluoxetine delayed-release form (Prozac Weekly) 90 mg once weekly<br>paroxetine (Paxil) 10–20 mg orally, usually in the morning; can be increased to a maximum of 50 mg/day<br>paroxetine controlled-release form (Paxil CR) 12.5–75 mg daily<br>sertraline (Zoloft) 25–50 mg orally once daily; maximum of 200 mg/day | • Work with the RN or other healthcare provider to screen all patients who are taking antidepressants for thoughts of suicide because they are at increased risk, particularly when starting to take antidepressants.<br>• Do not discontinue these drugs suddenly because the patient may experience withdrawal symptoms.<br>• Report any signs of agitation, irritability, or unusual behaviors to the RN or other healthcare provider because these drugs can trigger mania in some patients.<br>• Teach patients to contact their healthcare provider before beginning any over-the-counter or herbal drugs to avoid any harmful adverse effects, including serotonin syndrome.<br>• Remind patients that it may take several weeks for the drug to take effect, and they may not experience full benefit until 4–8 weeks after starting therapy.<br>• Until the drugs become effective, provide patients with resources to treat their depression by referral to community agencies, including the local crisis line or healthcare providers with expertise in the treatment of depression.<br>• Teach patients that they may experience sexual side effects while taking these drugs and to contact their healthcare provider to discuss alternative drugs that may be helpful.<br>• Monitor for signs of dizziness or changes in gait that may lead to falls. |

### Serotonin-Norepinephrine Reuptake Inhibitors

| | |
|---|---|
| venlafaxine (Effexor)<br>venlafaxine immediate-release form: 75 mg/day orally given in 2–3 divided doses; may be increased to 375 mg/day given in 3 divided doses<br>venlafaxine extended-release form (Effexor XR): 37.5–75 mg orally once daily; maximum 225 mg daily<br>duloxetine (Cymbalta) initially 20–60 mg by mouth daily in a single or divided doses; maximum 120 mg/day | • Work with the RN or other healthcare provider to screen all patients who are taking antidepressants for thoughts of suicide because they are at increased risk, particularly when starting to take antidepressants.<br>• Do not discontinue these drugs suddenly because the patient may experience withdrawal symptoms.<br>• Report any signs of agitation, irritability, or unusual behaviors to the RN or other healthcare provider because these drugs can trigger mania in some patients.<br>• Teach patients to contact their healthcare provider before beginning any over-the-counter or herbal drugs to avoid harmful adverse effects, including serotonin syndrome.<br>• Remind patients that it may take several weeks for the drug to take effect and they may not experience full benefit until 4–8 weeks after starting therapy.<br>• Until the drugs become effective, provide patients with resources to treat their depression by referral to community agencies, including the local crisis line or healthcare providers with expertise in the treatment of depression.<br>• Teach patients that they may experience sexual side effects while taking these drugs and to contact their healthcare provider to discuss alternative drugs that may be helpful. |

*Continued*

| Table 11.3 | Examples of Antidepressant Drugs—cont'd |
|---|---|
| **Tricyclic Antidepressants** | |
| amitriptyline (Elavil) usual dose between 50–150 mg/day orally at bedtime; hospitalized patients may need up to 300 mg/day; older adults may be prescribed lower doses with 10 mg orally three times a day and 20 mg orally at bedtime<br><br>imipramine (Tofranil) usual dose 30–150 mg in single or divided doses; maximum dose 200 mg/day for outpatients, 300 mg/day for hospitalized patients | • Watch for side and adverse effects, especially as the dosage is being increased.<br>• Remind patients that use of marijuana can cause serious cardiac problems if taken with TCAs.<br>• Teach patients that use of tobacco products can decrease the effectiveness of TCAs.<br>• TCAs should be avoided with MAOIs, SSRIs, and SNRIs because they can increase the risk of serotonin syndrome.<br>• Patients who are receiving TCAs for depression have often been through several trials of antidepressant agents without success. Make sure to assess the patient's history, current drugs, and mental status.<br>• Give doses at bedtime because most patients experience some drowsiness. This also helps prevent daytime sleepiness. In some cases, patients have difficulty sleeping after taking TCAs; if that is the case, the patient can take the drug in the morning.<br>• Teach patients to contact their healthcare provider if they have new or troublesome symptoms such as difficulty urinating, blurred vision, or shortness of breath because these can indicate adverse effects. |
| **Monoamine Oxidase Inhibitors** | |
| phenelzine (Nardil) usually starts with 15 mg orally three times daily; may increase to 60 mg/day; maximum dose 90 mg/day<br><br>isocarboxazid (Marplan) begins with 10 mg orally twice daily; may increase to 60 mg/day in 2 to 4 divided doses<br><br>selegiline (Eldepryl, Zelapar) 6–12 mg transdermal patch applied to the skin once daily | • These drugs are usually reserved for patients who have had multiple trials of other antidepressant agents without relief.<br>• Provide the patient with information regarding foods and beverages high in tyramine (see Box 11.3). They must be avoided because taking them with MAOIs can result in hypertensive crisis and even death.<br>• Remind the patient that it can take up to 2 to 6 weeks to feel the effects.<br>• Monitor vital signs carefully because this drug can cause hypertensive crisis if taken with certain foods, drinks, or drugs.<br>• To avoid serotonin syndrome, teach patients to wait at least 2 weeks after discontinuing an MAOI before taking any drugs with serotonin. |

*MAOI,* monoamine oxidase inhibitor; *SSRI,* selective serotonin reuptake inhibitor; *SNRI,* serotonin-norepinephrine reuptake inhibitor; *TCA,* tricyclic antidepressant.

Adverse effects include increased risk of suicide, particularly during the first few months of therapy. This risk is slightly higher among young adults and children. In most cases, the benefit of taking the SSRI to reduce symptoms of depression is greater than the risk of suicide. It is critically important for the healthcare provider to talk with the patient and his or her family about this risk to prevent this adverse effect.

Other adverse effects include bleeding, hyponatremia (low sodium level), and bone fracture, particularly in patients with osteoporosis. Skin reactions are rare but can be severe. These drugs can also cause changes in the electrical conduction system of the heart.

SSRIs should be avoided in pregnancy because the drugs affect the fetus. Infants can experience neonatal abstinence syndrome, a condition associated with physical symptoms of drug withdrawal.

Suddenly stopping an SSRI can cause a flulike syndrome. Tapering the drug dosage can decrease the risk for these symptoms.

### Drug Interactions

Any drug that affects serotonin can interact with SSRIs. These include a variety of other antidepressants such as MAOIs, SNRIs, and other SSRIs. Too much serotonin can lead to the adverse effect known as *serotonin syndrome* (Box 11.2). Serotonin syndrome is a life-threatening adverse effect, and it must be avoided. Use of the herbal drug St. John's wort (commonly used to treat mild to moderate depression) can significantly increase the risk of serotonin syndrome.

Other drugs that can potentially interact with SSRIs include those that affect clotting, such as anticoagulants, antiplatelet drugs, and nonsteroidal anti-inflammatory drugs (NSAIDs). Caution should be

| Box 11.2 | Signs and Symptoms of Serotonin Syndrome |
|---|---|

- Confusion
- Agitation
- Restlessness
- Stomach disturbances, diarrhea
- Sweating
- Extremely high blood pressure
- Seizures
- Dilated pupils
- Tremors

used in giving SSRIs to patients with certain cardiac dysrhythmias.

❖ **Nursing Implications and Patient Teaching**
◆ *Assessment.* A thorough assessment of mental health status is important for patients who are beginning treatment with antidepressants. RNs or other healthcare providers typically perform the assessment. Baseline measurements of depression are often collected using questionnaires.

Assessment of suicide risk is essential before beginning antidepressant drugs. If you are practicing in a psychiatric setting, you may be trained to use specific questions or tools to assess risk. Table 11.4 provides an example of a screening device for suicide assessment. One approach is to ask the patient whether he or she has any thoughts of suicide or of "hurting yourself." If so, immediately contact the RN or other healthcare team professional to further evaluate risk.

Ask the patient about current use of drugs, including herbal and OTC drugs. Knowledge of patients' drug use can help prevent serious complications of serotonin syndrome.

◆ *Planning and implementation.* After risk assessment, providing a safe environment for the patient is very important. Good communication and thorough monitoring can help you determine the effectiveness of therapy. Remind the patient that it may take several weeks for the drug to take effect. For treatment in the meantime, provide the patient with resources such as referral to community agencies or healthcare providers with expertise in treatment of depression. Provide the patient with the telephone numbers of local crisis lines. Teach patients that they may have thoughts of suicide early in therapy and that considering suicide or self-harm may be a side effect of the drug, not a logical action. Tell patients that if they do have such feelings, they should notify their healthcare provider or crisis line immediately.

Most SSRIs can be given without regard to meals. Giving the drugs in the morning helps decrease the risk of sleeping difficulties. Some patients may experience sedation while taking SSRIs; if this is the case, they can take the drug in the evening.

| Table 11.4 | Columbia-Suicide Severity Rating Scale (C-SSRS): Triage and Risk Identification |
|---|---|

Ask questions 1 and 2:
1. Have you wished you were dead or wished you could go to sleep and not wake up?
2. Have you actually had any thoughts about killing yourself?
If Yes to 2, ask questions 3, 4, 5, and 6. If No to 2, go directly to question 6.
3. Have you been thinking about how you might kill yourself?
4. Have you had these thoughts and had some intention of acting on them?
5. Have you started to work out or worked out the details of how to kill yourself? Do you intend to carry out this plan?
6. Have you ever done anything, started to do anything, or prepared to do anything to end your life? If Yes, ask: How long ago did you do any of these?
If the answer to question 1 or 2 on the scale is Yes, information related to the intensity of ideation is collected. Intensity is determined based on questions identifying suicidal ideation on a scale of 1 to 5 (1 is least severe, and 5 is most severe) for the past month and over the lifetime of the individual. Other follow-up question topics related to suicidal thinking include frequency, duration, controllability, deterrents, reasons for wanting to die, and a description of suicide attempts.

(From Halter, M. J. (2013). *Varcarolis' foundations of psychiatric mental health nursing: A clinical approach* (7th ed.). Saunders.)

Teach patients that it may take several attempts to get the best drug for their depression. Close work with healthcare providers helps the patient move toward best symptom relief.

◆ *Evaluation.* Patients typically begin to experience relief from symptoms within a few weeks of starting drug therapy. Maximum benefit may not occur until after the patient has taken the drug for 4 to 8 weeks. Compare symptoms with baseline measurements. Ask patients to describe any side effects they may be having. Ask whether they have had thoughts of suicide or of self-harm. If so, report this immediately to the RN or the healthcare provider.

◆ *Patient and family teaching.* Tell the patient and family:
- Take the drugs exactly as ordered by your healthcare provider. It may take several weeks before you feel better.
- Some patients experience sexual side effects. Before you decide if you want to stop taking the drugs, contact your healthcare provider to discuss any alternative drugs that may be helpful.
- Take these drugs in the morning because many can cause insomnia.
- Symptoms such as nausea, loss of appetite, and headache typically go away after several weeks of

treatment. Contact your healthcare provider if you have any questions.

- Do not take any herbal or OTC drugs without talking to your healthcare provider. Herbal drugs, particularly St. John's wort, can cause a dangerous adverse effect if taken with SSRIs.
- Talk to your healthcare provider if you are pregnant or are considering becoming pregnant because these drugs can affect the fetus.
- Some patients have increased thoughts of suicide or of hurting themselves when they first start taking these drugs. These may be side effects of the drug. If you have these feelings, contact your healthcare provider or call your local crisis line immediately.

 **Top Tip for Safety**

**SELECTIVE SEROTONIN REUPTAKE INHIBITORS**
SSRIs can cause thoughts of suicide, most likely in children and young adults. Remind patients and their families that this may be a side effect of the drug and should be reported to healthcare providers immediately.

 **Lifespan Considerations**

**Older Adults**

SSRIs can cause falls or fractures in older adults. Monitor for signs of dizziness or changes in gait that may lead to falls.

## SEROTONIN-NOREPINEPHRINE REUPTAKE INHIBITORS

### Action and Uses

A **serotonin-norepinephrine reuptake inhibitor (SNRI)** prevents reabsorption of serotonin and norepinephrine, increasing the concentration of both neurotransmitters available to postsynaptic receptors. These drugs are very similar to the SSRIs, and their response rates are also similar. They may be used to treat depression, hot flashes, premenstrual dysphoric disorder, fibromyalgia, and chronic pain. They can also be used for some patients with diabetic neuropathy. Table 11.3 lists the names, adult dosages, and nursing implications for the most common SNRIs. Check a drug reference or ask a pharmacist for information about other drugs in this category.

### Expected Side Effects and Adverse Reactions

Expected side effects of SNRIs include nausea, dry mouth, loss of appetite, fatigue, and drowsiness. Some patients experience a condition called *hyperhidrosis* (increased sweating).

Sexual side effects are more common in men than in women. These range from decreased sex drive to decreased ability to have an orgasm and erectile dysfunction. Some patients experience an elevation in blood pressure, particularly when starting an SNRI. Sudden discontinuation of an SNRI can cause withdrawal symptoms, and tapering is required.

Adverse effects include epistaxis (nosebleeds), GI bleeding, and liver damage. As with SSRIs, patients can experience hyponatremia, severe skin reactions, and an increased risk of suicide. SNRIs are avoided particularly late in pregnancy because the drugs affect the fetus. Infants can experience neonatal abstinence syndrome.

### Drug Interactions

Any drug that affects serotonin or norepinephrine can interact with SNRIs. This includes a variety of other antidepressants such as MAOIs, SSRIs, and other SNRIs. These combinations can increase the risk of serotonin syndrome or neuroleptic malignant syndrome.

The herbal drug St. John's wort (commonly used to treat mild to moderate depression) can significantly increase the risk of serotonin syndrome. Other drugs that can potentially interact with SNRIs include drugs that affect clotting, such as anticoagulants, antiplatelet drugs, and NSAIDs.

### ❖ Nursing Implications and Patient Teaching

◆ *Assessment.* A thorough assessment of mental health status is important for patients who are starting treatment with SNRIs. RNs or other healthcare providers typically conduct the formal assessment; however, you are a member of the team and can contribute your observations. Baseline measurements of depression are often collected using questionnaires.

Assessment of suicide risk is essential before beginning SNRIs. Ask the patient about current use of drugs, including herbal and OTC drugs. Knowledge of the patient's drug use can help prevent serious complications of serotonin syndrome.

◆ *Planning and implementation.* After risk assessment, providing a safe environment for the patient is very important. Good communication and thorough monitoring help you determine the effectiveness of therapy. Remind the patient that it may take several weeks for the SNRI to take effect. Provide the patient with resources to treat his or her depression in the meantime by referral to community agencies or healthcare providers with expertise in the treatment of depression. Provide the patient with the telephone numbers of local crisis lines.

Teach patients that it may take several trials of different drugs to find the best drug for their depression. Working closely with healthcare providers helps the patient move toward the best relief of symptoms.

◆ *Evaluation.* Patients typically begin to experience relief from symptoms within a few weeks after starting therapy. Maximum benefit may not occur until after the patient has taken the drug for 4 to 8 weeks. Ask patients whether they have had any thoughts of suicide or of "hurting yourself." If they have, report this immediately to the RN or the healthcare provider.

◆ *Patient and family teaching.* Tell the patient and family:
- Take the drugs exactly as ordered by your healthcare provider. It may take several weeks for you to feel better.
- Some patients experience sexual side effects. Before you decide if you want to stop taking the drugs, contact your healthcare provider to discuss alternative drugs that may be helpful.
- Take these drugs in the morning because many can cause insomnia.
- Symptoms such as nausea, loss of appetite, and headache typically go away after several weeks of treatment. Contact your healthcare provider if you have any questions.
- Do not take any herbal or OTC drugs without talking to your healthcare provider. Herbal drugs, particularly St. John's wort, can cause a dangerous adverse effect if taken with SNRIs.
- Talk to your healthcare provider if you are pregnant or are considering becoming pregnant because these drugs can affect the fetus.
- Some patients have increased thoughts of suicide or of hurting themselves when they first start taking these drugs. These are side effects of the drug. If you have these thoughts, contact your healthcare provider or call your local crisis line immediately.

## TRICYCLIC ANTIDEPRESSANTS

### Action and Uses
Tricyclic antidepressants (TCAs) are an older class of drugs first used in the 1950s to reduce depression. The precise action is unknown, but they are thought to interfere with the reuptake of norepinephrine and serotonin.

TCAs work as well as the SSRIs or SNRIs for treating mild to moderate depression, but they have more side effects. As a result, these drugs are usually reserved for patients with severe depression or people who do not respond to other treatments. You may see TCAs used for patients with illnesses such as migraine headaches, panic disorder, obsessive-compulsive disorder, or peripheral neuropathy. Table 11.3 lists the names, adult dosages, and nursing implications for the most common TCAs. Check a drug reference or ask a pharmacist for information about other drugs in this category.

### Expected Side Effects and Adverse Reactions
Common side effects of TCAs include dry mouth, drowsiness, constipation, nausea, and orthostatic hypotension. Some patients experience weight gain resulting from increased appetite; others may experience weight loss. TCAs can cause mild to severe vision problems. If this happens, the patient should contact his or her healthcare provider.

Adverse reactions include cardiac dysrhythmias, heart failure, and seizures. TCAs can trigger a manic episode in patients who have an underlying bipolar disorder. They can also cause delirium in older patients with cognitive impairment (decreased memory, language, or thinking ability). Like other antidepressants, TCAs can increase the risk for suicide in younger patients. TCAs should not be used in patients with glaucoma because these drugs can increase intraocular pressure.

### Drug Interactions
Avoid giving TCAs with drugs that depress the CNS, such as opioids, sedatives, or alcohol. These drugs can increase the risk for respiratory depression, sedation, and severe hypotension. TCAs can also interact with a wide variety of antidysrhythmic drugs, causing serious cardiac problems.

TCAs should be avoided with MAOIs, SSRIs, and SNRIs because of the risk of serotonin syndrome (see Box 11.2). Any drug that increases serotonin (including the herbal drug St. John's wort) can be dangerous in patients who are taking TCAs. Marijuana can cause serious cardiac problems if taken with TCAs. Use of tobacco products can decrease the effectiveness of TCAs.

### ❖ Nursing Implications and Patient Teaching
◆ *Assessment.* Patients who are taking TCAs for depression often have been through several trials of antidepressant agents without success. Assess the patient's history, current drug use, and mental status. A thorough history helps the healthcare provider make the best decisions for timing and dosages of the drugs. Assessment of suicide risk is essential before beginning or changing any antidepressant drugs.

Assess vital signs, including baseline weight. TCAs can cause hypotension and weight gain. Report any history of drug abuse to the provider.

◆ *Planning and implementation.* Reassess the patient's symptoms to determine his or her response to the drugs. Remind patients that the effects may not be felt for several weeks. Refer patients with a history of smoking to smoking-cessation resources in your community.

Teach patients about common drug side effects, including dry mouth, constipation, and orthostatic hypotension. Some patients may experience an increase in blood pressure. If this occurs, report it to the healthcare provider.

◆ *Evaluation.* Evaluate your patient's response to the antidepressant because symptom relief may take several weeks. Always assess the patient for suicidal ideation. Refer patients who have thoughts of suicide immediately to the healthcare provider or your local crisis line.

Patients who have taken TCAs for a long period need to taper them if they are going to be changing drugs. Tapering helps reduce the risk of withdrawal symptoms, including headache, nausea, or diarrhea.

◆ *Patient and family teaching.* Tell the patient and family:

- Do not stop taking your drug suddenly because it can cause you to have symptoms such as nausea, vomiting, or diarrhea. Your healthcare provider can help you taper the drug if you need to do so.
- Avoid alcohol, sedatives, opioid pain drugs, or any drugs that can cause drowsiness while you are taking TCAs.
- TCAs often cause dry mouth. Sugarless gum or candy, ice chips, or sips of water can help relieve this problem.
- You may be more sensitive to sunburn while taking these drugs and for several weeks after completing drug therapy. Use good skin protection, including sunscreen and protective clothing.
- TCAs can cause dizziness or lightheadedness with changes in position. Move slowly when you change from lying or sitting to a standing position.
- Most patients have some drowsiness, and you may want to take the drug at bedtime. That will help prevent daytime sleepiness. Some patients have difficulty sleeping after taking TCAs. If that is your experience, you can take the drug in the morning.
- Contact your healthcare provider if you have any new or troublesome symptoms, such as difficulty urinating, blurred vision, or shortness of breath, because these can indicate adverse effects.
- Wear a medical alert bracelet or necklace or carry a wallet medical identification card listing this drug to inform healthcare providers that you are taking it.

## MONOAMINE OXIDASE INHIBITORS

### Action and Uses

Monoamine oxidases (MAOs) are a family of enzymes located in cells throughout the body. The enzymes break down neurotransmitters, including dopamine, norepinephrine, and serotonin. A monoamine oxidase inhibitor (MAOI) blocks this enzyme, increasing the available neurotransmitters and reducing depressive symptoms.

---

⬆ **Top Tip for Safety**

MAOIs may cause hypertensive crisis if the patient ingests foods or drinks that contain tyramine. Examples of these foods include aged cheese, overripe fruit, cured or smoked meat, beer, and wine.

---

MAOIs are typically used to treat severe depression that is not controlled with other categories of antidepressants. This is because of the serious interactions that can occur with certain drugs, foods, and beverages, which can make taking MAOIs very challenging

---

**Box 11.3  High-Tyramine Foods to Avoid When Taking Monoamine Oxidase Inhibitors**

- Alcoholic beverages
  - Beer and ale
  - Wine
  - Alcohol-free beer
- Dairy products
  - Mature cheeses (e.g., cheddar, bleu cheese, mozzarella)
  - Sour cream
  - Yogurt
- Fruits and vegetables
  - Avocados
  - Bananas
  - Fava beans
  - Canned figs
  - Sauerkraut
- Meats
  - Bologna
  - Liver
  - Dried fish
  - Meat tenderizer
  - Pickled herring
  - Sausages
  - Salami
- Other foods
  - Caffeinated drinks (e.g., coffee, cola, tea)
  - Chocolate
  - Licorice

Adapted from Keltner, N., & Steele, D. (2015). *Psychiatric nursing* (7th ed.). Mosby.

and risky. Box 11.3 lists high-tyramine foods and drinks.

MAOIs can be used for cases of certain anxiety disorders that are not responsive to other drugs. Several can be used in the treatment of Parkinson's disease. Table 11.3 lists the names, adult dosages, and nursing implications for the most common MAOIs. Check a drug reference or consult a pharmacist for information about other drugs in this category.

### Expected Side Effects and Adverse Reactions

Side effects that can occur while taking MAOIs include constipation, headache, dizziness, drowsiness, and dry mouth. Some patients experience orthostatic hypotension. Weight gain occurs in more than 10% of patients, and it may be related to increased appetite and/or increased peripheral edema.

Adverse effects include the possibility of liver damage, a variety of blood disorders, and thoughts of suicide. Some patients who are receiving MAOI therapy may experience severe hyponatremia (severe loss of sodium).

### Drug Interactions

The combination of MAOIs and certain drugs or foods can result in severe high blood pressure, even hypertensive crisis (extremely high blood pressure that can lead to stroke, heart failure, renal failure, and death). Drugs that can cause this dangerous interaction include SSRIs, SNRIs, St. John's wort, and any drug that has stimulant qualities (e.g., beta-agonists, epinephrine, venlafaxine).

Drugs that decrease blood pressure can increase the hypotensive side effects. Use of MAOIs with drugs that depress the CNS, such as opioids, alcohol, and BNZs, can cause sedation, respiratory depression, and coma. Patients who are taking insulin or oral hypoglycemic drugs may be at risk for hypoglycemic reactions.

---

### 🔆 Top Tip for Safety

Do not give MAOIs and SSRIs within 2 weeks of each other. Combining these drugs can cause serotonin syndrome, a life-threatening adverse effect related to too much serotonin.

---

Most problematic for patients who are taking MAOIs is the risk of hypertensive crisis from ingesting foods or drinks high in tyramine. Tyramine is an amino acid that is involved in the release of norepinephrine. Tyramine is normally broken down by the enzyme MAO. When the patient is taking an MAOI, there can be an increase in norepinephrine that can lead to a significant increase in blood pressure and an increased risk of stroke. In addition, patients should avoid caffeine-containing products that can cause increased blood pressure and irregular heart rhythms. These substances should be avoided for up to 2 weeks after the patient stops taking the MAOI.

### ❖ Nursing Implications and Patient Teaching

◆ *Assessment.* Obtain a thorough drug history, including the patient's history of drugs used for depression or other mental health issues. This is very important because MAOIs are usually prescribed after other drug therapies have failed. Determine whether the patient has used any herbal drugs, including St. John's wort. This important information allows the healthcare provider to determine appropriate drugs and doses.

Obtain a diet history to assess food and drink preferences. Use of MAOIs requires restricting certain types of food and beverage. Detailed diet histories may need to be determined by your agency's RN or registered dietitian.

Assess baseline vital signs, weight, and laboratory values. These are important in assessing the patient's response to the drug. Determine whether the patient has any suicidal thoughts (see Table 11.4).

◆ *Planning and implementation.* MAOIs are typically used in patients who have not responded to the other, more commonly prescribed antidepressants. Remind patients that it may take 3 to 4 weeks to feel relief from depressive symptoms.

Patient teaching is vital for getting the best results from the drug and preventing adverse effects,

particularly hypertensive crisis related to eating foods high in tyramine. Beyond avoiding foods with tyramine, patients are at risk for weight gain while taking MAOIs. Refer patients to your agency dietician for follow-up.

Tell patients to use good oral hygiene while taking MAOIs because they can cause dry mouth. Sugar-free gums or candies or sips of water can also help to relieve symptoms.

Monitor vital signs and blood sugar levels carefully. Patients can experience hypotension while taking MAOIs. Diabetic patients who take insulin or other antidiabetic drugs are at increased risk for hypoglycemia.

◆ *Evaluation.* Ask patients about symptoms of depression. Have the symptoms decreased? Determine whether the patient has had any suicidal thoughts. If so, report it immediately to the RN or to the healthcare provider.

MAOIs continue to work on the body as long as 2 weeks after the drug is discontinued. Patients who have been taking these drugs should avoid all drugs, foods, and drinks that can increase serotonin or tyramine levels.

◆ *Patient and family teaching.* Tell the patient and family:
- Take the drug as prescribed. It may take several weeks for you to feel the benefit.
- Do not drink alcohol or use any sedating drugs while taking these drugs. They can cause severe sedation or a drop in blood pressure.
- Avoid coffee, colas, teas, and other drinks that have caffeine. These can cause a dangerous increase in your blood pressure.
- Do not take any herbal or OTC drugs while taking MAOIs without checking with your healthcare provider to avoid dangerous interactions.
- Remember that the effect of MAOIs can linger for up to 2 weeks after you stop taking the drug. Do not start eating foods or drinking beverages that contain tyramine or caffeine. Do not take any new herbal or OTC drugs without talking to your healthcare provider.
- Change positions slowly because these drugs can lower your blood pressure.
- These drugs can cause dizziness or drowsiness. Avoid driving, operating heavy machinery, or making important decisions. This feeling should improve with time.
- Notify your healthcare provider or call 911 if you experience a sudden fever, severe headache, nausea, vomiting, or chest pain or have a rapid heartbeat, because these can be signs of severe adverse effects.
- Use a medical alert bracelet or keep a drug list to alert healthcare providers that you are taking this drug.

**Box 11.4** **Symptoms of Mania**

- Abnormal or excessive elation
- Decreased need for sleep
- Grandiose notions
- Inappropriate social behavior
- Increased sexual desire
- Increased talking
- Markedly increased energy
- Poor judgment
- Racing thoughts
- Unusual irritability

From Workman, M., & LaCharity, L. (2016). *Understanding pharmacology: Essentials for medication safety* (2nd ed.). Saunders.

## MOOD STABILIZERS

Bipolar illness is characterized by extreme changes in mood that can lead to an inability to work, difficulty in maintaining social relationships, and inability to accomplish basic ADLs. A challenging aspect of this illness is that many times patients may function very well early in the manic stage.

Bipolar disease was once called *manic-depressive illness*. Patients can exhibit symptoms of mania such as rapid speech, flight of ideas, excessive activity, staying awake for hours, and having feelings of elation or superiority. They may spend money recklessly, engage in sex with multiple partners, or engage in other high-risk behaviors. Box 11.4 lists common symptoms of mania. Patients can also become extremely depressed, lose interest in events, feel sad or down, have feelings of hopelessness, and consider suicide.

**Mood stabilizers** are used primarily to treat patients with bipolar illness. They help manage or reduce the symptoms associated with mania and improve the symptoms of depression. The main drugs are lithium and a variety of anticonvulsant drugs used to treat epilepsy (e.g., lamotrigine, carbamazepine). Chapter 10 provides detailed information about anticonvulsant drugs.

Treatments are usually long term because the illness does not have a cure. Patients may have difficulty adhering long term to the therapies because of side effects and because of the loss of some of the "highs" associated with the manic phase.

### Action and Uses

Lithium is primarily used to treat patients with bipolar illness, including acute mania and during long-term maintenance therapy. Although the exact mechanism of action in stabilizing mood is not known, it is thought that the drug inhibits the synthesis, storage, release, and reuptake of monoamine neurotransmitters. An advantage of lithium is that it does not cause sedation, depression, or euphoria (intense excitement or exhilaration). The onset of action to treat mania is usually about 1 week, but it may take 2 to 3 weeks for the patient to experience the full benefit.

Lithium has a very narrow therapeutic range, which means that the dosage that improves symptoms is close to the dosage that can cause toxic effects. It is important to regularly monitor the lithium blood levels. The first blood level of lithium is usually measured about 3 days into therapy. The healthcare provider then adjusts the patient's dosage accordingly. Regular serum lithium measurements are required to keep the patient safe. Table 11.5 lists examples of mood stabilizers (including lithium) with their adult dosages and nursing implications. Check a drug reference or consult a pharmacist for information about other mood stabilizers.

### Expected Side Effects and Adverse Reactions

Expected side effects for lithium are mild weight gain, increased thirst, increased urine output, and dry skin. Some patients have mild drowsiness after starting lithium. Hand tremors occur in almost 50% of patients but usually decrease with continued use of the drug. At first, patients may have some nausea, vomiting, or diarrhea after starting lithium therapy. This is important to assess, particularly because if it occurs later in therapy, nausea and vomiting can be signs of lithium toxicity.

It is important to recognize the signs and symptoms of drug toxicity because of the narrow therapeutic range of lithium. Severity of symptoms increases with the lithium level. Table 11.6 details the symptoms associated with lithium blood levels.

 **Top Tip for Safety**

Early signs of lithium toxicity include increased nausea, vomiting, drowsiness, muscle weakness, coarse hand tremor, and incoordination. Later signs include ataxia (loss of control of body movements) and tinnitus (ringing in the ears).

Fluid balance is very important in patients who are taking lithium because any condition that leads to a drop in sodium levels or dehydration can increase the risk of lithium toxicity. These conditions include reduced salt intake, intensive exercise, and very hot environments.

Adverse reactions include hypothyroidism, renal failure, and diabetes insipidus (severe imbalance of water in the body). Other adverse reactions include neuroleptic malignant syndrome and serotonin syndrome.

**Top Tip for Safety**

Lithium has a very narrow therapeutic range. Knowledge of the signs of lithium toxicity and careful monitoring of lithium levels are essential.

### Drug Interactions

Diuretics, NSAIDs, antidepressants, and antipsychotic drugs can interact with lithium. Any drugs that affect the electrical conduction of the heart also can cause dangerous interactions. Drugs that affect sodium

Table 11.5 **Mood Stabilizers**

*Mood stabilizers* are used primarily to treat patients with bipolar illness. They help to reduce the symptoms associated with mania and improve the symptoms of depression. Several drugs in this category are also used as antiseizure drugs.

| DRUG/ADULT DOSAGE | NURSING IMPLICATIONS |
|---|---|
| **Mood Stabilizers** | |
| lithium carbonate, initially 300 mg orally three times daily; maintenance: 300–600 mg orally two or three times a day<br><br>lithium carbonate controlled-release tablet (Eskalith CR) 900 mg twice daily; maintenance dose 450 mg orally twice daily (range 900–1200 mg daily in divided doses)<br><br>lithium carbonate extended-release tablet (Lithobid) 900 mg twice daily or 60 mg orally three times a day<br><br>carbamazepine (Tegretol, Equetro) initially 200 mg orally twice daily; gradually increased; usual dosage 600–1600 mg/day orally in divided doses<br><br>divalproex sodium delayed release (Depakote) 750 mg orally daily in divided doses; maximum 60 mg/kg/day | • Lithium has a narrow therapeutic range. Monitor carefully for side effects and adverse reactions. See Table 11.6 for common symptoms of toxicity.<br>• Teach the patient to avoid conditions that result in severe sweating or potential for dehydration because these can result in low sodium and increase the risk of lithium toxicity.<br>• Diuretics can increase the risk for lithium toxicity.<br>• Teach the patient to avoid reducing salt intake. Sodium is needed in the diet to prevent lithium toxicity.<br>• Patients will need to have regular serum lithium levels measured to help prevent lithium toxicity, usually beginning within 3 days after starting therapy (draw sample 12 hours after the last dose given). The lithium level should range between 0.8 and 1.2 mEq/L initially, then between 0.8 and 1 mEq/L. Lithium levels are typically measured every 2 months while the patient is taking maintenance doses.<br>• Risk factors for lithium toxicity include older age, kidney disease, low sodium levels, dehydration, heart disease, debilitated state, and taking certain drugs such as angiotensin-converting enzyme inhibitors, diuretics, or NSAIDs.<br>• You can mix lithium oral solutions with fruit juice or flavored drinks to improve the taste. Do not mix lithium oral solution with other drugs because they can form an insoluble salt.<br>• As with lithium, the carbamazepine serum blood level should be carefully monitored to avoid drug toxicity. The normal serum carbamazepine level is 8–12 mcg/mL.<br>• Maintenance levels for divalproex (as valproic acid) typically range from 50–100 mcg/mL. In acute mania, maintenance levels may be up to 125 mcg/mL. |

*GI,* gastrointestinal; *NSAIDs,* nonsteroidal anti-inflammatory drugs; *RN,* registered nurse.

Table 11.6 **Symptoms Associated with Elevated Lithium Levels**

| THERAPEUTIC SERUM LEVELS | MILD TO MODERATE TOXICITY | MODERATE TO SEVERE TOXICITY | SEVERE TOXICITY |
|---|---|---|---|
| (0.6–1.2 mEq/L) | (1.5–2 mEq/L) | (2–3 mEq/L) | (>3 mEq/L) |
| Hand tremor (fine) | Diarrhea | Symptoms of lower drug levels *and* | Symptoms of lower drug levels *and* |
| Memory problems | Vomiting | Ataxia | Seizures |
| Goiter | Drowsiness | Giddiness | Organ failure |
| Hypothyroidism | Dizziness | Tinnitus | Renal failure |
| Mild diarrhea | Hand tremor (coarse) | Blurred vision | Coma |
| Anorexia | Muscular weakness | Large output of diluted urine | Death |
| Nausea | Lack of coordination | Delirium | |
| Edema | Dry mouth | Nystagmus | |
| Weight gain | | | |
| Polydipsia, polyuria | | | |

From Keltner, N., & Steele, D. (2015). *Psychiatric nursing* (7th ed.). Mosby, p. 177.

intake or fluid balance can increase the risk of lithium toxicity.

❖ **Nursing Implications and Patient Teaching**

◆ *Assessment.* Laboratory work is usually required to determine whether the patient is a candidate for lithium therapy. Complete blood count, blood urea nitrogen (BUN) and creatinine, serum electrolytes, and thyroid function tests provide baseline information to check patients for underlying health conditions.

A thorough assessment of mental status is important before beginning lithium therapy. In some cases, your patient may be having acute symptoms of bipolar illness, including hyperactivity, irritability, pacing, and rapid speech. Work with the RN and other healthcare team members to determine the best way to give the drug.

Assess normal dietary history. Adequate sodium and fluid intake is important for decreasing the risk of lithium toxicity. Physical exertion or exposure to extreme heat can increase sweating and fluid loss and increase the risk of elevated serum lithium levels.

Determine whether the patient has a history of alcohol use, thyroid problems, cardiac disease, or renal problems because they can increase the risk of health problems from taking lithium. In most cases, lithium is contraindicated in women who are pregnant or breastfeeding. Pregnant women with bipolar illness need to work very closely with their healthcare provider to choose the best alternatives to manage their symptoms.

◆ *Planning and implementation.* Monitor the patient for signs and symptoms of lithium toxicity, including nausea, vomiting, increased drowsiness, muscle weakness, severe hand tremor, and incoordination. Report these symptoms to the RN or healthcare provider immediately.

The serum lithium level needs to be monitored frequently while the patient is taking the drug. Blood levels are checked 4 days after the patient starts taking lithium. The desired level to treat acute mania is 0.8–1.2 mEq/L. Maintenance level is about 0.8–1.0 mEq/L. The healthcare provider adjusts dosages to keep the patient safe and to avoid toxicity. Any levels greater than 1.5 mEq/L are considered toxic (see Table 11.6). Levels greater than 3 mEq/L are associated with coma, organ failure, and death.

Teach patients to avoid making any significant increases or decreases in salt or fluid intake. Patients may experience increased thirst or increased urination. Tell the patient to contact his or her healthcare provider if these symptoms are severe.

Older adult patients are often more sensitive to lithium than younger patients. It is important to start these patients on lower doses and to monitor the therapeutic and adverse effects closely while increasing the dosage.

### Lifespan Considerations
#### Older Adults
Older adults may show signs and symptoms of lithium toxicity at lower serum levels. Dosages often start lower and are increased more slowly than with younger patients.

◆ *Evaluation.* Evaluate your patient's mental status regularly to determine the effect of the lithium. Emotional, cognitive, and behavioral symptoms of mania should diminish. As your patient is adjusting to the dose changes, evaluate for signs and symptoms of drug toxicity.

Blood levels are measured one to two times each week during the acute phase and then every 1 to 2 weeks until the dosage and blood levels are stable. After that, patients need blood levels checked every 6 to 12 weeks.

◆ *Patient and family teaching.* Tell the patient and family:
* Take your lithium as prescribed. It may take several weeks before you notice a change in your symptoms.
* If you are taking the oral liquid, you can mix it with fruit juices or other flavored drinks to improve the taste. Do not mix the liquid with other drugs.
* Avoid making any big increases or decreases in your salt or fluid intake. These can affect your drug levels and may increase the risk of adverse effects from the lithium.
* If you have excessive thirst or urination, notify your healthcare provider immediately because these symptoms can be related to adverse effects.
* Report significant nausea, vomiting, increased drowsiness, muscle weakness, severe hand tremor, and incoordination to your healthcare provider because they may indicate an adverse reaction.
* Do not use alcohol or any sedating drugs while you are taking this drug to avoid serious CNS side effects.
* Contact your healthcare provider if you are thinking of becoming pregnant. Lithium may be toxic to your baby.
* Physical exertion or exposure to extreme heat can increase sweating and fluid loss and increase the risk of high lithium levels.
* Keep all appointments to have your drug level monitored to avoid adverse actions to lithium. This is done frequently when first starting to ensure that you are getting the correct dosage, and later it will be done every 6 to 8 weeks.
* Wear a medical alert bracelet or necklace and carry a medical identification card stating the name of the drug to ensure that all healthcare providers are aware that you are taking this drug.

## ANTIPSYCHOTICS

Antipsychotic drugs are used to treat psychosis, which involves a loss of contact with reality. How the psychosis occurs and the types of symptoms produced vary. Psychosis may develop over a few hours or days (acute form) or over months or years (chronic form). It is important to distinguish between acute psychosis (delirium) and chronic psychosis (e.g., schizophrenia, bipolar illness) because you may see both conditions in clinical practice.

Delirium is an acute condition. Patients experience a sudden change in awareness and attention that is related to problems in the brain. Delirium can occur in a patient who has previously been alert and oriented but suddenly becomes confused after taking a new drug. It can occur in an older person who has a urinary tract infection. It can also occur in a patient who has been diagnosed with dementia and who suddenly has a change in symptoms after being moved from his or her home into a new setting. Family members may notice before you do as a nurse that the patient is confused or "different." A previously calm patient may be trying to pull out tubes or get out of bed without help. The patient is suddenly agitated and confused, may be unable to focus, or may seem frightened. The patient's awareness can change over the course of the day—sometimes oriented, sometimes confused. He or she may have more symptoms at night. Because delirium is often temporary, it may not be considered a big problem. However, delirium can increase the patient's length of stay, mortality risk, and risk of falls.

Patients with chronic mental illnesses such as schizophrenia have symptoms that increase over a long period. It may be months or years before the patient is accurately diagnosed. Families and friends may notice changes in behavior but may not be fully aware of the problems until the person develops delusions and hallucinations. Many of these symptoms can be effectively managed with antipsychotic drugs and other therapies. This chapter reviews drugs that are used in patients with mental illness. Drugs that can be used for delirium may be mentioned, but the focus is on drugs for chronic mental illnesses.

In the past, antipsychotic drugs were used in patients with dementia. Although patients with dementia may exhibit confusion or agitation, use of antipsychotic drugs in these cases can increase the risk of stroke, rate of cognitive impairment (decline in ability to think and remember), and risk of mortality.

Symptoms of psychosis are classified as positive or negative (Box 11.5). In mental health, the positive symptoms of psychosis are those that add to the person's normal behaviors. Positive symptoms include hallucinations (e.g., seeing things, hearing voices), delusions (e.g., ideas that he or she has special powers or is famous), and disorganized thoughts or speech (e.g., jumbled ideas or words that do not make sense to the listener). These are the conditions that we may think about right away when we hear the term *psychotic*.

Negative symptoms of psychosis are those that subtract from the person's normal behavior. Negative symptoms include poor hygiene, difficulty with social relationships, lack of interest in activities, and lack of motivation.

| Box 11.5 | Positive and Negative Symptoms Associated with Schizophrenia |
|---|---|
| **POSITIVE SYMPTOMS** | **NEGATIVE SYMPTOMS** |
| Hallucinations (visual or auditory) | Lack of motivation |
| Delusions (holding a belief without any evidence) | Flat affect (decreased facial expression or tone with emotion) |
| Disordered thinking (unusual ways of thinking, speaking) | Decrease in personal hygiene |
| Agitation or other bizarre behavior | Lack of social interest |

Drugs that treat symptoms of psychosis are grouped in two main categories: typical antipsychotics and atypical antipsychotics. These drugs are discussed here in terms of their use in the psychosis associated with schizophrenia.

## TYPICAL ANTIPSYCHOTIC DRUGS

### Action and Uses

The typical antipsychotics are the first generation of this drug type. In general, these drugs treat the positive symptoms of psychosis. Typical antipsychotics are thought to block dopamine receptors in the brain, which helps to treat the positive symptoms of psychosis such as hallucinations and delusions; they do not affect the negative symptoms.

Schizophrenia is thought to result from overstimulation of dopamine receptors by too much dopamine (recall that Parkinson's disease is caused by too little dopamine). The typical antipsychotic drug blocks dopamine and therefore can treat the positive symptoms of schizophrenia, but it also creates a series of side and adverse effects, including pseudoparkinsonism and other extrapyramidal symptoms (EPSs). The extrapyramidal system, the part of the nervous system involved in movement, normally helps to ensure smooth or flowing movements of the body. EPSs are associated with disordered movements.

The two main categories of typical antipsychotics are the phenothiazines and the nonphenothiazines. Phenothiazines block transmission of dopamine at the dopamine receptors and transmission of other neurotransmitters at acetylcholine and alpha-adrenergic receptors. These drugs reduce positive symptoms but have significant side and adverse effects. The nonphenothiazines are chemically different from the phenothiazines but have similar actions, side effects, and adverse effects. Which drug type is prescribed for long-term therapy depends on the patient's responses. Table 11.7 lists the names, adult dosages, and nursing implications for the most common typical antipsychotic drugs. Check a drug reference or ask a pharmacist for information about other typical antipsychotics.

### Expected Side Effects and Adverse Reactions

Expected side effects and adverse reactions of typical antipsychotics are primarily related to the blocking of key neurotransmitters. Examples of side effects include headache, drowsiness, nausea, constipation, and dry mouth.

The main adverse effects are described as drug induced movement disorders (DIMDs). DIMDs include pseudoparkinsonism, acute dystonia, and akathisia (also known as *extrapyramidal symptoms [EPS]*). A fourth DIMD is *tardive dyskinesia*. These DIMDs are related to the decrease in dopamine; many are severe, and some may be irreversible, and it is important to recognize them very early in treatment. They can occur

## Table 11.7   Examples of Common Antipsychotic Drugs

*Typical antipsychotics*, which block dopamine receptors in the brain, are primarily used to manage psychosis, including hallucinations, delusions, and paranoia or disordered thought. Blocking dopamine can also induce pseudoparkinsonism and other movement disorders.

*Phenothiazines* block signal transmission by dopamine at the dopamine receptors and other block neurotransmitters at the acetylcholine and alpha-adrenergic receptors.

*Nonphenothiazines* have similar actions, side effects, and adverse reactions but are chemically different from the phenothiazines. Drug selection depends on patients' responses.

*Atypical antipsychotics* usually are a combination of dopamine and serotonin blockers. They can reduce positive symptoms and improve negative symptoms without the severe extrapyramidal effects characteristic of the typical antipsychotics.

*Dopamine system stabilizers* affect dopamine and serotonin receptors slightly differently from other atypical antipsychotics. As a result, they have fewer motor side effects and adverse reactions than other atypical antipsychotics.

| DRUG/ADULT DOSAGE | NURSING IMPLICATIONS |
|---|---|
| **Typical Antipsychotics** | |
| **Phenothiazines**<br>chlorpromazine (Thorazine) for mild to moderate symptoms, 10 mg three to four times per day or 25 mg two to three times per day orally, then adjusted to patients' symptoms; IM: 25–50 mg every 4–6 hours; higher doses may be required for severe symptoms<br>fluphenazine (Prolixin) 2.5–10 mg/day orally in divided doses; maximum is 40 mg/day<br>fluphenazine immediate-release IM dose: 1.25–10 mg/day in divided doses<br>fluphenazine decanoate IM or subcutaneous route: usual initial dose 12.5–25 mg; IM or subcutaneously, maximum 100 mg as a depot injection; a single dose can last 3–6 weeks | • Recognize the signs of EPSs because many are severe and some may be irreversible. They can occur in as many as 10% of patients who take these drugs.<br>• Monitor blood pressure when using intramuscular forms of these drugs.<br>• Although it is rare, patients with a history of low white blood cell counts are at increased risk for agranulocytosis with chlorpromazine.<br>• Teach patients to avoid becoming dehydrated, participating in strenuous exercise, or experiencing extremes in temperature because these drugs may affect the body's ability to regulate core body temperature.<br>• Report sudden increases in blood pressure; increase in temperature and confusion may indicate signs of neuroleptic malignant syndrome.<br>• Know the specific onsets of action, peak effects, and durations when you are giving these drugs. Some injectable drugs are used for rapid treatment of symptoms, whereas others are designed for long-term management (i.e., long-acting injectables [LAIs]).<br>• Monitor changes in mental status with the healthcare team to determine the effectiveness of these drugs.<br>• Teach the patient to avoid activities that require alertness, particularly when first using the drug. This effect usually improves over time. |
| **Nonphenothiazines**<br>haloperidol (Haldol) 0.5–5 mg orally two to three times per day depending on symptoms<br>haloperidol IM route: 0.5–10 mg IM every 4–8 hours depending on level of agitation<br>haloperidol decanoate (depot preparation) initial injection not to exceed 100 mg; with average maintenance, typically 50–200 mg every 4 weeks | • Recognize the signs of EPSs because many are severe and some may be irreversible. They can occur in as many as 10% of patients who take these drugs.<br>• Teach patients to avoid becoming dehydrated, participating in strenuous exercise, or experiencing extremes in temperature because these drugs may affect the body's ability to regulate core body temperature.<br>• Report sudden increases in blood pressure; increase in temperature and confusion may be signs of neuroleptic malignant syndrome.<br>• Know the specific onsets of action, peak effects, and durations when you are giving these drugs. Some injectable drugs are used for rapid treatment of symptoms, whereas others are designed for long-term management (i.e., LAIs).<br>• Monitor changes in mental status with the healthcare team to determine the effectiveness of these drugs.<br>• Teach the patient to avoid activities that require alertness, particularly when first using the drug. This effect usually improves over time. |

| Table 11.7 | Examples of Common Antipsychotic Drugs—cont'd |
|---|---|
| **Atypical Antipsychotics** | |
| risperidone (Risperdal) initially 0.5–3 mg orally as a single or divided dose; usual is 4–16 mg/day orally<br>NOTE: Also available as orally disintegrating tablets (ODT; e.g., Risperdal M-tab) to be absorbed sublingually<br>IM route (Risperdal Consta) depot preparation: 25–50 mg every 2 weeks<br>Subcutaneous route (Perseris) depot preparation: 90–120 mg given by abdominal subcutaneous injection once monthly<br>ziprasidone (Geodon) initially 20–40 mg orally twice daily with food; maximum 80 mg orally twice daily with food<br>IM route: 10–20 mg per dose; do not give IM for more than 3 consecutive days; maximum dose 40 mg/day<br>quetiapine (Seroquel) initially 25–50 mg by mouth twice daily; may be increased to 300–400 mg/day in 2–3 divided doses; maximum dose is 800 mg daily<br>Extended-release form (Seroquel XR): 25–50 mg once or twice daily; maximum dose is 800 mg daily or in divided doses | • Watch for signs and symptoms of extrapyramidal effects. This is less common with atypical antipsychotics but must be monitored.<br>• Teach patients about good nutrition and physical activity because these drugs can cause weight gain.<br>• Monitor blood glucose levels for patients with diabetes and those at risk for diabetes because these drugs can increase blood glucose levels.<br>• Monitor vital signs because sudden changes in blood pressure or increase in temperature can indicate dangerous adverse effects.<br>• Remind patients that they should not drink alcohol or take any sedating drugs without talking to the healthcare provider. These drugs can cause drowsiness or insomnia.<br>• Encourage patients to maintain a diet high in fiber to avoid constipation, which is common with atypical antipsychotics.<br>• For patients who have difficulty adhering to oral drug schedules, IM depot drugs may allow less frequent dosing, up to 2 weeks or even longer.<br>• Work with healthcare team members to maintain a safe environment for patients who are experiencing symptoms of their psychosis.<br>• Teach patients to avoid extremes in temperature because these drugs can affect the body's ability to adjust to changes in temperature. |
| **Dopamine System Stabilizers** | |
| aripiprazole (Abilify, Abilify Mycite) 10–30 mg once daily by mouth<br>IM route: 30 mg/day for an immediate-release injection<br>Extended-release IM suspension (Abilify Maintena): 400 mg once per month | • Teach patients that oral doses can be given with or without food.<br>• Read drug packaging information carefully when giving aripiprazole intramuscular injection. Do NOT administer subcutaneously or intravenously. Several preparations are available in prefilled syringes.<br>• See also nursing implications for atypical antipsychotics. |

*EPSs*, extrapyramidal symptoms; *IM*, intramuscular.

in as many as 10% of patients who take these drugs. Fig. 11.4 describes these symptoms.

Onset of DIMDs varies, and treatment focuses on symptom management and altering the cause. Acute dystonia usually occurs within 1 to 4 days after the start of treatment. It is more common in younger men and in patients who are taking large doses. It may be managed with anticholinergic drugs and BNZs. Akathisia usually develops several days to several weeks into therapy. Management may include decreasing the drug dosage and/or adding a BNZ or beta-blocker. Pseudoparkinsonism usually occurs 1 to 2 weeks after beginning antipsychotic therapy. It is more common in women and older adults. Anticholinergics, antihistamines, and BNZs may be used to manage symptoms.

Unlike the earlier onset of other DIMDs, tardive dyskinesia can occur during long-term therapy or after stopping therapy. It occurs more frequently in older women. The disorder is characterized by involuntary movements of the tongue, jaw, mouth, or face. The patient's lips may be smacking, the cheeks puffing, or there may be other bizarre movements of the arms and shoulders. It is more likely to occur in patients with bipolar disorder than in patients with schizophrenia.

These drugs may affect the body's ability to regulate core body temperature. The risk increases if patients become dehydrated, participate in strenuous exercise, or are in very hot environments. In rare cases, patients may experience hypothermia. This usually occurs in the presence of other risk factors such as hypothyroidism, brain injury, or cold environmental temperature.

Neuroleptic malignant syndrome (NMS) is a potentially fatal adverse effect. NMS is characterized by hyperpyrexia (abnormally high body temperature, above 104°F [40°C]), confusion, changes in blood pressure (hypotension to hypertension), and EPSs; it can lead to coma and death. It occurs more often in men than in women. Box 11.6 lists the common signs and symptoms associated with NMS.

### Drug Interactions

Typical antipsychotics interact with a wide range of drugs, including acetaminophen, diuretics such as furosemide or hydrochlorothiazide, certain calcium channel blockers, and several antidiabetic agents. Consult a pharmacist or other healthcare provider if you have any questions.

### ❖ Nursing Implications and Patient Teaching

◆ *Assessment.* Determine the baseline level of consciousness. Is the patient agitated? Hallucinating? If you are in a behavioral health setting, you may be working

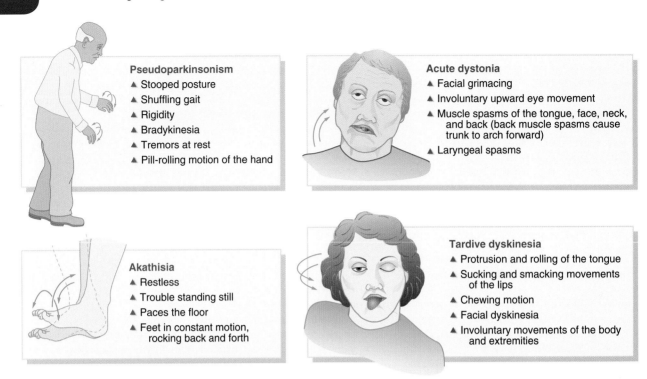

**Pseudoparkinsonism**
- ▲ Stooped posture
- ▲ Shuffling gait
- ▲ Rigidity
- ▲ Bradykinesia
- ▲ Tremors at rest
- ▲ Pill-rolling motion of the hand

**Acute dystonia**
- ▲ Facial grimacing
- ▲ Involuntary upward eye movement
- ▲ Muscle spasms of the tongue, face, neck, and back (back muscle spasms cause trunk to arch forward)
- ▲ Laryngeal spasms

**Akathisia**
- ▲ Restless
- ▲ Trouble standing still
- ▲ Paces the floor
- ▲ Feet in constant motion, rocking back and forth

**Tardive dyskinesia**
- ▲ Protrusion and rolling of the tongue
- ▲ Sucking and smacking movements of the lips
- ▲ Chewing motion
- ▲ Facial dyskinesia
- ▲ Involuntary movements of the body and extremities

**Fig. 11.4** Characteristics of drug-induced movement disorders: Pseudoparkinsonism, acute dystonia, akathisia, and tardive dyskinesia. (From McCuistion, L. E., DiMaggio, K. V., Winton, M. B., & Yeager, J. (2021). *Pharmacology* (10th ed.). Elsevier.)

| Box 11.6 | Signs and Symptoms of Neuroleptic Malignant Syndrome |
|---|---|

- Sudden elevated temperature
- Increased white blood cell count
- Muscle rigidity
- Unstable blood pressure
- Elevated serum creatine kinase level
- Hyperkalemia

with the RN who may conduct a formal mental status exam. Components of the mental status exam include factors such as the patient's appearance, behavior, mood, affect, and thought processes. This assessment is very helpful in determining a baseline from which to evaluate the effects of the drugs.

For patients requiring antipsychotic therapy, assessment for any symptoms of DIMDs will be important, particularly with beginning therapy or with any change in dose. For patients requiring long-term therapy, the provider may use the *Abnormal Involuntary Movement Scale (AIMS)* to assess and monitor symptoms.

◆*Planning and implementation.* Maintaining patient safety is vitally important in caring for patients who are experiencing psychosis. Whether the patient has acute delirium or chronic mental illness, he or she is at risk for injury to self or others. Keeping the patient, caregivers, and others free from injury is a priority. You will work with other members of the healthcare team to keep the milieu (social environment or surroundings) safe and calm. Review of the techniques for working with patients with psychosis is beyond the scope of this textbook. You should consult professional resources in mental health, such as experienced mental health nurses, mental health nursing textbooks, or continuing education.

 **Bookmark This!**

The National Institute of Mental Health (NIMH) is a great resource for nurses, patients, and families to learn more about mental health disorders: https://www.nimh.nih.gov. You can print or order free brochures, booklets, posters, and fact sheets for your agency.

Monitor vital signs carefully for any significant changes. Increase in temperature or drastic changes in blood pressure can indicate the severe adverse effect of NMS.

Recognize the classic characteristics of DIMDs (see Fig. 11.4). Early recognition is essential in reducing the risk of long-term consequences. Any changes in motor function, such as altered muscle tone, gait, or fine motor movement, can be warning signs of DIMDs, especially tardive dyskinesia. Report these symptoms to the RN or healthcare provider immediately. Treatment often requires discontinuing the drug and changing to another drug to treat the mental illness. In some cases, these problems are irreversible and will require treatment with medications to reduce the tardive dyskinesia symptoms.

Know the specific onsets of action, peak effects, and durations when you are giving these drugs. Some oral or injectable drugs are used for rapid treatment of symptoms, whereas others are designed for long-term management. For example, an oral form of haloperidol may take 4 to 6 hours to achieve for peak effect, whereas an oral form of chlorpromazine may take 6 weeks to 6 months. Some LAI antipsychotic agents are excellent for helping patients better adhere to treatment, particularly in managing symptoms associated with severe chronic mental illness. Understanding these facts will help you to plan your care and recognize whether the drug is effective.

◆ *Evaluation.* Has the patient had any changes in mental status since beginning this drug? Remember, these drugs affect only positive symptoms, and you may see a decrease in agitation, hallucinations, and delusions. Determine whether the patient has had any side effects from these drugs. For improvement in negative symptoms, the patient needs the addition of or substitution with an atypical antipsychotic. Typical antipsychotics are not used alone for an extensive period because of the possibility of EPSs.

◆ *Patient and family teaching.* Tell the patient and family:
- Continue to take the drugs as prescribed even if you do not start feeling better right away. It may take several weeks before significant changes occur. Suddenly stopping these drugs can result in nausea, dizziness, and tremors.
- To prevent deep sedation and other dangerous side effects, do not drink alcohol or use any sedatives while taking these drugs.
- Avoid activities that require alertness, particularly when first using the drug, because these drugs can reduce clear thinking and induce drowsiness. This usually improves over time.
- These drugs may affect your body's ability to adjust to changes in temperature. Avoid extremes of temperature and situations that can affect your temperature, such as dehydration or strenuous exercise.
- If you or your family member has difficulty remembering to take these drugs, check with your healthcare provider about long-acting injectable drugs.
- These drugs may cause dryness of your mouth. You can try sugarless gum, sugarless candy, sips of water, or ice chips to reduce this sensation.
- If you develop unusual muscle spasms or other types of movement problems, contact your healthcare provider right away.

- Avoid getting liquid forms of these drugs on your skin because they can cause irritation.
- You can take many of these drugs with food to avoid GI upset.
- Avoid using any herbal or other OTC drugs without first checking with your healthcare provider because they can interact with your prescription drugs.
- Wear a medical alert bracelet or carry a drug identification card to identify that you are taking these drugs.

## ATYPICAL ANTIPSYCHOTIC DRUGS
### Action and Uses
Atypical antipsychotics are also known as *second-generation antipsychotics*. Whereas typical antipsychotics block dopamine receptors in the brain, atypical antipsychotic drugs work in a variety of ways. Many block dopamine or other subtypes of dopamine receptor and certain subtypes of serotonin receptor. They are used primarily for schizophrenia but also can be used for bipolar illnesses and schizoaffective disorder.

The atypical antipsychotics have a lower risk of EPSs and have the benefit of treating negative and positive symptoms (see Box 11.5). Atypical antipsychotics are more commonly used for long-term management of chronic mental illnesses associated with psychosis. They are not recommended for any patient who has psychosis resulting from dementia.

The newest category of atypical antipsychotic drugs are called dopamine system stabilizers (DSSs). DSSs affect dopamine and serotonin receptors slightly differently from other atypical antipsychotics. As a result, they have even fewer motor side effects and adverse reactions than other atypical antipsychotics. The DSSs can be used in schizophrenia and bipolar disorders. They can also be used to relieve symptoms in some autistic disorders and in Tourette syndrome. Table 11.7 lists the names, adult dosages, and nursing implications for the most common atypical antipsychotic drugs. Check a drug reference or consult with a pharmacist for information about other atypical antipsychotics.

 **Memory Jogger**

Atypical antipsychotics are also known as *second-generation antipsychotics*.

### Expected Side Effects and Adverse Reactions
The most common side effects of atypical antipsychotics are insomnia and drowsiness. Although many of these drugs have sexual side effects, they are less common than with the typical antipsychotics. Other common side effects include dizziness, orthostatic hypotension, constipation, and dry mouth.

A major advantage of atypical antipsychotics is significantly lower rates of DIMDs than with the typical antipsychotics. This means a reduced risk of adverse effects such as acute dystonia, akathisia, pseudoparkinsonism, and tardive dyskinesia. Although the risk is not totally eliminated, the reduced risk makes atypical antipsychotic drugs preferable to the typical antipsychotics in most situations.

Weight gain is common with many of the atypical antipsychotics. Beyond weight gain, hypertriglyceridemia (increase in blood triglyceride levels) and a risk of insulin resistance and diabetes type 2 are associated with these drugs. These changes can significantly increase the risk of cardiovascular problems, even death. Use caution in starting these drugs for patients with preexisting hypertension, heart or cerebrovascular disease, heart failure, or any dysrhythmia.

Atypical antipsychotic drugs can also affect the ECG, prolonging the QT interval (part of the cardiac cycle). This is very important for patients with heart disease because it can result in severe cardiac dysrhythmias.

One drug, clozapine, is associated with agranulocytosis (decreased white blood cell count). This can result in a significantly increased risk of infection or death. As a result, clozapine is usually reserved for patients who do not experience symptom relief from other antipsychotics.

### Drug Interactions

Atypical antipsychotics interact with a wide range of drugs. Drugs that decrease dopamine, such as metoclopramide or any of the typical antipsychotics, increase the risk of DIMDs. Use of these drugs with any SSRI or with an SNRI can increase the risk of serotonin syndrome (see Box 11.2).

Alcohol and other CNS depressants increase the sedating and nervous system side effects of these drugs. These drugs also affect specific enzymes in the liver that metabolize drugs. Check drug references and contact your agency pharmacist or the patient's healthcare provider for other interactions with additional drugs the patient takes.

### ❖ Nursing Implications and Patient Teaching

◆ *Assessment.* It is important to determine the baseline level of consciousness for any patient prescribed an antipsychotic drug. Work with the RN and other healthcare team members to determine the patient's mental status. This includes assessment of appearance, behavior, mood, affect, and thought processes. A good baseline assessment is essential to determining whether the drugs are effective.

Determining baseline levels for vital signs, weight, and blood glucose is important for patients beginning therapy with atypical antipsychotic drugs. These data are useful in looking for side or adverse effects the patient may experience.

Thorough assessment of a history of hypertension, diabetes, cardiovascular or cerebral vascular disease, or dysrhythmia is needed. Assess prescriptions, OTC drugs, and herbal drugs the patient is taking.

◆ *Planning and implementation.* As with typical antipsychotics, maintaining patient safety is very important. Work with members of the healthcare team to keep the patient, caregivers, and others free from injury.

Monitor the patient carefully for side effects and adverse reactions. Sudden changes in vital signs, such as a drop in blood pressure or severe and sudden increase in temperature, can be indicators of complications of drug therapy. For patients who are taking clozapine, monitor white blood cell counts. Fewer white blood cells can indicate the life-threatening complication of agranulocytosis, which significantly affects the patient's ability to fight infection.

The risk of EPSs is much lower with atypical antipsychotics than with the typical antipsychotics, but these symptoms can still occur. It is important to recognize changes in fine motor movement, gait, or muscle tone as indicating a potential adverse effect. Report these to the healthcare provider immediately.

Monitor the patient's weight on a regular basis because weight gain is a very common side effect of drug therapy. You may need to consult your agency dietician or RN to help patients find strategies for managing their weight.

Atypical antipsychotics can cause dry mouth. Make sure the patient has good oral hygiene. Sugar-free gums or candies, ice chips, or sips of water may be helpful in moistening the mouth. Remind the patient to avoid extremes of cold or heat because the drug may affect the area of the brain that is responsible for temperature regulation.

◆ *Evaluation.* Determine whether the patient has had any changes in mental status since beginning the drug. Be sure of the drug's onset of action. Many of these drugs can take several weeks before they have significant impact on patient behaviors. Remember that these drugs can impact positive and negative symptoms. Assess whether the patient has had an increase in the ability to interact with others, more interest in activities, or improved hygiene and whether there has been a reduction in the positive symptoms of hallucinations and delusions.

◆ *Patient and family teaching.* Tell the patient and family:
- Continue to take the drugs as prescribed even if you do not start feeling better right away. It may take several weeks before significant changes occur. Suddenly stopping these drugs can result in nausea, dizziness, and tremors.
- To avoid oversedation and other dangerous nervous system side effects, do not drink alcohol or use any sedatives while using these drugs.
- Avoid activities that require alertness, particularly when first using the drug, because the drug increases drowsiness and interferes with clear thinking. This usually improves over time.

- These drugs may affect your body's ability to adjust to changes in temperature. Avoid temperature extremes and situations that can affect your temperature such as dehydration or strenuous exercise.
- If you or your family member has difficulty remembering to take these drugs, check with your healthcare provider about long-acting injectable drugs.
- These drugs may cause dryness of your mouth. You can try chewing sugarless gum, sucking on sugarless candy, or drinking sips of ice or water to reduce this problem.
- If you have unusual muscle spasms or other types of movement problems, contact your healthcare provider right away.
- You can take many of these drugs with food to avoid GI upset.
- Avoid using herbal or other OTC drugs without checking with your healthcare provider first because they can interact with your prescription drugs.
- Wear a medical alert bracelet or carry a drug identification card to identify that you are taking these drugs.

## VESICULAR MONOAMINE TRANSPORTER 2 (VMAT2) INHIBITORS

### Action and Uses

Vesicular monoamine transporter 2 (VMAT2) inhibitors are a newer category of drugs that are used to treat movement disorders (such as tardive dyskinesia). These drugs may be beneficial in patients who require long-term antipsychotic medications to manage their mental illness despite having symptoms of tardive dyskinesia. They work by decreasing dopamine available to stimulate dopamine receptors ultimately reducing the involuntary motor symptoms. Table 11.8 lists the names, adult dosages, and nursing implications for the most common VMAT2 inhibitors used to treat tardive dyskinesia.

### Expected Side Effects and Adverse Reactions

The most common side effects of VMAT2 inhibitors are drowsiness and fatigue. These usually improve with time and adjusting of doses if needed. Other side effects include dry mouth, nausea, constipation, mild dizziness, and urinary retention. Some patients may experience weight gain. Pseudoparkinsonism has occurred in some patients and may be severe. VMAT2 inhibitors have also been associated with depression and suicidal thoughts in some patients.

### Drug Interactions

VMAT2 inhibitors have multiple drug interactions including with digoxin, certain antidepressants, and mood stabilizers. They should be used cautiously in patients who require treatment for tuberculosis. Because they cause drowsiness, patients should avoid use of alcohol or other CNS depressants. Use of St. John's wort should be avoided.

❖ **Nursing Implications and Patient Teaching**

◆ *Assessment.* A good understanding of the patient's history of tardive dyskinesia and assessment of specific symptoms will be important. If available in your healthcare setting, review the results of the AIMS. This will give you a good baseline for the severity of the involuntary movements of the facial and oral muscles, extremities, and trunk. Also assess the level of the patient's distress with these movements: How much do the movements affect his or her quality of life?

◆ *Planning and implementation.* Because patients with tardive dyskinesia have involuntary movements, make sure they are evaluated carefully for fall risk. Patients may experience drowsiness, especially early in therapy, so carefully monitor their level of alertness. Remind patients to avoid driving or doing anything that requires mental alertness until they know how the medication affects them. Encourage a diet high in fruits and vegetables to help decrease constipation. For patients who have a dry mouth, encourage use of sugarless gum or sucking on hard candy.

| Table 11.8 | Examples of Common Drugs Used to Treat Tardive Dyskinesia |
|---|---|

*Vesicular monoamine transporter 2 inhibitors* reduce symptoms of tardive dyskinesia by decreasing dopamine leading to a decrease in involuntary movements.

| DRUG/ADULT DOSAGE | NURSING IMPLICATIONS |
|---|---|
| Valbenazine (Ingrezza) initially 40 mg orally once daily; after one week, increased to 80 mg orally once daily<br>Deutetrabenazine (Austedo) initially 6 mg orally once daily; increased weekly by 6 mg according to reduction of symptoms and tolerability. For doses 12 mg or more, given in two divided doses. Maximum dose 48 mg/day. | • Valbenazine may be given with or without food.<br>• Deutetrabenazine should be given with food.<br>• Encourage a balanced diet with fruits and vegetables to help decrease risk of constipation.<br>• Monitor symptoms of tardive dyskinesia for improvement. Report to the healthcare provider any increase in symptoms.<br>• Monitor the patient carefully for drowsiness or dizziness, particularly at the onset of therapy or with dosage changes. |

◆ *Evaluation.* The goal of therapy is to reduce symptoms of tardive dyskinesia. It may take several weeks to achieve noticeable effects, so maintaining good communication with the patient and the provider will be important. Report onset of any side effects or adverse effects.

◆ *Patient and family teaching.* Tell the patient and family:
- Take the medication as prescribed; do not stop taking without contacting your healthcare provider.
- This drug may cause drowsiness, especially early in treatment, so avoid driving, operating heavy machinery, or making major decisions until you understand how this drug affects you.
- Avoid drinking alcohol while taking this drug as it may increase dizziness and drowsiness.
- Avoid using herbal medications, including St. John's wort, as they may cause dangerous drug interactions.

- VMAT2 inhibitors may cause constipation. Be sure to include a diet rich in fiber with foods such as fruits, vegetables, and whole grains. Notify your provider if you go more than 3 days without a bowel movement.
- For a dry mouth, try chewing sugarless gum or sucking on hard candy and taking in plenty of fluids daily. Notify your provider if these symptoms are severe.
- Notify your provider for any increase in movements such as an increase in tremor or difficulty with walking. You may require a decrease in dose or change to another drug.
- Tell your patient that these drugs may increase depression or suicidal thinking. If they do, contact your healthcare provider or the emergency services in your area.

## Get Ready for the Next-Generation NCLEX® Examination!

### Key Points

- Mental illness is a condition in which the individual experiences significant changes in the ability to think, along with changes in behaviors and emotions. Patients can have problems in coping with normal stressors, interacting with others, and functioning within their own cultural norms.
- The main neurotransmitters affected by psychiatric drugs are serotonin, dopamine, norepinephrine, GABA, acetylcholine, and histamine.
- All sedatives depress the CNS to some degree.
- Flumazenil (Romazicon) is a benzodiazepine receptor antagonist; it is used as an antidote to reverse an overdose of a benzodiazepine (BNZ) or a BNZ agonist sedative.
- If a BNZ or BNZ agonist is taken with another CNS depressant, the CNS effects are more severe, and coma or death is possible.
- Major categories of antianxiety agents (also called *anxiolytics*) include BNZs, BNZ agonists, and certain antidepressants (selective serotonin reuptake inhibitors [SSRIs] and serotonin norepinephrine reuptake inhibitors [SNRIs]).
- BNZs act with GABA receptors to enhance GABA effects, leading to a reduction in anxiety and decrease in muscle tension.
- BNZs are recommended primarily for short-term use.
- Long-term use of BNZs can result in physical dependence and withdrawal symptoms if the drug is stopped suddenly.
- A newer drug from the BNZ agonist category, buspirone, reduces anxiety through a variety of actions that affect the neurotransmitters serotonin and dopamine.
- Certain drugs often considered antidepressants are commonly used to relieve symptoms of anxiety.

- BNZs should not be used to treat insomnia, agitation, or delirium in patients older than 65 years of age and should be avoided in all patients with cognitive impairment, dementia, or a history of falls or fractures.
- Most patients with depression require several trials of different drugs to determine which drug is the most effective to manage their symptoms.
- Screen for thoughts of suicide in all patients who are taking antidepressants.
- Patients should not stop taking antidepressants suddenly because this may cause withdrawal symptoms or a relapse of depressive symptoms.
- Maximum benefit of many antidepressants may take 4 to 8 weeks. Always make sure your patient has a referral to professional support services and information about local crisis lines.
- Teach patients not to take any herbal or OTC drugs, particularly St. John's wort, because they can cause a dangerous adverse effect if taken with SSRIs, SNRIs, TCAs, or MAOIs.
- SSRIs may cause thoughts of suicide (suicidal ideation) or self-harm; this occurs more often in children and young adults. Remind patients and their families that this is just a side effect of the drug and should be reported to the healthcare providers immediately.
- SSRIs and SNRIs can cause falls or fractures in older adults. Monitor for signs of dizziness or changes in gait that may lead to falls.
- TCAs work as well as SSRIs or SNRIs for treating mild to moderate depression but have more side effects. As a result, TCAs are usually reserved for patients with severe depression or those who do not respond to other treatments.
- TCAs should be avoided with MAOIs, SSRIs, and SNRIs because of the risk for serotonin syndrome.

- MAOIs may cause a hypertensive crisis if the patient ingests foods or drinks that contain tyramine. Examples of these foods include aged cheese, overripe fruit, cured or smoked meat, beer, and wine.
- Do not give MAOIs and SSRIs within 2 weeks of each other. Combining these drugs can cause serotonin syndrome, a life-threatening adverse effect related to too much serotonin.
- Lithium is used mainly to treat patients with bipolar illness, including acute mania, and for long-term maintenance therapy.
- Lithium has a very narrow therapeutic range (i.e., it can easily become toxic). Patients should have serum lithium levels assessed regularly to keep safe.
- Early signs of lithium toxicity include increased nausea, vomiting, drowsiness, muscle weakness, severe hand tremor, and incoordination. Later signs include ataxia (loss of control of body movements) and tinnitus (ringing in the ears).
- Fluid balance is very important in patients who are taking lithium because any condition that leads to lower sodium levels or dehydration can increase the risk of lithium toxicity.
- Symptoms of psychosis are classified as positive or negative. Typical antipsychotics treat positive symptoms, and atypical antipsychotics can treat both positive and negative symptoms.
- The main adverse effects of typical antipsychotics are extrapyramidal symptoms (EPSs). Early recognition can prevent long-term consequences.
- Neuroleptic malignant syndrome (NMS) is a potentially fatal adverse effect associated with antipsychotics and other drugs that affect dopamine.
- Atypical antipsychotics are also known as *second-generation antipsychotics* and have a lower risk of extrapyramidal effects.
- Patients who are taking atypical antipsychotics are at risk for weight gain, increase in blood triglycerides, and diabetes type 2.
- VMAT2 inhibitors are a newer category of drug that can be used for patients that have tardive dyskinesia as a result of taking their antipsychotic medications.

## Clinical Judgment and Next-Generation NCLEX® Examination-Style Questions

1. Which precaution is most important to teach a patient who is prescribed temazepam (Restoril)?

   1. Take this drug with a full glass of water, and remain upright for at least 30 minutes.
   2. Notify your healthcare provider if you become constipated or feel lightheaded.
   3. Avoid driving for 6 to 8 hours after taking this drug.
   4. Do not take this drug for longer than 1 week.

2. The patient is prescribed phenelzine (Nardil), a monoamine oxidase inhibitor, for depression. Which of the following meals would be a good choice for this patient?

   1. Ham and cheddar cheese sandwich on rye bread, 12 ounces beer
   2. Spaghetti with meatballs, tossed salad, glass of red wine
   3. Pancakes with maple syrup, banana, 2 cups of coffee
   4. Baked chicken with a whole grain roll, broccoli, and decaf coffee

3. A patient who started taking buspirone (Buspar) states that he has not felt any relief from his anxiety and it has been 2 days. What is the best response?

   1. "I will tell the healthcare provider the drug is not working and you should be started on a new one."
   2. "Call your healthcare provider and tell them that you need a higher dose."
   3. "You need to start psychotherapy to get the effect you need."
   4. "This antianxiety agent can take 1 to 2 weeks to take effect."

4. A patient who is taking atypical antipsychotic reports a 10-pound weight increase since starting the drug. Which of the following recommendations is appropriate by the LPN/VN?

   1. "This is common for patients taking these drugs. There is nothing you can do about it."
   2. "You should talk to your healthcare provider about starting one of the drugs that works only on positive symptoms."
   3. "Let me talk to your healthcare provider about setting up an appointment to meet with a nutritionist to help you with your diet."
   4. "People taking these drugs usually lose weight. You probably have a slow metabolism."

5. Which of the following symptoms are common in patients experiencing lithium toxicity? **Select all or any that apply.**

   1. Vomiting
   2. Dizziness
   3. Constipation
   4. Weight gain
   5. Tinnitus
   6. Coarse hand tremor

6. A patient has a history of major depression and has tried many different types of drugs. She will be starting a tricyclic antidepressant. Which of the following statements by the patient indicates a need for more teaching?

   1. "I will use sugar-free candy or gum to relieve my dry mouth."
   2. "I should let my healthcare provider know right away if I have any thoughts of suicide."
   3. "I will need to work carefully with my healthcare provider to get the right dosage for me."
   4. "If I have any nausea or a headache, I will stop taking my medication immediately."

7. Which complementary and alternative therapy is known to increase risk of serotonin syndrome if taken with an SSRI?

   1. Feverfew
   2. White willow
   3. Grape seed
   4. St. John's wort

8. Ms. T. is a 72-year-old who recently lost her husband to COVID-19. Since he died, she has experienced difficulty sleeping, decreased appetite, and feelings of hopelessness. Her primary care provider prescribed medications to help with sleep and to reduce her anxiety and depression. Her new drugs include these:

- Zolpidem 5 mg orally at bedtime PRN
- Paroxetine 10 mg orally once daily, increased to 20 mg orally once daily after 1 week

Choose the most likely options for information missing from the statement below by selecting from the options provided.

The nurse teaches the patient to take the zolpidem ____1____ and to take the paroxetine ____2____.

**Options**

- About 1 hour before bedtime
- With a large meal to increase absorption
- First thing in the morning
- With a small amount of grapefruit juice
- A second time if relief no achieved
- Immediately before bedtime
- For about 3 months

## Unfolding Case Study for Discussion

Allison R. is a 33-year-old woman with a history of bipolar illness. She has been taking combination therapy with lithium and valproate to manage her symptoms but stopped taking her medications about 2 weeks ago. Allison's mother states that Allison has become increasingly irritable, talking very rapidly with grandiose ideas, and has not slept in 3 days. After being evaluated in the emergency department, Allison is admitted to the psychiatric unit for observation and treatment.

1. What are your nursing priorities for a patient who is actively experiencing these symptoms?

2. The healthcare provider initially orders the typical antipsychotic haloperidol by mouth and restarted the lithium. What side effects do you expect for this patient in the acute care setting?

3. Approximately 24 hours after starting haloperidol, Allison shows signs of acute dystonia. Describe the symptoms.

At the time of discharge, the prescriber recommended that Allison begin a course of lithium carbonate 300 mg three times a day. Which of the following actions should the nurse take? **Select all or any that apply.**

1. Check the patient's serum sodium level prior to administration.

2. Draw the patient's lithium level as ordered 3 days after beginning therapy.

3. Mix liquid lithium solution with other liquid drugs to decrease patient stress from taking so many medications.

4. Immediately report to the prescriber symptoms of increased nausea, vomiting, drowsiness, coarse hand tremor, and incoordination.

5. Teach the patient to begin a low-salt diet.

6. Assess mental status before beginning lithium therapy.

7. Provide the family with the National Alliance on Mental Illness Web site (https://nami.org/Home) for information about support groups.

8. Teach the patient that it is safe to take over-the-counter drugs with lithium.

9. Monitor the lithium level and report ranges outside the expected range.

## Drug Calculation Review

1. A 36-year-old male patient with schizophrenia is to take ziprasidone 40 mg by mouth twice daily with food. The ziprasidone is available as 20 mg capsules. How many capsules will the patient require with each dose?

2. A 63-year-old patient diagnosed with chronic schizophrenia is prescribed fluphenazine decanoate 12.5 mg intramuscular (IM) every 2 weeks. Fluphenazine is supplied in a vial of 25 mg/mL. How many milliliters will the patient receive?

# Drugs for Analgesia and Anesthesia

## Learning Outcomes

1. List the names, actions, possible side effects, and adverse effects of opioid analgesics and anesthetics.
2. Explain what to teach patients and families about opioid analgesics and anesthetics.
3. List the names, actions, possible side effects, and adverse effects of non-opioid analgesics and anesthetics.
4. Explain what to teach patients and families about non-opioid analgesics and anesthetics.
5. List five common types of miscellaneous drugs used to help manage pain and the types of pain they most commonly relieve.

## Key Terms

**acute pain** Pain that is usually related to an injury, such as recent surgery, trauma, or infection, and ends within an expected time frame.

**analgesics** Drugs that have the specific purpose of relieving pain by changing the patient's perception of pain or by reducing painful stimulation at its source.

**anesthesia** A loss of feeling or awareness caused by drugs or other substances.

**breakthrough pain** A sudden increase in pain that may occur in patients who are already being treated with a long-acting pain medication.

**chronic pain** Any pain that continues beyond the expected time frame of an acute injury and does not trigger the stress response.

**corticosteroids** Drugs built on the structure of cholesterol that are able to prevent or limit inflammation and allergy by slowing or stopping production of the mediators histamine and leukotriene; chemically similar to the glucocorticoid hormones secreted by the adrenal glands.

**dependence** A state in which the body shows withdrawal symptoms when the drug is stopped or a reversing agent is given.

**drug misuse** The use of illegal drugs and/or the use of prescription drugs in a manner other than as directed by a doctor, such as use in greater amounts, more often, or longer than told to take a drug, or using someone else's prescription.

**miscellaneous analgesic** Drug that has specific purposes and actions for other health problems but can help provide relief for certain types of pain.

**neuropathic pain** Pain that results from nerve damage or from a nervous system that is not functioning properly.

**nociceptive pain** Pain caused by damage to body tissue, usually from some external injury.

**nonopioid centrally acting analgesic** Drug that works in the CNS to help manage pain but does not interact with opioid receptors to do so.

**opioid** Any substance derived from natural opium or chemically similar to opium that alters the perception of pain and has the potential to induce dependence and misuse; also called a *narcotic*.

**opioid agonist** Any drug that activates (turns on) opioid receptors to change a patient's perception of discomfort and pain; also refers to a class of antidiarrheals that do not have analgesic or opioid-like effects; they reduce GI motility and increase the ability of the intestine to absorb water.

**opioid agonist-antagonist analgesic** A pain-management drug that has mixed actions at opioid receptor sites.

**pain** An unpleasant sensory and emotional experience associated with or resembling that associated with actual or potential tissue damage.

**pain threshold** The smallest amount of tissue damage that makes a person aware of feeling pain.

**radicular pain** Pain that radiates from the back and hip into the legs through the spine.

**skeletal muscle relaxant** Drug that reduces muscle spasm by depressing the CNS.

**substance use disorder (addiction)** A psychological dependence in which there is a desperate need to have and use a drug for a nonmedical reason. The addicted person has a limited ability to control this drug craving or use.

**tolerance** A drug-related metabolism problem that causes the same amount of drug to have less effect over time.

**withdrawal symptoms** Changes in the body or mind, such as nausea or anxiety, that occur when a drug is stopped or reduced after regular use.

# PAIN

## DEFINITION OF PAIN

The experience of pain is the most common reason for visits to a healthcare provider. The International Association for the Study of Pain defines **pain** as "An unpleasant sensory and emotional experience associated with, or resembling that associated with, actual or potential tissue damage." Pain is experienced as an unpleasant sensation and can be described as sharp or dull, a tingling, stinging, stabbing, throbbing, burning, or aching. Pain can only be measured by the individual person experiencing it. *Pain is whatever the patient says it is, occurring whenever the patient says it occurs, and at the intensity the patient states.* All people experience the sensation of pain a little differently because pain perception also includes behavioral, psychological, and emotional factors. These factors include age, gender, ethnicity, genetics, comorbid disease, smoking status, fatigue, and sleep problems.

 **Memory Jogger**

- A person's report of pain is whatever the person says it is, occurring whenever and at whatever intensity reported.
- Pain can have adverse effects on physical function and social and psychological well-being.
- Pain is always a personal experience that is influenced by biological, psychological, and social factors.

The **pain threshold** is the minimum point at which tissue damage resulting from injury or disease causes pain. The pain threshold is different for every person and varies from one body site to another. For example, a small blister on a fingertip usually is perceived as more painful than the same-size blister on the back. Other factors, such as age and comorbid diseases, also affect the pain threshold. Most drugs used for pain management raise the patient's pain threshold.

Pain is initially classified as acute or chronic. **Acute pain** is usually related to an injury, such as recent surgery, trauma, or infection, and ends within an expected time frame. For example, acute pain can occur when you accidentally touch a hot stove that causes a burning sensation. One of the main features of acute pain is your body's physical response to it. Acute pain triggers the stress response (sometimes called the *fight-or-flight response*), resulting in increased heart and respiratory rates, increased blood pressure, sweating of the palms and soles of the feet, dry mouth, and dilated pupils. A person with acute pain is often restless and unable to concentrate.

**Chronic pain** is any pain that continues beyond the expected time frame of an acute injury process. Some definitions of pain suggest that pain must exist for 3 to 6 months to be considered chronic. People with cancer-related pain or chronic disorders (e.g., arthritis, shingles, lower back pain [sciatica]) experience chronic pain. It does not trigger the stress response because it has been present for a long time and the body has adapted to it. As a result, the person with chronic pain does not have the physical responses seen with acute pain. Chronic pain may hurt less on some days than others, but usually it is always present to some degree. This problem has often led to family members and healthcare workers not believing the patient's reports of pain or its intensity. Chronic pain is often hard to relieve; it may interfere with activities of daily living (ADLs) and greatly reduces quality of life.

**Neuropathic pain** results from nerve damage or from a nervous system that is not functioning properly. This damage changes nerve function both at the injured area and locations around it. Neuropathic pain is often described as a shooting or burning pain. Neuropathic pain is often chronic.

**Nociceptive pain** is caused by damage to body tissue, usually from some external injury such as bruises, burns, cuts, or fractures. Nociceptive pain feels sharp, aching, or throbbing.

**Radicular pain** is pain that radiates from the back and hip into the legs through the spine. The pain travels along the spinal nerve root. Radicular pain occurs when the spinal nerve gets compressed (pinched) or inflamed.

 **Memory Jogger**

- There are 5 types of pain: acute, chronic, neuropathic, nociceptive, and radicular.
- *Acute pain* is usually related to an injury, such as recent surgery, trauma, or infection, and it ends within an expected time frame. It triggers the stress response.
- *Chronic pain* is any pain that continues beyond the expected time frame of an acute injury process. It does not trigger the stress response because the body adapts to the pain sensation over time.

Pain is also classified by the duration of time, and the specific sensations and causes of the pain (Table 12.1). Some pain is present constantly, or pain can come and go (is *intermittent*). For example, cancer pain has many causes and sensations that can influence the times when pain is felt and how intense the pain sensation is. Cancer pain is complex and often requires more than one drug type to manage it.

## HOW PAIN IS PERCEIVED

Pain is recognized (felt or perceived) in the brain rather than in the body area where it occurs. When a body part is injured, such as when you drop a hammer on your toe, the toe is injured. This injury stimulates pain nerve endings in the toe that send (transmit) electrical nerve impulses as a signal from the toe along nerves to the spinal cord. At the spinal cord, the original signal is transferred to special pain nerve tracts and travels up the spinal cord to the area of the brain where toe activity is located. The signal is then transferred to the

## Table 12.1   Classification of Pain

| CATEGORY | CHARACTERISTICS | EXAMPLE |
|---|---|---|
| Acute | Sudden onset; has a specific cause; triggers the stress response with changes in breathing, heart rate, blood pressure; improves with time and healing | Postsurgical pain, traumatic injury, bone fracture, infection |
| Chronic | Continues beyond the usual course of an acute injury process; may not have an identifiable cause; does not trigger the stress response; is usually present continuously | Arthritis pain, sciatica, shingles |
| Continuous | Always present but may vary in intensity | Sciatica |
| Intermittent | Comes and goes | Abdominal cramping from constipation or intestinal irritation |
| Nociceptive | Specific to a body area that is easy to identify and describe; words used to describe often include *aching* and *throbbing* | Cuts, fractures, arthritis |
| Visceral | Hard to locate, may be referred to more distant sites than the cause of the pain; often described as continual aching | Pain under the right shoulder blade with gallstone disease |
| Radicular | Pain that radiates from the back and hip to legs through the spine, traveling along the spinal nerve root; leg pain can be accompanied by numbness, tingling, and muscle weakness | Herniated disc |
| Neuropathic | Sharp, shooting, stabbing, and burning sensations | Diabetic neuropathy, trigeminal neuralgia, pain with shingles |
| Cancer pain | Often includes all specific types of pain with multiple causes (e.g., organ compression, tissue stretching, nerve compression, bone pain); complex; requires multiple types of agents for best relief | Usually advanced cancers that have spread beyond the original site and are pressing on nerves and/or organs, putting pressure on the inside of bones, secreting chemicals that make pain receptors more sensitive, causing inflammation |

brain, and you become aware of (perceive or feel) the pain in your toe (Fig. 12.1).

You perceive pain only in the brain, and anything that interferes with transmission of the pain signal from your toe along the nerves to and within your brain can change how and whether you perceive the pain. So if you had a stroke that damaged the part of the brain where toe pain would be perceived, you would not feel the pain. If the pain nerve tracts in the spinal cord were severed, you would not feel the pain in your toe even though the injury is severe. Also, if the nerves in your leg were severed, the pain signals would not reach the brain and you would not feel the toe pain.

*Anxiety, depression, fatigue, and other chronic diseases may increase the perception of pain.* Activities that distract the patient, create positive attitudes, or provide support may reduce the perception of pain. These activities include listening to music, massage therapy, cold or hot packs, hydrotherapy, acupuncture, biofeedback, relaxation therapy, art therapy, hypnosis, therapeutic touch, Qigong or Reiki energy therapies, and use of transcutaneous electrical nerve stimulation (TENS) units. These nondrug therapy techniques typically are used together with analgesics for optimal pain management.

## PRINCIPLES OF PAIN MANAGEMENT

Based on the idea that pain is a very unpleasant sensation that requires relief, the Agency for Healthcare Research and Quality (AHRQ) has developed specific principles for pain management regardless of the source or type of pain:

- *Ask* about pain on a regular basis. Drugs are to be given regularly and are more effective if given *before* the patient is in severe pain and miserable. Substance use disorder (addiction) is usually not a concern for patients with a terminal illness.
- *Assess* pain systematically. Use pain intensity scales (Figs. 12.2, 12.3, and 12.4).
- *Believe* the patient and family's reports of pain, its occurrence and intensity, and what relieves it.
- *Choose* analgesic and nonpharmacological pain-management options that are appropriate for the patient, family, and setting. Discuss the wishes of the patient and family with the RN and healthcare provider.
- *Deliver* pain relief interventions in a timely, logical, and coordinated fashion.
- *Empower* patients and their families to discuss pain relief needs with the healthcare provider.
- *Enable* patients to manage their pain to the greatest extent possible.

## ANALGESIC DRUGS FOR PAIN MANAGEMENT

Many nerve paths carry the sensation of pain from the pain site to the brain. This means that there are different places to block or alter the sensation of pain. Some milder forms of pain may be relieved by nondrug therapies such as exercise, heat, ice or cold compresses, music, massage, diversion techniques, sedation, and rest; changing the room to be quieter, darker, or cooler; or other methods, such as herbal poultices or acupuncture. Severe pain often requires a management strategy using a combination of nondrug and drug therapies.

A wide range of drugs are used in managing pain. Some of these drugs are actual **analgesics**, drugs that have the specific purpose of relieving pain by changing the patient's perception of pain or by reducing painful stimulation at its source. The word *analgesia* means absence of the sensation of pain. The analgesic categories are *opioid agonists* (narcotics), *opioid agonist-antagonists*, *nonopioid centrally acting analgesics*, and *miscellaneous analgesics*, which include drugs with other purposes that also help reduce pain. The specific drug prescribed depends on the type of pain being experienced; its cause, intensity, and expected duration; and the patient's perception of the pain.

Opioid agonists are drugs that bind to opioid receptors and provide pain relief. An opioid antagonist is a drug that binds to the opioid receptors (i.e., mu-, kappa-, or delta-opioid receptors) and blocks opioid agonists from reaching them, preventing a response.

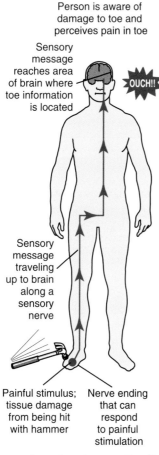

Fig. 12.1 A sensory pathway for pain perception. (From Workman, M. L., & LaCharity, L. A. (2016). *Understanding pharmacology* (2nd ed.). Elsevier.)

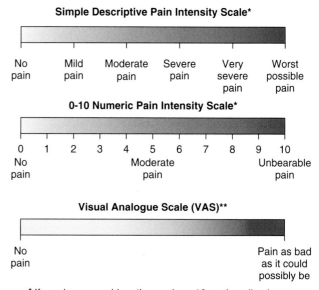

Fig. 12.2 Common pain measurement scales. (From Black, J. M., & Hawks, J. H. (2009). *Medical-surgical nursing: Clinical management for positive outcomes* (8th ed.). Elsevier.)

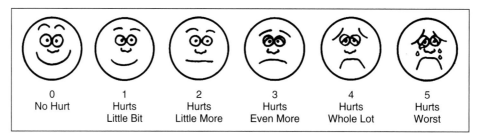

**Brief word instructions:** Point to each face using the words to describe the pain intensity. Ask the child to choose the face that best describes own pain and record the appropriate number.

Fig. 12.3 Wong-Baker FACES Pain Rating Scale. (Copyright 1983, Wong-Baker FACES Foundation, www.WongBakerFACES.org. Used with permission. Originally published in *Whaley & Wong's nursing care of infants and children*. © Elsevier Inc.)

| Category | Score | | |
|---|---|---|---|
| | **0** | **1** | **2** |
| Face | No particular expression or smile | Occasional grimace or frown, withdrawn, disinterested | Frequent-to-constant quivering chin, clenched jaw |
| Legs | Normal position or relaxed | Uneasy, restless, tense | Kicking, or legs drawn up |
| Activity | Lying quietly, normal position, moves easily | Squirming, shifting back and forth, tense | Arched, rigid, or jerking |
| Cry | No cry (awake or asleep) | Moans or whimpers, occasional complaint | Crying steadily, screams or sobs, or frequent complaints |
| Consolability | Content, relaxed | Reassured by occasional touching, hugging, or being talked to, distractible | Difficult to console or comfort |

Each of the five categories–(F) Face, (L) Legs, (A) Activity, (C) Cry, (C) Consolability–
is scored from 0-2, which results in a total score between 0 and 10.

**Fig. 12.4** The FLACC pain rating scale for infants and patients who are not alert. (From Workman, M. L., & LaCharity, L. A. (2023). *Understanding pharmacology* (3rd ed.). Elsevier.)

### Memory Jogger

There are four main categories of drugs used for pain management:
- Opioid agonists
- Opioid agonist-antagonists
- Nonopioid centrally acting analgesics
- Miscellaneous analgesics

## OPIOID AGONIST ANALGESICS

Many drugs used for managing severe pain are opioids. An **opioid** (also called a *narcotic*) is any substance derived from natural opium (extracted from the poppy plant) or chemically similar to opium that alters the perception of pain and has the potential to induce dependence and misuse. Opioid agonists include chemicals such as morphine, codeine, and heroin. In addition to natural opioids, synthetic opioids have been developed by drug companies. Both natural and synthetic opioids are useful for pain management. Morphine is the basic chemical from which the synthetic opioid analgesics hydrocodone, hydromorphone, fentanyl, and oxycodone have been developed. All natural and synthetic opioids are *high-alert drugs* because they have an increased risk of causing patient harm if given in error.

Opioids and opioid agonists have a relatively high potential for abuse. In efforts to limit the abuse of these drugs, the U.S. government has developed regulations that describe who may prescribe or give opioids (Chapter 2). In order to practice legally, you are responsible for knowing and following the regulations for LPN/VNs giving opioids in your state. Nurses have the responsibility for keeping opioids in a safe place, typically a locked cabinet, and accounting for their use in the hospital or long-term care setting.

As stated, morphine is the main opioid agonist analgesic, and it is the drug with which all other pain-management drugs are compared for effectiveness.

Table 12.2 shows the equianalgesic dosages needed for common opioid agonists to achieve equal pain relief. Although different opioid agonist analgesics vary by strength (some are stronger than morphine, and some are not as strong as morphine), they all work in the same way and have the same side effects and adverse reactions.

Morphine and other strong opioid agonists are used often in acute care, cancer care, and hospice settings for patients who have severe pain. Codeine, hydrocodone (Vicodin, Lortab), and oxycodone (OxyContin) are weaker than morphine and are often used in combination with acetaminophen in the outpatient setting. Hydromorphone (Dilaudid) is much stronger than morphine. Table 12.3 lists dosages and nursing considerations for common opioid agonists.

### Memory Jogger

Strong opioid agonist analgesics such as hydromorphone and fentanyl require less drug (lower doses given less often) to achieve the same level of pain relief as weaker opioid agonist analgesics.

### Action

The human brain has opioid receptors to make its own internal opioids to provide some pain relief and an increased sense of well-being when the person is physically stressed. The morphinelike chemicals produced in the brain are the *endorphins*, *enkephalins*, and *dynorphins*. Think about the jogger who runs for 10 miles, looks terrible, but feels wonderful. How is this possible? In response to the physical stress and hard work of running 10 miles, the brain makes much more of these substances, which then bind to and activate specific opioid receptors in the brain to change the runner's perception from discomfort and pain to comfort. These internal opioids are **opioid agonists** because

| Table 12.2 | Equianalgesic Adult Doses of Common Opioid Agonists and Opioid Agonist-Antagonists |
|---|---|
| **DRUG** | **EQUIANALGESIC DOSE[a]** |
| **Opioid Agonists** | |
| Morphine | 30 mg (oral) 10 mg (parenteral) |
| codeine (many brand-name combination drugs) | 200 mg (oral) NOT recommended 120 (parenteral) |
| fentanyl (Actiq, Apo-fentanyl ♣, Duragesic, Lazanda) | 0.2 mg (transdermal patch) 0.1 mg (parenteral) |
| hydrocodone (Hycet, Lortab, Norco, Vicodin, and many brand-name combination drugs) | 30 mg (oral) |
| hydromorphone (Dilaudid, Apo-Hydromorphone ♣) | 7.5 mg (oral) 1.5 mg (parenteral) |
| oxycodone (Endocodone, Oxaydo, OxyContin) | 20 mg (oral) |
| oxymorphone (Numorphan, Opana) | 10 mg (oral) 1 mg (parenteral) |
| **Opioid Agonist-Antagonists** | |
| buprenorphine (Buprenex, Probuphine) | 0.4 mg (parenteral) |
| butorphanol (Stadol) | 2 mg (parenteral) |
| nalbuphine (Nubain) | 10 mg (parenteral) |
| pentazocine (Talwin) | 150 mg (oral) 60 mg (parenteral) |

[a]Equianalgesic doses provide about the same degree of pain relief as 30 mg of oral morphine.

they activate (turn on) the opioid receptors to change a person's perception of discomfort and pain. External opioids that are given for pain relief also bind to opioid receptors and perform as agonists to activate the opioid receptors. (You may need to review the actions of agonists, antagonists, and receptors that were discussed in Chapter 3.)

Morphine and all opioid agonist analgesics work by binding to opioid receptor sites in the brain and other areas. The main opioid receptors are named *mu, kappa,* and *delta*. When an agonist drug binds to and activates mu receptors, the responses include pain relief, some degree of respiratory depression with slower breathing, some sleepiness or sedation, decreased intestinal motility with constipation, pupil constriction, lower blood pressure, and *euphoria* (feeling of emotional happiness). When an agonist binds to and activate kappa receptors, the responses include some pain relief, sedation, pupil constriction, and *dysphoria* (feeling of emotional or mental discomfort, restlessness, and anxiety). When an agonist binds to and activates delta receptors, the responses include some pain relief, dysphoria, and hallucinations.

### Memory Jogger

There are three types of opioid receptors:
- Mu
- Kappa
- Delta

Opioid receptor agonists act primarily at the mu receptors found in the brain, spinal cord, and sensory neurons.

| Table 12.3 | Examples of Common Opioid Agonists |
|---|---|
| **ALL *OPIOID AGONISTS* BIND MU-OPIOID RECEPTOR SITES (ACTIVATING THEM) IN THE BRAIN AND OTHER AREAS, CHANGING THE PERSON'S PERCEPTION OF PAIN.** | |
| **DRUG/ADULT DOSAGE** | **NURSING IMPLICATIONS** |
| codeine 15–60 mg every 4 hours (oral and parenteral) fentanyl (Actiq, Apo-fentanyl ♣, Duragesic, Lazanda) 50–100 mcg IM or by slow IV over 1–2 minutes; 12–100 mcg/hour by transdermal patch hydrocodone (Hycet, Lortab, Norco, Vicodin, and many brand-name combination drugs) 10–40 mg orally every 12 hours hydromorphone (Dilaudid, Apo-Hydromorphone ♣) 2–4 mg orally every 4–6 hours; 0.2–1 mg IV every 2–3 hours morphine 2–4 mg orally every 4–6 hours; 0.2–1 mg IV every 2–3 hours oxycodone (Endocodone, Oxaydo, OxyContin) 5–30 mg every 4 hours (immediate release); 10 mg every 12 hours (extended release) oxymorphone (Numorphan, Opana) 5–20 mg orally every 4–6 hours; 0.5–1.5 every 4–6 hours parenterally | • Reassess the patient's level of pain within 1 hour after giving an opioid to determine its effectiveness. <br> • During periods of acute pain, encourage the patient to take the drug on the prescribed schedule for best pain relief. Assess elimination status daily because all opioids cause constipation. <br> • Assess respiratory rate and pulse oximetry frequently because opioids can cause respiratory depression. <br> • If patients cannot be aroused, have respirations below 8 breaths/min, have severe hypotension, or develop hypothermia, notify the healthcare provider immediately to prevent coma or death. <br> • Patients may also be prescribed stimulant laxatives because of the high incidence of constipation common with opioids. <br> • Instruct patients who are taking extended-release tablets or capsules not to chew, open, crush, bite, or cut them to prevent rapid absorption of excess drug. <br> • Instruct patients not to drink alcohol or take other CNS depressants while taking an opioid analgesic because the CNS effects are intensified. <br> • Change fentanyl patches and rotate sites at least every 72 hours and wash the skin under the old patch to prevent excess drug absorption. |

*CNS,* central nervous system; *IM,* intramuscular; *IV,* intravenous.

Morphine binds most tightly and best to the mu receptor, acting as an agonist. This activates the mu receptors, and the person's perception of pain is changed. *Opioid agonists change only the perception of pain; they do nothing at the site of injured tissue to reduce the cause of pain.* Some drugs act as agonists at one type of opioid receptor but act as antagonists at another type of opioid receptor, producing mixed responses. The opioids that provide the best pain relief bind most strongly (tightly) to the mu receptors. Pain drugs that are strong opioid agonists include morphine, hydromorphone, oxymorphone, and fentanyl. Those that bind moderately well to the mu receptors and provide some degree of pain relief include codeine, hydrocodone, and oxycodone.

 **Memory Jogger**

Strong opioid agonist analgesics include:
- morphine
- hydromorphone
- oxymorphone
- fentanyl

## Uses

Opioid agonists are used to manage moderate to severe acute pain and chronic pain. They may be used preoperatively (before surgery), to treat pain from injury or other disease processes, for constant and severe cough (codeine), and for postoperative pain. Opioids are available as oral tablets, capsules, lozenges, and liquids; as intravenous and other parenteral solutions for injection; and some (e.g., fentanyl) as a slow, continuous-release transdermal (skin) patch.

Some opioids are commonly available as combination products along with drugs such as acetaminophen, aspirin, caffeine, and barbital. This allows a small dose of opioid to be combined with other chemicals to relieve symptoms or calm the patient. There are also long-acting (sustained or extended release) opioid drugs that are given every 12 hours to manage more severe, chronic pain, such as cancer-related pain. Even so, this type of pain often requires additional short-acting opioids to manage breakthrough pain. Breakthrough pain is a sudden increase in pain that may occur in patients who have chronic pain treated with a long-acting pain medication.

## Expected Side Effects

The two most common side effects of opioid agonists are *sedation* (sleepiness) and *constipation*. Other expected reactions to opioid agonist analgesics include *bradycardia* (slower heartbeat), hypotension (low blood pressure), decreased respirations, *anorexia* (lack of appetite), dry mouth, and *euphoria* (sense of happiness). Most patients, especially older adults, have decreased pupil size *(miosis)* and are at increased risk for falling. All patients beginning opioids should have orders for stool softeners and/or laxatives to prevent severe constipation from opioids.

## Adverse Reactions

Serious adverse reactions include very slow, shallow breathing *(bradypnea)*, also known as *respiratory depression*; severe hypotension; decreased urine output *(oliguria)*; below-normal body temperature *(hypothermia)*; excessive sedation or coma; and cool, clammy skin. These serious reactions may indicate overdose and require immediate medical attention. The drug dose should be lowered, or the drug discontinued when any serious reaction occurs.

 **Top Tip for Safety**

Serious adverse reactions and symptoms of overdose for opioid agonist analgesics require immediate medical attention:
- Respirations of 8 breaths/min or less
- Very low blood pressure
- Excessive sedation or coma
- Below-normal body temperature

If a serious adverse reaction or an overdose occurs with an opioid agonist, the effects can be reversed by giving an intravenous, intramuscular, or subcutaneous opioid antagonist such as naloxone (Narcan) or naltrexone (Revia, Vivitrol). They work by binding tightly to the mu-opioid receptors and blocking them, preventing opioid agonists from binding with them. In an emergency, these drugs can be given without a prescription. Naloxone is also available as an intranasal spray, but this route is not as reliable as the parenteral route.

## Opioid-Induced Constipation
- Opioids slow emptying of the stomach and peristalsis in the GI tract, resulting in hard stools and constipation.
- Symptoms of opioid-induced constipation include bloating, constipation alternating with diarrhea, nausea, vomiting, and impacted stool.
- Stool softeners (docusate) can prevent constipation, but they do not treat it.
- Laxatives such as bisacodyl can be prescribed for prevention and treatment of constipation from opioids.

 **Lifespan Considerations**

**Older Adults**

Older adults are more likely to have some degree of liver or kidney impairment that reduces their ability to metabolize and excrete opioid agonists. This makes them more sensitive to the drugs, and normal doses can cause serious adverse reactions. Older adults may require doses to be lowered or the drugs to be given less frequently. Constipation from opioids can be more severe in older adults because of decreased activity and lower fluid or fiber intake.

**Infants**

There is evidence to support the use of facial expressions, body movements, heart rate, and oxygen saturation to assess acute pain in infants.

## Tolerance, Dependence, and Substance Use Disorder (Addiction)

Tolerance is a condition that occurs when the body gets used to a medicine such that the same amount of drug has less effect over time and either more or different medicine is needed. Although tolerance can happen with any drug, it is most often seen with opioid agonists. Tolerance occurs because the body gradually increases the rate at which it degrades and eliminates the drug. In the case of pain, higher doses are needed for relief. Dependence can be physical, psychological, or both. In physical drug dependence, the body relies on the drug, so that withdrawal symptoms occur when the drug is stopped, or a reversing agent is given. Physical dependency requires higher levels of the drug to keep withdrawal symptoms away. Psychological dependence affects the person's mental and emotional well-being. Both physical and psychological dependence can present as drug cravings, restlessness, depression, irregular sleep, inability to stop taking the substance, obsessing about obtaining the drug or substance, and denial about the problem.

Withdrawal symptoms are changes in the body or mind, such as nausea or anxiety, that occur when a drug is stopped or reduced after regular use. Tapering off (slowly taking less of the drug) can reduce withdrawal symptoms. Psychological dependence, or substance use disorder (addiction), is the desperate need to have and use a drug for a nonmedical reason. The addicted person has a limited ability to control this drug craving or use. Drug misuse is the use of illegal drugs and/or the use of prescription drugs in a manner other than as directed by a doctor, such as use in greater amounts, more often, or longer than told to take a drug, or using someone else's prescription.

Tolerance and dependence result from regular use of an opioid for a certain length of time and should not be confused with or labeled as substance use disorder. Substance use disorder is a problem; however, a patient in pain should not be denied pain relief because of fear of substance use disorder. Before beginning opioid therapy for noncancer pain management, recent guidelines recommend obtaining thorough medical and social histories, including tobacco and alcohol use, and a family history of substance use disorder. All opioid agonists have the potential to cause tolerance and dependence, which are not the same as substance use disorder or abuse, when taken on a long-term basis.

*Opioid misuse disorder.* In recent years the use of opioid pain relievers has increased dramatically. Among people ages 12 or older in 2019, 3.7 percent (10.1 million people) misused opioids in the past year, with 9.7 million reporting misuse of prescription pain relievers. Risk factors for opioid misuse or addiction include past or current substance abuse, untreated mental health problems, younger age, and social or family environments that support misuse. Opioids are highly addictive because they induce euphoria (pleasure) and cessation of chronic use produces dysphoria (negative feelings). Chronic exposure to opioids results in changes in the part of the brain that controls impulse, reward, and motivation. The disease of opioid misuse arises from repeated exposure to opioids and can occur in individuals using prescription opioids to relieve pain and in nonmedical users of opioids. Many different strategies can be used to decrease opioid use. Drugs that have been effective for treating opioid misuse disorder include methadone (an opioid agonist), buprenorphine (a partial agonist), and naltrexone (an opioid antagonist). Methadone and buprenorphine act to decrease opioid withdrawal symptoms. Naltrexone works by blocking the mu-opioid receptor, preventing the action of any opioids used. Oral methadone has the strongest evidence for effective treatment of opioid misuse.

National medical societies have developed clinical practice guidelines for pain management that incorporate the use of patient education and nonopioid drugs to combat opioid abuse.

### Drug Interactions

Along with pain relief, decreased pupil size, sedation, dry mouth, and euphoria are the central nervous system (CNS) effects of opioid agonists. These effects can be intensified and made worse when the patient also uses certain other substances or drugs that act on the CNS, such as alcohol, antianxiety drugs, skeletal muscle relaxants, barbiturates, drugs used for psychiatric disorders, and other opioid agonists.

> **⌂ Top Tip for Safety**
>
> The sedation and slowed breathing caused by opioid agonist analgesics are intensified and made worse when the patient also drinks alcohol or uses antianxiety drugs, skeletal muscle relaxants, barbiturates, many of the drugs used for psychiatric disorders, or other opioid agonists. Determine which other prescription and nonprescription drugs the patient takes to prevent adverse drug interactions.

### ❖ Nursing Implications and Patient Teaching

◆ *Assessment.* The first step in addressing a patient's pain report is to determine the type and cause of the pain.

Ask the patient to describe the location of the pain, the type of pain (Table 12.1), pain characteristics (sharp, burning, stabbing, dull), and pain intensity. A pain scale is used to assess pain intensity (severity). Fig. 12.2 shows several examples of pain rating scales for patients who are alert to indicate how much pain they are having. Fig. 12.3 shows an example of a pain rating scale for children and adults who may have trouble expressing their thoughts. Ask the patient what drugs or other actions have been taken to relieve the pain, as well as what may make the pain better or worse. Ask the patient whether he or she has ever received morphine (or another opioid agonist) in the past and what, if any, problems occurred with its use. When opioids are first prescribed, ask the patient about current tobacco and alcohol use, past substance use disorder, drug misuse, or any family history of substance misuse.

---

### 🍃 Lifespan Considerations
#### Pediatric Patients: Pain Assessment

Children experience pain in the same way as adults, but young children may have difficulty communicating their level of discomfort. Use an age-appropriate rating scale to assess pain in younger pediatric patients. When assessing pain in infants, pay attention to the infant's position (especially whether the legs are drawn up), facial expression, crying pattern, sleep/rest cycles, interest in eating, and how easily he or she can be consoled (Fig. 12.4). Compare these observations with those obtained when the infant appears to be comfortable.

---

◆ *Planning and implementation.* Opioid agonists are used in the treatment of severe pain conditions. Opioid agonists work better when given on a schedule rather than waiting until the patient asks for them. Usually, oral opioid agonist analgesics begin to take effect in 15 to 30 minutes. For intramuscular (IM) preparations, the onset of action is about 8 minutes with a duration of about 2 hours. When opioid agonists are given intravenous (IV), it is immediately absorbed into the body and begins working to relieve pain almost instantly with a peak effect in 5 to 10 minutes. IV preparations have a duration of action of 2 to 4 hours—the reason for this is that scheduled dosing results in more stable opioid blood levels, better pain relief, fewer side effects, fewer pain behaviors, and lower addiction risk. When the patient asks for another dose of a prescribed opioid agonist, check to see when the patient received his or her most recent dose to determine whether another dose can be given at that time. If a patient taking a sustained-release or long-acting opioid agonist reports pain before the next scheduled dose, the patient may require a short-acting opioid agonist for breakthrough pain. Report your findings to the RN or healthcare provider.

Check the prescribed drug name and dose carefully before giving it to the patient. Opioid agonists are not interchangeable because drug strength varies across the different formulations. Only the prescribing healthcare provider can change the order. Be sure to sign out the dose as required by the Drug Enforcement Administration (DEA) of the U.S. government.

If this is the *first* dose of an opioid agonist the patient is to receive, check his or her respiratory rate and oxygen saturation before giving the drug because these drugs can cause respiratory depression. This action is especially important for older patients and those who are receiving higher doses.

Most patients become drowsy with opioid agonists, and it is important to ensure that the bed's upper side rails are raised and the call light is in reach. If the patient is in a chair, remind him or her to call for assistance to avoid falls from drowsiness or low blood pressure when moving from a sitting or lying position to standing.

◆ *Evaluation.* Be sure to check the patient for pain relief and for changes in respiratory rate and depth. Report any concerns about decreases in respiratory status to the RN or healthcare provider. Ask the patient to rate their pain intensity using a validated pain scale when pain relief may be expected. Recheck at least every hour. If pain relief is not obtained or is not sufficient to keep the patient comfortable, report this to the prescriber so that changes in pain management can be made. Higher doses and/or more frequent dosing may be needed.

Opioid agonist analgesics may slow the respiratory rate and decrease cough reflexes. Patients who have a history of smoking and who have had surgery may develop areas where the lungs do not inflate well (*atelectasis*) or where fluid may collect and pneumonia may develop. Therefore frequent position changes and encouraging patients to take deep breaths and ambulate as soon as possible are recommended.

If the patient will be receiving an opioid agonist for 2 days or longer, be sure the patient has an order for stool softener and/or a laxative and give the order as prescribed. Ask the patient daily about the presence of constipation because this is a very common side effect of these drugs

◆ *Patient and family teaching.* Tell the patient and family:
- It is important to only take this drug as prescribed. Do not change the frequency or dosage without consulting with your healthcare provider. For acute pain, it is most effective to take the drug before you have severe pain and on a regular schedule, if possible. Write down the time when the drug was last taken to prevent taking too much by accident.
- To avoid any adverse drug interactions, be sure to tell your healthcare provider about all the other drugs you are taking.
- Avoid drinking alcohol. Alcohol increases the effects of opioids, and taking both together may lead to serious adverse reactions.
- Report any unrelieved pain or new symptoms or problems to your healthcare provider.
- Change positions slowly to prevent dizziness and falling caused by a rapid drop in blood pressure.
- Do not drive, operate heavy machinery, or make important decisions while under the influence of opioids because your judgment may be impaired.
- Increase fluid (water) and fiber-rich foods (fruits, vegetables, bran) intake and, at the very least, maintain physical activity to prevent constipation. Use prescribed stool softeners or laxatives to prevent severe constipation.

- Take oral opioids with food to prevent nausea. If nausea persists, inform your healthcare provider as an antiemetic (drug that prevents vomiting) may be needed.
- If the opioid prescribed is an extended-release tablet or capsule, do not cut it in half, chew it, or crush it because the time-release feature will be ruined and too much drug may be absorbed too quickly, causing severe adverse reactions.
- If the drug is in a transdermal patch, place the patch on intact skin of the upper arm, cheek, or back. Be careful to avoid coming in contact with the drug. Remove any old patches. Wash your hands after applying the patch.
- Do not allow anyone else except the patient to use the drug, and keep all opioids out of the reach of children and others to prevent misuse and abuse.

## OPIOID AGONIST-ANTAGONIST ANALGESICS

An **opioid agonist-antagonist analgesic** is a pain-management drug that has mixed actions at opioid receptor sites. Although these drugs are not as strong as opioid agonist analgesics, they are thought to have a lower risk for substance use disorder or abuse because of some of the side effects.

### Action

Four opioid agonist-antagonists are available for pain relief (Table 12.4). An agonist-antagonist is a drug that binds to a receptor that produces pain relief (agonist effect) and binds another receptor that does not produce a physiologic effect (antagonist effect). Three of them (pentazocine, nalbuphine, and butorphanol) act as antagonists at mu-opioid receptors and as agonists at kappa-opioid receptors. This action makes them less effective for pain control than pure opioid agonists. They do provide pain relief because of activation of the kappa receptors along with sedation (see Opioid Agonist Analgesics).

The fourth drug, buprenorphine, is different because it acts as a partial agonist at mu receptors and as an antagonist at kappa receptors. This allows buprenorphine to have greater pain relief potential than the other three drugs and less dysphoria. The sensation of dysphoria, which is a state of emotional or mental discomfort, restlessness, and anxiety, is unpleasant and decreases the likelihood that patients would want to use these drugs when they are not in pain.

**Memory Jogger**

There are four opioid agonist-antagonist analgesics:
- pentazocine
- nalbuphine
- butorphanol
- buprenorphine

### Uses

Opioid agonist-antagonist analgesics are used to relieve mild to moderate pain. They are less useful for severe pain. Pentazocine is available in oral and parenteral forms. The three that are antagonists at the mu-opioid sites raise only limited concerns about respiratory depression. Buprenorphine also causes less respiratory depression than pure opioid agonists because it only partially binds mu receptors.

Nalbuphine and butorphanol are sometimes used to manage pain during labor and delivery. Butorphanol may be prescribed as a metered-dose nasal spray for management of migraine headaches.

### Expected Side Effects

Common mild side effects are similar to those for morphine. They include sedation, constipation, and constricted pupils.

### Adverse Reactions

Higher doses of opioid agonist-antagonist analgesics are associated with nightmares and hallucinations. The opioid agonist-antagonists can cause serious cardiac reactions. Pentazocine, nalbuphine, and butorphanol excite the cardiac system, making the heart work harder and elevating blood pressure. They should not

## Table 12.4   Examples of Common Opioid Agonist-Antagonist Analgesics

| MOST *OPIOID AGONIST-ANTAGONIST ANALGESICS* ANTAGONIZE (BLOCK) MU-OPIOID RECEPTORS AND CHANGE THE PERCEPTION OF PAIN BY ACTIVATING KAPPA-OPIOID RECEPTORS. BUPRENORPHINE IS A PARTIAL MU-RECEPTOR AGONIST. | |
| --- | --- |
| **DRUG/ADULT DOSAGE** | **NURSING IMPLICATIONS** |
| buprenorphine (Buprenex, Probuphine) 0–3 mg IM or IV every 6–8 hours<br>butorphanol (Stadol) 1–4 mg IM or 0.5–2 mg IV every 3–4 hours<br>nalbuphine (Nubain) 10 mg IM, IV, or subcutaneously every 3–6 hours<br>pentazocine (Talwin) 30 mg IV or 30 mg IM or subcutaneously every 3–4 hours | • Reassess the patient's level of pain within 1 hour after giving an opioid agonist-antagonist to determine its effectiveness.<br>• Assess the patient's emotional responses because butorphanol, nalbuphine, and pentazocine can cause dysphoria, anxiety, nightmares, and hallucinations.<br>• Assess blood pressure and heart rate and rhythm frequently because these drugs can excite the cardiac system and cause dysrhythmias.<br>• Avoid the use of butorphanol, nalbuphine, and pentazocine in a patient who is physically dependent on an opioid agonist because blocking the mu receptor can cause withdrawal symptoms. |

*IM,* intramuscular; *IV,* intravenous.

be used in patients with suspected myocardial infarction (heart attack), and they should be used carefully in those with heart failure. Buprenorphine can cause serious cardiac dysrhythmias and should not be used for patients who have other serious dysrhythmias. Although respiratory depression is possible with these drugs, it is not common.

Use of pentazocine, butorphanol, or nalbuphine in a patient who is *physically dependent* on morphine or other opioid agonists will cause withdrawal symptoms because they block mu receptors. Use of these three drugs in a patient who is physically dependent on opioid agonists should be avoided.

### Drug Interactions

The sedating effect of these drugs is made worse with alcohol, antianxiety drugs, skeletal muscle relaxants, barbiturates, many drugs used for psychiatric disorders, and pure opioid agonists. Be sure to determine and record all other drugs the patient takes.

### ❖ Nursing Implications and Patient Teaching

◆ *Assessment.* Assess the patient's pain in the same way as for opioid agonists or other pain-management drugs. Ask the patient whether he or she has ever taken any of these specific drugs and, if so, whether any problems resulted. Ask what other OTC (OTC) and prescribed drugs the patient has taken in the past 24 hours, especially opioid agonist analgesics. Monitor the patient for pain relief and any potential adverse effects.

◆ *Planning and implementation.* Planning, implementation, evaluation, and patient and family teaching activities are the same as for opioid analgesics.

### NONOPIOID CENTRALLY ACTING ANALGESICS

A nonopioid centrally acting analgesic is a drug that works in the CNS to help manage pain but does not interact with opioid receptors to do so. The two most commonly used drugs in this class are clonidine (Duraclon) and tramadol (Ultram, Ryzolt).

 **Memory Jogger**

There are two common nonopioid centrally acting analgesics:
• clonidine
• tramadol

### Action

Clonidine and tramadol have completely different mechanisms of action for pain relief. Clonidine is an antihypertensive drug most commonly used to lower blood pressure. It works for pain management by binding to specific receptors (alpha-adrenergic receptors) in the spinal cord and blocking their activity. This action keeps signals from the source of pain from traveling to the brain. As a result, fewer pain signals reach the brain to be perceived as pain. Clonidine does not change the conditions at the source of the pain.

Although it has a chemical structure similar to codeine, tramadol has only weak effects at opioid receptors. Instead, it works by blocking (inhibiting) the action of some neurotransmitters in the spinal cord and areas of the brain, which reduces pain signal transmission to areas of the brain that perceive pain. The usual adult dosage for tramadol ranges from 50 to 100 mg orally every 6 hours (immediate-release tablets) or from 100 to 200 mg every 12 hours (extended-release capsules).

### Uses

Clonidine formulated for pain management (Duraclon) is approved for severe pain (often cancer pain) and is given as a continuous epidural infusion. It is indicated as a combination with opioids for cancer patients experiencing severe pain that is not controlled with opioids alone. It is not a controlled substance because it is considered to have no potential for substance use disorder or abuse. The oral formulation (Catapres) is only for blood pressure control and does not have a role in pain management.

Tramadol is an oral drug used for moderate or moderately severe acute pain. It is only as effective as codeine (not as effective as morphine) and is often used along with acetaminophen. Tramadol is used to relieve moderate to moderately severe pain, including pain after surgery. The extended-release capsules or tablets are used for chronic ongoing pain.

### Expected Side Effects

Clonidine dilates blood vessels, which can lead to severe hypotension. It should not be used in patients who have low blood pressure. Tramadol has mild side effects of sedation, dizziness, dry mouth, and constipation.

### Adverse Reactions

Tramadol misuse or abuse has the potential to lead to severe adverse reactions, such as seizures. Seizures are most likely when large dosages are taken (usually 400 mg or more daily) for extended periods of time. Seizures are also more common when tramadol is taken with antidepressants. Tramadol should not be used in any patient who has epilepsy or any other neurologic disorder.

### Drug Interactions

Clonidine, because it is given for pain by the epidural route, has no direct drug interactions. However, if a patient also takes another drug for blood pressure management, epidural clonidine can make hypotension worse.

The sedating and other CNS effects of tramadol are made worse with alcohol, antianxiety drugs, skeletal muscle relaxants, barbiturates, many drugs used for psychiatric disorders, and opioid analgesics. Be sure to determine which other drugs the patient takes.

## ❖ Nursing Implications and Patient Teaching

◆ *Assessment.* Assess the patient's pain in the same way as for opioid agonists or other pain-management drugs. Ask the patient whether he or she has ever taken any of these specific drugs and whether any problems resulted from taking it. Ask what other over-the-counter and prescribed drugs the patient has taken in the past 24 hours. For tramadol, determine whether the patient has a known seizure disorder or other neurologic problem. If so, hold the dose and notify the prescribing healthcare provider.

Planning, implementation, evaluation, and patient and family teaching activities are the same as for opioid analgesics.

## MISCELLANEOUS DRUGS FOR PAIN MANAGEMENT

**Miscellaneous analgesics** are drugs that have specific uses for other health problems but can help provide relief for certain types of pain. These drugs can help reduce a person's perception of pain and often enhance the pain-management effectiveness of other analgesics. They may be used alone or in combination with opioids.

The most outstanding feature of nonopioid analgesics is that they are *not* chemically or structurally similar to opioids. As a result, they have less potential for dependence and misuse. Many nonopioid analgesics have other uses and are discussed in more detail elsewhere in this textbook. An overview of how they work and are used in pain control is provided in this section.

Regardless of category, nursing responsibilities when giving nonopioid analgesics are the same as those described for opioid agonists. Pain assessment and determination of effectiveness in managing pain are necessary.

 **Memory Jogger**

Several common miscellaneous drugs and classes of drugs are used for pain management:
- Acetaminophen
- Corticosteroids
- Nonsteroidal anti-inflammatory drugs
- Skeletal muscle relaxants
- Antidepressants
- Anticonvulsants

### ACETAMINOPHEN

Acetaminophen (Abenol, Atasol, Panadol, Tylenol, and many others) is a common drug used for pain relief. It can be purchased over the counter as a single drug or combined with other substances, such as acetaminophen with caffeine and aspirin (Excedrin). When combined with some pain-control drugs, especially opioid agonists, this acetaminophen formulation requires a prescription.

Acetaminophen can be given orally in chewable, tablet, capsule, or liquid form or given rectally in a suppository. A special formulation (Ofirmev) is available for intravenous infusion.

### Action

Acetaminophen acts only in the brain to reduce the production of prostaglandins, a chemical that can cause inflammation in other body areas. In the brain, prostaglandins increase the perception of pain. When the amount of prostaglandins in the brain is reduced, perception of pain is reduced. Acetaminophen does not act at the site of an injury that is causing pain and does not have anti-inflammatory effects.

### Uses

Acetaminophen alone is used to manage mild to moderate pain. It is often used for infants and children to reduce fever. In combination with other pain-controlling drugs, acetaminophen can help manage more severe pain. It is often used in place of aspirin or other nonsteroidal anti-inflammatory drugs (NSAIDs) for pain because acetaminophen does not increase the risk of bleeding. Children should not take aspirin because of its association with development of Reye's syndrome.

Acetaminophen comes in liquid, tablet, and capsule forms. The usual adult dose is 325 to 650 mg every 4 to 6 hours and should not exceed a total of 4 g per day. The usual dose for children weighing more than 60 kg (more than 132 lb) is 325 to 650 mg every 4 to 6 hours as needed for pain, not to exceed 4 g/day. For children weighing less than 60 kg give 10 to 15 mg/kg/dose orally every 4 to 6 hours as needed. For infants give 10 to 15 mg/kg/dose orally every 4 to 6 hours as needed. The maximum total daily dose for children varies with the child's weight. For neonates the dose is dependent on the age (in days) of the neonate.

 **Top Tip for Safety**

In adults, acetaminophen has a maximum total dose of 4 g per day to prevent liver damage.

### Expected Side Effects

Side effects of acetaminophen are rare when it is taken at the recommended dosages, although an allergic reaction is always possible. The most common side effects are nausea and skin rash.

### Adverse Reactions

Although acetaminophen is available without a prescription, it can have serious adverse effects. When taken at higher doses or for prolonged periods, acetaminophen is toxic to the liver, resulting in liver damage. The potential for liver toxicity is why there is a maximum total daily dose for this drug.

### Drug Interactions

Many common OTC drugs for sleep, colds, headaches, and allergies contain acetaminophen as one of the ingredients. These additional sources of acetaminophen must be added when calculating the total daily dose. Liver damage occurs more rapidly when acetaminophen is taken with alcohol.

 **Top Tip for Safety**

Acetaminophen can be toxic to the liver and should not be taken by anyone who already has liver damage.

Acetaminophen poisoning is among the most common causes of drug-related toxicity and death.

Acetaminophen poisoning can occur after taking one single overdosage or by taking repeated excessive doses over time.

N-acetylcysteine is the treatment for acetaminophen overdose. It works by binding the poisonous forms of acetaminophen that are formed in the liver.

### ❖ Nursing Implications and Patient Teaching

◆ *Assessment.* Assess the patient's pain location, severity, and frequency, and be sure to use a standardized pain scale. Ask the patient to report the dose and frequency of acetaminophen taken—you may have to use the most common brand name in your area, such as Tylenol—and ask whether any problems resulted from taking it. Ask what other OTC and prescribed drugs the patient has taken in the past 24 hours.

◆ *Planning and implementation.* Oral tablet or capsule acetaminophen comes in a variety of strengths. Liquid oral acetaminophen also comes in many strengths. Some liquid forms contain as few as 16 mg/mL, and others may contain as much as 70 mg/mL. *Carefully check the strength to ensure the correct dosage, especially for infants and children. If you are not sure of your dosage calculations, check with the healthcare provider or pharmacist.* Acetaminophen can be given with or without food because it does not increase the risk for stomach ulcers.

◆ *Evaluation.* Within 1 hour after giving acetaminophen, assess the patient's pain level to determine the effectiveness of the drug. Ask the patient about changes that may indicate sensitivity to acetaminophen, such as difficulty breathing or swallowing; swelling of the face, lips, throat, or tongue; hives; or severe itching.

◆ *Patient and family teaching.* Tell the patient and the family:
- Take acetaminophen as prescribed by your healthcare provider and not more often or at higher dosages.
- Many OTC sleep aids and drugs for colds, headache, and allergies contain acetaminophen, as do some other drugs prescribed for pain. The acetaminophen in these drugs must be figured into the total maximum daily dose of 3 g for an adult along with any separate acetaminophen sources.

- To prevent liver damage, do not drink alcoholic beverages on days when you take acetaminophen or any drug that contains acetaminophen.

**Lifespan Considerations**
**Pediatric Patients**

An infant or young child should never receive an adult dose of acetaminophen because it can cause severe liver toxicity. Teach parents to read the label on liquid acetaminophen bottles for infants and small children very carefully to ensure the correct dose for the child's size. Teach parents to call the nearest pharmacy and talk with the pharmacist to ensure that the dose is correct if they are unsure what dose to give.

### CORTICOSTEROIDS

When tissue injury occurs, the injured tissues release chemicals that start the inflammatory processes that causes pain. The released chemicals bind to pain receptors in the area and send pain signals along the nerve tracts to the brain. These chemicals also make the pain receptors more sensitive, so that even touching the inflamed area can increase the pain.

**Corticosteroids** are drugs with powerful anti-inflammatory actions that are chemically similar to the glucocorticoid hormones secreted by the adrenal glands. These drugs can greatly inhibit the production of mediators that result in the actions and symptoms of inflammation. However, they have many side effects and adverse reactions that limit their use for pain. The two most common oral corticosteroids used for pain are prednisone and methylprednisolone. Corticosteroids can be given intravenously, topically, or as an epidural injection (usually for acute back pain). Chapter 13 provides a complete discussion of the actions and uses of corticosteroids and the nursing responsibilities associated with their use.

### NONSTEROIDAL ANTI-INFLAMMATORY DRUGS

NSAIDs are nonopioid analgesics that have the main action of reducing inflammation. NSAIDs can help manage pain associated with inflammation, bone pain, cancer pain, and soft tissue trauma. Like corticosteroids, NSAIDs act in the tissue where pain starts, and they do not change a person's perception of pain.

NSAIDs help stop tissue production of the chemicals of inflammation and reduce the symptoms of inflammation (pain, warmth, redness, swelling, and reduced use) to the injured area. With inflammation reduced, pain also is reduced. Many NSAIDs are available over the counter and are commonly used for mild to moderate pain. Some of these same NSAIDs may also be formulated at higher doses per tablet or capsule; they and the stronger NSAIDs require a prescription and are used for pain for a limited period.

Mild NSAIDs include salicylic acid (aspirin), ibuprofen (Advil, Motrin), and naproxen (Aleve, Anaprox, Naprosyn). Stronger NSAIDs include oxaprozin (Daypro), indomethacin (Indocin), nabumetone (Relafen), ketorolac (Toradol), piroxicam (Feldene), celecoxib (Celebrex), and meloxicam (Mobic). All NSAIDs work in much the same way and have many of the same adverse effects. Chapter 13 discusses the actions and uses of NSAIDs and the associated nursing responsibilities.

The most common NSAID in use today is salicylic acid (aspirin), which is available over the counter. A side effect of aspirin and many other NSAIDs is increased risk of bleeding. Aspirin affects blood clotting longer than other NSAIDs. Aspirin should never be given to infants or children because of its association with the very serious health problem known as *Reye's syndrome*. The U.S. Federal Drug Administration (FDA) has issued a warning concerning certain NSAIDs, including ibuprofen, naproxen, and cyclooxygenase 2 (COX-2) inhibitors such as celecoxib (Celebrex), due to the increased risk of heart attack or stroke. This warning does not apply to aspirin, which is used as prevention for heart attack and some strokes. Other adverse effects include irritation of the stomach and intestinal tract, allergic reactions, and asthma. Stronger NSAIDs can raise blood pressure, increase the risk of heart failure, cause fluid retention, and damage kidneys.

 **Lifespan Considerations**

**Pediatric Patients**

Aspirin should never be given to infants or children because of its association with development of a very serious health problem known as *Reye's syndrome*. This disorder often leads to mental deficits, coma, or death.

## SKELETAL MUSCLE RELAXANTS

Skeletal muscles contract in response to nerve stimulation to allow you to move. When you want to stand up from a sitting position, the motor area of your brain triggers the nerves that specifically control the muscles of your legs so that only those muscles contract to enable you to straighten the legs enough to lift you to a standing position. If for some reason the nerves connecting your brain to your leg muscles are not working, the muscles will not contract, and no movement will occur.

A *skeletal muscle spasm* is an unwanted overcontraction of one or more muscles. This often occurs when nerves controlling contraction of a muscle send an inappropriate signal to that muscle. Common causes of inappropriate nerve signals include pressure on the nerve, swelling along the nerve path, and low blood calcium levels. Spasms also occur when a muscle is irritated or damaged. Pain from a spasm in a large muscle can be intense. A charley horse in the calf is an example of a painful muscle spasm.

### Action

A **skeletal muscle relaxant** is a drug that reduces muscle spasm by depressing the CNS. This action slows signal transmission along motor nerves, resulting in fewer muscle spasms and less muscle pain. The most commonly prescribed muscle relaxants are methocarbamol (Robaxin) and cyclobenzaprine (Flexeril) (Table 12.5).

### Uses

Skeletal muscle relaxants are used for pain and insomnia when excessive skeletal muscle contractions or spasms contribute to these problems in adults. They are not typically used for children.

### Expected Side Effects

Common side effects of methocarbamol are flushing, low blood pressure, slow heart rate, and fainting. Common side effects of cyclobenzaprine are dizziness, headache, dry mouth, blurred vision, and urinary retention.

### Adverse Reactions

Serious adverse effects of methocarbamol are a high risk of allergic reactions and temporary memory loss *(amnesia)*. It lowers the seizure threshold. Serious adverse effects of cyclobenzaprine are cardiac dysrhythmias and prolonged cardiac conduction. Cyclobenzaprine is not to be used in a patient who is recovering from a heart attack or who has a heart rhythm problem. It also should not be given to a patient who takes a monoamine oxidase inhibitor drug (which is usually used for psychiatric disorders) because of the risk of severe high blood pressure and high fever. Cyclobenzaprine also lowers the seizure threshold.

| Table 12.5 | Examples of Common Skeletal Muscle Relaxants |
|---|---|
| | *SKELETAL MUSCLE RELAXANTS* RELIEVE THE PAIN ASSOCIATED WITH MUSCLE SPASMS BY SLOWING CONTRACTION SIGNAL TRANSMISSION IN MOTOR NERVES. |
| **DRUG/ADULT DOSAGE** | **NURSING IMPLICATIONS** |
| methocarbamol (Robaxin) 1.5 g orally every 6 hours or 1 g IM/IV every 8 hours<br>cyclobenzaprine (Flexeril) 5–10 mg orally every 8 hours | • Before giving the first dose of either skeletal muscle relaxant, ask whether the patient has a seizure disorder, because these drugs lower the seizure threshold.<br>• Check the dose of methocarbamol carefully because it is in grams, not milligrams.<br>• Instruct patients who are taking extended-release tablets or capsules not to chew, open, crush, bite, or cut them to prevent rapid absorption of excess drug.<br>• Instruct patients not to drink alcohol or take other CNS depressants while taking a skeletal muscle relaxant because the CNS effects are intensified. |

*CNS*, central nervous system; *IM*, intramuscular; *IV*, intravenous.

**Top Tip for Safety**

Methocarbamol and cyclobenzaprine should not be given to anyone who has a seizure disorder because these drugs lower the seizure threshold.

## Drug Interactions

The sedating and other CNS effects of these drugs are made worse with the use of alcohol, antianxiety drugs, skeletal muscle relaxants, barbiturates, many drugs used for psychiatric disorders, and opioid analgesics because skeletal muscle relaxants affect the brain and spinal cord. Be sure to determine which other drugs the patient takes.

## ❖ Nursing Implications and Patient Teaching

◆ *Assessment.* Before giving a muscle relaxant to a patient for the first time, assess the level of consciousness, cognition, and skeletal muscle reactivity. Ask the patient whether he or she has a seizure disorder or has ever had a seizure because these drugs lower the seizure threshold.

Before giving the first dose of cyclobenzaprine, assess the patient's blood pressure for the presence of hypotension and radial and apical pulses for any skipped beats, extra beats, or other type of irregular heartbeat.

 **Top Tip for Safety**

Assess patients for cardiac irregularities before giving cyclobenzaprine. If you find any persistent heartbeat irregularity, notify the healthcare provider before giving the drug.

◆ *Planning and implementation.* After giving either muscle relaxant, assess for level of consciousness and degree of muscle relaxation or muscle weakness. Patients often become very drowsy and may fall. Raise the side rails and remind the patient to call for help before getting out of bed.

Help the patient change position slowly because these drugs can cause a sudden lowering of blood pressure. Teach the patient to sit for a few minutes on the side of the bed before attempting to get up. Help the patient during walking to prevent falling.

Methocarbamol and cyclobenzaprine can cause urinary retention. If a patient who is receiving one of these drugs has an enlarged prostate gland or is also taking a drug for overactive bladder, assess for signs or symptoms of urine retention. Symptoms include difficulty starting the urine stream, weak urine stream, and bulge in the lower abdomen.

◆ *Evaluation.* After giving the first dose of cyclobenzaprine, assess the patient's radial and apical pulses hourly for any skipped beats, extra beats, or other type of irregular heartbeat. If you find a persistent irregularity, notify the healthcare provider. Assess the patient's

degree of comfort and muscle reflexes to determine effectiveness.

◆ *Patient and family teaching.* Tell the patient and family:
- Skeletal muscle relaxants are to be taken only on a short-term basis. The drugs usually are prescribed for 2 to 3 weeks because of their potential for abuse.
- As for any substance that causes sedation, avoid operating dangerous equipment, driving a car, or making critical decisions while under the influence of these drugs.
- Avoid alcohol because the sedation effect of these drugs is potentiated by alcohol.
- If you are taking cyclobenzaprine, take your pulse daily, and report new-onset, persistent irregularities to your healthcare provider. Go to the nearest emergency department or call 911 if you develop shortness of breath or chest pain.

## ANTIDEPRESSANTS

Antidepressant drugs that improve a long-term sense of sadness can also reduce some types of chronic pain and cancer pain, especially *neuropathic* pain (which results from injury to the nervous system and causes tingling and burning sensations). The most common antidepressants used for pain management are amitriptyline (Elavil), nortriptyline (Pamelor), paroxetine (Paxil), and sertraline (Zoloft).

The oral doses of these drugs for pain management are often different from the doses used to manage depression. Antidepressants work for pain management by increasing the amount of natural opioids (endorphins and enkephalins) in the brain and by reducing the depression that often occurs with chronic pain. Patients usually must take an antidepressant for 1 or 2 weeks before they feel any relief from pain. Chapter 11 discusses the actions and uses of antidepressants and the associated nursing responsibilities.

 **Memory Jogger**

Several common antidepressants are used for pain management:
- amitriptyline
- nortriptyline
- paroxetine
- sertraline

## ANTICONVULSANTS

Anticonvulsants are drugs that work in the brain to reduce seizures. Some have been found to reduce neuropathic pain (nerve pain with tingling and burning) and migraine headaches. The two most common anticonvulsants used for pain management are gabapentin (Neurontin) and pregabalin (Lyrica). They appear to reduce the rate of pain signal transmission along sensory nerves and may also affect pain perception. The doses for pain management are often higher than those used to manage seizure disorders. Chapter 10 discusses the actions and nursing responsibilities associated with anticonvulsants.

 Memory Jogger

Two common antidepressants are used for pain management:
- gabapentin
- pregabalin

## ANESTHESIA

Anesthesia is a state of controlled, temporary loss of sensation or awareness that is produced for medical purposes. Patients can experience pain relief, paralysis, amnesia (memory loss), and unconsciousness. A patient who receives anesthetic drugs is referred to as being *anesthetized*. Three types of anesthetics are used: local anesthetics, regional anesthetics, and general anesthetics. To achieve anesthesia, one or more different drugs can be used in combination, depending on the patient's condition and the procedure being done. Generally, anesthesia consists of three major components used individually or together. These components are analgesia, temporary amnesia/unconsciousness, and muscle relaxation.

### How Anesthesia Works

The mechanism of action differs for each of the three types of anesthesia used. Local anesthesia works by blocking the nerves from a specific part of the body so that nerves cannot transmit pain signals to the brain. When nerves are blocked in this way, the affected part of the body will feel numb. The numbing effect usually occurs within minutes and may last for a few hours. Regional anesthesia numbs larger areas of the body for pain relief or for surgical procedures. Types of regional anesthesia include spinal anesthesia, epidural anesthesia, and nerve blocks. General anesthesia usually consists of a combination of intravenous drugs and inhaled gasses (anesthetics) to achieve a state of unconsciousness. General anesthesia works by interrupting nerve signals in the brain to prevent the brain from processing pain and from remembering what happened during a procedure or surgery.

The LPN/VN does not give any anesthetic drugs, with the possible exception of applying a topical anesthetic cream to the skin or mucous membrane as ordered. In general, LPNs play a supporting role in caring for patients in the immediate postsurgical recovery period. However, the role of the LPN/VN in the postanesthesia care unit (PACU) or in ambulatory surgery is far less clear and varies by state. The LPN/VN can work in a limited capacity in these areas under the supervision of a registered nurse. You are responsible for knowing the scope of practice for the LPN/VN in your state regarding patient care in the PACU or ambulatory surgery center.

### Drugs for Anesthesia

Common local and regional anesthetics include lidocaine, prilocaine, bupivacaine, and etidocaine (Table 12.6). Local anesthetics can be given topically or by injection. Intravenous drugs such as propofol, etomidate, and ketamine are considered sedative-hypnotic agents commonly used to induce general anesthesia. In the induction state, the patient begins to feel the effect of the IV drug but has not yet become unconscious. Adjuvant drugs such as opioids, lidocaine, or midazolam are often used to enhance the effects of the primary induction agent. Adjuvant drugs, when co-administered with local anesthetic agents, can work to improve the pain control of local anesthetics. Inhaled gasses such as isoflurane, desflurane, and sevoflurane

**Table 12.6**   Examples of Common Local and Regional Anesthetic Drugs

| LOCAL AND REGIONAL ANESTHETIC AGENTS WORK BY BLOCKING THE NERVES FROM A SPECIFIC PART OF THE BODY SO THAT NERVES CANNOT TRANSMIT PAIN SIGNALS TO THE BRAIN. | |
| --- | --- |
| **DRUG/ADULT DOSAGE** | **NURSING IMPLICATIONS** |
| lidocaine 0.5 mg injected into skin 1–3 minutes before nonurgent procedures such as suturing, venipuncture, etc.<br>lidocaine regional dosage typically, 30–50 mg (3–5 mL of a 1% solution); can range up to 300 mg depending on the area to be anesthetized | All local or regional anesthetic drugs are given by a physician or advanced healthcare provider (nurse practitioner, physician assistant). |
| prilocaine regional dosage initially 1–2 mL (40–80 mg) of a 4% solution subcutaneously; for children < 10 years: no more than 1 mL (40 mg) of a 4% solution subcutaneously | Prilocaine can cause hypotension in geriatric patients, especially in those receiving antihypertensive drugs. Monitor blood pressure. |
| bupivacaine local anesthesia in adults and children 12 to 17 years up to 70 mL (up to 175 mg) by subcutaneous, intradermal, or submucosal injection; not to exceed 400 mg/day<br>bupivacaine regional anesthesia dosage varies with the anesthetic procedure | Monitor circulation (regional block) and respirations and blood pressure throughout and follow the procedure as ordered. |

are used in conjunction with regional anesthetics or other drugs to induce general anesthesia.

### Memory Jogger
The most commonly used local and regional anesthetics are these:
- Lidocaine
- Prilocaine
- Bupivacaine

## Action
Local/regional anesthetics, such as bupivacaine or lidocaine, act by blocking the generation and the conduction of nerve impulses. By applying the anesthetic topically or injecting it subcutaneously, intradermally, or submucosally around the nerve blockade results in a reduction in pain, temperature, and touch sensation.

## Uses
Local/regional anesthetics are used for topical anesthesia of skin and mucous membranes for nonurgent painful procedures or for regional nerve block or spinal anesthesia prior to surgery or a procedure. Lidocaine transdermal patches are also available for pain control.

## Expected Side Effects
The skin at the site of treatment may develop pain, erythema, or swelling.

## Adverse Reactions
Adverse reactions are rare because of the small amount absorbed after appropriate application of topical or transdermal preparations. However, excessive absorption can occur when applied over large skin areas, or if heat, bandages, or plastic wrap is also applied to treated skin areas. Skin with open or irritated areas may also absorb more topical medication than healthy skin. Cardiac toxicity (low blood pressure, decreased heart rate, or cardiac arrest) and CNS toxicity (seizures, respiratory depression, or coma) are the adverse effects when too much of the local/regional anesthetic is absorbed through the skin.

## Drug Interactions
Drugs such as beta-blockers that decrease heart rate reduce blood flow through the liver, decreasing lidocaine clearance that could lead to overdosage. Giving lidocaine with acetaminophen or aspirin may increase the risk of developing a rare blood disorder that affects how red blood cells deliver oxygen throughout your body, which is known as *methemoglobinemia*. Excessive dosing can also occur when lidocaine transdermal patches are applied to larger areas or for longer than recommended. Bupivacaine has no known serious interactions with other drugs.

### Top Tip for Safety
When lidocaine is applied to the oral mucosa, it can interfere with swallowing and increase the risk of aspiration. Patients should not eat or drink for at least 1 hour after the use of anesthetic agents in the mouth or throat.

Lidocaine should be used cautiously in patients with cardiac or liver disease.

### Lifespan Considerations
**Pregnant and Breast-feeding Patients**

When given as a nerve block, lidocaine can cross the placenta, but animal studies did not show harm to the fetus. However, the use of local anesthetics during the birth process can cause bradycardia (slow heart rate) and CNS depression in the infant. Lidocaine can pass into breast milk in tiny amounts, which are very unlikely to cause side effects.

❖ **Nursing Implications and Patient Teaching**
◆ *Assessment.* Assess the patient's current prescription and OTC drugs and report potential drug interactions to the healthcare provider. Understand the reason for the patient to be getting local or regional anesthetics to prepare the patient for a procedure, such as suturing. Assess for open areas or irritation the area where the anesthetic will be applied or injected. Determine if the patient has any reported cardiac or liver diseases that can pose a risk of adverse effects to the patient. Ask the patient if she could be pregnant or is breast-feeding. Once local anesthetic is applied, assess for expected pain relief or numbness to the area. Assess for adverse effects from application or potential overdosage.

◆ *Planning and implementation.* Prepare the patient for injectable local/regional anesthetics as ordered by cleaning the injection site and positioning the patient. Remain with the patient for the procedure as required. Once the local or regional anesthetic is given, assess the skin or mucous membranes for redness, swelling, numbness, and pain relief as expected.

Put on gloves before applying an anesthetic cream to prevent transfer of the drug to your skin. Clean the skin before applying an anesthetic cream, and only apply the prescribed amount to the specified area. Before applying a new lidocaine transdermal patch, make sure all old patches are removed and the skin is cleaned. Do not give a patient food or drink for 1 hour after a local anesthetic is applied to the oral mucous membranes.

Monitor the patient's heart rate and blood pressure. Report any symptoms of bradycardia, hypotension, excessive drowsiness, or seizure activity to the supervising RN or healthcare provider. For patients receiving spinal anesthesia, keep the patient in a supine position for 12 hours to minimize headaches.

◆ *Evaluation.* If the purpose of the local or regional anesthetic is pain relief, check the patient's response to the treatment using a standard pain scale, and report the results to the supervising RN or healthcare provider as needed. Report any concerns about decreases in respiratory status to the RN or healthcare provider. Spinal anesthesia can result in headaches or urinary retention. Evaluate CNS symptoms and the ability of the patient to urinate.

◆ *Patient and family teaching.* Tell the patient and family:

- The effects of an injectable local/regional anesthetic usually last only a few hours.
- During the time that local/regional anesthetics are active, assist the patient with activities to ensure safety.
- Monitor the injected area for any signs of excessive inflammation or irritation.
- Use the prescribed local anesthetic cream or transdermal patches only as prescribed.
- Remove all old transdermal patches and residue of anesthetic creams before applying a new patch or dose.
- Tell the patient or family to report any symptoms of dizziness, fainting, or seizure activity.
- Report severe headaches or inability to urinate following spinal anesthesia.

## GENERAL ANESTHESIA

As previously stated, general anesthetics are intravenous drugs or inhaled gasses used to produce pain relief, loss of sensation to touch or temperature, and a state of unconsciousness. General anesthetics are used for surgical and other medical procedures. Inhalation anesthetics consisting of drugs such as nitrous oxide, halothane, isoflurane, desflurane, and sevoflurane are used in combination with IV anesthetics for induction and maintenance of general anesthesia in the operating room.

While the exact mechanism of action of inhaled anesthetics is unknown, they are thought to work within the central nervous system by enhancing some CNS pathways while depressing the transmission of excitatory neurotransmitters. Excitatory neurotransmitters "excite" neurons and cause them to transmit or pass along a message to the next cell. Inhalation anesthetics are given through a face mask, laryngeal mask airway, or tracheal tube (Table 12.7).

The most common adverse effect of inhaled anesthetic agents is postoperative nausea and vomiting. A more severe adverse effect of inhalation anesthetics is malignant hyperthermia. Malignant hyperthermia is most often a genetic or inherited condition. Symptoms of malignant hyperthermia includes a dangerously high body temperature, rigid muscles or spasms, a rapid, irregular heart rate, and excessive sweating. This condition can be fatal if untreated. Treatments for malignant hyperthermia include the drug dantrolene, ice packs, and other measures to cool body temperature, as well as supportive care.

Intravenous anesthetics such as propofol, ketamine, and etomidate are also used as part of general anesthesia. These drugs can be used alone or with inhalation anesthetics, depending upon the specific surgical or medical procedure. When combined with inhalation anesthetics, IV drugs have an additive effect in producing anesthesia and allow for a lower dose of the inhalation agent used.

### Inhalation Agents for General Anesthesia

Nursing care for patients receiving general anesthesia occurs primarily in the pre- and postoperative period, so this chapter includes assessment, planning, implementation, evaluation, and patient and family teaching related only to this time frame.

Table **12.7**  Examples of Common General Anesthetic Drugs

| *GENERAL ANESTHETIC DRUGS* ARE THOUGHT TO WORK WITHIN THE CENTRAL NERVOUS SYSTEM BY ENHANCING SOME CNS PATHWAYS WHILE DEPRESSING THE TRANSMISSION OF EXCITATORY NEUROTRANSMITTERS. | |
| --- | --- |
| **DRUG/ADULT DOSAGE** | **NURSING IMPLICATIONS** |
| sevoflurane usual maintenance dose 0.5%–3% with or without nitrous oxide to maintain surgical anesthesia | All general anesthesia is given by an anesthesiologist or certified registered nurse anesthetist (CRNA) only. |
| desflurane usual maintenance dose 2.5%–8.5% by inhalation with or without nitrous oxide<br>Neonates, children, and adolescents: usual maintenance dose 5.2%–10% via inhalation, with or without nitrous oxide; use of desflurane contraindicated for anesthesia induction | Monitor arterial blood gas results.<br>Monitor potassium levels as hyperkalemia may occur.<br>Monitor for seizure activity.<br>Monitor heart rate and blood pressure.<br>Monitor behavior as in children desflurane may cause agitation as they emerge from anesthesia. |
| isoflurane usual maintenance dose 1%–2.5%, individualized based on the desired effect for patient's age and clinical status<br>Infants, children, and adolescents: 1%–2.5% isoflurane | Advise patients that performance of activities requiring mental alertness, such as driving or operating machinery, may be impaired for some time after general anesthesia. |

*CNS,* central nervous system.

Memory Jogger

The most commonly used inhalation agents for general anesthetics are these:
- sevoflurane
- desflurane
- isoflurane

## Action

For all inhaled drugs used for general anesthesia, the precise mechanism to induce and maintain general anesthesia is unknown but thought to work within the central nervous system by enhancing some CNS pathways while depressing the transmission of excitatory neurotransmitters.

## Uses

Inhalation anesthetics are used to cause general anesthesia (loss of consciousness) before and during surgical procedures.

## Expected Side Effects

Side effects of inhalation anesthetics such as cough, nausea, vomiting, and headache are common.

## Adverse Reactions

Inhalation anesthetics reduce blood pressure, resulting in hypotension by peripheral vasodilation. Another potential adverse effect is respiratory depression characterized by slow, ineffective breathing.

## Drug Interactions

There are many drug–drug interactions for inhalation anesthetics, so a through drug history, including OTC preparations, should be gathered before any surgery or procedure is done.

### 🔖 Top Tip for Safety

- Notify the surgeon or anesthetist if a patient reports malignant hyperthermia in their medical history.
- Malignant hyperthermia is a potentially fatal condition.
- Symptoms of malignant hyperthermia include dangerously high body temperature; rigid muscles or spasms; a rapid, irregular heart rate; and excessive sweating.

## ❖ Nursing Implications and patient teaching

◆ *Assessment.* Prior to surgery, ask the patient/family if any of them have had an adverse reaction to anesthesia. Verify the prescription and OTC drugs the patient is currently taking. Once the patient has returned from surgery, assess for expected side effects and adverse effects of general anesthesia.

◆ *Planning and implementation.* Monitor the patient's condition before and after surgery. Monitor vital signs, especially respiration depth and rate as ordered. Monitor for nausea or vomiting. Give antiemetics as ordered and assess for response.

◆ *Evaluation.* Check the patient's response to postoperative pain control using a standard pain scale and report the results to the supervising RN or healthcare provider as needed. Report any concerns about decreases in respiratory status or hypotensive episodes to the RN or healthcare provider.

◆ *Patient and family teaching.* Tell the patient and family:
- Ask for assistance when ambulating or other activities to ensure safety.
- Report symptoms of headache, nausea, and vomiting.
- Report any symptoms of dizziness or fainting that may be signs of hypotension.
- Review all postoperative instructions and drugs to be continued at home.
- Provide teaching on what symptoms and complications should be reported to the surgeon.

# Get Ready for the Next-Generation NCLEX® Examination!

## Key Points

- Pain is whatever the patient says it is, occurs whenever the patient says it occurs, and is the intensity the patient states.
- Opioid agonists change only the *perception* of pain; they do nothing at the site of injured tissues to reduce the cause of pain.
- Opioid agonist analgesics work by binding tightly to the mu-opioid receptor in the brain and activating it.
- Strong opioid agonist analgesics (e.g., hydromorphone, fentanyl) require less drug (lower dosages) to result in the same level of pain relief than weaker opioid agonist analgesics.

- All opioid drugs are considered high-alert drugs because they have an increased risk for causing patient harm when given in error.
- Tolerance to and dependence on opioid agonist analgesics are common and are not the same as misuse.
- Pain is best relieved when any type of analgesic is given on a schedule before the patient's pain becomes severe.
- Older adults may require opioid agonist doses to be lower or the drugs to be given less frequently because of age-related changes in liver and kidney function.
- Do not give tramadol to any patient who has a seizure disorder (epilepsy) or other neurologic disorder, because this drug can induce seizures.

- A variety of drugs that are used as therapy for other health problems, such as inflammation, seizures, psychiatric disorders, and muscle spasms, can also help relieve some types of pain.
- Acetaminophen can be toxic to the liver and should not be taken by anyone who already has liver health problems.
- An infant or young child should never receive an adult dose of acetaminophen because of its severe liver toxicity.
- Corticosteroids have many side effects and adverse reactions that limit their use in pain management.
- Aspirin and other NSAIDs interfere with blood clotting and increase the risk of excessive bleeding.
- Aspirin should never be given to infants or children because of its association with development of Reye's syndrome, a very serious health problem.
- Methocarbamol and cyclobenzaprine should not be given to anyone who has a seizure disorder because these drugs lower the seizure threshold.
- Antidepressants and anticonvulsants can help reduce some types of pain, especially neuropathic pain.
- When antidepressants or anticonvulsants are used in pain management, the dosages are usually different from those used to manage depression or seizures.
- Anesthesia is a state of controlled, temporary loss of sensation or awareness that is produced for medical purposes.
- Common local and regional anesthetics include lidocaine, prilocaine, bupivacaine, and etidocaine. Local anesthetics can be given topically or by injection.
- Inhaled gasses such as isoflurane, desflurane, and sevoflurane are used in conjunction with regional anesthetics or other drugs to induce general anesthesia.
- Topical or transdermal anesthetics can be excessively absorbed when applied over large skin areas, or if heat, bandages, or plastic wrap is applied to treated skin areas.
- Giving lidocaine with acetaminophen or aspirin may increase the risk of developing a rare blood disorder known as *methemoglobinemia*.
- When lidocaine is applied to the oral mucosa, it can increase the risk of aspiration.
- The most common adverse effect of inhaled anesthetic agents is postoperative nausea and vomiting.
- Symptoms of malignant hyperthermia includes a dangerously high body temperature, rigid muscles or spasms, a rapid, irregular heart rate, and excessive sweating.
- Inhaled anesthetics can cause hypotension and respiratory depression.

## Clinical Judgment and Next-Generation NCLEX® Examination-Style Questions

1. Some analgesics are considered strong opioid agonists. Indicate which of the following analgesics are considered strong opioid agonists. **Select all or any that apply.**
   1. codeine
   2. fentanyl
   3. hydrocodone
   4. hydromorphone
   5. morphine
   6. oxycodone

2. A 45-year-old woman has returned to the unit following a right breast mastectomy for breast cancer. The patient states her pain level is a 7/10. The patient has an order for morphine 1 mg IV for postoperative pain, which you are preparing to administer to her.

Place an X (or drag and drop) to indicate which client assessment findings are indications of serious adverse reactions and symptoms of opioid agonist analgesics overdose requiring immediate medical attention:

| ASSESSMENT FINDING | ADVERSE REACTIONS REQUIRING IMMEDIATE ATTENTION |
|---|---|
| Constipation | |
| Drowsiness | |
| Respiratory rate of 8 breaths/min | |
| Blood pressure of 80/60 | |
| Decreased pupil size | |
| Cool, clammy skin | |
| Temperature of 98.2°F (36.8°C) | |

3. A postoperative patient reports feeling nauseated after taking an oral opioid agonist for pain. What is your best response?
   1. "Make sure to take this drug with food."
   2. "I will ask the surgeon to change the order to an injectable form of the drug."
   3. "Once you take a few doses, the nausea will go away."
   4. "Since you just had surgery, nausea is less of a problem than is the sensation of acute pain."

4. A patient who is prescribed extra-strength acetaminophen for pain has been taking this drug at the maximum dose for 4 months. What laboratory test should be monitored for adverse effects of this drug?
   1. Complete blood count
   2. Cardiac enzymes
   3. Liver function tests
   4. Lipid profile

5. The patient is prescribed an antidepressant for neuropathic pain. The patient tells you that this must be a mistake because he does not have depression. What is your best response?
   1. Explain that the antidepressant was prescribed because it is less likely that he will become addicted to it than to other painkillers.
   2. Remind him that all patients who are having significant pain are depressed to some degree even if he does not recognize it.
   3. Explain that the antidepressant works by increasing chemicals in the brain that are helpful in relieving pain.
   4. Reassure him that you will contact his healthcare provider and report that he is not depressed.

6. Which class of drugs for pain management is used with caution due to the potential for misuse?
   1. Corticosteroids
   2. Skeletal muscle relaxants
   3. Opioid agonists
   4. NSAIDs

7. Among the following, what are the most important actions to take after giving the *first dose* to a patient who is newly prescribed cyclobenzaprine for pain?

| NURSING ACTION | EFFECTIVE | INEFFECTIVE | UNRELATED |
|---|---|---|---|
| Assess the patient's extremities for fluid retention. | | | |
| Assess the patient for seizures. | | | |
| Assess skeletal muscle reactivity. | | | |
| Assess the patient for visual changes. | | | |
| Assess for understanding of patient teaching. | | | |
| Assess the radial pulse. | | | |
| Assess the sense of touch. | | | |

8. The patient taking a prescribed NSAID for chronic arthritis pain has all of the following symptoms. Which one will you report to the prescriber immediately? **Select all or any that apply.**

1. Rapid heart rate
2. Increased headaches
3. Bloody stools
4. Joint pain
5. Difficulty sleeping
6. Excessive fatigue

**Rationale:** A side effect of aspirin and many other NSAIDs is increased risk of bleeding that can present as bloody stools. If the bleeding continues, the patient may show signs of anemia such as fatigue and rapid heart rate.

9. How much oral codeine would be needed for a patient to obtain the same degree of pain relief that 30 mg of oral morphine would provide?

1. 20 mg
2. 75 mg
3. 150 mg
4. 200 mg

10. What is the most important action to take after giving any analgesic for pain?

1. Assess the patient's likelihood for substance use disorder.
2. Assess the patient for nightmares or hallucinations.
3. Ask the patient to rate his or her degree of pain relief.
4. Ask the patient to count backward by threes to assess cognition.

**Drug Calculation Review**

1. An infant is to receive 80 mg acetaminophen (Tylenol). The liquid you have on hand has a concentration of 100 mg/mL.

    1. How many mL is the correct dose for this infant?
    2. How many mL is the correct dose if the liquid has a concentration of 120 mg/5 mL?

2. A patient is to receive 15 mg of morphine IM for pain. The available drug is morphine sulfate 10 mg/mL. How many mL is the correct dose for this patient?

**Case Study**

Mr. B is a 62-year-old man who lives alone. He was admitted for care and rehabilitation 4 days ago to an extended care facility on his third postoperative day after a right total knee replacement until he can safely care for himself at home. He is prescribed hydrocodone with acetaminophen (Vicodin) for pain control. The prescription reads: "Vicodin (5 mg hydrocodone; 300 mg acetaminophen) one to two tablets every 4 to 6 hours as needed for pain." He tells you that overall his pain is not bad except when he comes back from physical therapy. The pain is "much worse" after therapy. He also tells you that he tries to take the drug only when he really needs it.

1. What type of pain is Mr. B having?
2. How will you know the severity of the pain when it becomes much worse?
3. What specific type of drug is Vicodin?
4. What type of change or changes could be made in drug delivery for the current prescription to help relieve his pain more effectively?
5. If he were to receive two Vicodin tablets every 4 hours around the clock, what would his total dose of acetaminophen be for the day?

# 13 | Drugs for Inflammation, Arthritis, and Gout

## Learning Outcomes

1. List the names, actions, and possible adverse effects of nonsteroidal anti-inflammatory drugs (NSAIDs).
2. Explain what to teach patients and families about NSAIDs.
3. List the names, actions, and possible adverse effects of corticosteroid-based anti-inflammatory drugs.
4. Explain what to teach patients and families about corticosteroid-based anti-inflammatory drugs.
5. List the names, actions, and possible adverse effects of disease-modifying antirheumatic drugs (DMARDs)

for management of arthritis and other inflammatory disorders.
6. Explain what to teach patients and families about DMARDs for management of arthritis and other inflammatory disorders.
7. List the names, actions, and possible adverse effects of antigout drugs.
8. Explain what to teach patients and families about antigout drugs.

## Key Terms

**anti-inflammatory drug** Drug that has as its primary purpose to prevent or limit the tissue and blood vessel responses to injury or pathogen invasion.

**corticosteroids** Drugs built on the structure of cholesterol that are able to prevent or limit inflammation and allergy by slowing or stopping production of the mediators histamine and leukotriene; chemically similar to the glucocorticoid hormones secreted by the adrenal glands.

**disease-modifying antirheumatic drug (DMARD)** Drug that reduces the progression and tissue destruction of

the inflammatory disease process, especially rheumatoid arthritis, by inhibiting tumor necrosis factor (TNF).

**inflammation** A response to injury or infection caused by white blood cells (leukocytes) and their products that results in a predictable set of tissue and blood vessel actions.

**nonsteroidal anti-inflammatory drug (NSAID)** Drug that is not based on the chemical structure of cholesterol but can prevent or limit the tissue and blood vessel responses to injury by slowing the production of one or more inflammatory mediators.

## INFLAMMATION CAUSES AND ACTION

Inflammation occurs as a result to injury, infection, or a wide range of chronic diseases. When inflammation occurs, white blood cells (leukocytes) and their by-products cause reactions in tissues and blood vessels. These reactions result in the five major symptoms of inflammation: pain, redness, warmth, swelling, and loss of function. For example, a person with a severely sprained ankle can have redness, warmth, and pain. Swelling can prevent walking well on the ankle (i.e., loss of function).

Inflammation is generally considered to be a normal, protective reaction of the body to tissue injury. However, when inflammation occurs without tissue injury or infection, and occurs over a long time period, an overreaction of the inflammatory process can occur that can damage or destroy tissues.

 **Memory Jogger**

The five main symptoms of inflammation are pain, redness, warmth, swelling, and loss of function.

When an injury occurs, the damaged tissues and white blood cells (WBCs) in the injured area release inflammatory chemical mediators that cause certain actions to occur. These chemical mediators, which are important in starting and continuing inflammation, include kinins, prostaglandins (PGs), histamine, and tumor necrosis factor (TNF). Some mediators, especially histamine, act on blood vessels in the injured area, causing them to dilate and leak fluid from the capillaries. This results in redness and warmth of the tissues. Increased blood flow brings more WBCs to injured tissues, and the leaking capillaries cause swelling. Released kinins trigger pain receptors in nerve endings, which makes the area painful. Pain is the response to an injury and forces the person to move carefully to protect themselves from more harm.

As more and more WBCs come to the injured area to fight possible pathogens, the inflammatory response is increased by the arachidonic acid cascade (Fig. 13.1). It begins by converting fat from injured cell membranes into arachidonic acid (AA). The enzyme cyclooxygenase (COX) then converts AA into many mediators, especially different types of PGs.

There are two forms of the COX enzymes: COX-1 and COX-2. COX-1 is present in all cells and makes PGs that are helpful and protective; you can think of COX-1 as "good COX." For example, COX-1 in the cells of the stomach lining makes PGs that produces thick mucus. The mucus *protects* the stomach lining from being harmed by the gastric acids needed for food digestion. COX-2 is present mainly in areas of inflammation. COX-2 is responsible for the types of PGs and other mediators that start and continue the inflammation response; you can think of COX-2 as "bad COX." This distinction will be important as you consider some of the expected side effects and adverse reactions caused by anti-inflammatory drugs.

Although inflammation responses may be uncomfortable or painful, these responses help injured tissue to regain function. WBCs release growth factors that (1) trigger repair of damaged tissues and cells, (2) stimulate healthy cells in the injured area to divide and replace dead or damaged cells, and (3) promote scar tissue formation in tissues that can no longer divide. Remember that scar tissue does not act or function like normal tissue.

Although inflammation is mostly a protective process that helps prevent infection and promote healing, it can cause serious and sometimes painful tissue damage if it continues too long or occurs when it is not needed. For example, some people develop autoimmune diseases such as rheumatoid arthritis, in which the immune system fails to recognize normal body tissue and attacks tissue of the joints, releasing mediators such as TNF, causing inflammation and resulting in painful deformity and immobility, especially in the fingers, wrists, feet, and ankles.

 Bookmark This!

Here are some useful Web sites regarding inflammatory disorders and their treatment:

- National Institute of Arthritis and Musculoskeletal and Skin Diseases, https://www.niams.nih.gov
- The Arthritis Foundation, http://www.arthritis.org
- Centers for Disease Control and Prevention (Arthritis), https://www.cdc.gov/arthritis

## INFLAMMATION MANAGEMENT

Many acute problems that cause inflammation, such as sprains, fractures, or tears, require short-term therapy with anti-inflammatory drugs. An **anti-inflammatory drug** has as its primary purpose to reduce pain and prevent or limit the tissue and blood vessel responses to injury or infection. Many chronic inflammatory disorders, such as arthritis, can require long-term therapy with anti-inflammatory drugs. Long-term therapy is prescribed to reduce the symptoms of inflammation and prevent tissue-damaging complications.

It is important to recognize that most of the drugs used to treat short-term or long-term inflammation can have serious adverse reactions. The patient's response to therapy must be monitored closely.

A variety of drug categories are useful in managing acute and chronic inflammatory conditions: nonsteroidal anti-inflammatory drugs (NSAIDs), corticosteroids, disease-modifying antirheumatic drugs (DMARDs), and antigout drugs. As described in Chapter 12, one of the symptoms of inflammation is pain. When inflammation is managed, pain is also relieved to some

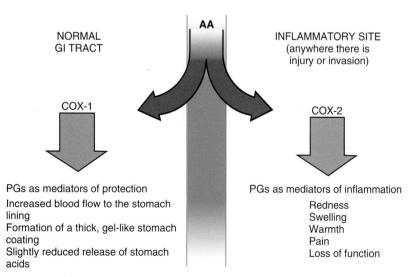

Fig. **13.1** Arachidonic acid cascade resulting from injured cells. You can see the influence of the cyclooxygenase enzymes. *AA*, arachidonic acid; *PGs*, prostaglandins; *COX-1*, cyclooxygenase 1; *COX-2*, cyclooxygenase 2.

degree, which is why anti-inflammatory drugs are prescribed for pain management. For inflammation caused by gout, management also includes drugs that reduce the production of uric acid, which forms crystals that deposit in joints and cause gout.

## NONSTEROIDAL ANTI-INFLAMMATORY DRUGS

### Actions

A nonsteroidal anti-inflammatory drug (NSAID) slows the production of one or more inflammatory mediators, thereby preventing or limiting the tissue and blood vessel responses to injury. NSAIDs are divided into two categories: (1) nonselective NSAIDs that inhibit the actions of COX-1 and COX-2 and (2) selective NSAIDs that have more inhibitory effects on the COX-2 enzyme and lesser effects on COX-1 (Fig. 13.2).

NSAIDs that are classified as COX-1 inhibitors are more likely to cause gastrointestinal side effects. Those that inhibit COX-2 have a higher risk of cardiovascular effects but less risk of gastrointestinal effects. Nonselective COX inhibitors such as aspirin, ibuprofen, and other NSAIDs disrupt COX-1 and COX-2 enzymes (see Fig. 13.2). The nonselective COX inhibitors also can block the protective and helpful cellular COX-1 effects (i.e., they block the "good COX") and reduce the inflammation associated with activation of COX-2 (i.e., they block the "bad COX"). As a result,

nonspecific NSAIDs (those that inhibit both COX-1 and COX-2) have more side effects than selective COX-2 inhibitor NSAIDs (those that affect only COX-2).

Selective and nonselective NSAIDs have the same anti-inflammatory actions: They reduce the production of PGs, kinins, histamine, TNF, and other inflammation mediators derived from AA. These effects produce the analgesic, anti-inflammatory, and antipyretic (fever-reducing) effects associated with NSAIDS.

The oldest NSAID still in use today is aspirin (ASA), which has a salicylate chemical structure. This chemical was first extracted from the bark and root of the white willow tree and has been used as an anti-inflammatory agent for centuries. More is known about aspirin due to its long history of use, so it is considered the classic NSAID with which all other NSAIDs are compared. Aspirin is a salicylate, but different chemicals are used as the drug base for other NSAIDs. They work in the same way as aspirin but have different strengths and different expected side and adverse effects.

Some earlier nonspecific NSAIDs were more potent than aspirin but also had some very harsh side effects that limited their use. For example, colchicine and indomethacin are rarely prescribed today. Newer NSAIDs and other types of targeted therapies have also reduced the need to use these drugs. Table 13.1 lists the NSAIDS most commonly used today.

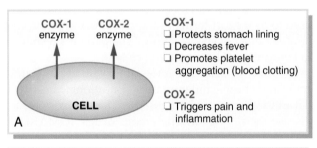

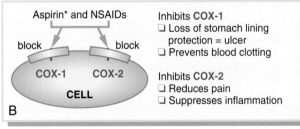

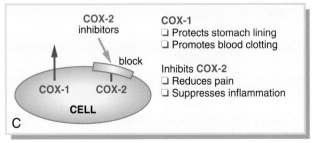

*Aspirin is only one of the NSAIDs.

Fig. 13.2 (A) Actions of selective and nonselective nonsteroidal anti-inflammatory drugs *(NSAIDs)*. (B) Inhibition of COX-1 and COX-2. (C) Selective inhibition of COX-2. *COX*, cyclooxygenase.

### Uses

NSAIDs are typically the first drugs used to treat a variety of inflammation-based problems that are often associated with pain and fever. Pain in the muscles, nerves, and joints (myalgias, neuralgias, and arthralgias, respectively); headache; and dysmenorrhea are commonly treated with NSAIDs. Various forms of arthritis, such as rheumatoid arthritis, osteoarthritis, and psoriatic arthritis, may be responsive to NSAIDs for pain and other symptoms of inflammation. NSAIDs are also used short-term for the management of pain related to dental extractions, minor surgeries, or athletic soft tissue injuries.

Although many NSAIDs are available over the counter (OTC), they are still potentially dangerous drugs, and great care should be taken to avoid overdose. Larger doses must be obtained by prescription from a healthcare provider and monitored very carefully.

Nonselective NSAIDS, particularly aspirin, inhibit platelet aggregation (clumping). This effect is very helpful, when these drugs are used in low doses, to prevent clotting in patients with coronary heart disease. However, the effect on platelets can also lead to an increased risk of bleeding, particularly when NSAIDs are given at higher doses. For NSAIDs other than aspirin, platelet inhibition is dose related and reversible. Patients who take aspirin must be monitored for bleeding due to irreversible platelet inhibition for the lifespan of the platelet (which is 7 to 8 days). This

## Table 13.1   Common NSAIDs for Inflammatory Problems

*Cyclooxygenase 1 and 2 inhibitors* decrease the activity of cyclooxygenase 1 (COX-1) and cyclooxygenase 2 (COX-2) to reduce the formation of inflammatory mediators from arachidonic acid. These drugs also disrupt the normal functions of other products derived from arachidonic acid that are helpful and protective.

*Cyclooxygenase 2 (COX-2) inhibitors* are selective and mostly inhibit the COX-2 pathway for arachidonic acid production of inflammatory mediators. Although the same side effects are possible as with the COX-1/COX-2 inhibitors, they usually occur only at higher doses or with prolonged use.

| DRUG/ADULT DOSAGE | NURSING IMPLICATIONS |
|---|---|
| **Cyclooxygenase 1 and 2 Inhibitors** | |
| aspirin (Bayer aspirin, Bufferin, Ecotrin, Entrophen ♣, many others) 325–650 mg orally three to four times daily<br>ibuprofen (Advil, Motrin, Actiprofen ♣) 200–800 mg orally three to four times daily<br>ketorolac (Toradol) oral 10–60 mg every 6 hours<br>ketorolac (Toradol) parenteral 15–30 mg every 6 hours<br>nabumetone (Relafen) 500–1000 mg orally once or twice daily<br>naproxen (Aleve, Anaprox, Naprosyn, Naxen ♣) 220–440 mg orally every 12 hours<br>oxaprozin (Daypro) 600–1800 mg orally once daily<br>piroxicam (Feldene, Novopirocam ♣) 20 mg orally once daily | • All COX-1/COX-2 inhibitors have more side effects at lower doses than selective COX-2 inhibitors have.<br>• Teach patients that all NSAIDs increase the risk of bleeding because they interfere with the platelet function of the clotting process.<br>• Remind patients to stop taking aspirin 1 week before dental or surgical procedures and other COX-1/COX-2 inhibitors at least 2–4 days before dental or surgical procedures because of the increased risk of bleeding from the procedure.<br>• Tell patients to report to their healthcare provider stomach or abdominal pain or any signs of bleeding from the gums or blood in the stool to because these drugs increase the risk of GI ulcer formation.<br>• Teach patients not to take NSAIDs while taking warfarin because the risk of bleeding is then so severe that hemorrhage and stroke are likely.<br>• Teach patients taking any NSAID except aspirin to weigh themselves at least twice weekly and keep a record because these drugs increase salt and water retention, which can worsen heart failure and raise blood pressure.<br>• Instruct patients to take any NSAID with food to help prevent stomach irritation.<br>• Teach patients to drink 2 to 3 liters of fluid daily while taking NSAIDs to ensure good blood flow to the kidneys because all of these drugs except aspirin can cause kidney damage.<br>• Instruct patients who have diabetes to check blood sugar levels more often because these drugs increase the risk of hypoglycemia (low blood sugar) in patients who take oral antidiabetic drugs.<br>• Teach patients to take the prescribed NSAIDs on a regular schedule because inflammation is better relieved when there is a stable blood level of the drug. |
| **Cyclooxygenase 2 (COX-2) Inhibitors** | |
| celecoxib (Celebrex) 100–400 mg orally per day<br>meloxicam (Mobic) 7.5–15 mg orally once daily<br>etodolac (Lodine) 600 mg orally per day<br>etodolac extended release (Lodine XL) 400–1000 mg orally per day<br>diclofenac (Voltaren) 50 mg orally two to three times daily<br>diclofenac extended release (Voltaren XR) 100 mg orally daily<br>diclofenac (also available in a topical gel; use as directed) | • Before the first dose of celecoxib, ask whether the patient has an allergy to sulfa-based antibiotics because a patient who is allergic to sulfa is likely to also be allergic to celecoxib (it contains a chemical similar to sulfa).<br>• Tell patients they do not have to stop these drugs before dental or surgical procedures because COX-2 inhibitors do not interfere with platelets and blood clotting.<br>• Teach patients to take a COX-2 inhibitor exactly as prescribed because higher doses will result in the same side effects and adverse reactions as the COX-1/COX-2 inhibitors.<br>• Avoid giving these drugs to anyone who has angina, smokes, or has severe coronary artery disease, because of the risk of heart attacks. |

is very important if a patient is scheduled for an invasive dental or surgical procedure. The healthcare provider must be made aware of the situation so that the aspirin can be discontinued 1 week before the procedure.

### Memory Jogger

Nonselective NSAIDs inhibit the COX-1 and COX-2 enzymes. Selective NSAIDs primarily inhibit COX-2 and so have fewer side effects and adverse reactions.

### Expected Side Effects

Common side effects of nonselective NSAIDs are heartburn, nausea, vomiting, dizziness, headache, and increased risk of bleeding and bruising. The gastrointestinal (GI) effects may be minimized or avoided if the drug is taken with at least a full glass of water. If the medication does cause mild GI upset, the patient may take the medication with a small amount of food or milk. All NSAIDs except aspirin can cause some degree of fluid retention, edema formation, and increased blood pressure. This is particularly important to note because

NSAIDs should be avoided in patients who have high blood pressure, heart failure, or renal failure. Selective NSAIDs (i.e., COX-2 inhibitors) have fewer gastrointestinal (GI) effects because they do not impact the protective effects associated with the COX-1 enzyme.

## Adverse Reactions

Although expected side effects are often bothersome to the patient, they typically can be managed, and the patient can continue taking the medication. Adverse reactions, however, must be recognized and reported to the healthcare provider immediately, and the drug will most likely be discontinued. Several adverse reactions may occur in patients taking NSAIDs, including allergy (ranging from mild symptoms of rash and shortness of breath to anaphylaxis), renal failure, upper or lower GI bleeding, and blood disorders. Patients taking COX-2 inhibitors may have an increased risk of heart attack (myocardial infarction) and stroke, and it is important to recognize symptoms associated with those disorders. Finally, hypertension due to fluid retention is an adverse response of NSAIDs.

While generally rare, patients who are allergic to one nonaspirin NSAID may also be allergic to another due to cross-sensitivity. It is important to note all allergies in the medical record and report them to the healthcare provider before giving the NSAID.

---

 **Top Tip for Safety**

- NSAIDs increase the risk of serious cardiovascular events, including myocardial infarction and stroke, which can be fatal. Cardiovascular events can occur early in treatment, and their incidence may increase with the length of NSAID use.
- NSAIDs increase the risk of serious gastrointestinal (GI) adverse events, including bleeding, ulceration, and perforation of the stomach, which can be fatal. Elderly patients and patients with a prior history of peptic ulcer disease and/or GI bleeding are at greater risk for serious GI events.

---

Aspirin has been associated with the occurrence of Reye's syndrome when given to children with a viral infection such as varicella (chickenpox) or influenza. In Reye's syndrome, symptoms may affect all organs of the body, but most seriously affected are the brain and liver. It can lead to permanent brain damage and death. Therefore the use of aspirin is avoided in children, especially those who have an acute illness.

---

 **Lifespan Considerations**
### Pediatric Patients

Aspirin should not be given to infants or children who have an acute illness because of its association with the development of Reye's syndrome, a rare but serious condition that causes swelling in the liver and brain. Reye's syndrome most often affects children and teenagers recovering from a viral infection. This disorder can lead to mental deficits, coma, or death.

---

Too much aspirin can lead to toxicity and can be life-threatening. Symptoms of aspirin toxicity may progress from mild to severe, beginning with tinnitus (ringing in the ears), hyperventilation, diaphoresis (sweating), thirst, headache, drowsiness, skin eruptions, and electrolyte imbalance. Symptoms can progress to central nervous system (CNS) depression, stupor, convulsions and coma, tachycardia (rapid heartbeat), and respiratory insufficiency. If patients exhibit any of these symptoms, it is important to notify the healthcare provider early.

---

 **Lifespan Considerations**
### Older Adults

Older adults taking NSAIDs have a higher incidence of excessive bleeding and perforated ulcer compared with younger adults. Older adult patients who have some degree of renal impairment are at higher risk for damage to the liver and kidneys caused by NSAIDs. These drugs should be avoided in older adults. If prescribed, they should be administered with a proton-pump inhibitor (PPI), such as omeprazole (Prilosec), to reduce risks of GI effects.

---

## Drug Interactions

Alcohol taken with any of the NSAIDs increases the risk of GI bleeding. The effects of anticoagulants, sulfonylureas, and sulfonamides are increased if they are used at the same time as aspirin. NSAIDs interact with each other, which increases the risks of side effects, adverse reactions, and toxicities. Patients should not be taking more than one type of NSAID at any one time.

Different NSAIDs interact differently with other drugs, and interactions are common. Consult a pharmacist or drug handbook for a complete discussion of the interactions associated with a particular NSAID. These are examples of common interactions:

- Aspirin and other NSAIDs should not be given to treat vaccination-associated fever and pain because they can prevent the normal immune response and its protection.
- NSAIDs (except for aspirin) decrease the effectiveness of many antihypertensive drugs, especially angiotensin-converting enzyme inhibitors (ACE-Is), angiotensin II receptor blockers (ARBs), beta-blockers, and most diuretics.
- All NSAIDs increase the risk of bleeding for patients who take any type of anticoagulant.
- All NSAIDs increase the risk of hypoglycemia (low blood sugar) in patients with diabetes who take oral antidiabetic drugs.

## ❖ Nursing Implications and Patient Teaching
◆ *Assessment.* Ask patients whether they are using any other OTC or prescribed NSAIDs because patients sometimes do not report or may forget occasional use of aspirin or other OTC NSAIDs. Many

forms of NSAIDs are available OTC, and it is important to assess whether patients are taking more than one kind.

Check for a history of allergy to aspirin or other NSAIDs, asthma, blood disorders, GI problems or ulcer disease, or other liver or kidney problems. These conditions are precautions for or contraindications to the use of NSAIDs and should be reported to the healthcare provider before giving the drug. Assess which other prescribed and OTC drugs the patient takes daily because NSAIDs interact with many other drugs. Check with the pharmacist to determine whether or how the NSAID is expected to interact with the patient's other drugs.

◆ *Planning and implementation.* The dosages for different NSAIDs vary widely. Ensure that you give a dose that is within the correct dosage range for the specific NSAID.

There are many forms of NSAIDs, including tablets, capsules, eye drops, chewable preparations, suppositories, and injectables. Several NSAIDs may be applied topically. The healthcare provider considers the best form for the patient's individual needs.

Give the NSAID with a full glass of water to reduce the risk of GI disturbances. If the patient has a stomach upset, try giving the drug with food or milk to reduce the symptoms. If the patient continues to have GI upset, notify the healthcare provider. If the drug is given in suspension form, shake the container well so that the dosage is accurate. The patient should be well hydrated before taking the drug, to reduce the risk of kidney damage.

◆ *Evaluation.* Monitor the patient to be sure that symptoms resolve (e.g., pain level decreased, temperature reduced to 101°F [38.3°C] or lower). Pain typically decreases after administration of the drug, but a reduction of inflammation may take up to 1 to 2 weeks. The dosage of the NSAID should be reduced or the drug stopped if tinnitus (ringing in the ears) develops. Observe for symptoms such as pain or fever that do not respond to the drug, which suggests that the patient is getting worse, and notify the healthcare provider. The patient may need a larger dose, a more potent drug, or alternative therapy.

Assess the patient for signs of increased bleeding, especially of the gums and mucous membranes. Check the skin for large bruises or areas of bruising that flow together. Assess for petechiae (pinpoint purple or reddish spots) on the torso or extremities.

Examine the gums, stool, urine, and vomitus for blood. When blood counts are performed, assess whether the numbers of red blood cells and platelets are normal or low. Report low counts to the healthcare provider immediately.

◆ *Patient and family teaching.* Tell the patient and family:

- These drugs may cause stomach upset, and NSAIDs should be taken with a full glass of water and/or food.
- Contact your healthcare provider right away if ringing in the ears, abnormal bleeding or bruising, or bloody or black tarry stools are noted.
- Go the emergency room immediately if you experience chest pain, shortness of breath, or other signs of a heart attack.
- For some chronic problems, you may need to take your prescribed NSAID for longer than 1 to 2 weeks before noticing a decrease in symptoms.
- Drink at least 8 to 10 glasses of water per day to stay well hydrated while taking the NSAID.
- For best effect to reduce inflammation, take the prescribed NSAID on a regular schedule to keep a stable blood level of the drug. Do not take more than the prescribed dose.
- Do not take any other drugs, including OTC drugs (especially aspirin or another NSAID), at the same time as this drug without telling your healthcare provider.
- Contact your healthcare provider if your fever does not come down in 24 to 48 hours.
- Keep aspirin and all other NSAIDs out of the reach of children because wrong doses may be toxic to a child.
- If you are unable to take the drug in the form prescribed (e.g., difficulty with swallowing), contact your healthcare provider so that another form of the drug may be prescribed.

## CORTICOSTEROIDS

**Corticosteroids**, also known as *glucocorticoids*, are drugs that prevent or limit inflammation by slowing or stopping the pathways of inflammatory cytokine production. The corticosteroids are similar to the natural cortisol hormones secreted by the adrenal gland that are necessary for life. These drugs may be given to replace missing or low hormone levels in cases of adrenal insufficiency (Addison disease). They are most commonly used, however, to reduce the inflammatory response. Common systemic corticosteroid drugs include prednisone, methylprednisolone, hydrocortisone, and dexamethasone (Table 13.2).

 **Do Not Confuse**

Do not confuse prednisone with prednisolone. They are not the same drug. Although both drugs are corticosteroids, their strengths, dosages, and routes of administration differ.

## Actions

Corticosteroids are useful for managing severe or chronic inflammation. These powerful drugs can decrease the production of all known mediators that trigger inflammation. Corticosteroids inhibit enzymes and proteins that allow the COX-1 and COX-2 enzyme

| Table 13.2 | Common Corticosteroid Drugs |
| --- | --- |

*Corticosteroids* inhibit enzymes and proteins that allow the COX-1 and COX-2 enzyme systems to produce inflammatory mediators from arachidonic acid. They are very powerful in decreasing the production of all known mediators that trigger inflammation. The systemic forms of these drugs also disrupt the normal functions of other products derived from arachidonic acid that are helpful and protective.

| DRUG/ADULT DOSAGE | NURSING IMPLICATIONS |
| --- | --- |
| Oral Corticosteroids<br>dexamethasone (Decadron, Apo-dexamethasone ♣) 2–20 mg orally once daily<br>prednisolone (Medrol ♣, Millipred) 5–40 mg orally once daily<br>prednisone (Apo-prednisone ♣, Deltasone, Rayos) 5–60 mg orally daily in divided doses<br>Parenteral Corticosteroids<br>cortisone acetate 20–300 mg IM once daily<br>dexamethasone (Decadron, Dexasone ♣, Solu-Medrol) 1–80 mg IM or IV once daily<br>hydrocortisol (Solu-Cortef) 25–125 mg IM two to four times daily<br>methylprednisolone (Duralone, Solu-Medrol) 10–60 mg IM or IV two to four times daily<br>Topical Corticosteroids<br>betamethasone (Beta Derm, Del-Beta) 0.5%–1%<br>hydrocortisone (Dermacort, Lanacort) 0.1%–1%<br>triamcinolone (Kenalog, Triderm) 0.5%–1% | • Check the order carefully because different types of corticosteroids come in different strengths and are not interchangeable.<br>• Warn patients not to stop taking the oral drug suddenly (without the guidance of their healthcare provider) to prevent possible adrenal insufficiency.<br>• Oral drugs should be taken with food or milk to reduce the risk of gastric ulcers.<br>• Check the patient's blood pressure and weight when giving oral or parenteral corticosteroids because these drugs cause water retention and raise blood pressure.<br>• Assess for infection because these drugs reduce the immune response and increase the susceptibility to infection.<br>• When patients are taking these drugs for a long period, be sure to handle the patient carefully and not apply tape to the skin because these drugs increase bruising and thin the skin.<br>• Never apply a topical corticosteroid cream, ointment, or lotion to a skin area that has indications of infection because the infection will spread.<br>• Apply topical corticosteroids in a thin layer to help prevent systemic absorption.<br>• Make sure to follow directions very carefully when drugs are pre-packaged in a dose pack to ensure proper dosage and tapering.<br>• Make sure to monitor blood sugar regularly for patients with diabetes or prediabetes because corticosteroids reduce the sensitivity of insulin receptors and increase blood glucose levels. Patients may need adjustments in their oral antidiabetic drug or insulin.<br>• Patients may experience a change in mood while taking corticosteroids. Notify the healthcare provider if these changes are significant to reduce psychotic reactions. |

*COX*, cyclooxygenase; *IM*, intramuscular; *IV*, intravenous.

systems to start and continue the production of inflammatory mediators from AA. They also slow the production of WBCs in the bone marrow. This action helps reduce inflammation because WBCs usually are the source of the mediators that trigger inflammation. The actions of corticosteroids occur in all cells, not just those involved in inflammation. As a result, their therapeutic effects, side effects, and adverse effects are widespread. These problems limit how and when they can be used.

## Uses

Corticosteroids are most commonly given to reduce inflammatory, allergic, or immunologic responses. Examples of when corticosteroids might be used include acute adrenal emergencies, allergic states, acute brain injury, severe respiratory disease or asthma, and any condition in which chronic inflammation could lead to tissue damage, such as osteoarthritis, rheumatoid arthritis, inflammatory bowel diseases, systemic lupus erythematosus, and a wide variety of other inflammatory and autoimmune diseases.

Corticosteroids can be injected locally for problems related to joints (intraarticular injection), soft tissues, or bursae (fluid-filled sacs located near muscles and tendons that reduce friction resulting from movement). They can also be injected into lesions or subcutaneous dermatologic problem areas. Topical corticosteroids may be prescribed for acute and chronic dermatoses, rectal problems, and some eye (ophthalmic) or ear (otic) problems. Inhaled corticosteroids are commonly used to manage inflammation associated with asthma.

### Expected Side Effects

The side effects of systemic corticosteroids in pharmacologic doses are predictable exaggerations of the actions of the natural corticosteroids produced by the adrenal glands, or they can result from reduced function of the hypothalamic-pituitary-adrenal axis. Box 13.1 lists the short-term and long-term effects of corticosteroid use.

Common side effects of corticosteroids that occur even when they are used for relatively short periods include sodium retention, increased blood pressure, weight gain, bruising, and reduced immunity. It is not unusual for patients, particularly diabetics, to have an elevated blood sugar level, and doses of insulin or an oral hypoglycemic agent may need to be adjusted

| Box 13.1 | Common Side Effects of Systemic Corticosteroids |
|---|---|

**SIDE EFFECTS OCCURRING AS SOON AS 1 WEEK OF THERAPY**
- Acne
- Sodium and fluid retention
- Elevated blood pressure
- Sensation of "nervousness"
- Difficulty sleeping
- Emotional changes, crying easily

**SIDE EFFECTS OCCURRING WITHIN A MONTH AFTER THERAPY**
- Weight gain
- Fat redistribution (moon face and "buffalo hump" between the shoulders)
- Increased risk for gastrointestinal ulcers and bleeding
- Fragile skin that bruises easily
- Loss of muscle mass and strength
- Thinning scalp hair
- Increased facial and body hair
- Increased susceptibility to colds and other infections
- Stretch marks

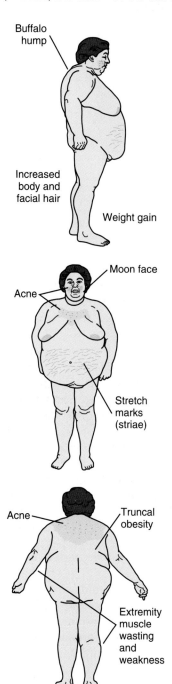

Fig. 13.3 Physical changes resulting from long-term corticosteroid therapy, known as a *Cushingoid appearance.*

while the patient is receiving steroid therapy. Patients may experience a change in mood while taking corticosteroids; some experience mild euphoria, whereas others experience some depression. These drugs also increase the risk of bleeding in general and especially in the gastrointestinal tract. Although many of these effects may be expected, if they become severe, it is very important to notify the healthcare provider.

Fig. 13.3 shows the physical changes associated with long-term corticosteroid use, known as *Cushing syndrome.* The changes may reverse after the patient stops taking the drug, but reversal can take several months to a year.

### Adverse Reactions

Many effects of systemic corticosteroids can cause serious problems if not managed carefully. These issues are not problematic for topical corticosteroids. The most important problems are associated with long-term use and include adrenal gland suppression and reduced immunity. Thus long-term use of corticosteroids is limited to the treatment of severe inflammation that cannot be managed in any other way.

Adrenal suppression occurs when circulating blood levels of corticosteroids are higher than the amount of cortisol normally made by the adrenal glands (Fig. 13.4). This causes the adrenal glands to quit making and secreting natural cortisol because the body appears to not need it. As a result, the cells of the adrenal glands shrink (atrophy) and cannot quickly start making cortisol again. This becomes a problem if the patient suddenly stops taking corticosteroids because it may take weeks or even months for the adrenal glands to produce normal levels of cortisol again.

Because cortisol is necessary to maintain life, the patient who suddenly stops taking systemic corticosteroids has no circulating cortisol and could die from acute adrenal insufficiency. Symptoms include anorexia, nausea and vomiting, lethargy, headache, fever, joint pain, skin peeling, myalgia (widespread muscle pain), weight loss, and hypotension. Abruptly stopping the drug may also result in a rebound of symptoms of the condition being treated. Patients who have been taking any corticosteroid daily for 1 week or longer need to slowly decrease the dose over time (tapering) instead of just stopping the drug suddenly. Tapering of the drug allows the atrophied adrenal gland cells to gradually begin producing cortisol again and prevents acute adrenal insufficiency. Fig. 13.5 provides an example of a dose pack that can be used to assist the patient

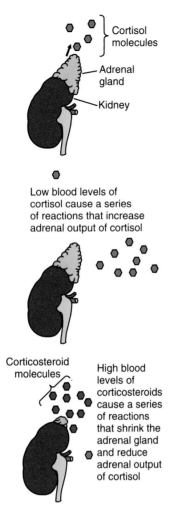

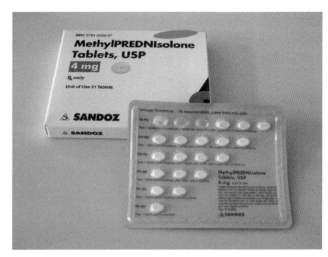

Fig. 13.5 Oral corticosteroid dose pack. Patients begin on day 1, taking six tablets. As the patient goes through the week, the drug dosages taper down daily until the sixth day.

## Drug Interactions

Corticosteroids increase the effects of barbiturates, sedatives, narcotics, and anticoagulants. They decrease the effects of insulin and oral hypoglycemics, isoniazid, and broad-spectrum antibiotics. Drugs that *increase* the effects of corticosteroids include other NSAIDs and oral contraceptives, especially estrogen. Drugs that *decrease* the effects of corticosteroids include ephedrine, barbiturates, phenytoin, antihistamines, chloral hydrate, rifampin, and propranolol. The effect of corticosteroids on warfarin anticoagulants varies; in some cases they may increase the effect, and in other cases they decrease it.

Some drugs produce exaggerated side effects when given with corticosteroids. They include alcohol, NSAIDs, amphotericin B, thiazides and other potassium-wasting diuretics, anticholinergics, cardiac glycosides, and stimulants such as adrenaline, amphetamines, and ephedrine. Because NSAIDs can cause GI distress, the use of aspirin or any other drug should be avoided while taking corticosteroids.

## ❖ Nursing Implications and Patient Teaching

◆ *Assessment.* There are many contraindications to and precautions for the use of corticosteroids, and it is important to obtain an accurate drug history, including OTC drugs, herbal agents, and any topical or inhaled drugs. The most important contraindication for corticosteroids is the presence of infection because corticosteroids can increase the risk of more severe infections. Assess the patient for any signs or symptoms of local or systemic infection before starting the drug. These include fever, drainage, foul-smelling urine, productive cough, and redness around a wound or other open skin area.

Corticosteroids tend to thin the skin, and their use increases the risk of skin tears. Corticosteroids can also slow wound healing and therefore must be carefully assessed in patients who are to have any kind of

Fig. 13.4 Corticosteroid influence on adrenal production of cortisol.

with dosing on days 1 through 6, each day tapering the dose.

Any use of corticosteroids also reduces the number of WBCs, which can decrease inflammation but also decreases the immune response. The longer the patient has been taking a corticosteroid and the higher the dose, the more immunity is reduced. This greatly increases the patient's risk of infection. Because inflammation is reduced, the usual symptoms of infection, especially fever and pus formation, may not be present. It is especially important to monitor patients for other signs of infection such as cough, changes in color of any sputum or other drainage, and symptoms such as headache or behavior changes.

Other adverse effects associated with long-term corticosteroid use include osteoporosis, cataracts, hypertension, and ocular hemorrhage. Delirium or extreme changes in behavior such as mania may warrant reduction of the dose or cessation of the corticosteroid in affected patients.

 **Memory Jogger**

To prevent adrenal insufficiency, doses of systemic corticosteroids must be tapered rather than stopped abruptly.

surgery. Report symptoms of infection to the healthcare provider because corticosteroids reduce immunity and can make an existing untreated infection worse.

◆ *Planning and implementation.* Corticosteroids come in many forms and may be administered by the following routes: oral, inhalation, intranasal, intravenous, intramuscular (IM), subcutaneous, intrabursal, intradermal, intrasynovial, intralesional, soft tissue injection, topical using creams or gels, with ophthalmic (eye) and otic (ear) preparations, and per rectum. Only corticosteroid preparations with specific labels should be used for ophthalmologic or otic administration. Topical steroids should not be applied to open wounds. Topical steroids should be avoided if there are any signs of infection because they may increase the risk of spreading the infection due to their effect on the immune/inflammatory response.

It is vitally important to confirm the proper form of the drug and the proper route of administration of corticosteroids. State nurse practice acts indicate which route of drug administration is appropriate for the LPN/VN. Even if the LPN/VN does not give the drug, it will be important for you to monitor for expected side effects, adverse reactions, and effectiveness.

Corticosteroid dosages vary, and the dose is determined for each patient based on the specific problem or diagnosis, severity, prognosis, and estimated length of treatment. The general rule for prescribing corticosteroids is to prescribe as high a dose as necessary initially to get a favorable response and then to decrease the amount gradually to the lowest level that can maintain the therapeutic effect but not produce complications. It is critical to check the specific drug name, the route, and the dose carefully because there are different strengths. Do not exchange one type of systemic corticosteroid for another because the dosages may not be equivalent.

It is recommended that doses of oral corticosteroids be taken with meals or a light snack to help reduce the chance of GI distress and peptic ulcer. Systemic corticosteroids are typically given orally, except for patients who are acutely ill or unable to take oral drugs. The onset of action is typically 2 to 8 hours, and the effects are seen after 12 to 24 hours, depending on the drug. Oral corticosteroids are almost completely absorbed in the GI tract. For corticosteroids injected into a muscle or joint, it may take several days to weeks for onset of effects.

When corticosteroids are given orally to patients with functioning adrenal glands, the total dose should be taken first thing in the morning. This is the time when the adrenal glands are normally secreting the most cortisol, and the corticosteroid dose more closely mimics the body's usual actions at that time.

◆ *Evaluation.* All patients receiving systemic corticosteroids should be monitored carefully, and the dosage may be adjusted by the healthcare provider to reflect reduced or increased symptoms, the patient's response, and any periods of stress in the patient's life (e.g., injury, infection, surgery, emotional crisis). Patients who require high-dose or long-term treatment should be monitored carefully for up to 1 year after the drug is stopped for symptoms of adrenal insufficiency.

### Top Tip for Safety

While transferring or positioning patients who are taking corticosteroids, carefully protect their skin to prevent skin tears.

Corticosteroids can hide the usual symptoms of infection, and they also increase the patient's risk of infection. This makes it essential for you to monitor the patient for any unusual symptoms that might suggest infection. For example, corneal fungal infections are particularly likely to develop with extensive ophthalmologic corticosteroid use. If the patient has any new onset of blurred vision, discoloration of the eye, or tearing, the healthcare provider should be contacted. Corticosteroids are particularly dangerous to use in patients with a history of tuberculosis because the disease can be reactivated, and it is important to monitor for cough or shortness of breath in these patients.

◆ *Patient and family teaching.* Tell the patient and family:
- Keep all appointments to monitor therapy while taking corticosteroids.
- Heavy smoking may add to the expected action of a corticosteroid because nicotine raises the blood level of naturally secreted cortisol.
- Avoid alcohol during the course of therapy because it enhances the risk of GI ulcers.
- Report any signs and symptoms of infection (e.g., fever, cough, pain or burning on urination, foul-smelling drainage, generally feeling unwell) to your healthcare provider immediately because corticosteroids reduce resistance to infection.
- Inform other healthcare providers, including your dentist, that a corticosteroid is being taken.
- Report any of the following signs and symptoms to the healthcare provider immediately because they indicate a life-threatening problem of the adrenal glands: malaise, weakness, hypotension, anorexia, nausea and vomiting, aching of bones and muscles, headache, increased temperature, and diarrhea.
- Do not stop taking corticosteroids suddenly. Consult with your healthcare provider.
- During and after corticosteroid treatment, wear a medical alert bracelet (e.g., MedicAlert) or necklace, or carry a medical identification card with the name of the drug.
- Do not receive any immunizations without consulting the nurse or other healthcare provider first.
- Take oral corticosteroids with a meal or light snack to minimize stomach upset.

- Eat a diet that is rich in potassium and low in sodium to replace lost potassium and prevent excessive water retention.
- If you forget to take a prescribed dose, take a dose as soon as possible and then follow the prescribed schedule.
- Call the nurse or other healthcare provider if any of the following develop: rapid weight gain; black or tarry stools; unusual bleeding or bruising; or signs of hypokalemia (decreased potassium level in the blood), including anorexia, lethargy, confusion, nausea, and muscle weakness.

## DISEASE-MODIFYING ANTIRHEUMATIC DRUGS

A disease-modifying antirheumatic drug (DMARD) reduces the progression and tissue destruction of the inflammatory disease process by inhibiting TNF. DMARDs are classified as either conventional or biologic agents. Commonly used conventional DMARDs include methotrexate, leflunomide, hydroxychloroquine, and sulfasalazine. Biologic DMARDs are usually prescribed after the failure of conventional DMARD therapy with disease progression. Common biologic agents include adalimumab, etanercept, and tocilizumab.

DMARDs are prescribed for treatment of rheumatoid arthritis, psoriatic arthritis, and ankylosing spondylitis. DMARDs prevent or limit bone destruction, and they are used only in diagnosed cases of rheumatoid arthritis or another chronic inflammatory disorder that worsened despite other treatments. In addition to their anti-inflammatory effects, DMARDs work to suppress specific pathways of the immune system.

DMARDs can result in significant risk and toxic effects. Patients taking these drugs need regularly scheduled follow-up and evaluation to assess for any adverse effects.

### Actions

DMARDS work through a variety of actions to decrease or suppress the inflammatory response and, in cases of rheumatoid arthritis, slow down the progression of disease and preserve joint function. The most commonly used DMARDS inhibit the inflammatory mediator TNF—they do this by binding to the TNF molecules produced by WBCs, which keeps them from binding to TNF receptor sites on inflammatory cells and other cells. This prevents the cells with TNF receptors from continuing to produce more TNF and other substances that enhance the inflammatory response and cause direct tissue destruction. As a result, pain is relieved, physical function improves, and tissue damage is reduced or delayed. DMARDs can take several weeks or months to demonstrate a clinical effect.

Most DMARDs are given by injection, although there are a few oral formulations. The two most common DMARDs are adalimumab and etanercept (Table 13.3).

### Uses

DMARDs are used to treat many types of chronic inflammatory disorders that involve severe tissue destruction caused by excessive amounts of TNF. In addition to rheumatoid arthritis, other autoimmune disorders that respond to DMARDs include ankylosing spondylitis, psoriasis, psoriatic arthritis, Crohn's disease, and ulcerative colitis.

### Expected Side Effects

The most common side effect from injected DMARDs is a reaction at the injection site. Reactions include pain, swelling, itching, and redness at the site for about 1 week. Many patients also have headache and nausea. Because these drugs reduce bone marrow production of red blood cells and platelets, patients may develop anemia and have an increased risk for bleeding.

### Adverse Reactions

Severe adverse reactions are possible and relatively common in patients taking DMARDs. It is important to monitor patients very carefully and to teach patients the symptoms to report.

All DMARDs reduce the patient's immune response to some degree, increasing the risk of infection. Patients who have had tuberculosis or a viral infection such as shingles or hepatitis in the past are at high risk for reactivation of the old infection. Although reduced immunity is an expected result of therapy with DMARDs, it is considered an adverse reaction that must be monitored for severity. If reduced immunity is severe enough or severe infection develops, DMARD therapy must be stopped.

 **Top Tip for Safety**

All DMARDs reduce immunity and increase the risk of infection. It is important to assess the patient for any signs or symptoms of infection.

DMARDs can cause heart failure that may be new or more severe while taking the drug. DMARDs should not be given to anyone who has severe heart failure.

Patients taking injectable DMARDs may be at greater risk for allergic reaction, even anaphylaxis, because the solutions may contain some animal proteins. Fortunately, these reactions are not common.

### Drug Interactions

If the patient is taking any other type of drug that reduces immunity, taking a DMARD will make immunosuppression more severe, greatly increasing the risk of infections. It is not recommended to give two types of DMARDs that interfere with TNF at the same time.

Some immunizations contain live vaccines. For the patient receiving DMARDs, live vaccine immunizations are avoided because the patient may develop the disease that the immunization is supposed to prevent.

Table **13.3**   Disease-Modifying Antirheumatic Drugs

| DRUG/ADULT DOSAGE | NURSING IMPLICATIONS |
|---|---|
| *Disease-modifying antirheumatic drugs (DMARDS) reduce progression and tissue destruction of the inflammatory disease process by inhibiting tumor necrosis factor (TNF). As a result, pain is relieved, physical function improves, and tissue damage is reduced or delayed.* | |
| **CONVENTIONAL AGENTS** | |
| methotrexate 7.5–15 mg orally once weekly<br><br>leflunomide 10–20 mg orally once daily<br><br>hydroxychloroquine 400–600 mg orally once daily<br><br>sulfasalazine 500 to 1,000 mg orally once or twice daily | • Administer enteric-coated tablets whole; do not crush or chew.<br>• Tell patients the importance of carefully following all drug instructions, including taking the recommended dose as directed. Serious reactions have been reported with medication errors.<br>• Monitor complete blood count (CBC) and liver enzymes for patients taking methotrexate, as this drug can cause severe bone marrow suppression and liver failure.<br>• Tell patients taking sulfasalazine to take this drug with a full glass of water after meals or with food to minimize indigestion or gastrointestinal irritation.<br>• Review safe handling precautions for administering these drugs.<br>• Tell patients that hydroxychloroquine can be toxic to the retina. An initial and annual routine eye exam is recommended. |
| **BIOLOGIC AGENTS** | |
| adalimumab (Humira) 40 mg subcutaneously every 2 weeks<br><br>etanercept (Enbrel) 50 mg subcutaneously once per week<br><br>tocilizumab 162 mg subcutaneously every other week | • Tell patients that injection-site reactions, including redness, pain, swelling, and itchiness, may occur but typically subside within a few days.<br>• Rotate injection sites on the front of the thighs and the abdomen to ensure best absorption and prevent skin problems. Avoid giving within 2 inches of the umbilicus because this area has many blood vessels and absorption can be too rapid.<br>• Do not shake the vial, prefilled pen, or prefilled syringe because shaking may damage the drug.<br>• To prevent bleeding and bruising at the site, do not rub the site after giving the injection.<br>• Monitor the CBC for low white blood cell count (neutropenia).<br>• For patients with psoriasis, make sure not to inject in any lesions because drug absorption is delayed in these areas and the lesions may mask skin reactions to the drug.<br>• Do not administer these drugs to patients with an active infection, including local infections, because the drugs reduce the immune response and can make infections worse.<br>• Teach patients to report any signs of infection to the healthcare provider immediately because these drugs reduce the immune response and can make infections worse.<br>• Patients who take these drugs before surgery may have greater risk of infection postoperatively because the drug reduces the immune response.<br>• Patients may need to undergo testing for tuberculosis (TB) infection before starting therapy to prevent reactivation of the disease or worsening of existing disease. If latent TB is present, the patient may need to undergo TB treatment.<br>• Monitor patients carefully for any symptoms of allergic reaction so that interventions can begin quickly.<br>• Instruct patients to avoid vaccination with live viruses while taking DMARDs; the vaccine may not be fully effective because of a reduced immune response.<br>• So that patients will not be alarmed by this side effect, teach them that it is not unusual to experience a mild headache while taking these drugs. |

Because DMARDs reduce immunity, the patient may not have an accurate response to tuberculosis testing with the purified protein derivative (PPD) test. The response may be negative even if the person has active tuberculosis.

 **Top Tip for Safety**

Always ask patients about whether they have a current infection or have had any of the following infections in the past: tuberculosis, hepatitis, shingles, HIV infection, pneumocystis pneumonia, or any type of opportunistic infection.

❖ **Nursing Implications and Patient Teaching**

◆ *Assessment.* Before giving a DMARD, ask the patient to list every drug he or she is currently taking. Ask about symptoms of infection, such as fever, cough, foul-smelling drainage, pain or burning on urination, and general malaise, as well as any recent exposure to people who are ill. Ask whether the patient has received an immunization within the past month. All patients must be tested for tuberculosis before starting a DMARD.

◆ *Planning and implementation.* The first dose of an injectable DMARD must be given by a physician or registered nurse in a setting that can handle severe allergic reactions. It cannot be started in an extended care facility or in the home. Take the patient's vital signs, especially pulse, blood pressure, and oxygen saturation, before giving the first dose. Use this information as a baseline to assess for an adverse drug reaction.

Keep an emergency cart close to the patient during the first injection and for 2 hours afterward. After the first dose is given, observe the patient every 15 minutes for any type of allergic or adverse reaction for at least 2 hours. These observations include respiratory rate, ease of respirations, blood pressure, pulse oximetry, and rash or hives at the injection site.

After the first therapeutic dose is given and no adverse reactions have occurred, LPN/VNs can administer subsequent doses. Some patients can be taught to self-inject subcutaneous doses. Carefully read the specific directions for administration of the drugs before giving them. For example, adalimumab should not be shaken before giving it because damage to the drug may occur. The drug can be left at room temperature for 15 to 30 minutes before injecting it, but the cap or cover must be left on the drug bottle while allowing it to warm to room temperature.

◆ *Evaluation.* Closely monitor the injection site and the whole patient for signs of an adverse reaction. Document the patient's responses, even if no problems occur. Document any symptoms or injection-site responses that do occur.

◆ *Patient and family teaching.*
 • Check for and report the signs and symptoms of infection (e.g., fever, cough, malaise, foul-smelling drainage, pain or burning on urination) to the healthcare provider immediately.
 • Teach patients how to inject themselves, and obtain a return demonstration of proper techniques for self-injection before discharge to ensure proper drug delivery.
 • Report any nausea, vomiting, loss of appetite, severe fatigue, or changes in color of the urine because these may be symptoms of problems with the liver.
 • To avoid dangerous drug interaction, do not take any OTC drugs without contacting the healthcare provider.

## GOUT

Gout is a metabolic disorder that causes a person to produce or accumulate too much uric acid crystals from the proteins they eat or to not eliminate the crystals in the urine. The crystals are deposited in joints, tendons, and surrounding tissue, causing the arthritis symptoms of pain, redness, and swelling (gouty arthritis) and causing progressive joint damage with loss of function. Although the metabolic disorder is always present, the symptoms of gout come and go.

### MANAGEMENT OF INFLAMMATION AND GOUT PAIN

About 10% of people who have gout can control the problem with lifestyle changes that involve eating less of the foods that produce uric acid, including shellfish, herring, sardines, salmon, haddock, and anchovies; red meat, organ meats, and pork; beer and wine; and drinks made with high-fructose corn syrup. The other 90% of patients with gout are unable to eliminate uric acid well through the kidneys. Losing weight if obese, avoiding alcohol, and including low-fat dairy products and complex carbohydrates in the diet may reduce the risk of flare-ups.

When patients have symptoms of gout, general anti-inflammatory drugs can help reduce the pain and inflammation but do not address the uric acid problem. These drugs also do not prevent progressive joint damage. Specific drugs for pain management may be prescribed during acute attacks (see Chapter 12). Drugs that lower uric acid levels can prevent gout attacks and reduce symptoms during an attack.

### ANTIGOUT DRUGS

The most common drugs used to reduce the uric acid levels associated with gout are uric acid synthesis inhibitors. The two drugs in this class are allopurinol and febuxostat (Table 13.4).

### Actions
Allopurinol and febuxostat help prevent gout attacks by reducing the amount of an enzyme that converts purines into uric acid. As a result, there is less uric acid available to form irritating and inflammatory deposits in joints. These drugs help patients maintain a lower blood uric acid level.

### Uses
The main use of antigout drugs is to prevent gout and shorten gout attacks. For gout prevention, they must be taken daily. Allopurinol (but not febuxostat) is also used to lower uric acid levels that occur when rapid cell destruction (e.g., with effective cancer chemotherapy) results in a huge release of purines from inside the cancer cells.

### Expected Side Effects
The most common side effects of allopurinol and febuxostat are headache, rash, and minor nausea. Rare side effects include breast development in men and erectile dysfunction. There is a risk of gout flare with the start of therapy. Teach patients to report increased gout symptoms. Gout flare may be managed with NSAIDs or colchicine.

### Adverse Reactions
Adverse reactions to allopurinol and febuxostat are rare and occur only with very long-term use. They include kidney stone formation, liver failure, heart failure, and stroke. Rarely, depression and cardiac dysrhythmias have been reported.

### Drug Interactions
Aluminum-based antacids inhibit absorption of allopurinol. Antigout drugs also interfere with the

| Table 13.4 | **Common Antigout Drugs** |
|---|---|

*Uric acid synthesis inhibitors* prevent gout, reduce gout symptoms, and lower blood uric acid levels by inhibiting the enzyme that converts the purines into uric acid.

| DRUG/ADULT DOSAGE | NURSING IMPLICATIONS |
|---|---|
| **Uric Acid Synthesis Inhibitors** | |
| allopurinol (Aloprim, Zyloprim) 200–800 mg orally daily; intravenous (IV) 200–400 mg/m² daily<br>febuxostat (Uloric) 40–120 mg orally daily | • Take allopurinol after a meal to prevent gastrointestinal side effects.<br>• Wait at least 3 hours after taking an aluminum-based antacid before taking allopurinol because the antacid inhibits its absorption.<br>• Patients who also take warfarin need more frequent monitoring of their international normalized ratio (INR) because allopurinol interferes with warfarin metabolism.<br>• When giving the IV form of allopurinol, do not give it in the same port or tubing as other drugs because many drugs are incompatible with it.<br>• Do not give either of these drugs to a breast-feeding woman because the drugs do enter breast milk and their effects on the baby are not known.<br>• Febuxostat can be taken at any time of day regardless of meals.<br>• Teach patients to drink plenty of fluids to dilute uric acid and prevent kidney complications of the drug.<br>• Teach patients to keep all appointments for laboratory tests to monitor for drug effectiveness and toxicities. |

metabolism and action of warfarin. Febuxostat interacts with many chemotherapy drugs to form other metabolic products that can damage kidneys, which is why it is not used for the hyperuricemia (elevated uric acid level) associated with cancer therapy.

 Lifespan Considerations

**Pregnancy and Lactation**

Drugs to treat gout are not recommended for breast-feeding women because they can be passed to the infant in breast milk.

❖ **Nursing Implications and Patient Teaching**

Patients are rarely hospitalized for gout. The most important action is to teach patients how to take these drugs to prevent and control gout.

◆ *Patient and family teaching.* Tell the patient and family:
• Take allopurinol after a full meal.
• Drink 8 to 16 glasses of liquids, especially water, throughout the 24-hour day.
• Wait at least 3 hours to take allopurinol after using an aluminum-based antacid.
• Febuxostat can be taken with or without meals and is not affected by antacids.
• If you are breast-feeding, do not take these drugs.
• Avoid foods that are high in purines because those foods may precipitate an acute attack.
• Keep all appointments for laboratory tests of uric acid levels and for liver and kidney function tests while taking these drugs.
• Many drugs can trigger gouty flare-ups, and it is important to let the provider know if you have gout.

# Get Ready for the Next-Generation NCLEX® Examination!

## Key Points

- Acute inflammatory reactions are common and may be helpful or protective.
- Chronic inflammatory reactions can cause tissue damage and destruction.
- All NSAIDs have the same mechanism of action, although their chemical structures, strengths, interactions, and adverse reactions may vary.
- All NSAIDs increase the risk of bleeding, especially in older patients and patients who take any type of anticoagulant.
- NSAIDs (except for aspirin) decrease the effectiveness of many antihypertensive drugs, especially the ACE-Is, ARBs, beta-blockers, and most diuretics.
- Patients who take corticosteroids must not suddenly stop the drug; rather, the dose must be tapered by the healthcare provider to avoid adrenal insufficiency.
- Corticosteroids have a wide range of side effects and adverse reactions, and patients must be monitored very carefully.
- Always ask patients who are to receive a DMARD about whether they have a current infection or have had any of the following infections in the past: tuberculosis, hepatitis, shingles, HIV infection, pneumocystis pneumonia, or any type of opportunistic infection.
- Anti-inflammatory drugs do not prevent gout or the associated joint damage of gout.
- Use of drugs for gout should be combined with patient teaching about weight loss and avoiding high-purine foods and alcohol.

## Clinical Judgment and Next-Generation NCLEX® Examination-Style Questions

1. A patient is taking an anti-inflammatory drug and calls the clinic to tell the LPN/VN that he missed some of the doses last week. The LPN/VN instructs the patient about what to do in this situation.

   **Place an X next to the appropriate response from the nurse.**

   | | |
   |---|---|
   | Skip all missed drug doses | |
   | If it is close to the next time the drug is due, skip the missed dose. | |
   | All missed doses of the drug should be returned to the pharmacy. | |
   | Never take a double dose of this drug. | |
   | If possible, take the missed dose within an hour of the scheduled time. | |
   | Once you miss a dose, you should double up on the drug dose at the next time it is due. | |

2. A nursing home resident has been prescribed 20 mg of prednisolone orally to be given immediately. The facility does not have prednisolone, only prednisone. What is your best action?

   1. Substitute prednisone for prednisolone because they are both corticosteroids.
   2. Hold the dose until the pharmacy opens the next day.
   3. Notify the healthcare provider immediately about this problem.
   4. Give the parenteral form of the drug.

3. A patient who has been taking the NSAID etodolac for osteoarthritis for 1 year calls the clinic to report chest pain and shortness of breath. What is your best response?

   1. "Mild chest pain and shortness of breath are expected side effects after taking etodolac over time."
   2. "Call an ambulance and go directly to the emergency department."
   3. "This symptom of heartburn can be caused by this drug. Make sure you take it with food."
   4. "Come into the office today so we can check your blood pressure."

4. Corticosteroids are a class of drugs that are used to manage inflammation. What are the properties or actions associated with corticosteroids? Select all or any that apply.

   1. Corticosteroids decrease inflammatory mediators.
   2. Corticosteroids act only within the cells that are inflamed.
   3. Corticosteroids can be used to manage chronic inflammation.
   4. Corticosteroids slow the production of WBCs in the bone marrow.
   5. Corticosteroids have few adverse effects due to their localized action.
   6. Corticosteroids increase arachidonic acid production of inflammatory mediators.

5. A patient prescribed an NSAID contacts the clinic to say she has noticed that her bowel movements have become very dark, like tar. What will the LPN/VN say to the patient?

   1. "This is an adverse effect of the drug. You need to come to the clinic today."
   2. "This is an expected side effect of the drug. You can try taking an antacid when you take the NSAID."
   3. "You should stop taking NSAIDs. You are probably allergic."
   4. "The healthcare provider will switch the drugs to a less irritating type."

6. A 37-year-old woman diagnosed with rheumatoid arthritis has been managing her symptoms with NSAIDs and now is starting a DMARD. You are planning an education session for the patient and her family about this new drug.

   **Place an X next to the actions that you will take in the educational session.**

   | | |
   |---|---|
   | Ask whether the patient has received an immunization within the past month. | |
   | Instruct the patient to take the first dose at home right before bedtime. | |
   | Instruct the patient to report the signs and symptoms of infection to the healthcare provider immediately. | |
   | Instruct the patient to avoid drinking cold or cool liquids. | |
   | Instruct the patient to prevent sun exposure with hats, long sleeves, and sunscreen. | |
   | Teach the patient the principles of self-injection. | |
   | Ask the patient if she has had shingles or hepatitis in the past. | |
   | Instruct the patient to report symptoms of excessive bleeding. | |
   | Instruct the patient to get tested for TB before starting a DMARD. | |

7. **What is the main difference between a nonselective COX inhibitor and a COX-2 inhibitor?**

   1. COX-2 inhibitors have fewer GI side effects than nonselective COX inhibitors.
   2. COX-2 inhibitors are less effective than nonselective COX inhibitors.
   3. COX-2 inhibitors can be taken with any OTC drugs without risk.
   4. COX-2 inhibitors are safe in children with Reye's syndrome.

8. A 72-year-old patient has been taking prednisone for an autoimmune disease for 10 weeks. She is concerned about the side effects and tells the LPN/VN that she has decided to stop taking the drug. What is the LPN/VN's best response?

   1. "Make sure to notify your healthcare provider that you stopped taking the prednisone."
   2. "Call the healthcare provider first because it is very important that you do not stop prednisone suddenly but rather taper the drug."
   3. "There are very few side effects to prednisone, so it must be another drug."
   4. "Do not stop taking the drug because you will increase your risk of infection."

9. **Which of the following symptoms is associated with aspirin toxicity?**

   1. Tinnitus
   2. Respiratory depression
   3. Constipation
   4. Abdominal pain

10. **What category contains the drugs that reduce the progression and tissue destruction of the inflammatory disease process, especially rheumatoid arthritis, by inhibiting tumor necrosis factor (TNF)?**

    1. Corticosteroids
    2. Nonsteroidal anti-inflammatory drugs
    3. Disease-modifying antirheumatic drugs
    4. Purine-reducing drugs

11. **You are to administer 6 mg of IM dexamethasone after consulting the package label shown. How many mL will you give?**

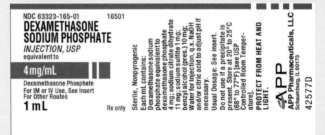

## Next-Generation NCLEX® (NGN) Examination–Style Question

### History and Physical
### 1 week ago, 0900

A 2-year-old, female client presents to the clinic with their parent. The parent provides the history and states the child woke up 2 days ago with a fever, cough, and fatigue.

Physical Exam:

General: flushed. Awake and alert but resting quietly on parent's shoulder

HEENT: oropharynx clear, mucous membranes moist. TM tubes intact, no drainage.

Respiratory: faint wheezing bilaterally

Cardiovascular: S1, S2, no murmur

### Today, 0900

The client's parent states, "They got better from the visit last week, but then got sick again today. I had been alternating ibuprofen, baby aspirin, and acetaminophen to help the fever, which finally went away 2 days ago only to return this morning." The parent reports that the client has been profusely vomiting all morning and cannot keep fluids down.

Physical Exam:

General: slow to arouse, lethargic

HEENT: oropharynx clear, mucous membranes moist. TM tubes intact, no drainage.

Respiratory: bilateral breath sounds clear

Cardiovascular: S1, S2, no murmur

### Laboratory Results
### 1 week ago, 0900

| TEST/PANEL | RESULT | NORMAL |
|---|---|---|
| Influenza A | positive | negative |
| Influenza B | negative | negative |
| Hemoglobin | 13.2 g/dL | 9.5–14 g/dL |
| Creatinine | 0.2 mg/dL | 0.2–0.5 mg/dL |
| Aspartate aminotransferase (AST) | 40 units/L | 15–60 units/L |
| Alanine aminotransferase (ALT) | 30 IU/L (30 units/L) | 4–36 IU/L or 4–36 units/L |

### Today, 0900

| TEST/PANEL | RESULT | NORMAL |
|---|---|---|
| Influenza A | negative | negative |
| Influenza B | negative | negative |
| Hemoglobin | 14.2 g/dL | 9.5–14 g/dL |
| Creatinine | 0.6 mg/dL | 0.2–0.5 mg/dL |
| Aspartate aminotransferase (AST) | 66 units/L | 15–60 units/L |
| Alanine aminotransferase (ALT) | 40 IU/L (40 units/L) | 4–36 IU/L or 4–36 units/L |

### Flow Sheet
### 1 week ago, 0900

Heart Rate: 114/min
Respiratory Rate: 30/min
Temperature: 101.8°F (38.7°C)
Weight: 27 pounds (12.2 kg)

### Today, 0900

Heart Rate: 120/min
Respiratory Rate: 22/min
Temperature: 102.2°F (39°C)
Weight: 26.5 pounds (12.0 kg)

### Orders
### 1 week ago, 0930

Oseltamivir 30 mg BID x 5 days
The nurse is caring for the client in an outpatient pediatrician's office.

**Choose the most likely options for the information missing from the statement(s) by selecting from the lists of options provided.**

The nurse suspects the client may have developed ____1____ as evidenced by the client's ____2____.

| OPTIONS FOR 1 | OPTIONS FOR 2 |
|---|---|
| Aspirin toxicity | Heart rate |
| Reye's syndrome | AST/ALT |
| Gastrointestinal bleed | Hemoglobin |
| Acute kidney injury | Creatinine |

See answer on Evolve at http://evolve.elsevier.com/Visovsky/LPNpharmacology/.

# Drugs for Gastrointestinal Problems

14

## Learning Outcomes

1. List the names, actions, possible side effects, and adverse effects of antiemetics and promotility drugs.
2. Explain what to teach patients and families about antiemetics and promotility drugs.
3. List the names, actions, possible side effects, and adverse effects of antacids and histamine $H_2$ receptor blockers.
4. Explain what to teach patients and families about antacids and histamine $H_2$ receptor blockers.
5. List the names, actions, possible side effects, and adverse effects of proton-pump inhibitors and cytoprotective drugs.
6. Explain what to teach patients and families about proton-pump inhibitors and cytoprotective drugs.
7. List the names, actions, possible side effects, and adverse effects of laxatives and antidiarrheals.
8. Explain what to teach patients and families about laxatives and antidiarrheals.

## Key Terms

**antacid** Drug that reduces symptoms of indigestion and heartburn by neutralizing hydrochloric acid (HCl) in the stomach.

**antidiarrheal** Drug that reduces or stops loose, watery stools (diarrhea) and helps restore normal bowel movements.

**antiemetic** Drug used to prevent and treat nausea and vomiting.

**cannabinoids** Natural or synthetic forms of tetrahydrocannabinol (THC) that reduce nausea and vomiting by binding to cannabinoid receptors in the chemoreceptor trigger zone (CTZ) and by preventing serotonin ($5\text{-}HT_3$) from binding to its receptors in the CTZ.

**chloride channel activators** These are used for patients with chronic constipation or irritable bowel syndrome with constipation. They act by increasing water and chloride in the lumen of the intestine.

**cytoprotective drugs** A class of drugs that protect the lining of the stomach and prevent further damage from stomach acid.

**guanylate cyclase-C agonists** A class of drugs used for chronic constipation and irritable bowel syndrome with constipation (IBS-C) that can decrease abdominal pain, decrease inflammation, and increase fluids in the intestinal lumen.

**histamine $H_2$-receptor blocker** A class of drugs that inhibit the binding of histamine to $H_2$ receptors on the parietal cells in the stomach, thereby decreasing gastric acid secretions.

**irritable bowel syndrome (IBS)** A chronic bowel disorder characterized by symptoms of abdominal pain and changes in bowel movements. Patients may have primary symptoms of diarrhea (IBS-D) or constipation (IBS-C). Some patients may have symptoms of both diarrhea and constipation.

**laxatives** A class of drugs that promote bowel movements by stimulating peristalsis, increasing the bulk of the stool, or softening the stool. They are typically used to relieve constipation.

**opioid agonists** A class of antidiarrheals that are effective for diarrhea but do not have analgesic or opioid-like effects. They reduce GI motility and increase the ability of the intestine to absorb water.

**phenothiazines** A class of antiemetic drugs that reduce nausea and vomiting by blocking dopamine ($D_2$) receptors in the CTZ of the brain. These drugs are also called *dopamine antagonists*.

**promotility drugs** A class of drugs that increase contraction of the upper GI tract, including the stomach and small intestines, to move contents more quickly through the tract. They do this by blocking dopamine ($D_2$) receptors in the CTZ and in the intestinal tract.

**proton-pump inhibitors (PPIs)** A class of drugs that bind to the proton pump of the gastric parietal cells, which blocks acid secretion into the stomach.

**select serotonin receptor agonists** A class of drugs that stimulates peristalsis in the GI tract. It can be used only in women younger than 65 years of age for irritable bowel syndrome with constipation (IBS-C).

**serotonin ($5\text{-}HT_3$) receptor antagonists** A class of antiemetic drugs that reduce or halt nausea and vomiting by blocking $5\text{-}HT_3$ receptors in the intestinal tract and in the CTZ so that serotonin cannot activate these receptors.

**substance P/neurokinin 1 (NK1) receptor antagonists** A class of antiemetic drugs that block substance P/neurokinin 1 (NK1) receptors in the chemoreceptor trigger zone (CTZ). This prevents substance P and neurokinin, which are released from cells exposed to chemotherapy and from tissues that are traumatized during surgery, from binding to and triggering the CTZ.

## THE DIGESTIVE SYSTEM

The digestive system is composed of the mouth, esophagus, stomach, intestines, and accessory structures (Fig. 14.1). This system performs the mechanical

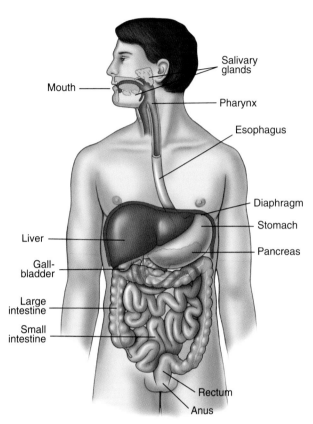

Fig. 14.1 The digestive system. (Modified from Herlihy, B. (2014). *The human body in health and illness* (5th ed.). Elsevier.)

and chemical processes of digestion, absorbs nutrients, and eliminates waste (Fig. 14.2). Although it is located inside the body, the digestive system is in constant contact with the external environment. It is open at both ends, and unlike other internal body areas, substances placed in it do not need to be sterile. In addition to problems that arise within the digestive system, being open to the environment increases the number and types of problems that can occur anywhere along the gastrointestinal (GI) tract.

Digestion begins in the mouth, where food is chewed and mixed with enzyme-rich saliva secreted by salivary glands. The food passes from the mouth to the anus through the digestive tract. During this passage, the complex compounds that enter the mouth as food are reduced to smaller dissolvable particles and their carriers (see Fig. 14.2). Usable food particles are absorbed, whereas indigestible pieces and waste materials are eliminated. *Accessory digestive glands* (salivary glands, gallbladder, and pancreas) secrete enzymes and other chemicals that are required to break down food substances and promote absorption into the bloodstream.

In the stomach, digestion requires a strong acid (i.e., hydrochloric acid [HCl]) to break down protein and other substances. However, this gastric acid is so strong (has a low pH) that it could erode the cells lining the stomach and form open sores (ulcers). Think of the burning sensation you feel in your mouth, throat, and nose when you vomit. Fortunately, several factors work together to protect the GI tract mucosa from injury. One protective substance secreted by stomach-lining parietal cells is a type of prostaglandin. This substance triggers the production of thick mucus that

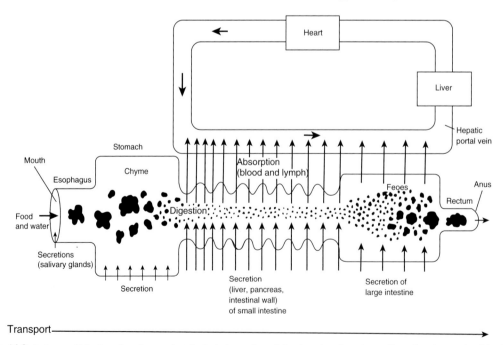

Fig. 14.2 Actions within the digestive system include ingestion of food and water, absorption of water and nutrients, secretion of aids to digestion, and removal of waste products. (From Vander, A. J., Sherman, J. H., & Luciano, D. S. (1990). *Human physiology* (5th ed.). McGraw-Hill. Used with permission.)

forms a gel-like layer in the stomach that helps prevent stomach acid and enzymes from coming into direct contact with and damaging the lining. *Prostaglandins* also maintain good blood flow to the stomach, which keeps these tissues well oxygenated and allows the immune system to help keep them healthy.

As partially digested food and liquid leave the stomach and enter the *duodenum* (first 12 to 18 inches of the small intestine), the stomach contents are still very acidic. The duodenum does not have the mucous protection that the stomach has, and it could easily develop ulcers from exposure to acid and digestive enzymes. However, the pancreas produces copious amounts of bicarbonate and secretes it into the duodenum to neutralize the acid in the partially digested contents from the stomach.

Two of the more common GI problems are nausea and vomiting as well as peptic ulcer disease. Other problems include the movement of stomach contents back into the esophagus *(gastric reflux)*, abnormally slow movement of contents through the intestinal tract *(constipation)*, and abnormally fast movement of contents through the intestinal tract *(diarrhea)*. *Irritable bowel syndrome (IBS)* is a chronic bowel disorder that is characterized by symptoms of abdominal pain and changes in bowel movements. This chapter focuses on drug therapy to prevent or manage these problems. The digestive tract can become infected with bacteria, viruses, fungi, and parasites, and drug therapy for these infections is described in Chapters 5, 6, and 7.

## ANTIEMETIC DRUGS

Nausea and vomiting are common GI problems that occur as a result of infection, fever, motion, certain foods, anesthesia, and exposure to one or more of a wide range of drugs, including cancer chemotherapy drugs. Nausea and vomiting often occur together, or vomiting follows nausea. However, nausea can occur without vomiting and is still an unpleasant sensation. Vomiting also can occur without the sensation of nausea.

Although we tend to think of nausea and vomiting as problems of the digestive tract, they result from a complex set of interactions that involve the brain, nervous system, inner ear, stomach, and intestines (Fig. 14.3). Messages from the cerebral cortex (e.g., fear, anxiety), the sensory organs (e.g., sights, odors, pain), or the vestibular apparatus in the inner ear (e.g., motion sickness) can be sent to the vomiting center in the brain. These are called *direct-acting stimuli* because the message goes directly to the vomiting center. *Indirect-acting stimuli* involve the chemoreceptor trigger zone (CTZ). For example, opioids, alcohol, certain antibiotics, and types of anesthesia can stimulate the CTZ. The CTZ then sends messages to the vomiting center. Signals from the stomach or small intestine can send messages to the CTZ, such as after a big meal or a food that "does not agree" with you. Think of the last time

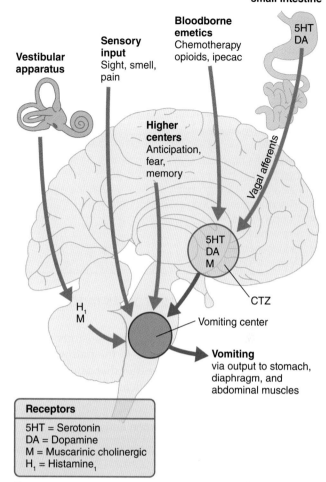

**Fig. 14.3** Vomiting is a complex reflex. It involves stimulation of the vomiting center directly or indirectly through the chemoreceptor trigger zone *(CTZ)*. Many types of receptors are involved in vomiting. By understanding that there are different types of receptors, you can understand different types of antiemetics and how they work. For example, some affect dopamine, some serotonin, some histamine, and some acetylcholine.

you felt nauseated and vomited. Was it a direct or indirect stimulus that caused the nausea and vomiting?

> **Top Tip for Safety**
>
> Patients with nausea and vomiting are at risk for dehydration, weight loss, and electrolyte imbalance. Monitor and report any changes in fluid balance or food intake and laboratory abnormalities.

An **antiemetic** is a drug used to prevent and treat nausea and vomiting, regardless of the cause. There are many classes of antiemetic drugs, including serotonin receptor antagonists, substance P antagonists, phenothiazines, cannabinoids, promotility drugs, nonphenothiazines, and anticholinergics. Most work in the brain, stomach, and intestinal tract to change the sensation of nausea and to reduce the stomach contractions that make vomiting occur. Which class of drug is used depends on the severity of the problem and the patient's individual response. Some patients require a combination of two or more types of antiemetic drugs for effective management of nausea and vomiting. The first five categories of antiemetic drugs are discussed here. The nonphenothiazines and anticholinergic drugs are discussed in Chapters 11 and 8, respectively.

 **Memory Jogger**

These are the major categories of antiemetic drugs:
- Serotonin (5-HT$_3$) receptor antagonists
- Substance P antagonists
- Phenothiazines (dopamine antagonists)
- Cannabinoids
- Promotility drugs
- Nonphenothiazines
- Anticholinergics

## SEROTONIN (5-HT$_3$) RECEPTOR ANTAGONISTS

### Action and Uses

A *neurotransmitter* is a chemical that transmits signals from one nerve to the next nerve in the pathway or to the brain. A major neurotransmitter that causes nausea and vomiting when it binds to its receptors in the CTZ or the GI system is a form of serotonin, known as *serotonin 5-hydroxytryptamine type 3 (5-HT$_3$)*.

The serotonin (5-HT$_3$) receptor antagonists are a class of antiemetic drugs that reduce or halt nausea and vomiting by blocking 5-HT$_3$ receptors in the intestinal tract and the CTZ so that serotonin cannot activate these receptors. These antiemetics are used to reduce or prevent the nausea and vomiting resulting from cancer chemotherapy, radiation therapy, and anesthesia-induced nausea and vomiting after surgery. These drugs may be called *setrons* for short because their generic names typically end in the suffix *-setron*. Table 14.1 lists the names, dosages, and nursing implications for common serotonin (5-HT$_3$) receptor antagonists. Consult a drug reference book for more information about specific drugs.

 **Memory Jogger**

All of the serotonin (5-HT$_3$) receptor antagonists have the suffix *-setron* in their generic names.

### Expected Side Effects

Common central nervous system (CNS) side effects of serotonin (5-HT$_3$) receptor antagonists include dizziness, headache, and drowsiness. Some patients

| Table 14.1 Examples of Common Antiemetics |
|---|
| *Serotonin (5-HT$_3$) receptor antagonists* reduce or halt nausea and vomiting by blocking 5-HT$_3$ receptors in the intestinal tract and the chemoreceptor trigger zone (CTZ) so that serotonin cannot activate these receptors. |
| *Substance P/neurokinin 1 receptor antagonists* reduce or prevent immediate and delayed nausea and vomiting by blocking the substance P/neurokinin 1 receptors in the CTZ, preventing both substances from binding to and triggering the CTZ. |
| *Phenothiazines* reduce nausea and vomiting by blocking dopamine (D$_2$) receptors in the CTZ. |
| *Cannabinoids* are natural or synthetic forms of THC that reduce nausea and vomiting by binding to cannabinoid receptors in the CTZ and by preventing serotonin 5-HT$_3$ from binding to its receptors in the CTZ. |
| *Promotility drugs* increase contraction of the upper GI tract, including the stomach and small intestine, by blocking dopamine (D$_2$) receptors in the CTZ and the intestinal tract. |

| DRUG/ADULT DOSAGE | NURSING IMPLICATIONS |
|---|---|
| **Serotonin (5-HT$_3$) Receptor Antagonists** | |
| ondansetron (Zofran, Zuplenz) 16 mg orally 1 hour *before surgery* as a single dose; *after surgery* 4 mg intramuscular (IM) as a single dose if the patient has nausea and vomiting *or* 8 mg orally disintegrating tablets (ODT) as a single dose at the end of surgery; may also give 4 mg IM as a single dose before anesthesia or once postoperatively if nausea and vomiting after surgery<br><br>ondansetron (Zofran, Zuplenz) 8 mg orally 30 minutes *before chemotherapy*, with doses 8 hours after the initial dose; may give doses every 12 hours for 1–2 days after chemotherapy is completed; doses may be higher for highly emetogenic chemotherapy agents | • Make sure the patient has a call light available because these drugs can cause dizziness.<br>• Give the drug before the patient has an episode of vomiting because it can prevent or relieve nausea before the patient vomits.<br>• ODTs dissolve in seconds after being placed on the tongue. After the tablet is dissolved, the patient may swallow. It does not need to be given with water.<br>• Contact the healthcare provider if the patient is also taking drugs that affect serotonin levels because the interaction can cause serious adverse effects.<br>• These drugs may be given for postoperative nausea and vomiting but typically are delivered intravenously rather than orally.<br>• Follow the hospital protocols carefully if given for chemotherapy-induced nausea and vomiting. Protocols vary according to the potential of the chemotherapy drugs to cause nausea and vomiting. More emetogenic chemotherapy drugs may require more frequent dosing. |

Table **14.1**   **Examples of Common Antiemetics—cont'd**

**Substance P/Neurokinin 1 Receptor Antagonists**

| | |
|---|---|
| aprepitant (Emend-oral) on day 1, 125 mg orally 1 hour before chemotherapy; on days 2 and 3, 80 mg orally 1 hour before chemotherapy, or if no chemotherapy is scheduled on days 2 and 3, give in the morning; available as capsule or oral suspension<br><br>rolapitant (Varubi) 180 mg orally on day 1, given 1–2 hours before chemotherapy; follow hospital protocols for dosages | • Always double-check doses of substance P/neurokinin 1 receptor agonists because protocols vary according to the potential of the chemotherapy drugs to cause nausea and vomiting. More emetogenic chemotherapy drugs may require more frequent dosing.<br>• In some cases this drug may be combined with a corticosteroid to further reduce symptoms of nausea and vomiting. |

**Phenothiazines**

| | |
|---|---|
| prochlorperazine (Compazine, Compro) 5–10 mg orally three to four times daily as needed; IM 5–10 mg every 3–4 hours as needed; rectally 25 mg twice daily as needed<br><br>promethazine (Phenergan, Promethegan) 12.5–25 mg orally every 4–6 hours as needed; IM 12–25 mg every 4–6 hours as needed; rectal 12.5–25 mg every 4–6 hours as needed<br><br>promethazine (Phenergan) for motion sickness 25 mg orally or rectally 30–60 minutes before departure, then every 12 hours as needed | • Teach patients to change position slowly because these drugs can cause orthostatic hypotension.<br>• Give IM injections deeply into large muscle.<br>• Remind patients that alcohol may increase drowsiness and risk of injury.<br>• Watch carefully for side or adverse effects related to these drugs and their effects on dopamine. Contact the healthcare provider for any Parkinson's disease–like tremors or gait changes, muscle spasms, or changes in motor movement such as tongue rolling or lip smacking because these are serious adverse reactions.<br>• Monitor the patient carefully for any sudden increase in temperature because this can be an indication of neuroleptic malignant syndrome, a rare but life-threatening adverse effect. |

**Cannabinoids**

| | |
|---|---|
| dronabinol (Marinol, Syndros) 5 mg/m$^2$ orally as liquid-filled capsules given 1–3 hours before chemotherapy and then every 2–4 hours afterward for a total of four to six doses per day; 4.2 mg/m$^2$ as oral solution (rounded to the nearest 0.1 mg) given 1–3 hours before chemotherapy and then every 2–4 hours after chemotherapy for a total of four to six doses per day Follow hospital protocols carefully.<br><br>nabilone (Cesamet) 1–2 mg orally twice daily; the initial dose is given 1–3 hours before chemotherapy; a dose of 1–2 mg the night before chemotherapy may be useful Follow hospital protocols carefully | • Cannabinoids are typically reserved for patients who continue to have nausea and vomiting that does not respond to other antiemetics.<br>• These drugs are typically given as an oral solution or in liquid-filled capsules with the dosage individualized according to *body surface* area calculations (e.g., a person who is 6 feet tall and weighs 225 pounds would receive 11.2 mg of the drug). The dosage is determined by the healthcare provider in conjunction with the pharmacist.<br>• For liquid drugs, always use the proper measuring device (e.g., oral syringe) to ensure accuracy.<br>• Advise patients to avoid alcohol, sedatives, and other central nervous system depressants because they may increase the risk of sedation.<br>• Monitor the patient carefully for changes in mental status. Cannabinoids can cause confusion, sedation, and sometimes feelings of euphoria or a "high." These responses typically decrease after a few days of use. |

**Promotility Drugs**

| | |
|---|---|
| metoclopramide (Reglan) for postoperative nausea and vomiting or prevention of them, 10 mg IM intravenous every 4-6 hours as needed<br><br>trimethobenzamide (Tigan) 300 mg orally three or four times daily PRN; IM 200 mg three or four times daily PRN | • Monitor the patient carefully for any mood changes or restlessness because these are common side effects.<br>• Check vital signs regularly to assess for changes in blood pressure (decrease) because there is a risk of orthostatic hypotension.<br>• When giving IM, use large muscle mass. |

experience changes in taste, heartburn, constipation, or diarrhea. Rarely, a patient may experience chills with shivering.

### Adverse Reactions
Adverse reactions include allergic reactions, dysrhythmias, and renal or liver damage. Serotonin syndrome can occur if the patient is taking other drugs that increase serotonin (e.g., certain antidepressants, St. John's wort). For more information about serotonin syndrome, see Chapter 11.

### Drug Interactions
These drugs can interact with a variety of drugs that contain the neurotransmitter serotonin or are similar to serotonin. Examples include monoamine oxidase inhibitors (MAO-Is), morphine, and serotonin reuptake inhibitors. If 5-HT$_3$ receptor antagonists are combined with phenothiazine drugs, patients may experience cardiac dysrhythmias.

### ❖ Nursing Implications and Patient Teaching
◆ *Planning and implementation.* In addition to the general nursing considerations related to care of the patient with antiemetic drugs described in Box 14.1, the following issues and actions are important. Follow protocols very carefully to ensure adequate timing before the patient receives chemotherapy. Monitor vital signs before and after giving the drug. Ask the patient about any abdominal pain. Severe pain can indicate

infection, bleeding, or other severe problems in the GI tract. Follow up with your patients to make sure they are getting relief from their nausea.

◆ *Patient and family teaching.* Tell the patient and family:
- To avoid possible interactions, do not take any herbal agents without checking with a pharmacist or other healthcare provider while taking any of the serotonin 5-HT$_3$ receptor antagonists.
- Tell your healthcare provider if you are taking serotonin 5-HT$_3$ receptor antagonists because these drugs interact with a variety of other drugs.
- Avoid driving, operating heavy machinery, or participating in critical decision making while taking this drug because it may impair your judgment and reflexes.
- It is best to take the drug before you have vomited rather than waiting until after you have had an episode of vomiting.
- Do not use alcohol or other drugs with sedating effects while taking this drug.

## SUBSTANCE P/NEUROKININ 1 RECEPTOR ANTAGONISTS

### Action and Uses
Another receptor in the CTZ that can cause nausea and vomiting when activated is the substance P/neurokinin 1 (NK1) receptor. *Substance P* is produced by many normal cells all over the body when they have been traumatized by inflammation and pain or exposed to noxious stimuli. Substance P enters the bloodstream

---

| Box **14.1** | General Nursing Considerations for Antiemetic Drug Therapy |

- Assess heart rate, blood pressure, respiratory rate, and level of consciousness before giving any antiemetic agent.
- Remove any foods, smells, or images that may make nausea worse.
- Ask the patient to describe his or her nausea, and if the patient vomits, record the color, consistency, and amount.
- Give the antiemetic drug for nausea rather than waiting until the patient vomits.
- Vomiting can result in dehydration and electrolyte imbalance, so make sure to monitor weight, skin turgor, and intake and output. Review serum electrolytes and report abnormal results to the healthcare provider.
- If the patient is taking an antiemetic for chemotherapy, carefully review the prescribed protocol to ensure good timing of drug administration.
- Determine the effectiveness of the antiemetic by monitoring the patient's report of relief from nausea and no further vomiting.
- Tell the patient to ask for help when getting out of bed or out of the chair because these drugs can cause dizziness and drowsiness. Be sure to have the call light within the reach of the patient.
- Immediately report to the healthcare provider any symptoms of severe abdominal pain or signs of

abdominal distention because these may be signs of complications.
- Immediately report to the healthcare provider emesis that looks like coffee grounds or is red-tinged because this may indicate bleeding in the gastrointestinal tract.
- Tell the patient to avoid driving or use of heavy machinery while taking antiemetics because they can cause dizziness and drowsiness.
- Teach the patient to contact the healthcare provider before adding any over-the-counter drugs or herbal drugs because they can increase the risk for drug interactions.
- Remind the patient to avoid alcohol, sedatives, and tranquilizers unless specifically advised by the healthcare provider.
- Many of these drugs cause increased sun sensitivity, and patients must avoid direct sunlight without sunscreen and protective clothing.
- Teach the patient to rinse his or her mouth carefully with clear liquids after vomiting. Ice chips or mild-flavored popsicles may be soothing.
- Teach the patient to contact his or her healthcare provider if nausea and/or vomiting lasts more than 2 days or he or she is unable to take any fluids or has fever.

and crosses into the brain, where it can bind to the substance P/NK1 receptors that are present in many parts of the brain, including the CTZ and areas that perceive pain. Activating these receptors in the CTZ stimulates immediate and delayed nausea and vomiting. **Substance P/neurokinin 1 (NK1) receptor antagonists** are a class of drugs that block the substance P/NK1 receptors in the CTZ. This prevents substance P and neurokinin, which are released from cells exposed to chemotherapy and from tissues injured during surgery, from binding to and triggering the CTZ.

The most common uses for drugs in this class are to reduce or prevent the nausea and vomiting that result from cancer chemotherapy and occur after surgery. These drugs are especially effective at managing the delayed nausea and vomiting that often starts 24 to 72 hours after chemotherapy. The oldest drug in this class is aprepitant (Emend). These drugs are most effective when used in combination with the serotonin (5-HT$_3$) receptor antagonists. Table 14.1 lists the names, dosages, and nursing implications for the substance P/NK1 receptor antagonists. Be sure to consult a drug reference book for more information about specific drugs.

## Expected Side Effects

Fatigue, diarrhea, headache, and dizziness are side effects of the substance P/NK1 receptor antagonists. The patient may experience mild hiccups, flatulence, and sweating.

## Adverse Reactions

Neutropenia is one of the most common adverse reactions associated with substance P/NK1 receptor antagonists. Angioedema, severe allergic reactions, and respiratory depression may occur. Other blood abnormalities include anemia and thrombocytopenia, and you should monitor laboratory values carefully.

## Drug Interactions

Substance P/NK1 receptor antagonists interact with a variety of drugs. In particular, they interact with opioid drugs, causing increased dizziness, drowsiness, and sedation. Use of these drugs with certain benzodiazepines can increase the effect of the benzodiazepines, and they should be used together with caution.

❖ **Nursing Implications and Patient Teaching**

◆ *Planning and implementation.* In addition to the general nursing considerations related to care of the patient with nausea and vomiting listed in Box 14.1, the following issues and actions are important. Carefully review the drug instructions to ensure that the drug is prepared properly. For example, the oral form of aprepitant should not be opened until you are ready to prepare it. At that time, the mixing cup provided in the drug kit should be filled with room-temperature drinking water. After you have added the precise amount of water to the mixing cup as directed, pour the contents

of the drug into the cup and then snap the lid shut. Gently swirl the solution 20 times to mix it, and then invert the cup. To prevent foaming, do not shake the cup. Be sure there are no clumps or foam in the solution. At that time, you can measure the solution to give it to the patient. Discard any remaining solution.

As for the oral liquid aprepitant, injectable fosaprepitant must be carefully prepared. Do not shake the drug. You may gently swirl the drug or invert the solution to gently mix it. Follow directions specifically for proper mixing and rate of administration.

◆ *Patient and family teaching.* Tell the patient and family:
- If you are taking the oral solution, avoid shaking the mixture. You can gently swirl and turn over the measuring cup or syringe.
- After the drug is mixed, it can be stored in the refrigerator for up to 30 days.
- To prevent side effects, avoid alcohol and any sedating drugs while you are taking these drugs.
- Do not take any over-the-counter (OTC) or herbal drugs without checking with your healthcare provider or pharmacist because drugs from this category can interact with other drugs.

## PHENOTHIAZINES
### Action and Uses

**Phenothiazines** are a class of antiemetic drugs that reduce nausea and vomiting by blocking select dopamine receptors in the CTZ of the brain. For this reason, drugs in this class are also called *dopamine antagonists*. Dopamine receptors are present in many areas of the brain and the body. As a result, these drugs have many other effects in the body in addition to antiemetic effects. Dopamine antagonists are approved to reduce nausea and vomiting from many problems except for the morning sickness associated with pregnancy. Table 14.1 lists the names, dosages, and nursing implications for the phenothiazines. Be sure to consult a drug reference book for more information about specific drugs.

## Expected Side Effects

Common side effects of phenothiazines include drowsiness, blurred vision, dry mouth, and dizziness. Some phenothiazines can cause urine to change to a pinkish-red color. Sensitivity to sun exposure is common.

## Adverse Reactions

Adverse reactions to phenothiazine drugs are most common at higher doses. As a result of blocking dopamine, the patient can experience extrapyramidal symptoms (EPSs), as discussed in Chapter 11. The effects include tardive dyskinesia, acute dystonia, and neuroleptic malignant syndrome. Blood abnormalities are also possible while the patient is taking phenothiazines. These drugs should be avoided in patients with cardiovascular disease because they can cause patients to experience angina, tachycardia, and/or orthostatic hypotension.

### Drug Interactions

Phenothiazines interact with a wide variety of drugs. They should not be given with the promotility drug metoclopramide (Reglan), which also affects dopamine levels. Phenothiazines can increase the effects of other drugs that affect dopamine, including monoamine oxidase inhibitors and several other antidepressants. Benzodiazepines can increase drowsiness. Phenothiazines should be avoided in patients who are taking levodopa/carbidopa (a combination medicine) for Parkinson's disease (see Chapter 10).

### ❖ Nursing Implications and Patient Teaching

◆ *Planning and implementation.* In addition to the general nursing considerations related to antiemetic drug therapy listed in Box 14.1, the following issues and actions are important.

Carefully assess the vital signs in patients who are taking phenothiazines because these drugs can decrease blood pressure and increase the heart rate in some patients. Avoid giving a phenothiazine antiemetic to any patient who has low blood pressure or is dehydrated. Make sure the patient has the call light available to ask for help when getting out of bed after receiving this drug because it can cause orthostatic hypotension.

Assess for any occurrence of EPSs, as detailed in Chapter 11. If the patient demonstrates unusual muscle movements or has abrupt changes in temperature, heart rate, or blood pressure, notify the healthcare provider immediately.

◆ *Patient and family teaching.* Tell the patient and family:
- You may experience dizziness, drowsiness, or blurred vision while taking this drug. Avoid driving, using any heavy equipment, or participating in any dangerous activity.
- Change position slowly to avoid dizziness.
- Do not drink alcohol while taking this drug. Alcohol may increase the side effects.
- You may notice a slight change in your urine to a pinkish-red color. This is an expected side effect.
- If you have any muscle spasms (particularly of the neck muscles); involuntary movements of the face, tongue, or upper or lower extremities; or any unusual restlessness, notify your healthcare provider immediately.
- The drug may decrease your ability to sweat, so make sure to avoid becoming overheated during physical activity or very hot weather.
- For relief of dry mouth, try sugarless gum or candy, or use ice chips to moisten your mouth.
- These drugs can cause your skin to be more sensitive to light, so avoid direct sunlight and, if needed, wear protective eyewear and clothing. Wear sunblock while outside to avoid sunburn.

## CANNABINOIDS

### Action and Uses

Marijuana, a common street drug approved in some states for use in the medical treatment of certain health problems, has been used to help control the nausea and vomiting associated with cancer chemotherapy. Although many chemicals are present in marijuana, the one that has antiemetic actions is tetrahydrocannabinol (THC). All humans have THC receptors in many areas of the brain, including the CTZ and pleasure centers.

Cannabinoids are natural or synthetic forms of THC that reduce nausea and vomiting by binding to cannabinoid receptors in the CTZ and by preventing serotonin 5-HT$_3$ from binding to its receptors in the CTZ. Because of the potential for addiction (rare but possible) and other side effects, use of cannabinoids as antiemetics is typically reserved for patients with severe nausea and vomiting that have not been relieved by other antiemetics.

According to the National Council of State Boards of Nursing (NCSBN), no nurse may administer cannabis unless authorized by jurisdiction law. *It is critical for you to have a working knowledge of state and agency protocols guiding clinical practice before giving any cannabinoid.* Table 14.1 lists the names, dosages, and nursing implications for the cannabinoids. Consult a drug reference book for more information about specific drugs.

### Expected Side Effects

The most common side effects are related to the actions of cannabinoids in the CNS. Some patients experience a dose-related "high" (easy laughing, elation, and increased awareness). Other CNS effects are dizziness, anxiety, insomnia, difficulty concentrating, and mood changes. Some patients may experience *emotional lability* (wide swings in emotion). These side effects may decrease after 2 weeks of treatment. Some patients have GI side effects such as nausea, vomiting, and abdominal pain. Orthostatic hypotension is more common in older adults.

### Adverse Reactions

Acute confusion, hypersensitivity, and seizurelike activity have occurred in some patients. Rarely, hallucinations, excessive sweating, or fainting can happen, and it is important to carefully monitor the patient. Cannabinoids should be used with caution in patients who have a history of substance abuse (including alcohol) because of the increased risk of abuse of the drug.

### Drug Interactions

Cannabinoids can interact with a variety of drugs. Examples include warfarin, calcium channel blockers, opioid agonists, and a variety of antiretroviral drugs used to treat human immunodeficiency virus (HIV). Patients who take dronabinol should avoid grapefruit juice because it can increase adverse effects.

### ❖ Nursing Implications and Patient Teaching
◆ *Planning and implementation.* In addition to the general nursing considerations related to antiemetic drug therapy listed in Box 14.1, the following issues and actions are important.

These drugs can be given using standard tablets and capsules or as a liquid or in liquid-filled capsules with the dosage individualized according to *body surface area* (measure of the total external surface area of the body). The dosage is determined with the use of body surface area calculations by the healthcare provider in conjunction with the pharmacist.

If you are giving a dose of the liquid drug, use the proper measuring device (e.g., an oral syringe) to ensure accuracy. Give the first dose on an empty stomach 30 minutes before a meal. After the first dose, these drugs can be given with food.

Carefully monitor the patient for changes in mental status. Cannabinoids can cause confusion, sedation, and sometimes feelings of euphoria or a "high." These typically decrease after a few days to weeks of use. Advise patients to avoid alcohol, sedatives, and other CNS depressants because they may increase the risk of sedation.

◆ *Patient and family teaching.* Tell the patient and family:
- Avoid using alcohol, sedatives, or any antianxiety drugs with cannabinoids without talking to your healthcare provider.
- Take the dose as prescribed; do not increase it without talking to your healthcare provider.
- This drug may cause you to feel slightly "high," with feelings of easy laughing, mood changes, elation, and increased awareness. These feelings decrease in a few days to a few weeks.
- Do not drive, operate heavy machinery, or participate in important decision making while taking this drug.
- Ask family members to stay with you when you first start taking the drugs in case you have some confusion or dizziness.

### PROMOTILITY DRUGS
#### Action and Uses
**Promotility drugs** (also called *prokinetic drugs*) increase contraction of the upper GI tract, including the stomach and small intestines, and move contents more quickly through the tract. They do this by blocking dopamine ($D_2$) receptors in the CTZ and the intestinal tract. They work in a fashion similar to the phenothiazines but do not have the sedating side effect.

Promotility drugs may be used in patients with postoperative nausea and vomiting, chemotherapy-induced nausea and vomiting, or gastroesophageal reflux disease (GERD). They may also be used in patients who have difficulty emptying the stomach, such as a patient with diabetic gastroparesis. Table 14.1 lists the names, dosages, and nursing implications of common drugs from the promotility class. Consult a drug reference book for more information about specific drugs.

#### Expected Side Effects
The most common side effects of promotility drugs are drowsiness, fatigue, and restlessness. Others are visual impairment, urinary incontinence, and insomnia.

#### Adverse Reactions
Promotility drugs should be used with caution in patients with a history of depression because they can cause depression and suicidal ideation, seizures, blood disorders, cardiac dysrhythmias, and heart failure. Other adverse effects are related to decreased levels of the neurotransmitter dopamine. This can result in symptoms similar to Parkinson's disease, including tremor, bradykinesia (slow movement), and masklike faces. These symptoms decline in 2 to 3 months after stopping the drug. More severe adverse effects include tardive dyskinesia, akathisia, and acute dystonia. Neuroleptic malignant syndrome is a rare, life-threatening reaction to drugs that decrease dopamine levels. These problems are discussed further in Chapter 11.

#### Drug Interactions
Promotility drugs are contraindicated in patients who are taking phenothiazine drugs, typical or atypical antipsychotics (see Chapter 11), or levodopa/carbidopa (see Chapter 10). Use of these drugs with certain antidepressants can increase the risk of serotonin syndrome, which is discussed in greater detail in Chapter 11.

### ❖ Nursing Implications and Patient Teaching
◆ *Planning and implementation.* In addition to the general nursing considerations related to antiemetic drug therapy listed in Box 14.1, the following issues and actions are important.

Carefully monitor the patient for symptoms of restlessness, dizziness, and fatigue. This is especially important for the older adult who may be at greater risk for confusion or falls. Monitor the patient for Parkinson's disease–like symptoms such as tremor, slower gait, or masklike facial appearance. If the patient experiences these side effects, notify the healthcare provider because the drug may need to be discontinued.

◆ *Patient and family teaching.* Tell the patient and family:
- Avoid driving, using heavy machinery, or making important decisions while using this drug until you are aware of the effects.

- To avoid severe side effects, do not drink alcohol while taking this drug.
- If you have any depression or thoughts of suicide, notify your healthcare provider immediately.
- Inform your healthcare provider immediately if you have any sudden increase in fever, muscle spasms, or difficulty with movement because these may be signs of a more serious health issue.
- Some men may experience erectile dysfunction or *gynecomastia* (enlargement of the breasts); some women may experience menstrual irregularities. These effects are usually reversible within a few weeks to a few months.

## DRUGS FOR PEPTIC ULCER DISEASE AND GASTROESOPHAGEAL REFLUX DISEASE

The lining of the stomach is usually strong enough to resist the powerful digestive juices and acids that aid normal digestion. Gastric distress may be caused when stress or disease produces excess secretion of gastric acids or when alcohol, chemicals, drugs, or disease damages the protective mucosal lining. If the protective lining is not repaired or the gastric acid level is not reduced, duodenal and gastric ulcers are produced. This is known as *peptic ulcer disease (PUD)*, as shown in Fig. 14.4. PUD is associated with inflammation, pain, bleeding, reduced nutrition, and reduced quality of life.

 **Memory Jogger**

Prostaglandins maintain good blood flow to the stomach, which keeps these tissues well oxygenated and allows the immune system to help keep them healthy. This is why drugs that decrease prostaglandins, such as corticosteroids and NSAIDs, can be harmful to the stomach.

For many people, another problem is GERD, a condition in which the highly acidic stomach contents move backward *(reflux)* into the esophagus (Fig. 14.5). The esophagus has no protection against this acidity and therefore can be damaged very easily. Drug therapies for PUD and GERD are essentially the same. Commonly used drug therapies include antacids, histamine $H_2$-receptor blockers, proton-pump inhibitors (PPIs), and cytoprotective drugs. Table 14.2 lists the names, dosages, and nursing implications of common drugs for PUD and GERD. More than one drug type may be used at the same time to help in healing the initial problem.

 **Memory Jogger**

These common drugs are used to manage peptic ulcers and GERD:
- Antacids
- Histamine $H_2$-receptor blockers
- Proton-pump inhibitors (PPIs)
- Cytoprotective drugs

Some peptic ulcers may be caused by *Helicobacter pylori (H. pylori)*. *H. pylori* infections are typically treated by a combination of antimicrobial drugs and PPIs. Patients with *H. pylori*–associated ulcers are treated for about 10 to 14 days with a standard triple therapy consisting of a PPI and two selected antimicrobials. Alternatively, a standard quadruple therapy with a PPI and three antimicrobials may be considered. The *H. pylori* bacteria must be eradicated for successful treatment of the peptic ulcer. Chapter 5 discusses the patient teaching issues and nursing implications for antimicrobial therapy.

### ANTACIDS

#### Action and Uses

An **antacid** is a drug that reduces symptoms of indigestion and heartburn by neutralizing hydrochloric acid (HCl) in the stomach. This increases gastric pH (makes the stomach's pH less acidic), which reduces gastric irritation. Antacids are typically formulated with at least

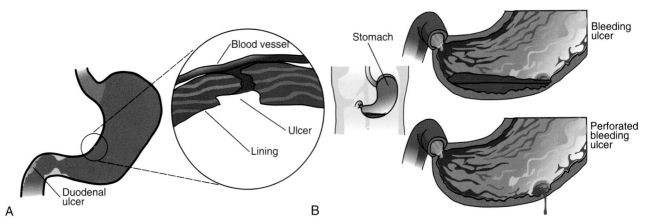

**Fig. 14.4** (A) Peptic ulcer pathophysiology. The mucosa breaks down, and an open sore develops. (B) A peptic ulcer may lead to bleeding, perforation, or other emergencies. (From Workman, M. L., & LaCharity, L. A. (2016). *Understanding pharmacology: Essentials for Medication Safety* (2nd ed.). Elsevier.)

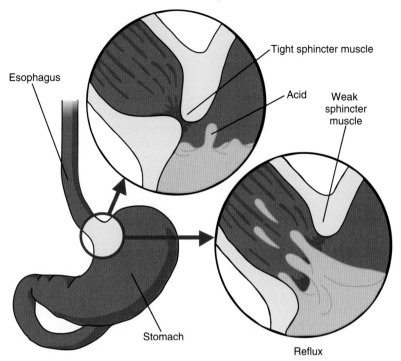

**Fig. 14.5** Pathophysiology of gastroesophageal reflux disease (GERD). Acid refluxes into the esophagus through the lower esophageal sphincter. (From Workman, M. L., & LaCharity, L. A. (2016). *Understanding pharmacology: Essentials for Medication Safety* (2nd ed.). Elsevier.)

| Table **14.2** | Common Drugs for Peptic Ulcer Disease and Gastroesophageal Reflux Disease |
|---|---|

*Antacids* neutralize stomach acids to help relieve heartburn and indigestion.

*Histamine H_2-receptor blockers* bind to the H_2 receptors in stomach cells, which decreases production of basal and nighttime gastric acid. They also decrease the amount of gastric acid that is released with meals and substances such as caffeine.

*Proton-pump inhibitors* help heal gastric ulcers and reduce symptoms of GERD by stopping the acid secretory pump that is located in the gastric parietal cell membrane, which reduces the amount of acid secreted into the stomach.

*Cytoprotective drugs* protect the lining of the stomach and prevent further damage.

| DRUG/ADULT DOSAGE | NURSING IMPLICATIONS |
|---|---|
| **Antacids** | |
| aluminum hydroxide (Alternagel, Alu-Cap) dosages vary depending on the formulation; make sure to check your drug handbook<br>calcium carbonate (Rolaids Extra Strength, Tums, Caltrate, Maalox) dosages vary depending on the formulation; make sure to check your drug handbook<br>magnesium hydroxide (Milk of Magnesia) regular suspension, 5–15 mL orally up to four times per day | • Antacids are often available as combination drugs, so review drug information carefully before giving.<br>• Timing of antacids related to meals and other drugs is important. Many drugs bind with antacids and lose effectiveness. In general, antacids should be given 1 hour before any other drugs and 2 hours after any other drugs.<br>• Patients with heart failure or other cardiac diseases should avoid antacids that are high in sodium. |
| **Histamine H_2-Receptor Blockers** | |
| famotidine (Pepcid AC) OTC for prevention, 10 mg orally 15 minutes to 1 hour before eating a meal that is expected to cause symptoms (maximum 20 mg/day); for treatment, 10 mg orally, may repeat one time to maximum of 20 mg/day<br>famotidine (Pepcid) 20 mg orally twice daily for up to 6 weeks; may be up to 40 mg twice daily for 12 weeks; for acute peptic ulcer disease 40 mg orally once daily at bedtime or 20 mg IV every 12 hours; for maintenance therapy in duodenal ulcer 20 mg once daily at bedtime<br>nizatidine (Axid) capsules 150 mg orally twice daily for up to 12 weeks; OTC to prevent heartburn, 75 mg immediately or up to 60 mg before food or beverages expected to cause symptoms; for treatment, 75 mg orally once or twice daily; for active ulcer 300 mg orally at bedtime or 150 mg orally every 12 hours for 8 weeks | • OTC doses are typically about one-half of the prescription drug doses. Patients who are taking OTC histamine H_2-receptor blockers should not take them for more than 2 weeks without seeing a healthcare provider because they may have a more significant health issue.<br>• Monitor the patient for signs of restlessness or confusion because these side effects may increase the risk for falls. Patients with impaired renal function will typically receive lower doses or have increased time between doses. |

*Continued*

| Table **14.2**  Common Drugs for Peptic Ulcer Disease and Gastroesophageal Reflux Disease—cont'd | |
|---|---|
| **Proton-Pump Inhibitors** | |
| esomeprazole (Nexium) 20–40 mg orally one to two times daily given 60 minutes before first meal of the day for up to 8 weeks<br>lansoprazole (Prevacid) 15–30 mg orally once daily 30–60 minutes before first meal of the day for up to 8 weeks<br>omeprazole (Prilosec) 20–40 mg orally once daily with full glass of water 60 minutes before first meal of the day for 2–12 weeks<br>pantoprazole (Protonix) 20–40 mg orally once daily for 2–16 weeks | • Give with a full glass of water 30–60 minutes before the first meal of the day for maximum benefit. Read drug information carefully.<br>• OTC PPIs should not be taken for more than 2 weeks because failure to relieve symptoms may indicate a more severe health problem.<br>• PPIs may be prescribed long term depending on the patient's presenting condition.<br>• Teach patients that it may take several days to experience relief after beginning a PPI.<br>• If the patient has *H. pylori* bacteria in the stomach, the PPI will be combined with specific antibiotics to treat the infection. Remind the patient to take the full prescription. |
| **Cytoprotective Drugs** | |
| sucralfate (Carafate, Sulcrate) 1 g orally two to four times daily 1 hour before meals and at bedtime for 4–8 weeks<br>bismuth subsalicylate (Pepto-Bismol) for relief of gastric distress:<br>Chewable or caplets: 2 tablets orally every 30–60 minutes PRN; do not exceed eight doses per day<br>Liquid regular strength: 30 mL orally every 30–60 minutes PRN; do not exceed eight doses per day<br>Liquid maximum strength: 30 mL orally every 60 minutes as needed: do not exceed four doses/day<br>misoprostol (Cytotec) 50–200 mcg orally four times per day, with meals and at bedtime | • Do not give antacids within 30 minutes before or 1 hour after sucralfate because they decrease the drug's effectiveness.<br>• Do not crush or chew the tablets. The tablets are scored, and they may be cut in half for easier swallowing. For patients who are unable to swallow the half or whole tablet, dissolve the tablet in 10 mL of water (called a *slurry*) and allow it to stand for 10–20 minutes.<br>• To achieve a consistent dose of drug in solution, shake the oral suspension well before giving it.<br>• Carefully review dosages for bismuth subsalicylate before giving because this drug can be used for several conditions besides gastric distress (e.g., treatment of diarrhea, prevention of traveler's diarrhea). It can also be used for its antibiotic properties.<br>• If patients do not receive relief from the recommended doses, make sure to contact the patient's healthcare provider in case there is a significant underlying condition that needs treatment.<br>• Teach patients that bismuth subsalicylate can turn stools dark brown or black while taking the drug.<br>• Taking too much bismuth subsalicylate can result in symptoms of aspirin toxicity because of the salicylate components of the drug.<br>• Encourage the patient to drink at least 2–3 L of liquid daily unless contraindicated because this drug can cause constipation.<br>• Remember that misoprostol must never be given to pregnant women because it can cause uterine contractions. |

*GERD*, gastroesophageal reflux disease; *IV*, intravenous; *OTC*, over-the-counter; *PPI*, proton-pump inhibitor.

one of the following ingredients: calcium, magnesium, and aluminum.

Antacids are most often used in combination with other drugs to treat a number of GI conditions, including PUD, gastritis, gastric ulcer, peptic esophagitis, hiatal hernia, gastric hyperacidity, and GERD. In most cases, antacids are not used as the primary treatment for these disorders because they provide only temporary relief and do not prevent any future attacks. Table 14.2 lists the names, dosages, and nursing implications of common antacids. Consult a drug reference book for more information about specific drugs.

## Expected Side Effects

Use of antacids as directed rarely results in significant side effects. In general, brands with magnesium can cause diarrhea; brands with calcium or aluminum can cause constipation. Other side effects include loss of appetite, frequent burping, nausea and vomiting, fatigue, and weight loss.

## Adverse Reactions

Adverse reactions are usually specific to the type of antacid. For example, if the patient is taking a magnesium-based antacid, adverse effects are usually related to hypermagnesemia, such as muscle weakness, low

| Box 14.2 | General Nursing Considerations for the Patient with Peptic Ulcer Disease or Gastroesophageal Reflux Disease |
|---|---|

- Teach patients to avoid eating within 3 hours of bedtime to reduce the risk of reflux while lying flat in bed.
- Recommend that the patient stop smoking because nicotine increases stomach acid.
- Recommend that the patient eat smaller portions at mealtimes.
- Tell patients to notify their healthcare provider if they have taken H$_2$-receptor blockers for longer than 2 weeks, because these drugs can lose their effectiveness over time and the patient may need different drugs.
- GERD and PUD have symptoms similar to those of cancer of the stomach, and overuse of OTC drugs can mask symptoms of other health problems.
- For patients with PUD, monitor vital signs regularly. Notify the healthcare provider of any increase in heart rate or decrease in blood pressure that may indicate internal bleeding.
- Monitor level of consciousness while the patient is taking drugs for GERD and PUD because these drugs often cause confusion or restlessness, particularly in older adult patients.
- Teach patients to avoid driving, using heavy machinery, or making important decisions while taking these drugs because they can cause drowsiness or confusion in some cases.
- Tell the patient to report severe dizziness or changes in stool color (black) because these may be an indication of bleeding.

*GERD*, gastroesophageal reflux disease; *OTC*, over the counter; *PUD*, peptic ulcer disease.

blood pressure, and low heart rate. Adverse effects of calcium-containing antacids include bone pain, kidney stones, and—in severe cases—cardiac dysrhythmias. Aluminum-containing antacids can cause mood changes, confusion, osteoporosis, and hypercalcemia.

### Drug Interactions

A major concern about all antacids is their impact on absorption of other drugs. For this reason, timing of administration of the antacids related to meals and other drugs is very important. Always consult your drug reference before you give an antacid.

### ❖ Nursing Implications and Patient Teaching

◆ *Planning and implementation.* In addition to the general nursing considerations related to care of the patient with PUD or GERD listed in Box 14.2, the following issues and actions are important. Antacids are available OTC and in a variety of flavors and forms to help make them more palatable to the patient. Depending on the brand, antacids can come as liquids, as chewable tablets or gummies, or as tablets that dissolve in water. The neutralizing abilities of antacids vary, and one type of antacid does not necessarily produce the same results as another. The sodium content of various antacids must be carefully assessed before giving them to patients who are on restricted sodium intake. These patients include pregnant women and patients with heart failure (HF) or other cardiac conditions, hypertension (high blood pressure), edema (fluid buildup in the body tissues), or renal failure.

◆ *Patient and family teaching.* Tell the patient and family:

- Antacids neutralize gastric acids and are typically most beneficial if given between meals and at bedtime.
- Take the drug exactly as prescribed. Antacids are generally taken 1 hour after meals and before bedtime.
- If you are taking other drugs, it is usually best to take them 1 hour before or 2 hours after taking the antacid. Consult your pharmacist or healthcare provider if you have any questions.
- Diarrhea and constipation are common side effects of different antacids. Contact your healthcare provider if they are severe.
- To avoid adverse effects, never take more than the recommended amount.
- Antacids are used for short-term treatment only; they do not prevent future attacks.
- If you are taking a chewable antacid, chew it thoroughly before swallowing, and take it with a full glass of water.
- Shake any liquid antacid well before taking it, to ensure that the dosage is correct.

### HISTAMINE H$_2$-RECEPTOR BLOCKERS

#### Action and Uses

A **histamine H$_2$-receptor blocker** decreases gastric acid secretions by inhibiting the binding of histamine to H$_2$ receptors on the parietal cells in the stomach. This leads to a decrease in production of basal gastric acid (the minimum amount of acid your body needs throughout the day) and nighttime gastric acid. It also decreases the amount of gastric acid released with meals and substances such as caffeine. The drugs may be used intravenously before and during long, major surgical procedures to prevent ulcer formation resulting from the physiologic stress of surgery.

Table 14.2 lists the names, dosages, and nursing implications of common H$_2$-receptor blockers. Consult a drug reference book for more information about specific drugs.

**Memory Jogger**

All the H$_2$-receptor blockers have the suffix *-tidine* in their generic names.

## Expected Side Effects

Expected side effects include headache, nausea, diarrhea or constipation, and mild abdominal pain. Some patients have mental status changes, including confusion, anxiety, or depression. These usually resolve when the drug is stopped.

## Adverse Reactions

Severe adverse reactions to H$_2$-receptor blockers are rare and include severe allergic reactions, a variety of blood disorders, and cardiac dysrhythmias. Although the reason is not fully known, patients may also be at risk for pneumonia.

## Drug Interactions

H$_2$-receptor blockers can affect certain enzymes in the liver that metabolize drugs. This can result in changes in how certain drugs are metabolized in the body, including warfarin, beta-blockers, benzodiazepines, calcium channel blockers, and alcohol. Contact the healthcare provider or pharmacist if there is any concern about interactions.

## ❖ Nursing Implications and Patient Teaching

◆ *Planning and implementation.* In addition to the general nursing considerations related to care of the patient with PUD or GERD listed in Box 14.2, the following issues and actions are important. Assess the complete blood count and check for unusual bleeding or signs of infection. After patients begin H$_2$-receptor blockers, monitor them for changes in mental status, such as confusion or anxiety. For best effects, these drugs should be given with meals and at bedtime.

◆ *Patient and family teaching.* Tell the patient and family:
- Once-daily dosing of H$_2$-receptor blockers is best at bedtime to reduce symptoms of acid reflux at night.
- Avoid cigarette smoking because it increases gastric acid production and can decrease the effectiveness of H$_2$-receptor blockers.
- Take H$_2$-receptor blockers only for occasional episodes of heartburn because they can lose their effectiveness. If symptoms continue, contact your healthcare provider for diagnosis and treatment.
- Do not drive or operate heavy machinery until you see how the drug affects you. These drugs may cause dizziness in some people.
- Use handrails when you are using stairs in case you have any dizziness.
- Ask your family members to observe you for any changes in mental status, such as confusion or anxiety and depression.

 **Lifespan Considerations**
### Older Adults

Older adults are more likely than younger adults to experience confusion and dizziness as side effects of H$_2$-receptor blockers.

## PROTON-PUMP INHIBITORS
### Action and Uses

**Proton-pump inhibitors (PPIs)** are a class of drugs that help heal gastric ulcers and reduce symptoms of GERD by stopping the acid secretory pump that is located within the gastric parietal cell membrane. They bind to the proton pump of the gastric parietal cell, which blocks acid secretion into the stomach.

PPIs are used to reduce gastric acid in a variety of conditions, including GERD and PUD, or in combination with other drugs to treat *H. pylori* infection. They also may be used in acute care settings to decrease the risk for stress ulcers in critically ill patients. Length of treatment varies according to the type of illness but typically is about 4 to 8 weeks. In some cases, longer-term treatment may be indicated for patients who produce excessive amounts of gastric acid (e.g., Zollinger-Ellison syndrome). Some patients may need the drug for as long as 5 years. Table 14.2 lists the names, dosages, and nursing implications of common PPIs. Consult a drug reference book for more information about specific drugs.

 **Memory Jogger**

All the PPIs have the suffix *-prazole* in their generic names.

## Expected Side Effects

Common side effects include headache, mild abdominal pain, nausea and vomiting, flatulence (passing gas), and diarrhea or constipation. Many patients experience increased sensitivity to light (photosensitivity). Less common side effects include dizziness, anxiety, and mild rash. Low vitamin B$_{12}$ (cobalamin) levels leading to anemia may develop in patients who have taken PPIs for more than 1 year.

## Adverse Reactions

Possible adverse reactions include severe allergic reactions, pancreatitis, and blood abnormalities including thrombocytopenia and hemolytic anemia. Sustained gastric acid suppression by PPIs has been associated with other adverse effects, including increased risks of *Clostridium difficile* infection, low magnesium and iron levels, and chronic kidney disease. There is some concern that decreased calcium absorption in the stomach may place the patient at risk for osteoporosis and bone fractures with long-term use.

## Drug Interactions

PPIs inhibit certain enzymes in the liver that are involved in metabolizing other drugs. This is important because PPIs can increase or decrease the effectiveness of those drugs. Examples include warfarin, alprazolam, drugs given to treat tuberculosis, and certain drugs used to decrease blood cholesterol.

### ❖ Nursing Implications and Patient Teaching

◆ *Planning and implementation.* In addition to the general nursing considerations related to care of the patient with PUD or GERD listed in Box 14.2, the following issues and actions are important. Give PPIs about 30 to 60 minutes before the first meal of the day (usually breakfast). This helps decrease the amount of acid secreted while eating. It may take 1 to 3 days for the patient to experience any relief from symptoms. For patients with or at risk for osteoporosis, manage their bone-density status according to the healthcare providers' recommendations from current clinical practice, and ensure adequate vitamin D and calcium supplementation.

◆ *Patient and family teaching.* Tell the patient and family:
- Avoid driving or using heavy machinery while taking this drug because it may cause dizziness.
- Contact your healthcare provider for recommendations about calcium and vitamin D because this drug can increase your risk of osteoporosis.
- Do not use OTC PPIs for longer than 2 weeks. If symptoms continue, contact your healthcare provider.
- If you are taking prescription PPIs, take the full prescription even if you feel better.
- These drugs do not cure ulcers, but they do reduce acid in your stomach so that the ulcer can heal.
- Wear sunscreen and protective clothing because your skin may be more sensitive to light.

## CYTOPROTECTIVE DRUGS

### Action and Uses

**Cytoprotective drugs** protect the lining of the stomach and help prevent further damage from stomach acid. When taken properly, some of these drugs can stick to the ulcerated areas in the stomach or duodenum to protect them from further damage and allow them to heal.

Sucralfate aids in the healing of ulcers by forming a protective layer at the ulcer site, providing a barrier to injury caused by gastric acids. Misoprostol is a synthetic prostaglandin with both an antisecretory and a mucosal protective action. Although it has other drug classifications, it is a cytoprotective drug for the GI tract. It is indicated for gastric distress or ulceration due to NSAID use. Names, usual adult dosages, and nursing implications of these drugs are listed in Table 14.2. Consult a drug reference book for more information about specific cytoprotective drugs.

## DRUGS FOR CONSTIPATION AND DIARRHEA

Constipation is not considered a specific disease; rather, it is a condition associated with other health problems. Normal bowel patterns vary widely, with some people having a bowel movement several times per day and others no more than three per week. Decreased frequency of bowel movements is one factor associated with constipation. Others include hard or dry stools, pain with a bowel movement, feeling bloated, and straining with a bowel movement. Fig. 14.6 shows how constipation occurs.

Patients experience constipation for multiple reasons, such as a low-fiber diet, low levels of physical activity, ignoring the urge to have a bowel movement, pregnancy, and aging. Other causes include certain drugs, dehydration, certain bowel disorders, depression, and other medical problems. Most episodes of constipation are mild and do not require drugs or input from a healthcare provider. Some are relieved with the use of an OTC laxative. However, if constipation becomes severe, the patient experiences bleeding or abdominal pain, or constipation lasts longer than a few weeks, the patient should contact his or her healthcare provider.

 Memory Jogger

These are signs and symptoms of constipation:
- Fewer than three bowel movements per week
- Sudden decrease in frequency of bowel movements
- Harder stools than normal
- Bowels still feeling full after a bowel movement
- Feeling bloated
- Straining to have a bowel movement

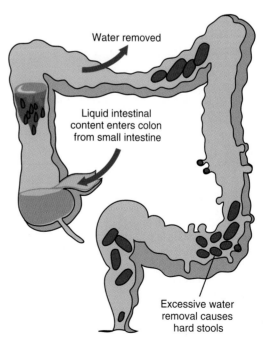

**Fig. 14.6** How constipation occurs. (From Workman, M. L., & LaCharity, L. A. (2016). *Understanding pharmacology: Essentials for Medication Safety* (2nd ed.). Elsevier.)

Like constipation, diarrhea is a symptom of other health conditions. Diarrhea is caused by an increase in the amount of water in the stool. This increased water results from an imbalance between the amount of fluid secreted from the intestines and the amount of fluid absorbed back into the body. If the amount of fluid secreted is greater than the amount reabsorbed, water will remain in the colon, and the stool will be loose and watery (Fig. 14.7). This may be a result of infection, drugs that change the bacteria in the colon, inflammatory bowel disorders, food poisoning, or other medical conditions. Box 14.3 lists common causes of diarrhea.

Episodes of diarrhea are usually self-limited, lasting no more than a few days. However, in certain conditions, diarrhea can be severe and long-lasting. The term *acute diarrhea* is used when it lasts 14 days or less; *chronic diarrhea* is considered when it lasts more than 2 to 4 weeks. Whatever the cause or length of time, the major risks of prolonged diarrhea are dehydration and electrolyte imbalance.

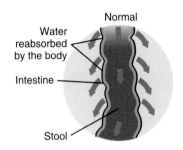

Normal

Water reabsorbed by the body

Intestine

Stool

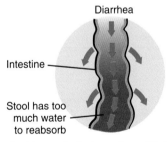

Diarrhea

Intestine

Stool has too much water to reabsorb

Fig. 14.7 Pathophysiology of diarrhea. (From Workman, M. L., & LaCharity, L. A. (2016). *Understanding pharmacology: Essentials for Medication Safety* (2nd ed.). Elsevier.)

---

Box **14.3**    **Common Causes of Diarrhea**

- Drugs (e.g., antibiotics, laxatives, chemotherapy)
- Food poisoning/traveler's diarrhea
- Gastrectomy (partial removal of the stomach)
- High-dose radiation therapy
- Medical conditions (e.g., malabsorption, inflammatory bowel diseases such as Crohn's disease or ulcerative colitis, irritable bowel syndrome, celiac disease)
- Nerve disorders (autonomic neuropathy, diabetic neuropathy)
- Other infections (bacteria, parasites)
- Viral gastroenteritis (most common cause)
- Zollinger-Ellison syndrome

From Workman, M. L., LaCharity, L., & Kruchko, S. (2016). *Understanding pharmacology: Essentials for medication safety* (2nd ed.). Saunders.

---

Irritable bowel syndrome (IBS) is a chronic bowel disorder characterized by symptoms of abdominal pain with defecation and changes in frequency and types of bowel movements. In general, patients have primary symptoms of diarrhea *(IBS-D) or* constipation *(IBS-C)*. Some patients have symptoms of both diarrhea and constipation. At one time, IBS was thought to be related to psychological problems. Now, researchers are learning that IBS is a complex disorder which can be related to factors such as infection, immune reactions to certain foods, inflammation, and even certain drugs. Drugs used to treat IBS are prescribed to reduce the primary symptoms.

Of special consideration are cases of infection from certain bacteria and parasites; drugs to reduce diarrhea may be contraindicated because they slow down or hamper the body's ability to eliminate the organism that is causing the problem. In this situation, the focus is on keeping the patient well hydrated and providing good skin care to reduce irritation to the anus and surrounding area of the skin.

## DRUGS FOR CONSTIPATION

**Laxatives** are a class of drugs that promote bowel movements by stimulating peristalsis, increasing the bulk of the stool, or softening the stool. They are typically used to relieve constipation. Laxatives are also used to cleanse the bowel in preparation for surgery involving the GI tract, certain x-ray studies, and endoscopic procedures such as colonoscopy or proctoscopy. They can be used as part of bowel care for individuals who have lost neurogenic control of the bowel.

Although laxatives can be very helpful for short-term treatment of constipation, they are not a substitute for healthy diet, adequate hydration, and physical activity. There are five major categories of laxatives based on the mechanism of action (Fig. 14.8): bulk-forming drugs, stool softeners, lubricants, osmotic laxatives (also called *saline laxatives*), and stimulants (also called *irritant laxatives*), plus a combination of stool softener and stimulant.

### Action and Uses

*Bulk-forming laxatives* relieve constipation by absorbing water in the GI tract, which alters intestinal fluid and electrolytes. Absorption of fluid expands the stool (increases the bulk). The increased bulk stimulates peristalsis, and the absorbed water softens the stool. Bulk-forming laxatives are used for treatment and prevention of constipation. They can also be used in the management of irritable bowel syndrome or diverticulosis. Laxative effects can occur as soon as 12 hours after the dose or as long as 3 days later.

*Stool softeners* relieve constipation by reducing surface tension of the stool so that water and lipids can enter the stool and soften the feces, which makes it easier to pass the stool. These drugs are helpful after surgery and for patients who should avoid straining. Softening of the stool typically takes between 1 and 3 days after starting the drug.

*Lubricant laxatives* relieve constipation by creating a barrier between the feces and the colon wall that prevents the colon from reabsorbing fecal fluid, softening the stool. The lubricant effect also eases the passage of feces through the intestine. Lubricant laxatives are used to soften stool in conditions in which straining should be avoided, such as myocardial infarction, aneurysm, stroke, hernia, as well as after abdominal or rectal surgery. They can help prevent pain and decrease the risk of tearing or laceration of hemorrhoids or anal fissures.

*Osmotic laxatives* (also called *saline laxatives*), such as lactulose and glycerin, relieve constipation by producing an osmotic effect and drawing water into the intestinal lumen of the small intestine and colon. The increased fluid helps soften the stool and increases stool volume, which helps stimulate peristalsis.

*Osmotic laxatives* are typically used to cleanse the bowel in preparation for colonoscopy, x-ray studies, or GI surgery. They can work very rapidly (30 minutes to 6 hours) and can work effectively to help empty the bowel. One of these drugs, lactulose, can also be used in patients with liver failure because it reduces ammonia levels by almost 50%. It can be helpful for some patients to reduce the confusion associated with liver failure.

When rapid relief of constipation is desired, stimulant (irritant) laxatives may be used. They are often used to treat acute constipation resulting from prolonged bed rest or poor dietary habits and constipation induced by other drugs. They may be used in combination with osmotic laxatives as part of bowel preparation for surgery. *Stimulant laxatives* increase peristalsis by several mechanisms, depending on the agent. These drugs can stimulate sensitive nerve fibers in the intestine, irritate the mucosa in the intestine, and affect water and electrolyte secretion in the bowel. The result is increased peristalsis and stimulation of a bowel movement, usually within 6 to 8 hours. Some drugs may act more rapidly, so carefully read the drug information before giving stimulant laxatives.

In the past, it was thought that stimulant laxatives could cause physical dependence on laxatives. Recent evidence suggests that this is not the case. Nevertheless, frequent use of stimulant laxatives should be avoided in favor of improving diet and physical activity. When long-term constipation relief is needed, bulk-forming laxatives are more likely to be recommended because of the low incidence of side effects. Table 14.3 lists the names, dosages, and nursing implications of selected laxatives from each of the categories. Consult a drug reference book for more information about specific drugs.

### Expected Side Effects

The most common side effects of laxatives are GI symptoms such as nausea, abdominal cramping, bloating,

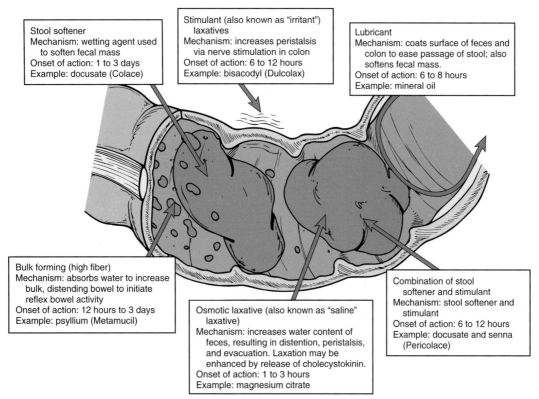

**Fig. 14.8** Sites of action for different types of laxatives. (From Fulcher, E., Fulcher, R., & Soto, C. (2012). *Pharmacology: Principles and applications* (3rd ed.). Elsevier.)

Table **14.3** **Common Drugs for Diarrhea and Constipation**

*Anticholinergic drugs* reduce diarrhea and associated symptoms by selectively blocking the neurotransmitter acetylcholine from binding to its receptors in nerve cells. The nerve fibers of the parasympathetic system affect the involuntary movement of smooth muscle in the gastrointestinal (GI) tract, lungs, and urinary tract.

*Antispasmodic drugs* reduce muscle contraction in the GI tract, which causes decreased cramping, bloating, and diarrhea.

*Synthetic opioid agonists* block mu-opioid receptors in the gut and decrease motility of the smooth muscle of the bowel. They are combined with atropine to decrease the mood-elevating effects of the opioid and reduce the potential for abuse.

*Bulk-forming drugs* absorb fluids in the GI tract, forming a mixture that leads to softening and increased bulk of the stool. The increased bulk stimulates peristalsis, resulting in increased bowel mobility and more rapid transit time through the GI tract. Stools are easier to pass. These drugs also help patients with watery diarrhea by increasing the bulk and consistency of the stool.

*Emollients/stool softeners* lower the surface tension of the stool, allowing water and lipids to permeate it. The stool is softer and easier to pass. It typically takes 1 to 3 days for the patient to receive benefit.

*Stimulants* stimulate peristalsis by irritating the mucosal lining of the intestine, and they increase the amount of fluid in the intestine, relaxing the bowel and easing the passage of stool.

*Osmotic laxatives* increase fluid absorption by the stool. As a result, the stool is softer and distends the colon, leading to peristalsis and easier passage of the stool.

| DRUG/ADULT DOSAGE | NURSING IMPLICATIONS |
|---|---|
| **Anticholinergic Drugs** | |
| dicyclomine (Bentyl) initially 20 mg orally four times per day; after the first week, the dose may be increased as tolerated; maximum of 40 mg orally four times daily <br> Intramuscular (IM) route: 10–20 mg IM four times per day for no longer than 1–2 days if the patient cannot take orally | • Do not give this drug within 2 hours of giving an antacid because absorption of this drug may be decreased. <br> • To avoid local skin reaction with local pain and swelling, inject this drug into a large muscle mass. |
| **Antispasmodic Drugs** | |
| atropine, hyoscyamine, phenobarbital, scopolamine (Donnatal) 1–2 tablets orally three to four times per day <br> Elixir: 5–10 mL orally three to four times per day <br> Extended release: 1 tablet orally every 12 hours; may give 1 tablet every 8 hours if needed | • Teach patients that while taking these drugs they should not use contact lenses because the drugs can cause dry eyes and blurred vision. <br> • These drugs decrease GI motility and should not be used for infectious diarrhea. <br> • Monitor the patient's vital signs carefully because these drugs can cause significant changes in heart rate (bradycardia or tachycardia). <br> • These drugs are not recommended for older adults because they can cause confusion and other adverse effects even at low doses. <br> • See nursing implications for anticholinergic drugs; these drugs contain atropine, which is an anticholinergic drug. |
| **Synthetic Opioid Agonists** | |
| loperamide (Imodium) 4 mg orally initially, followed by 2 mg orally after each unformed stool; do not exceed 16 mg/day <br> diphenoxylate with atropine (Lomotil) initially, 5 mg (2 tablets) orally three to four times per day; discontinue as soon as possible; do not exceed 20 mg/day orally; discontinue after 10 days if improvement not observed. | • Remind patients to avoid sedatives, tranquilizers, and opioid pain drugs because they may increase the risk of central nervous system effects. <br> • Teach patients to follow directions carefully because overuse can result in constipation. <br> • Drugs with atropine may cause side effects such as dry mouth or blurred vision. Use caution when taking the drug. Patients may find that ice chips or sugar-free candy may help keep their lips and mouth moist. |
| **Bulk-Forming Drugs** | |
| methylcellulose (Citrucel) 1 rounded tablespoon orally one to three times daily with 240 mL (8 ounce) of fluid; 2 caplets orally with at least 240 mL (8 ounces) of liquid, up to six times per day as needed <br> psyllium (Karacil, Metamucil) 1 rounded teaspoon, tablespoon, or premeasured packet in 8 ounces of fluid orally, one to three times per day (see directions for the specific product chosen) <br> Wafer form: give 2 wafers orally one to three times per day with 240 mL (8 ounces) of fluid | • Teach patients that these drugs typically work within 12 hours to 3 days. <br> • Instruct patients to drink at least one full glass of water with each dose to avoid blockages in the esophagus. <br> • These drugs can be mixed with water, fruit juices, or other cool liquid for better flavor. <br> Psyllium should be taken 2 hours before or 2 hours after other oral drugs. |

| Table 14.3 | Common Drugs for Diarrhea and Constipation—cont'd |
|---|---|
| **Emollients/Stool Softeners** | |
| docusate (Colace, Sulfolax, Surfak) capsules 50–300 mg/day orally given in single or divided doses; oral solution (containing 10 mg/mL docusate sodium) 50–200 mg/day orally given in single or divided doses; rectal dosage (283 mg enema) 1 to 3 enemas daily as needed. Do not use for longer than 1 week. | • Teach patients that they may experience a change in urine color from pinkish red to yellow-brown, depending on the alkalinity or acidity of the urine.<br>• Teach patients that these drugs typically have an effect in 1–3 days. They are not used to treat acute constipation but to prevent constipation from occurring. |
| **Stimulants** | |
| bisacodyl (Dulcolax, Doxidan, Feen-a-mint) 5–15 mg single oral dose *or* 10 mg rectally; rectal suppository or oral tablet(s) may be used for up to three times per week; rectal dosage (enema) 10 mg (1 retention enema) as a single dose or once daily | • These drugs are available over the counter and may be used for occasional constipation. Higher doses can be used as bowel preparation for x-rays of the colon or for colonoscopy.<br>• Inform patients regarding the expected onset of action. Oral tablets can work within 6–12 hours; rectal suppositories can work within 15 minutes to 1 hour. |
| **Osmotic Laxatives** | |
| polyethylene glycol (MiraLAX) 17 g of powder in 120–240 mL of fluid given orally once daily<br>sodium phosphate monobasic monohydrate/sodium phosphate dibasic anhydrous (Fleet Saline Rectal Enema) 1 bottle rectally (volume depends on product chosen); taking more than the recommended dose in 24 hours can be harmful<br>*Note*: each 118-mL bottle contains 4400 mg of sodium. | • Follow directions very carefully when these drugs are used as part of bowel preparation for colonoscopy or other procedures. Protocols may vary among prescribers. The goal is to have the best visibility of the lower intestine during the examination.<br>• Instruct patients not to use these drugs more than recommended to avoid severe fluid and electrolyte imbalance.<br>• Some preparations include high amounts of sodium, and they should be avoided in patients who require low-sodium intake.<br>• These drugs work very quickly, with onset of action within 1–3 hours. Teach patients that they should be near a place that has a bathroom or commode available. |

and diarrhea. Table 14.4 lists side effects associated with specific types of laxatives.

## Adverse Effects

Bulk-forming laxatives are the safest laxatives. Nevertheless, inhaling psyllium dust particles can cause hypersensitivity reactions. These reactions can be as severe as bronchospasm and anaphylaxis. Caution should be taken for patients with respiratory illnesses. Patients who do not take the drug with enough water (at least 8–12 ounces of fluid) are at risk for esophageal obstruction. Swelling of the throat or choking may occur. If patients do have severe difficulty swallowing, chest pain, or difficulty breathing, they should contact a healthcare provider immediately.

Stool softeners rarely cause adverse events; however, severe allergic reactions are possible. Lubricant laxatives may decrease absorption of nutrients and fat-soluble vitamins. Rarely, a condition called *lipid pneumonia* can result from inhalation of fat-containing substances such as mineral oil. The risk can be reduced by avoiding giving lubricant laxatives at bedtime or before lying down. Lubricant laxatives should also be avoided in patients who are at risk for aspiration. Osmotic laxatives can produce a fluid and electrolyte

disturbance if used daily or in patients with renal or cardiac impairment. Stimulant laxatives may produce muscle weakness (after excessive use), dermatitis, pruritus, alkalosis, and electrolyte imbalance (with excessive use).

 Memory Jogger

These common drugs are used to manage constipation:
• Bulk-forming laxatives
• Stool softeners
• Lubricants
• Osmotic laxatives
• Stimulant laxatives

## Drug Interactions

Laxatives in general may reduce absorption by increasing GI motility, and they may bind to certain drugs, reducing their effectiveness. In particular, loop diuretics, warfarin, salicylates (e.g., aspirin), and digoxin must be separated from administration of laxatives by at least 2 hours. Patients who take loop diuretics and digoxin are at risk for hypokalemia if they use laxatives frequently. Some laxatives given with foods that have high potassium or sodium content can increase the risk of hyperkalemia or hypernatremia.

| Table 14.4 | Summary of Common Side and Adverse Effects of Laxatives |
| --- | --- |
| **DRUG** | **COMMON SIDE AND ADVERSE EFFECTS** |
| **Bulk-Forming Drugs (onset of action 12 hours to 3 days)** | |
| psyllium (Metamucil) | Abdominal cramping, nausea, vomiting |
| **Stool Softeners** | |
| docusate (Colace, Surfak) | Mild abdominal cramping, nausea, cramps, throat irritation, rashes; with some stool softeners, urine can have a color change varying from pink-red to yellow-brown, depending on the acidity of the urine |
| **Lubricants (onset of action 6–8 hours)** | |
| glycerin suppository (Sani-Supp) | Abdominal cramping, hyperemia (increased blood flow) of rectal mucosa, rectal discomfort |
| **Osmotic Laxatives (onset of action 1–3 hours)** | |
| lactulose (Cephulac, Cholac, Constilac) | Abdominal distention, belching, diarrhea, flatulence, gastrointestinal (GI) cramps, hypoglycemia in patient with diabetes |
| lubiprostone (Amitiza) | Abdominal pain and distention, diarrhea, dizziness, dry mouth, gas, headache, nausea, peripheral swelling, reflux |
| magnesium hydroxide (Phillips' Milk of Magnesia) | Diarrhea, flushing, sweating |
| polyethylene glycol (MiraLAX) | Abdominal bloating, cramping, flatulence (gas), nausea |
| sodium phosphate (Fleet Enema) | Abdominal bloating, abdominal pain, dizziness, electrolyte imbalances (hyperphosphatemia, hypocalcemia, hypokalemia, sodium retention), GI cramping, headache, nausea, vomiting |
| **Stimulants (onset of action 6–12 hours)** | |
| bisacodyl (Dulcolax) | Abdominal cramps, diarrhea, hypokalemia (low potassium), muscle weakness, nausea, rectal burning |

Modified from Workman, M. L., LaCharity, L., & Kruchko, S. (2016). *Understanding pharmacology: Essentials for medication safety* (2nd ed.). Saunders.

## ❖ Nursing Implications and Patient Teaching

◆ *Planning and implementation.* In addition to the general nursing considerations related to care of the patient with constipation listed in Box 14.4, the following issues and actions are important. Some bulk-forming drugs are high in sugars. Suggest to patients with diabetes that sugar-free drugs are less likely to interfere with diabetes therapy. Although allergic reactions are rare, certain patients may be allergic to dust particles when the drug is mixed or poured. Report symptoms of allergy, such as rash, hives, or difficulty breathing, to the healthcare provider immediately. Bulk-forming drugs may become dry, thick, and hardened in the throat or intestine if they are swallowed without sufficient water, and thus they can cause GI obstruction. The drugs should never be chewed or swallowed without one or more full glasses of water.

Laxatives that are high in sodium should be avoided in patients with edema, pregnancy, heart failure, or sodium-restricted diets. Overuse of stimulant laxatives may cause excessive fluid and electrolyte imbalance, particularly dehydration and hypokalemia. Laxatives are available without prescription, and it is therefore especially important to teach the patient about risks associated with laxative use.

### 🔄 Top Tip for Safety

Make sure your patient has a call light available, particularly after giving osmotic or stimulant laxatives, because some of these drugs can cause a sense of urgency to have a bowel movement within 15 minutes to 1 hour after administration.

◆ *Patient and family teaching.* Tell the patient and family:
- Drink a full glass of fluid with each dose of bulk-forming laxative to avoid blockage in the esophagus.
- Most laxatives are recommended for short-term use only. Contact your healthcare provider if you require laxatives on a regular basis or do not have relief with the OTC drugs.
- Some laxatives are high in sodium or sugar. Read the labels carefully if you are on a low-sodium diet or have diabetes.
- Laxatives are not a substitute for good bowel habits, including regular physical activity and a diet that includes high-fiber foods such as whole grains, fruits, and fresh vegetables.
- Many types of drugs increase the risk of constipation. If you are taking a drug that causes constipation, contact your healthcare provider to determine the best type of laxative for you.

| Box **14.4** | General Nursing Considerations for Drugs for Constipation |

- Never give any type of laxative to a patient with severe abdominal pain, nausea and vomiting, or fever unless that patient has been thoroughly assessed by a healthcare provider or nurse practitioner. These symptoms may indicate a serious illness.
- Normal bowel function varies among individuals. Some patients may have one to three stools per day, others only three stools per week. Ask patients about their normal bowel history and whether they have had additional symptoms of diarrhea, including difficulty passing stool, straining at bowel movement, or hard, dry stools. Check to see if they have had mucus or blood with a bowel movement.
- For patients who are unable to communicate clearly (e.g., after stroke or with cognitive impairment), keep accurate records of when the patient has a bowel movement.

- Ask the patient about any chronic disease (especially heart failure), allergies, edema, any other drugs being taken, and whether he or she has been prescribed a sodium-restricted diet.
- Laxatives are not a substitute for adequate hydration and nutrition to maintain adequate bowel function.
- Make sure to include a variety of fruits and vegetables in the diet every day. The recommended fruit intake for adults is 1½ to 2 cups per day. The recommended vegetable intake is 2 to 3 cups per day.
- Assess the patient's drug list because many drugs can cause constipation, including some iron supplements, opioids, certain antacids, and anticholinergic drugs.
- Assess the patient's use of over-the-counter laxatives or herbal laxatives because some may cause electrolyte imbalances if used improperly or too often.

- Never take a laxative to treat severe abdominal pain because the drug may cause conditions such as appendicitis or diverticulitis that make the pain worse.
- The onset of action of laxatives varies according to the specific drug category. These drugs can work in as soon as 1 hour or as long as 2 to 3 days. Knowing the expected time of onset will help you plan.

## DRUGS FOR DIARRHEA

*Gastric motility* is the spontaneous but unconscious or involuntary movement of food through the GI tract. Much of the discomfort of GI disease is caused by increased intestinal peristalsis (bowel muscle contraction) and the resulting symptoms. Abdominal cramping, bloating, and pain may be related to acute minor illnesses associated with diarrhea and increased gas or to chronic diseases such as ulcers or colitis. Many drugs have both diarrhea and increased bowel motility as common side effects or adverse reactions.

An **antidiarrheal** is a drug that reduces or stops loose, watery stools (diarrhea) and helps restore normal bowel movements. Three general drug classes are used to treat these problems: anticholinergics, antispasmodics, and opioid agonists. Their actions are somewhat different, although they are often used in combination.

## Action and Uses

The *anticholinergic drugs* reduce diarrhea and associated symptoms by selectively blocking the neurotransmitter acetylcholine from binding to its receptors in nerve cells. The nerve fibers of the parasympathetic system affect the involuntary movement of smooth muscle in the GI tract, lungs, and

urinary tract. Anticholinergics reduce GI tract spasm and intestinal motility, acid production, and gastric motility, which reduces the associated pain. Gastric emptying time is slowed, and acid production is reduced. Anticholinergic drugs are rarely used alone but rather are used in combination with other drugs to reduce diarrhea.

The *antispasmodic drugs* reduce muscle contraction in the GI tract. This decreases cramping, bloating, and diarrhea. These drugs are typically combination drugs that affect the autonomic nervous system and the CNS. Antispasmodic drugs are used primarily to treat symptoms of irritable bowel syndrome. They can also be used to treat acute inflammation of the small bowel and colon or duodenal ulcer.

### Memory Jogger

When diarrhea is caused by infection, the healthcare provider may not give antidiarrheals. This allows the patient's body to get rid of the infection. In those cases, nursing support can prevent dehydration and provide excellent skin care.

Some antidiarrheals are categorized as **opioid agonists**. These drugs are effective for diarrhea but do not have the analgesic or opioid-like effects of the drugs discussed in Chapter 12. They reduce GI motility and increase the ability of the intestine to absorb water. Feces then increase in bulk, and the patient loses less fluid and electrolytes.

The cytoprotective drug bismuth subsalicylate (see Table 14.2), another antidiarrheal, is a salicylate drug. Although its action is not fully understood, bismuth subsalicylate may prevent the attachment of certain organisms to the intestinal mucosa and provide a protective coating for the intestinal mucosa. These drugs can be used to treat nonspecific diarrhea or diarrhea caused by antibiotics. Bismuth subsalicylate may be used to prevent traveler's diarrhea.

## Expected Side Effects

The most common side effects of antidiarrheals are nausea, vomiting, dry mouth, and constipation. Other side effects are dizziness and drowsiness.

## Adverse Reactions

Anticholinergics have many drug interactions (see Chapter 8 for additional discussion). Opioid agonists may interact with other opioid drugs to increase the opioid effect. Many of these drugs are combination drugs, so be sure to consult your nursing reference before giving them.

### ❖ Nursing Implications and Patient Teaching

◆ *Planning and implementation.* In addition to the general nursing considerations related to care of the patient with diarrhea discussed in Box 14.5, the following issues and actions are important. Anticholinergic drugs should not be given to patients with a history of GI obstruction, benign prostatic hypertrophy, or glaucoma because the drugs worsen these conditions. Some of the antispasmodic drugs contain phenobarbital (sedating drug and CNS depressant). Although the dosage is very small, these drugs should be avoided in patients with a history of sensitivity to barbiturates. They also should be avoided in patients with a history of substance abuse or alcoholism.

Physical dependence on opioid agonists contained in some antidiarrheal drugs is rare. Nevertheless, patients who use high doses of these drugs may experience withdrawal symptoms if they stop taking them suddenly. Table 14.3 summarizes anticholinergic, antispasmodic, and antidiarrheal drugs.

◆ *Patient and family teaching.* Tell the patient and family:
- Take this drug exactly as ordered by your healthcare provider.
- Notify your healthcare provider if any new or troublesome problems occur, especially if increased abdominal pain or fever is associated with diarrhea.
- The antidiarrheal drugs are used to relieve symptoms and to prevent dehydration until the underlying cause can be found and treated.
- Diarrhea that persists for more than 48 hours should not be self-treated. Return to your healthcare provider for further evaluation and diagnosis.
- Some antidiarrheal drugs contain habit-forming drugs, and they should be used only at the dosage recommended and for the length of time prescribed.

## DRUGS FOR IRRITABLE BOWEL SYNDROME

Diagnosis of irritable bowel syndrome (IBS) is generally based on a combination of factors, including pain with defecation, changes in frequency of bowel movements, and changes in consistency of bowel movements. Healthcare providers work with the patient to determine whether the majority of stools are hard or lumpy and/or loose or watery. Whatever symptoms the patient is experiencing, IBS can be very distressing to the patient and can affect their overall quality of life. Drugs are prescribed to help reduce the symptoms. Drugs to treat IBS with primary symptoms of constipation (IBS-C) include chloride channel activators, guanylate cyclase-C agonists, and selective serotonin (5-HT$_4$) agonists. Drugs used to treat IBS with the primary symptom of diarrhea include opioid agonists and antispasmodics such as dicyclomine (Table 14.5).

| Box 14.5 | General Nursing Considerations for Drugs for Diarrhea |

- Wash your hands between contacts with all patients. Wear gloves when directly caring for patients.
- Follow agency protocol to determine the need for isolation of a patient.
- Never give any type of antidiarrheal agent to a patient with severe abdominal pain, nausea and vomiting, or fever unless that patient has been thoroughly assessed by the registered nurse or healthcare provider. These symptoms may indicate a serious illness.
- Assess the patient's normal bowel pattern, including frequency, consistency, and regularity.
- Ask the patient about any underlying health conditions that may be causing the diarrhea.
- Check the patient's drug history because many drugs (e.g., antibiotics, laxatives, statin drugs, lithium, NSAIDs) have diarrhea as a side effect. Remind the patient to include OTC and herbal drugs on the list.
- Determine whether the patient has cramping or abdominal pain with defecation.

- Monitor stools for color, consistency, and presence of blood or mucus. If blood or mucus is present, report it to the registered nurse or healthcare provider.
- Report fever, abdominal distention, or severe pain to the registered nurse or healthcare provider.
- Track intake and output and daily weight to help prevent dehydration.
- Give oral (or intravenous) fluids to replace fluid losses from diarrhea.
- Maintain adequate nutrition, including complex carbohydrates such as rice, toast, and cereal as tolerated.
- Teach patients to avoid alcohol or other CNS depressants while taking these drugs.
- Special consideration should be given to older adults and children because of their increased risk of dehydration (symptoms include orthostatic hypotension, increased heart rate, poor skin turgor, and decreased urine output).
- Monitor laboratory values for changes in electrolytes (particularly hypokalemia).

*CNS,* central nervous system; *NSAIDs,* nonsteroidal anti-inflammatory drugs; *OTC,* over the counter.

## CHLORIDE CHANNEL ACTIVATORS

### Action and Uses

Chloride channel activators work by increasing secretion of intestinal fluids in the lumen of the bowel. This helps to increase motility of the bowel and decrease symptoms of IBS-C. They are used both for IBS-C and for patients with chronic constipation. They can also be used for patients who have opioid-induced constipation. An example of a chloride channel activator is lubiprostone.

### Expected Side Effects/Adverse Effects

The most common side effect of chloride channel activators are nausea, headache, and mild diarrhea. Some patients may have mild abdominal distention or increased flatulence. Severe diarrhea is an adverse reaction and should be reported to the healthcare provider.

### ❖ Nursing Implications and Patient Teaching

◆ *Planning and implementation.* Oral forms of chloride channel activators are typically given with food or milk to decrease nausea. Monitor the patient's reports of pain with defecation as well as the consistency and frequency of stools. The patient should report decreased straining with bowel movements.

◆ *Patient and family teaching.*
- Take the drug at the same time every day as directed.

---

| Table **14.5** | Common Drugs for Irritable Bowel Syndrome |
| --- | --- |

| | |
| --- | --- |
| *Chloride channel activators* are used for patients with chronic constipation or irritable bowel syndrome with constipation. They act by increasing water and chloride in the lumen of the intestine. | |
| *Guanylate cyclase-C agonists* decrease abdominal pain, decrease inflammation, and increase fluids in the intestinal lumen. They are used for chronic constipation and irritable bowel syndrome with constipation (IBS-C). | |
| *Selective serotonin (5-HT$_4$) agonists* stimulate peristalsis in the gastrointestinal (GI) tract. They can be used only in women younger than 65 years of age for irritable bowel syndrome with constipation (IBS-C). | |
| *Opioid agonists* block mu-opioid receptors in the gut and decrease motility of the smooth muscle of the bowel. | |
| *Antispasmodic drugs* reduce muscle contraction in the GI tract, which causes decreased cramping, bloating, and diarrhea. | |

| DRUG/ADULT DOSAGE | NURSING IMPLICATIONS |
| --- | --- |
| **Chloride Channel Activators** | |
| lubiprostone (Amitiza) for chronic constipation 24 mcg orally twice daily; for IBS-C 8 mcg orally twice daily | • Give with food and water to decrease drug-induced nausea. Patient should swallow the capsule whole without breaking or chewing it.<br>• Teach patients to report if they experience severe diarrhea. |
| **Guanylate Cyclase-C Agonists** | |
| linaclotide (Linzess) for treatment of chronic constipation 72–145 mcg orally once daily on an empty stomach; for IBS-C 290 mcg orally once daily on an empty stomach | • Give at least 30 minutes before the first meal of the day.<br>• If the patient has difficulty swallowing, the drug may given by sprinkling capsule contents onto 1 teaspoon of applesauce. See accompanying literature for specific instructions, if needed, to administer via nasogastric or gastric feeding tube. |
| **Selective Serotonin (5-HT$_4$) Agonists** | |
| Tegaserod 6 mg orally twice daily | • Tegaserod is only for adult females younger than age 65.<br>• Teach patients to contact their healthcare provider if they do not have symptom relief after 4-6 weeks of treatment. |
| **Opioid Agonists for IBS-D** | |
| eluxadoline (Viberzi) 75–100 mg orally twice daily | • Teach the patient to report increasing constipation as the drug may need to be discontinued<br>• This drug has lots of drug interactions. Teach patients to avoid taking any OTC drugs or herbal drugs and to report all drugs taken to their healthcare provider and pharmacist. |
| **Anticholinergic/Antispasmodic Drugs Used in IBS-D** | |
| dicyclomine (Bentyl) initially 20 mg orally four times per day; after the first week, the dose may be increased as tolerated; maximum of 40 mg orally four times daily; intramuscular (IM) route: 10–20 mg IM four times per day for no longer than 1–2 days if the patient cannot take it orally | • Do not give this drug within 2 hours of giving an antacid because absorption of this drug may be decreased.<br>• To avoid local skin reaction with local pain and edema, inject this drug into a large muscle mass. |

- Results may take up to 1 week to notice any change; however, some patients had benefit within 24 hours.
- Make sure to notify your healthcare provider if you have any severe diarrhea resulting from taking these drugs.
- Notify your provider if symptoms do not improve or worsen when taking these drugs.

## GUANYLATE CYCLASE-c AGONISTS

### Action and Uses

Guanylate cyclase-C (GC-C) agonists are used for patients with chronic constipation and with IBS-C. They help to increase intestinal fluid and increase GI motility. An additional advantage is that they can decrease the abdominal pain associated with IBS-C. The main is example is linaclotide.

### Expected Side Effects/Adverse Effects

The main side effect associated with linaclotide is diarrhea. It can also cause mild abdominal pain, flatulence, and headache. Severe diarrhea and loss of bowel control are rare.

### ❖ Nursing Implications and Patient Teaching

◆ *Planning and implementation.* Linaclotide is best administered at least 30 minutes before the first meal of the day. Avoid giving the med after a high-fat breakfast, which can result in loose stools and greater frequency of stools. This drug is recommended for adults only. Do not give it if there is extreme abdominal pain or indications of bowel obstruction.

◆ *Patient and family teaching.*
- Linaclotide should be given on an empty stomach. Take the drug about 30 minutes before your first meal of the day for best results.
- If you have difficulty swallowing, linaclotide can be given with a teaspoon of applesauce. Capsules can be opened and sprinkled into the applesauce and taken immediately.
- If you have severe diarrhea, notify your healthcare provider.

## SEROTONIN 5-HT₄ RECEPTOR AGONISTS

### Action and uses

Selective serotonin type 4 (5-HT$_4$) *agonists* are used to stimulate peristalsis in the GI tract. It is currently only recommended for females younger than 65 years of age who have IBS-C. An example is tegaserod.

### Expected Side Effects/Adverse Effects

The most common adverse effect associated with tegaserod is diarrhea. This usually improves after 1 to 2 weeks. If severe, notify the healthcare provider. In addition, tegaserod is associated with cardiovascular effects, including stroke and myocardial infarction. It is not recommended for anyone over the age of 65. Rarely, tegaserod can cause depression and suicidal thinking.

### ❖ Nursing Implications and Patient Teaching

◆ *Planning and Implementation.* Tegaserod should be given 30 minutes before meals to help absorption. Monitor the patient's response to this drug. Some patients may have mild diarrhea after beginning tegaserod. If diarrhea is severe, contact the healthcare provider.

◆ *Patient and family teaching.*
- Take the drug at the same time every day at least 30 minutes before breakfast.
- Follow up with your healthcare provider to monitor effectiveness of this drug.
- Notify your healthcare provider if you have any changes in mood or symptoms of depression or suicidal thoughts. While these are rare, they should be taken seriously and reported to your healthcare provider.
- If you have any chest pain, arm pain or weakness, dizziness, numbness of the face or extremities, difficulty speaking, or any other unusual symptoms, notify your healthcare provider or 911 immediately.

## OPIOID AGONISTS

### Action and Uses

Certain opioid agonists can be used to treat IBS-D. These drugs work on certain opioid receptors that are responsible for GI motility. The main example of an opioid agonist that works for IBS-D is eluxadoline.

### Expected Side Effects/Adverse Effects

The most common side effects associated with eluxadoline are nausea, mild abdominal pain, and dizziness. Moderate constipation can occur infrequently. Adverse effects include bronchospasm and pancreatitis. Severe constipation requiring hospitalization is rare but has been reported.

### ❖ Nursing Implications and Patient Teaching

◆ *Planning and implementation.* Eluxadoline should be taken with food twice a day. Patients taking opioid agonists to treat IBS-D should be monitored carefully for constipation.

◆ *Patient and family teaching.*
- Take eluxadoline with food twice a day. It may be easiest to take with breakfast and dinner.
- Notify your healthcare provider if you become constipated.
- Stop eluxadoline and notify your healthcare provider if you have severe abdominal pain that radiates to the back or shoulder as it may be a sign of pancreatitis.
- Avoid any other drugs that can cause constipation.
- Avoid alcohol as it can increase the risk of pancreatitis.

# Get Ready for the Next-Generation NCLEX® Examination!

## Key Points

- Nausea and vomiting result from a complex set of interactions that involve the brain, nervous system, inner ear, stomach, and intestines.
- All antiemetic drugs affect the CNS and cause various degrees of drowsiness.
- Antiemetic drugs are used to prevent and treat nausea and vomiting that occur with any problem.
- The class of antiemetic used depends on the severity of the problem and the patient's individual response. Some patients require a combination of two or more types of antiemetic drugs for effective management of nausea and vomiting.
- Serotonin (5-HT$_3$) receptor antagonists reduce or halt nausea and vomiting by blocking 5-HT$_3$ receptors in the intestinal tract and in the CTZ, preventing serotonin from activating these receptors.
- The major use of serotonin (5-HT$_3$) receptor antagonists is to reduce or prevent the nausea and vomiting resulting from cancer chemotherapy or radiation therapy and postoperative nausea and vomiting.
- Serotonin (5-HT$_3$) receptor antagonists are called *setrons* for short because their generic names end in the suffix *-setron*.
- Common CNS side effects for serotonin (5-HT$_3$) receptor antagonists include dizziness, headache, and drowsiness.
- Serotonin syndrome can occur if the patient is taking other drugs that increase serotonin (e.g., certain antidepressants, St. John's wort) with serotonin (5-HT$_3$) receptor antagonist drugs.
- Substance P/NK1 receptor antagonists are drugs that block the P/NK1 receptors in the CTZ. This prevents both substance P and neurokinin, which are released from cells exposed to chemotherapy and tissues injured during surgery, from binding to and triggering the CTZ.
- Fatigue, diarrhea, headache, and dizziness are side effects of the substance P/NK1 receptor antagonists.
- To avoid foaming or clumping, carefully review the drug instructions for making the oral or injectable forms of substance P/NK1 receptor antagonists.
- Phenothiazines are a type of antiemetic drug that reduces nausea and vomiting by blocking dopamine (D$_2$) receptors in the CTZ of the brain. For this reason, drugs in this class are also called *dopamine antagonists*.
- Some phenothiazines cause urine to change to a pinkish-red color. Sensitivity to sun exposure is common.
- High doses of phenothiazine drugs can cause serious extrapyramidal symptoms (EPSs), including tardive dyskinesia, acute dystonia, and neuroleptic malignant syndrome.
- Patients with nausea and vomiting are at risk for dehydration, weight loss, and electrolyte imbalance. Monitor and report any changes in fluid balance or food intake and laboratory value abnormalities.
- Cannabinoids reduce nausea and vomiting by binding to cannabinoid receptors in the CTZ and preventing serotonin 5-HT$_3$ from binding to its receptors in the CTZ. Use of cannabinoids as antiemetics is typically reserved for patients with severe nausea and vomiting that have not been relieved by other antiemetics.

- Some patients who are taking cannabinoids experience a dose-related "high" (easy laughing, elation, and increased awareness).
- Promotility drugs are used to increase contraction of the upper GI tract, including the stomach and the small intestines. They may be used in patients with postoperative nausea and vomiting, chemotherapy-induced nausea and vomiting, or GERD.
- Promotility drugs should be used with caution in patients with a history of depression because they can cause depression and suicidal ideation.
- Monitor the patient who is taking promotility drugs for any Parkinson's disease–like symptoms, such as tremor, slower gait, or masklike facial appearance. If the patient experiences these side effects, notify the healthcare provider because the drug may need to be discontinued.
- Drug therapy for PUD and GERD are essentially the same. Commonly used drug therapies include antacids, histamine H$_2$-receptor blockers, PPIs, and cytoprotective drugs.
- Some peptic ulcers may be caused by *H. pylori*. *H. pylori* infections are typically treated by a combination of antimicrobial drugs and PPIs.
- Antacids are drugs that neutralize HCl and increase gastric pH, which makes the stomach's pH less acidic and reduces gastric irritation.
- Antacids are typically formulated with at least one of the following ingredients: calcium, magnesium, and aluminum. They are most often used in combination with other drugs to treat several GI conditions, including PUD, gastritis, gastric ulcer, esophagitis, hiatal hernia, gastric hyperacidity, and GERD.
- In most cases, antacids are not used as the primary treatment for these disorders because they provide only temporary relief and do not prevent future attacks.
- Use of antacids as directed rarely results in significant side effects. In general, brands with magnesium can cause diarrhea; brands with calcium or aluminum can cause constipation.
- Antacids neutralize gastric acids and are typically most beneficial if given between meals and at bedtime.
- H$_2$ receptor blockers bind to the H$_2$ receptors in the stomach cells, which decreases production of basal gastric acid (the minimum amount of acid your body needs throughout the day) and nighttime levels of gastric acid.
- All H$_2$-receptor blockers have the suffix *-tidine* in their generic names.
- Some patients who are taking H$_2$-receptor blockers may have mental status changes, including confusion, anxiety, or depression. These usually resolve when the drug is stopped.
- H$_2$-receptor blockers given once daily are best taken at bedtime to reduce symptoms of acid reflux at night.
- Patients should avoid cigarette smoking because it increases gastric acid production and can decrease the effectiveness of H$_2$-receptor blockers.
- H$_2$-receptor blockers should be given only for occasional episodes of heartburn because they can lose their effectiveness.

- Older adults are more likely to experience confusion and dizziness as side effects of $H_2$-receptor blockers compared with younger adults.
- PPIs help heal gastric ulcers and reduce symptoms of GERD by stopping the acid secretory pump that is located in the gastric parietal cell membrane. This helps reduce the amount of acid secreted into the stomach.
- All of the PPIs have the suffix *-prazole* in their generic names.
- Give PPIs 30 to 60 minutes before the first meal of the day (usually breakfast). This will help decrease the amount of acid secreted while eating. It may take 1 to 3 days for the patient to experience any relief from symptoms.
- Cytoprotective drugs protect the lining of the stomach from further damage. When taken properly, some of these drugs can "stick" to the ulcerated areas in the stomach or duodenum to protect them from further damage and allow them to heal.
- Signs and symptoms of constipation include fewer than three bowel movements in a week, sudden decrease in frequency of bowel movements, harder stools than normal, bowels still feeling full after a bowel movement, feeling bloated, and straining to have a bowel movement.
- Laxatives are a class of drugs that promote bowel movements by stimulating peristalsis, increasing the bulk of the stool, or softening the stool.
- Bulk-forming laxatives absorb water in the GI tract, altering intestinal fluid and electrolyte levels. The increased bulk stimulates peristalsis, and the absorbed water softens the stool. They are the safest laxatives and can be used to prevent constipation.
- Stool softeners reduce surface tension of the stool so that water and lipids can enter the stool and soften the feces. This makes it easier to pass the stool, and they are helpful in postsurgical patients and patients who should avoid straining.
- Lubricant laxatives create a barrier between the feces and the colon wall that prevents the colon from reabsorbing fecal fluid, which softens the stool.
- Osmotic laxatives (also called *saline laxatives*) work rapidly and are typically used to cleanse the bowel in preparation for colonoscopy, x-ray studies, or GI surgery.
- When rapid relief of constipation is desired, stimulant or irritant laxatives can be used.
- Frequent use of stimulant laxatives should be avoided in favor of improving diet and physical activity.
- The most common side effects of laxatives are GI symptoms such as nausea, abdominal cramping, bloating, and diarrhea.
- Laxatives in general may reduce absorption (due to increased GI motility) or bind to certain drugs.
- Bulk-forming laxatives should be given with a full glass of water to prevent obstruction in the esophagus.
- Laxatives that are high in sodium should be avoided in patients with edema, pregnancy, heart failure, or sodium-restricted diets.
- Overuse of stimulant laxatives may cause excessive fluid and electrolyte imbalance, particularly dehydration and hypokalemia.
- Laxatives are available without a prescription; therefore it is especially important to teach the patient about risks associated with laxative use.

- Make sure your patient has a call light available, particularly after taking osmotic or stimulant laxatives because they may cause a sense of urgency to have a bowel movement.
- Antidiarrheals are drugs that reduce or stop loose, watery stools and help to restore normal bowel movements.
- Anticholinergic drugs reduce GI tract spasm and intestinal motility, acid production, and gastric motility, which reduces the associated pain.
- Anticholinergic drugs are rarely used alone but, rather, are used in combination with other drugs to reduce diarrhea.
- Antispasmodic drugs reduce muscle contraction in the GI tract. This decreases cramping, bloating, and diarrhea.
- When diarrhea is caused by infection, the healthcare provider may not give antidiarrheals in order to allow the patient's body to get rid of the infection.
- Opioid agonists are effective for diarrhea but do not have analgesic or opioid-like effects. They reduce GI motility and increase the ability of the intestine to absorb water.
- Physical dependence on opioid agonists as contained in antidiarrheal drugs is rare.
- Irritable bowel syndrome (IBS) is a chronic bowel disorder. In general, patients have primary symptoms of diarrhea (IBS-D) *or* constipation (IBS-C). Some patients have symptoms of both diarrhea and constipation.
- Diagnosis of IBS is generally based on a combination of factors including pain with defecation, changes in frequency of bowel movements, and changes in consistency of bowel movements.
- Drugs to treat IBS with primary symptoms of constipation (IBS-C) include chloride channel activators, guanylate cyclase-C agonists, and selective serotonin (5-$HT_4$) agonists.
- Drugs used to treat IBS with the primary symptom of diarrhea include opioid agonists and antispasmodics such as dicyclomine.
- Chloride channel activators work by increasing secretion of intestinal fluids in the lumen of the bowel. They are used both for IBS-C, chronic constipation, and opioid-induced constipation.
- Guanylate cyclase-C (GC-C) agonists are used for patients with chronic constipation and with IBS-C. They help to increase intestinal fluid and increase GI motility. An additional advantage is that they can decrease the abdominal pain associated with IBS-C.
- Selective serotonin type 4 (5-$HT_4$) agonists are used to stimulate peristalsis in the GI tract. They are currently only recommended for females younger than age 65 who have IBS-C.
- Certain opioid agonists can be used to treat IBS-D. These drugs work on certain opioid receptors that are responsible for GI motility.

## Clinical Judgment and Next-Generation NCLEX® Examination-Style Questions

1. The patient, who has been taking a docusate as a stool softener, tells the nurse she has a pinkish-red color to her urine. Which is the most appropriate response from the nurse?

    1. "This is an expected response to the drug."
    2. "This is evidence of a toxic dose of the drug."
    3. "This is an allergic response to the drug."
    4. "This response is not related to the drug."

2. **A 72-year-old man had recent episodes of confusion. The LPN discovers that the man recently started taking over-the-counter famotidine (Pepcid) for his "heartburn." What is the best action for the LPN?**

   1. Recommend that the patient's daughter increases the dosage of famotidine.
   2. Suggest that the daughter research placement of her father into a long-term care facility.
   3. Tell the daughter to contact the patient's healthcare provider because confusion is a common adverse effect of famotidine.
   4. Remind the daughter that her father is older and may have early signs of Alzheimer's disease.

3. **A patient with chemotherapy-related nausea and vomiting is prescribed ondansetron (Zofran). When you are giving morning drugs, you notice that she is taking a selective serotonin reuptake inhibitor for chronic depression. What is your best action?**

   1. Give the ondansetron and tell the patient she should stop taking her antidepressant.
   2. Hold the ondansetron and contact the healthcare provider to notify him or her that the patient takes the antidepressant.
   3. Give both the ondansetron and the antidepressant and monitor the patient for signs of serotonin syndrome.
   4. Hold the ondansetron and give it later in the day so it does not interact with the antidepressant.

4. **A patient with chronic constipation is prescribed psyllium (Metamucil). Which of the following statements should the nurse include in the teaching plan? Select all or any that apply.**

   1. Make sure to take this drug with a full glass of water to prevent blockage in your esophagus.
   2. Psyllium usually takes between 12 hours and up to 3 days to be effective.
   3. You may feel some nausea and abdominal cramping when you start taking this drug.
   4. Psyllium should be taken with all of your other medications to decrease nausea.
   5. This drug will replace your need for dietary fiber so you do not need to eat as many fruits and vegetables.
   6. This drug turns your urine pinkish-red.
   7. To improve the taste of psyllium powder, you may want to mix the dose with water, fruit juice, or other cool liquids.

5. **Which of the following patients are most likely to require a stool softener for management of bowel movements? Select all or any that apply.**

   1. An 84-year-old woman who has moved into a skilled nursing facility after having a stroke
   2. A 64-year-old patient who states she has not had a bowel movement in a week and needs relief immediately
   3. A 62-year-old patient who recently underwent open heart surgery to replace a heart valve
   4. A 34-year-old pregnant woman with constipation who has a prescription from her healthcare provider
   5. A 55-year-old man who comes to the emergency room with severe abdominal pain and feels like he has to have a bowel movement

6. **A nurse is teaching a patient about the loperamide prescribed for acute diarrhea. Which of the following statements should be included in the patient teaching? Select all or any that apply.**

   1. "Loperamide will reduce the number of liquid stools that you are experiencing."
   2. "Make sure you take 4 mg (2 tablets) initially, then 2 mg by mouth after each unformed stool. Do not exceed 8 tablets per day."
   3. "This drug has an effect like opioid drugs, so you may have a 'high' feeling while taking it."
   4. "If your diarrhea does not stop after 48 hours, notify your healthcare provider."
   5. "Loperamide helps decrease the motility of your bowel so there is more time for the body to absorb water and you will have a more formed stool."

7. **A 47-year-old patient tells the nurse that he has been taking OTC lansoprazole for over 2 weeks without relief of symptoms of reflux. What is the best action for the nurse?**

   1. Tell the patient that OTC lansoprazole can be used for a maximum of 2 weeks only.
   2. Tell the patient to contact his healthcare provider for evaluation of the symptoms.
   3. Suggest to the patient adding an antacid to reduce gastric acid.
   4. Recommend to the patient avoiding spicy foods and maintain a normal weight.

8. **While studying for a test, a nursing student asks the nurse why misoprostol should not be given to pregnant women. What is the best response by the nurse?**

   1. "Misoprostol can increase the risk for severe nausea and vomiting early in pregnancy."
   2. "Misoprostol can induce uterine contractions and miscarriage if given during pregnancy."
   3. "Misoprostol is designed only for older people with gastric ulcers."
   4. "That is not true—misoprostol may be given in pregnant women."

9. **The LPN/VN is caring for a patient who is prescribed a calcium carbonate-based antacid. Which of the following statements by the patient suggests a need for more teaching?**

   1. "I should drink plenty of fluids and eat foods high in fiber to prevent constipation."
   2. "I should take my antacid with my other pills to decrease irritation to my stomach."
   3. "My antacid neutralizes the acid in my stomach."
   4. "I should avoid calcium antacids if I have a history of kidney stones."

10. **A patient is prescribed oral nabilone for symptoms of nausea and vomiting secondary to chemotherapy. What is the first essential action for the LPN/VN before giving the nabilone?**

    1. Be fully aware of the state and agency policies for administering cannabinoids before giving any medically based marijuana (natural or synthetic).
    2. It is safe to give the nabilone as long as the patient requests the drug.
    3. Nabilone is okay to give because it is a synthetic-based marijuana product.
    4. Double-check the dose with another nurse prior to giving.

## Drug Calculation Review

1. A patient is to receive nizatidine 150 mg orally twice daily to treat gastroesophageal reflux disease (GERD). The drug is available in 75-mg tablets. How many tablets should the patient receive with each dose?

2. A patient is to receive 4 mg of ondansetron (Zofran) orally 30 minutes before the start of chemotherapy to help prevent nausea and vomiting. Ondansetron is available in oral solution as 4 mg/5 mL. How many milliliters will the patient receive? ____mL

3. A patient is to receive sucralfate (Carafate) 1 g per gastrostomy tube four times daily. Sucralfate is available as an oral suspension containing 1 g/10 mL. How many milliliters will the patient receive each day? ____mL

4. A 59-year-old patient is to receive docusate sodium oral syrup 90 mg daily. The oral syrup is available as 60 mg/15mL. How many milliliters will the patient receive with each dose (round to the nearest tenth)? ____mL

### Case Study 1

M.K. is an 80-year-old female who has been taking over-the-counter (OTC) famotidine for indigestion for 2 weeks without significant relief. She decided to contact her healthcare provider because the symptoms were worsening. She is admitted to the hospital with increasing abdominal pain for the last 5 days. Her admission diagnosis is GERD, and she is scheduled for an esophagogastroduodenoscopy (EGD) to rule out peptic ulcer disease. She is to begin therapy with the oral proton-pump inhibitor omeprazole. The LPN documents these findings as part of her admission assessment.

**Highlight or place a check mark next to the assessment findings that require follow-up by the LPN/VN.**

- __ Temperature = 98.6°F (37°C)
- __ Heart rate = 106 beats/min and regular
- __ Respirations = 22 breaths/min
- __ Blood pressure = 96/52 mm Hg
- __ Skin cool and moist to touch
- __ Reports feeling unusually tired today
- __ Oriented to person, place, and time
- __ States that her abdominal pain is currently a 7 (on a 0-to-10 pain intensity scale)

### Case Study 2

S.Y. is a 37-year-old female with a history of irritable bowel syndrome with constipation (IBS-C). The healthcare provider prescribes lubiprostone 8 mcg orally twice daily. Which of the following statements should be included in patient teaching? **Select all or any that apply.**

- __ A. "Lubiprostone can be used in patients with IBS-C and chronic constipation."
- __ B. "Common side effects include nausea, headache, and mild diarrhea."
- __ C. "Take this drug with food to decrease nausea."
- __ D. "Lubiprostone works by turning on opioid receptors."
- __ E. "IBS-C is a psychological illness, so it is important to decrease stress."
- __ F. "Contact your healthcare provider if you experience severe abdominal pain or diarrhea."
- __ G. "Lubiprostone may change the color of urine a pinkish-red to a yellow-brown."

# Drugs for Immunization and Immunomodulation

**15**

## Learning Outcomes

1. Explain the differences between innate immunity and acquired immunity.
2. Describe the role of antibodies in providing true immunity.
3. Explain how vaccination affects acquired immunity.
4. Describe the recommended vaccination schedules for children, adults, and older adults.
5. Describe where to find current vaccination schedules for COVID-19.
6. Discuss the difference in the mechanism of action for the mRNA COVID-19 vaccinations versus the viral vector or adenovirus COVID-19 vaccination.
7. List issues for vaccination during pregnancy.
8. List the names, actions, possible side effects, and adverse effects of selective immunomodulating suppressant drugs (immunosuppressants).
9. Explain what to teach patients and families about selective immunomodulating suppressant drugs (immunosuppressants).

## Key terms

**acquired immunity** A long-acting and "learned" protective response in which B lymphocytes produce antibodies that are directed against specific microorganisms; also called *specific* or *adaptive immunity*.

**active immunity** Acquired immunity in which the body makes antibodies to specific antigens it has encountered; can be natural or artificial.

**antibody** A blood protein that is produced in response to and binds with any substance that the body's white blood cells consider foreign, such as bacteria, viruses, and foreign substances in the blood.

**antibody titer** A test that detects and measures the amount of a specific antibody in the blood to determine the strength of a person's immunity against a specific microorganism.

**antigen** Any substance that the body's white blood cells recognize as foreign and that causes lymphocytes to produce an antibody against it.

**antiproliferative drugs** Drugs that slow the growth of those lymphocytes most responsible for autoimmune diseases and for transplant rejection.

**antirejection drugs** Drugs that suppress the cells and factors of the immune system that are responsible for the patient's rejection of transplanted tissues and organs.

**artificially acquired active immunity** The type of immunity that develops against a specific microorganism when a form of that organism is deliberately ingested or injected into the body as a vaccine.

**artificially acquired passive immunity** The type of immunity that is transferred as premade antibodies made in other persons or animals into the body to provide immediate protection against a specific dangerous infection.

**attenuated vaccine** A vaccine containing live organisms that have been weakened and rendered harmless so that they are not capable of causing disease but are still able to produce an immune response; also called a *live vaccine*.

**biosynthetic vaccine** A vaccine composed of human-made substances that resemble the parts of a virus or bacterium that cause disease.

**calcineurin inhibitors** A class of drugs that works by forming a complex around the normal calcineurin present inside T lymphocytes, preventing calcineurin from activating those cells.

**immunity** The body's physical resistance to becoming ill every time it comes into contact with pathogenic (disease-causing) microorganisms.

**immunization** The result of successful vaccination that causes a person to develop antibodies that provide immunity against the substance in the vaccine. Often used in the same way as the term *vaccination*.

**immunomodulation** A process in which an immune response is altered. Immunomodulating drugs can stimulate or suppress the immune system.

**immunosuppressant drugs** Drugs that subdue or decrease the strength of the body's immune system.

**inactivated vaccine** A vaccine in which the organisms have been killed or inactivated by heat, radiation, or chemicals to prevent them from reproducing and causing disease, but they can still trigger antibody production and immunity Also called a *killed vaccine*.

**innate immunity** The body's intact protective barriers and the cellular responses of inflammation; also called *nonspecific* or *general immunity*.

**mRNA vaccine** Laboratory-created mRNA that instructs the body cells to make either a protein or a piece of a protein that will trigger an immune response.

**299**

**naturally acquired active immunity** The type of immunity that develops when a microorganism invades a person's body, usually causing illness and triggering the immune system to make antibodies against it.

**naturally acquired passive immunity** The immunity provided by the antibodies that a woman transfers to her fetus during pregnancy and to her infant during breast-feeding.

**passive immunity** Acquired immunity in which antibodies made in another person or an animal are given to a patient whose body had no part in making them; can be natural or artificial.

**toxoid** A pathogenic microorganism that is modified chemically so it is no longer toxic and can be used as a vaccine.

**vaccination** Injection or ingestion of a harmless form of bacteria or virus to stimulate antibody production against a certain disease.

**vaccine** A preparation of a synthetic, killed, or weakened form of a bacteria or virus that can be injected or ingested to stimulate antibody production against a certain disease.

**viral vector vaccine** Envelops a viral protein within a harmless virus to give the immune system instructions for making antigens from the disease-causing virus and inserting them into cells, thereby activating immunity.

## OVERVIEW OF IMMUNITY

**Immunity** is the body's physical resistance to becoming ill every time it comes into contact with pathogenic (disease-causing) microorganisms. It consists of the immune system working with the protective barriers of intact skin and mucous membranes and with the body's normal flora. The immune system has two main divisions: *innate immunity* (also called *nonspecific* or *general immunity*) and *acquired immunity* (also called *specific* or *adaptive immunity*).

When all of these protections are working well, we are healthy and well more often than we are sick, even when exposed to invading bacteria, viruses, and other organisms. Think of all the times someone in your family caught a cold, influenza, or some other contagious illness but not everyone in the family got sick.

### INNATE IMMUNITY

**Innate immunity** includes the body's intact protective barriers and the cellular responses of inflammation. *Inflammation* is a predictable set of tissue and blood vessel actions caused by white blood cells (WBCs) and their products when the body is injured or invaded by microorganisms. When microorganisms enter the body, many WBCs recognize them as foreign and take nonspecific actions to kill, neutralize, or eliminate them to prevent illness.

WBCs can recognize invading organisms as foreign because your cells have a unique code on the surface that works like a universal product code. Invading pathogens have different cell surface codes, and WBCs normally recognize this difference and take action against only the invaders, not your own cells. These protective inflammatory responses are nonspecific and can be overwhelmed, such as when you are heavily exposed to thousands of one type of streptococcal bacteria and develop a strep throat infection. If innate immunity were the only type of immunity you had, you would probably get another strep throat infection the next time the same type of streptococcal bacteria heavily invaded your body. This general part of innate immunity helps keep you well from day to day, but

it does not provide the long-lasting immunity that acquired immunity does.

**Memory Jogger**

Innate immunity helps protect you from smaller, day-to-day exposures to pathogenic organisms, but it cannot provide long-term immunity to a specific disease-causing microorganism.

### ACQUIRED IMMUNITY

**Acquired immunity** is a long-acting and "learned" protective response in which B lymphocytes produce antibodies. The antibodies are directed against specific microorganisms, which are considered foreign substances known as *antigens*. An **antigen** is any substance that the body's WBCs recognize as foreign and that causes lymphocytes to produce an antibody against it. An **antibody** is a blood protein that is produced in response to and binds with any substance that the body's WBCs consider foreign, such as bacteria, viruses, and foreign substances in the blood. Exposure to antigens is the trigger for the B cells to begin producing antibodies. T cells provide cellular immunity and assist the B cells with an antibody response. T cells also recognize and directly destroy cells infected with viruses and protozoans.

The B lymphocytes produce antibodies in high numbers. When you are re-infected by the same microorganism, the B cells attack and destroy it or rid the body of it before it can make you sick again. For example, if you were overwhelmingly infected with thousands of "*Streptococcus*-234" bacteria (this is a made-up type) and developed a strep throat from the infection, your lymphocytes would be learning how to make antibodies to *Streptococcus*-234. The next time you were heavily exposed to *Streptococcus*-234, your body would make so many anti–*Streptococcus*-234 antibodies that the bacteria would be killed or eliminated before you could get sick from them again. You would then be immune to *Streptococcus*-234.

Unfortunately, there are many different types of streptococci. Acquired immunity is specific, which in our example means that antibodies to *Streptococcus*-234 probably will not recognize and attack *Streptococcus*-422 (another made-up type). Until your body is exposed to type 422 and learns to make anti–*Streptococcus*-422 antibodies, you could still get sick from being infected with the new organism.

Acquired immunity has two major forms—*natural* and *artificial*—either of which can be active or passive. Both types involve the production of specific antibodies in response to exposure to an antigen. One difference between these two types is *how* you are exposed to the antigen. The immune system cannot make an antibody against a specific antigen unless the antigen enters the body and the immune system is exposed to it.

Whether immunity is active or passive depends on who made the antibodies. **Active immunity** (natural or artificial) occurs when the body makes antibodies to specific antigens it has encountered. In **passive immunity**, antibodies made in another person or an animal are given to you, and your body had no part in making them. Fig. 15.1 shows how the four different types of acquired immunity develop.

 **Memory Jogger**

A person's immune system can make antibodies *only* to antigens that have entered his or her body.

## Naturally Acquired Active Immunity

**Naturally acquired active immunity** is the type of immunity you develop to a microorganism that invades your body naturally, usually making you sick and triggering the immune system to make antibodies against it.

After the immune system learns to make the specific antibodies, every reexposure to the same microorganism produces more and more antibodies against it. As a result, you continually "self-boost" your immunity to the organism. This self-boosting part of naturally acquired active immunity makes it the most long-lasting type of immunity to a specific microorganism. Naturally acquired active immunity is *true immunity*.

## Naturally Acquired Passive Immunity

**Naturally acquired passive immunity** is provided by the antibodies that a woman transfers to her fetus during pregnancy and to her infant during breast-feeding. This immunity is short term but critically important in preventing young infants from developing illnesses during the first 6 months after birth.

## Artificially Acquired Active Immunity

**Artificially acquired active immunity** is the type of immunity that develops against a specific microorganism when a form of the organism is deliberately injected into you as a vaccine. It is considered active immunity because the body must learn how to make the antibodies, and it is artificial because the microorganisms were deliberately injected or ingested. Although this is a common type of immunity and usually works well, it wears off faster than naturally acquired active immunity because fewer microorganisms are injected than the amount that would have entered your body naturally to make you sick. As a result, you need periodic booster shots to help your immune system remember how to make the antibodies to these specific microorganisms.

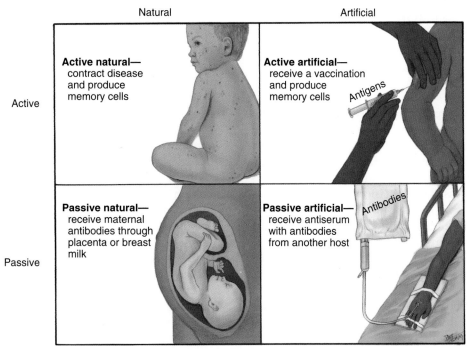

**Fig. 15.1** Examples demonstrate how different types of immunity develop. (From Applegate, E. J. (2011). *The anatomy and physiology learning system* (4th ed.). Saunders.)

### Artificially Acquired Passive Immunity

**Artificially acquired passive immunity** is the type of immunity that transfers as premade antibodies from one person or persons and even from animals to a person. It is considered to be passive because the person's body did not actively make the antibodies. This type of immunity is used only when a person is exposed to and most likely infected with a microorganism that can cause serious disease and he or she has no immunity against it. The purpose of giving a person a lot of these specific antibodies is to have the antibodies rid the body of the dangerous microorganisms before the person becomes sick with the disease.

Rabies is an example of a disease for which this type of immunity is needed. Most people have never received a rabies vaccination and have no antibodies to it. After the disease occurs, it is almost always fatal. If a person is bitten by an animal with rabies, immediate use of passive immunity can help prevent him or her from developing rabies and dying. As soon as possible, the exposed person is given a series of injections of rabies antibodies that were made by other people or animals. The injected antibodies attack and destroy the rabies virus before the disease can develop.

This immunity is immediate but temporary. Within a few weeks, the person's immune system will destroy the "foreign" antibodies. Other highly dangerous infections and disorders that can be managed with artificially acquired passive immunity include poisonous snakebites, tetanus, and Ebola.

> **Memory Jogger**
> Artificially acquired passive immunity is produced through the transfer of premade antibodies from another person or animal and provides only very short-term protection against a specific infectious disease.

## VACCINATION

Vaccinations can prevent life-threatening infections. If a person acquires an infection naturally, he or she becomes immune to that microorganism; however, death or complications of the disease can still occur. For instance, polio can cause paralysis, and measles can cause blindness. The first vaccine developed was for smallpox; it was created in 1796 by Dr. Edward Jenner. Today, more than 20 infectious diseases can be prevented with vaccines.

**Vaccination** is the injection or ingestion of a vaccine. A **vaccine** is a preparation of a synthetic, killed, or weakened form of a bacteria or virus that is given to stimulate antibody production by B lymphocytes against a certain disease. B cells are the only type of WBC that can form antibodies in response to exposure to a specific antigen. The antibodies provide immunity to the disease caused by the antigen. Although some vaccines, such as the one for polio, can be taken orally, most are injected.

Vaccination is not as efficient in stimulating antibody-mediated immunity as the natural acquisition of active immunity that occurs when one becomes sick with the disease. For full immunity to develop from vaccination, more than one injection with the same vaccine over time may be needed. This type of immunity wears off eventually, and the person requires a periodic booster shot (revaccination) to ensure continued production of enough antibodies to maintain immune resistance against the organism.

Many people use the terms *vaccination* and *immunization* interchangeably. However, **immunization** is the result of successful vaccination which causes a person to develop antibodies that provide immunity against the substance in the vaccine.

> **Memory Jogger**
> Successful vaccination causes immunization to develop with the production of antibodies against the organism in the vaccine, leading to immunity.

## VACCINE USE

### Types of Vaccines

Vaccines are prepared in different ways for different organisms. Inactivated viruses or bacteria are often used. **Inactivated vaccines** are composed of organisms that could cause disease but have been killed or inactivated by heat, radiation, or chemicals to prevent them from reproducing and causing disease. Diseases for which inactivated vaccines are commonly used include influenza, cholera, hepatitis A virus (HAV), and rabies.

An **attenuated vaccine** (also called a *live vaccine*) contains live organisms that have been weakened and rendered harmless so that they are not capable of causing disease but are still able to produce an immune response. Modifying the organisms through attenuation usually makes them noncontagious to people who have normal immune systems. Diseases for which attenuated vaccines are commonly used include measles, mumps, rubella, polio, and chickenpox.

**Toxoids** are pathogenic microorganisms that are modified chemically so that they are no longer toxic and can therefore be used as a vaccine. Diseases for which toxoid vaccines are commonly used include tetanus, diphtheria, pertussis (whooping cough), human papilloma virus (HPV), and hepatitis B virus (HVB).

**Biosynthetic vaccines** are those made by genetic engineering processes and contain a synthetic or natural extract of the virus or bacterium that causes disease. HVB is an example of this type of vaccine.

**mRNA vaccines** use laboratory-created mRNA to instruct the body cells to make either a protein or a piece of a protein that will trigger an immune response.

**Viral vector vaccines** (adenovirus vaccine) envelop a viral protein within a harmless virus to give the immune system instructions for making antigens from the disease-causing virus and inserting them into the cells, activating protective immunity. Viral vector vaccines are being used for Ebola as well as COVID-19.

**Memory Jogger**

6 types of vaccines are available:
- Inactivated vaccines
- Attenuated vaccines
- Toxoids
- Biosynthetic vaccines
- mRNA vaccines
- Viral vector vaccine (adenovirus vaccine) envelope a viral protein within a harmless virus to give the immune system instructions for making antigens from the disease-causing virus into the cells, activating protective immunity. Viral vector vaccines are being used for Ebola as well as COVID-19

## Vaccination and Booster Schedules

Vaccinations for artificially acquired active immunity usually require more than one injection to ensure that there are enough B cells that are sensitized to the specific antigen and can make antibodies against it. Additional vaccinations (boosters) that contain smaller doses of the original antigens are needed to continue immunity. For example, DTaP vaccinations, which contain antigens for diphtheria, tetanus, and pertussis combined in one injection, are given to infants three times, usually at 2, 4, and 6 months of age. Boosters of this vaccination are repeated once between the ages of 15 and 18 months and again between the ages of 4 and 6 years. Another booster with a different formulation of these same three antigens (tetanus, diphtheria, and acellular pertussis [Tdap]) should be given once to children between the ages of 11 and 12 years and to women during each pregnancy. It is also recommended that all adults older than 19 years receive this booster vaccination every 10 years.

Other common vaccinations recommended during childhood to prevent severe complications of contagious diseases include HVB, *Haemophilus influenza* type b (Hib), pneumonia, polio, measles, mumps, rubella, HVA, varicella, rotavirus, HPV, meningitis, and seasonal influenza. Fig. 15.2 presents the 2022 recommendations by the Centers for Disease Control and Prevention (CDC) for vaccination of children from birth through 6 years. The schedule includes ages for catch-up vaccinations and recommended ages for certain high-risk groups.

Also new is a schedule for Dengue in endemic areas. Dengue is common in the US territories of Puerto Rico, the US Virgin Islands, and American Samoa. Dengue is a virus carried by the same mosquitoes that carry Zika and chikungunya.

In addition to immunizing to prevent disease and complications of disease in individuals, it is necessary to immunize to protect the population. When a significant portion of the public is immunized against a specific contagious disease, most people in that population are protected against the disease because an outbreak has little chance of occurring. People who cannot receive certain vaccines, such as pregnant women and those who are immunocompromised, are still protected because exposure to the disease is limited or nonexistent. This is known as *herd immunity* and is the principle used to promote vaccination yearly for seasonal influenza. It is also the reason polio has been eradicated in the United States since 1979.

**Bookmark This!**

To deliver high-quality care to patients needing or requesting information about vaccinations, check the Centers for Disease Control and Prevention (CDC) Web site for up-to-date vaccination information: https://www.cdc.gov/vaccines/schedules/index.html. The CDC site includes a schedule for those who fall behind on vaccinations or who start late. There are also separate schedules for those who are immunosuppressed and those undergoing chemotherapy.

**Top Tip for Safety**

Tdap and DTaP vaccines have similar names but are used in different patients and under different circumstances. DTaP is used for active immunization in infants and children, and Tdap is used as a booster vaccine for older children and adults.

Vaccination and immunization are needed in adulthood, not just in childhood. Vaccines are recommended to stimulate protection for adults against common infectious diseases, especially older adults and those who have chronic health problems. For them, even less serious contagious diseases, especially pneumonia and influenza, can have fatal consequences. Additional vaccinations are recommended to prevent shingles (varicella), HVA, HVB, and pertussis. Recommendations for adults against other childhood diseases vary, depending on whether the adult had the diseases as a child. The CDC Web site includes adult vaccination schedules. Fig. 15.3 shows the CDC's 2022 recommended vaccinations for adults from ages 19 to 65 years.

Additional vaccinations may be recommended for adults depending on the person's history, job exposure, or travel. For example, the rabies vaccine is not part of a recommended set of vaccinations, but the vaccine is readily available for veterinarians and other animal handlers. Military personnel and others who travel to areas of the world where

**Table 1**  Recommended Child and Adolescent Immunization Schedule for ages 18 years or younger, United States, 2022

**These recommendations must be read with the notes that follow.** For those who fall behind or start late, provide catch-up vaccination at the earliest opportunity as indicated by the green bars. To determine minimum intervals between doses, see the catch-up schedule (Table 2).

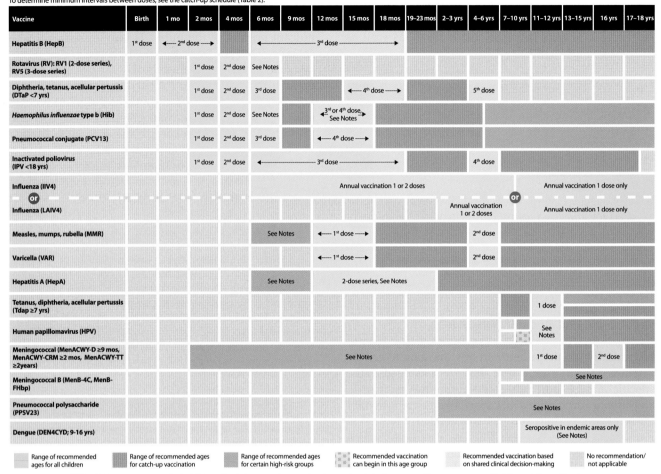

| Vaccine | Birth | 1 mo | 2 mos | 4 mos | 6 mos | 9 mos | 12 mos | 15 mos | 18 mos | 19–23 mos | 2–3 yrs | 4–6 yrs | 7–10 yrs | 11–12 yrs | 13–15 yrs | 16 yrs | 17–18 yrs |
|---|---|---|---|---|---|---|---|---|---|---|---|---|---|---|---|---|---|
| Hepatitis B (HepB) | 1st dose | ←— 2nd dose —→ | | | ←———————— 3rd dose ————————→ | | | | | | | | | | | | |
| Rotavirus (RV): RV1 (2-dose series), RV5 (3-dose series) | | | 1st dose | 2nd dose | See Notes | | | | | | | | | | | | |
| Diphtheria, tetanus, acellular pertussis (DTaP <7 yrs) | | | 1st dose | 2nd dose | 3rd dose | | ←—— 4th dose ——→ | | | | | 5th dose | | | | | |
| Haemophilus influenzae type b (Hib) | | | 1st dose | 2nd dose | See Notes | | 3rd or 4th dose, See Notes | | | | | | | | | | |
| Pneumococcal conjugate (PCV13) | | | 1st dose | 2nd dose | 3rd dose | | ←—— 4th dose ——→ | | | | | | | | | | |
| Inactivated poliovirus (IPV <18 yrs) | | | 1st dose | 2nd dose | ←———— 3rd dose ————→ | | | | | | | 4th dose | | | | | |
| Influenza (IIV4) | | | | | | | Annual vaccination 1 or 2 doses | | | | | | | Annual vaccination 1 dose only | | | |
| **or** | | | | | | | | | | | | | | | | | |
| Influenza (LAIV4) | | | | | | | | | | | Annual vaccination 1 or 2 doses | | | Annual vaccination 1 dose only | | | |
| Measles, mumps, rubella (MMR) | | | | | See Notes | | ←—— 1st dose ——→ | | | | | 2nd dose | | | | | |
| Varicella (VAR) | | | | | | | ←—— 1st dose ——→ | | | | | 2nd dose | | | | | |
| Hepatitis A (HepA) | | | | | See Notes | | 2-dose series, See Notes | | | | | | | | | | |
| Tetanus, diphtheria, acellular pertussis (Tdap ≥7 yrs) | | | | | | | | | | | | | | 1 dose | | | |
| Human papillomavirus (HPV) | | | | | | | | | | | | | | See Notes | | | |
| Meningococcal (MenACWY-D ≥9 mos, MenACWY-CRM ≥2 mos, MenACWY-TT ≥2years) | | | | | | | See Notes | | | | | | | 1st dose | | 2nd dose | |
| Meningococcal B (MenB-4C, MenB-FHbp) | | | | | | | | | | | | | | | See Notes | | |
| Pneumococcal polysaccharide (PPSV23) | | | | | | | | | | | | See Notes | | | | | |
| Dengue (DEN4CYD; 9-16 yrs) | | | | | | | | | | | | | | Seropositive in endemic areas only (See Notes) | | | |

Range of recommended ages for all children  ·  Range of recommended ages for catch-up vaccination  ·  Range of recommended ages for certain high-risk groups  ·  Recommended vaccination can begin in this age group  ·  Recommended vaccination based on shared clinical decision-making  ·  No recommendation/ not applicable

**FIG. 15.2** Recommended child and adolescent immunization schedule for ages 18 or younger. (Retrieved from Centers for Disease Control and Prevention. https://www.cdc.gov/vaccines/schedules/hcp/imz/child-adolescent.html#note-hib.)

contagious diseases are common may be vaccinated against diseases such as yellow fever, cholera, typhoid, malaria, anthrax, and many others, depending on which area of the world they enter. Many of the less common vaccinations require more than one injection on a specific schedule to ensure effective immunity. Vaccine guidelines and schedules for these contagious diseases can be found on the CDC Web site.

 **Bookmark This!**

For vaccination guidelines and schedules for contagious diseases: https://www.cdc.gov/vaccines/hcp/acip-recs/index.html.

It is important to properly store, handle, and give vaccines so that potency and safety are maintained. Box 15.1 lists important nursing responsibilities and actions for vaccine handling, storage, and administration.

### Antibody Titer

A vaccination does not always result in successful immunization. A person's immunity to a specific organism can be assessed by measuring a blood titer for that antibody. An **antibody titer** is a test that detects and measures the amount of specific antibody in the blood to determine the strength of a person's immunity against a specific organism.

The antibody titer can be used to determine the effectiveness of vaccination or to determine whether a person has retained immunity to a disease he or she once had. For example, a person who has a 0 titer for antibody to the organism that causes chickenpox (varicella zoster virus [VZV]), called *anti-VZV antibody*, has no antibodies to the chickenpox virus and is highly likely to develop the disease if he or she is heavily exposed to the organism. A person who has a positive antibody titer of 32 against that organism has so much antibody that it is still detectable even when the blood has been diluted to a ratio of 1 part blood to

**Table 1**  Recommended Adult Immunization Schedule by Age Group, United States, 2022

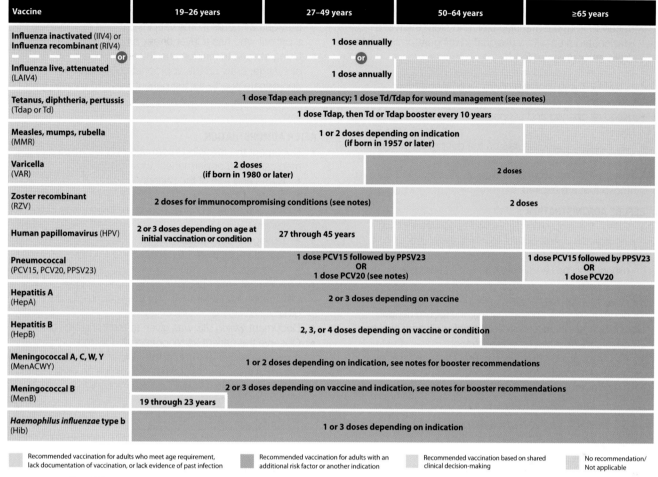

| Vaccine | 19–26 years | 27–49 years | 50–64 years | ≥65 years |
|---|---|---|---|---|
| **Influenza inactivated** (IIV4) or **Influenza recombinant** (RIV4) | 1 dose annually | | | |
| *or* | | | | |
| **Influenza live, attenuated** (LAIV4) | 1 dose annually | | | |
| **Tetanus, diphtheria, pertussis** (Tdap or Td) | 1 dose Tdap each pregnancy; 1 dose Td/Tdap for wound management (see notes) | | | |
| | 1 dose Tdap, then Td or Tdap booster every 10 years | | | |
| **Measles, mumps, rubella** (MMR) | 1 or 2 doses depending on indication (if born in 1957 or later) | | | |
| **Varicella** (VAR) | 2 doses (if born in 1980 or later) | | 2 doses | |
| **Zoster recombinant** (RZV) | 2 doses for immunocompromising conditions (see notes) | | 2 doses | |
| **Human papillomavirus** (HPV) | 2 or 3 doses depending on age at initial vaccination or condition | 27 through 45 years | | |
| **Pneumococcal** (PCV15, PCV20, PPSV23) | 1 dose PCV15 followed by PPSV23 OR 1 dose PCV20 (see notes) | | | 1 dose PCV15 followed by PPSV23 OR 1 dose PCV20 |
| **Hepatitis A** (HepA) | 2 or 3 doses depending on vaccine | | | |
| **Hepatitis B** (HepB) | 2, 3, or 4 doses depending on vaccine or condition | | | |
| **Meningococcal A, C, W, Y** (MenACWY) | 1 or 2 doses depending on indication, see notes for booster recommendations | | | |
| **Meningococcal B** (MenB) | 2 or 3 doses depending on vaccine and indication, see notes for booster recommendations | | | |
| | 19 through 23 years | | | |
| ***Haemophilus influenzae* type b** (Hib) | 1 or 3 doses depending on indication | | | |

Recommended vaccination for adults who meet age requirement, lack documentation of vaccination, or lack evidence of past infection

Recommended vaccination for adults with an additional risk factor or another indication

Recommended vaccination based on shared clinical decision-making

No recommendation/ Not applicable

**Fig. 15.3** Recommended immunization schedule for adults ages 19 years and older. (Retrieved from Centers for Disease Control and Prevention. https://www.cdc.gov/vaccines/schedules/hcp/imz/adult.html.)

31 parts diluent. This result indicates good immunity to the chickenpox virus.

Overall, this test can indicate whether you have ever had a specific infectious disease or have been vaccinated against it and how much immunity you had to it at the time the test was performed. Interpretation of antibody titers is guided by laboratory reference values that are specific to the disease.

### Seasonal Influenza Vaccination

It is recommended that adults and children receive a seasonal influenza vaccination every year. There are many strains of the influenza virus, and each strain is different and has a unique code. If you get sick with one specific strain this year, you will develop active immunity to it. However, each year a different strain may come to your community. Last year's antibodies do not provide immunity to this year's strain, and you will get sick if sufficiently infected with the new strain of influenza.

The situation with flu shots is the same. When you receive the current year's seasonal flu shot, the vaccination contains antigens for the three or four virus strains that are predicted by the CDC to be the most common ones prevalent that year. Receiving the vaccination helps you develop active immunity to these particular influenza strains, which protects you against them for a long time. However, the predicted most common strains next year may not be the ones you were vaccinated against this year. If you skip next year's vaccination, you may not have any immunity to the different strains of influenza and could become sick if you are heavily exposed to one or all of them.

It is advisable and in most cases mandated for healthcare workers to receive a flu shot every year to prevent individual sickness and to prevent giving the flu to an already sick patient population, which could make them sicker and even lead to untimely death. It takes about 2 weeks to develop antibodies after being vaccinated.

## Box 15.1   Nursing Responsibilities and Actions for Vaccine Administration

### STORAGE

- Immediately unpack vaccines as soon as they are received from the manufacturer, and store them in a designated area with a designated refrigerator, separate from other drugs or food.
- Ensure that the refrigerator is labeled "DO NOT UNPLUG" and is plugged into an outlet that has emergency power.
- Keep all opened and unopened vials in their original boxes.
- Do not place vaccine vials on the door of the refrigerator or in the freezer.
- Check the vials weekly for expiration dates, and discard those that are expired.

### BEFORE ADMINISTRATION

- Check the recommended schedule for whether the vaccination is appropriate for the patient.
- Check the expiration date on the vaccine vial, and if a diluent is to be used, check the expiration date on the diluent vial.
- Read the package insert to determine all vaccine components (i.e., preservatives); the recommended dosage, techniques, and solutions for dilution; and any special instructions for administration.
- Ask the patient (or parent) whether he or she has ever had a reaction to the vaccine or its components.
- Ask the patient (or parent) when he or she last received this or any other vaccine.

- Ask the patient (or parent) about any known allergies.
- Ask whether the patient is ill or has been ill within the previous 24 hours (some vaccines should *not* be given to a patient who has a fever or any type of infection).
- Using aseptic technique and the recommended type of syringe, draw up the appropriate dose. Use an appropriate needle for the patient size and vaccine type.
- Inject the drug using the recommended technique and site.

### AFTER ADMINISTRATION

- Document the following information in the patient's medical record or permanent vaccination log:
  - Name and age of the patient
  - Name of the vaccine
  - Manufacturer, lot number, and expiration date of the vaccine
  - Dosage of the vaccine
  - Site of vaccination
  - Condition of the site
- Give the patient or parent a copy of the Vaccine Information Statement (VIS) for the specific vaccine given.
- Document which VIS was given to the patient or parent.
- Observe the patient as recommended by the manufacturer for any immediate reaction.
- Tell the patient or parent what side effects to expect and which ones require immediate attention.

Note: Follow individual manufacturer instructions for COVID-19 vaccination storage.

 **Memory Jogger**

Some infectious organisms have many strains with different codes. Immunity to each requires becoming sick with each strain or being vaccinated against each strain.

 **Lifespan Considerations**

**Pediatric Vaccination**

For best effect, the recommended pediatric vaccination schedules must be followed closely. Most vaccinations given before 6 months of age require multiple doses over time because more time is needed for the infant's immature immune system to learn to make antibodies.

 **Lifespan Considerations**

**Vaccination and Pregnancy**

Some, but not all, vaccinations can be safely given during pregnancy, but live virus vaccinations—such as those for chickenpox, polio, measles, mumps, and rubella—are *not* recommended during pregnancy. Vaccinations that are recommended during pregnancy include seasonal influenza and Tdap.

 **Lifespan Considerations**

**Vaccinations and Older Adults**

As a person ages, previously acquired immunity slowly declines. As a result, older adults gradually lose immunologic protection, even natural active immunity. They need to receive scheduled booster shots for immunizations they have already received and new immunizations for other organisms such as influenza, pneumonia, and VZV (the virus that causes chickenpox). Many older adults are not aware of their loss of immunologic protection and the need for additional vaccinations. Urge all older adults to follow the recommended schedules for vaccination and revaccination.

### Expected Side Effects

All vaccines can cause side effects, but they are usually minor. A sore arm and minor swelling and redness at the injection site or low-grade fever are common and subside within a few days. Fever can be relieved by keeping the patient cool or administering age-appropriate doses of acetaminophen or ibuprofen. Applying cool compresses to the injection area can relieve minor swelling and discomfort. Fever higher than 101°F (38.3°C) should be reported to the healthcare provider because it may indicate an infection.

## Adverse Reactions

Vaccines are constantly monitored for safety, but just like all other drugs, they can cause adverse effects. However, the risk of rare complications from vaccines is outweighed by the serious problems that disease can cause for the patient and all others who come in contact with the patient. Minor adverse effects include a fever, hives, and joint discomfort. Severe side effects include a fever greater than 103°F (39.4°C), anaphylactic shock, seizures, and neuropathy.

The CDC monitors all vaccines licensed in the United States. Expected side effects and any adverse reactions associated with each of them can be found on the CDC Web site.

 **Bookmark This!**

Consult this Web site for adverse side effects of individual vaccinations: https://www.cdc.gov/vaccines/vac-gen/side-effects.htm.

## ❖ Nursing Implications and Patient Teaching

◆ *Assessment.* Obtain a medical history, in particular a history of any immunodeficiency disease such as HIV; any specific congenital immunodeficiency disease; pregnancy; or a plan to become pregnant because these conditions prohibit vaccination with a live virus. Some vaccines can be given during pregnancy, but other vaccines—such as the measles, mumps, and rubella (MMR) vaccines—must be given a month or more before pregnancy occurs.

Obtain a drug history, including use of immunosuppressant drugs, immune globulins, and blood products. Some drugs may interfere with the antibody response to vaccines. Intervals between receiving live vaccines and blood product transfusions are recommended because live vaccines must replicate to initiate an immune response; antibodies against injected live vaccine antigens in transfused blood may interfere with replication.

People who are immunocompromised are at increased risk for adverse reactions after administration of live attenuated vaccines because they have less ability to build up an effective immune response. Ask whether there is an immunocompromised person living in the same household with the person who is to be vaccinated. Before giving a live vaccine, consult the household member's healthcare provider because the person with reduced immunity may be at increased risk for contracting the virus that the vaccine is designed to prevent.

A complete allergy history that includes drugs, foods, vaccines, and environmental allergens should be obtained. An updated CDC recommendation for people with egg allergy can be found at https://www.cdc.gov/flu/prevent/egg-allergies.htm#recommendations. Two vaccinations are available that do not use eggs and are considered egg free. Studies examining the use of injectable influenza vaccine in egg-allergic persons indicate that severe allergic reactions are highly unlikely. The only contraindication for allergic individuals is a previous severe allergic reaction to flu vaccine for any reason.

Assess the patient for symptoms of illness with or without fever that may require a delay in giving the vaccination until symptoms have subsided. Take a complete immunization history so that current vaccination needs can be determined. Ask about family and household members who are immunocompromised or unvaccinated so that their health and safety also can be assessed.

◆ *Planning and implementation.* Adhere to vaccine storage recommendations (see Box 15.1 for nursing responsibilities and actions) to ensure that the vaccination will be effective. *Never mix vaccines in the same syringe.* Keep epinephrine or an anaphylactic kit readily available for immediate use in case of an anaphylactic reaction.

◆ *Evaluation.* Observe the patient for signs and symptoms of adverse reactions. Provide the patient with a record of the vaccination (see Box 15.1).

◆ *Patient and family teaching.*
- Teach the parent or patient that localized reactions to the injection can occur. The discomfort can be relieved with cool compresses on the site and age-appropriate acetaminophen or ibuprofen as directed by the healthcare provider.
- Advise the parents or patient to notify the healthcare provider if fever greater than 101°F (38.3°C), rash, itching, or shortness of breath occurs.
- Tell the parent or patient to keep a current record of all immunizations. It is advisable to keep two copies in case one is lost.
- Teach the parent or patient the risks of contracting the disease that the vaccine is designed to prevent.
- Tell female patients that they should not become pregnant for at least 1 month after receiving the MMR vaccine.
- Remind the parent or patient to bring the immunization record to all visits.
- Give the parent or patient information and an appointment date to return for the next vaccination.

## COVID-19 Vaccinations

COVID-19 is an infectious disease caused by a new coronavirus called *SARS-CoV-2* or *novel coronavirus*. The World Health Organization (WHO) identified the virus in January 2020, and the virus has spread worldwide (see Chapter 7). In December 2020 the first mRNA vaccine for COVID-19, made by Pfizer-BioNTech, was administered. Since that time, two other vaccines have been manufactured; an mRNA vaccine by Moderna and an adenovirus vaccine manufactured by Johnson & Johnson (Janssen). In May of 2023 The Johnson & Johnson (Janssen) vaccine was discontinued in the United States.

The mRNA vaccines "message" instructions that tell cells in the body what to do. The vaccines teach the body how to make a protein (spike protein) that will help the immune system prevent and/or lessen the disease. Once the mRNA directs the making of the protein, it does not stay in the body long and does not change the DNA in any way. In every cell of every living organism since life began mRNA exists. The mRNA vaccines are safe with few serious adverse reactions.

COVID-19 vaccinations are recommended for all eligible women regardless of pregnancy status, which includes those who are pregnant, trying to get pregnant, or may become pregnant in the future. COVID-19 vaccinations are also recommended for women who are breast-feeding. If multiple vaccines are given at a single visit, administer each injection in a different injection site; if possible, separate injection sites by 1 inch or more.

A contraindication to receiving an mRNA vaccine is an allergy to polyethylene glycol or PEG. PEGs are widely used in cosmetics and as an ingredient when making drugs. MiraLAX or polyethylene glycol 3350 is an example of such a drug.

Recommendations are different for immunosuppressed and immunocompromised patients. For complete information regarding all COVID vaccinations, For complete information regarding COVID vaccinations it is best to refer to the CDC as COVID vaccines update frequently to keep up with viral changes. (https://www.cdc.gov/vaccines/covid-19/downloads/COVID19-vaccination-recommendations-most-people.pdf).

Nursing responsibilities for storage and handling of these vaccines are different from those for traditional vaccines and from the storage responsibilities in Box 15.1. Some vaccines require very cold storage and special thermal devices and thermometers. The nurse must always read the manufacturer's storage directions once the product has arrived.

## IMMUNOMODULATING THERAPY

**Immunomodulation** is a process in which an immune response is altered. Immunomodulating drugs can stimulate or suppress the immune system. Immunosuppressants are used to hinder the response in organ transplantation and in autoimmune diseases such as arthritis. Immunostimulants stimulate the immune response when it is deficient. Vaccines are an example of immunostimulants.

### SELECTIVE IMMUNOSUPPRESSANTS FOR AUTOIMMUNE DISEASES

Although the immune system is protective most of the time, it can sometimes overreact in certain tissues as a result of an autoimmune disorder (e.g., rheumatoid arthritis, psoriasis). In these cases, the immune

system wrongly sees normal body tissue as foreign and attacks it. These problems can become chronic and destructive, requiring the immune responses to be selectively modified or suppressed. Immune modification is also needed after organ transplantation to prevent destruction of the transplanted organ by an immune system that sees it as foreign. In both cases, management involves suppression of the immune response.

Some **immunosuppressant drugs** are nonselective and cause such general immune suppression that the patient is at high risk for life-threatening infections. General immunosuppressive drugs include corticosteroid anti-inflammatories and some types of cancer chemotherapy, such as methotrexate. Their use has decreased, and even when they are used today, the dosages are lower because they are used along with more selective immunosuppressants. The actions, effects, nursing implications, and other information specific for corticosteroids are detailed in Chapter 13.

Some drug therapies for autoimmune disorders use selective immunosuppressants that affect only the cells and products of the immune system that are most directly involved in tissue-damaging actions. The most commonly used selective immunosuppressants are the disease-modifying antirheumatic drugs (DMARDs). The actions, effects, nursing implications, and other information specific for DMARDs are detailed in Chapter 13.

### SELECTIVE IMMUNOSUPPRESSANTS TO PREVENT TRANSPLANT REJECTION

The immune system of a person who receives a transplanted organ (from anyone who is not an identical sibling) recognizes the transplanted organ as foreign and tries to attack it. For a transplanted organ to remain healthy in the recipient, the parts of his or her immune system that usually attack it must be suppressed for the rest of his or her life.

Drug therapy to prevent solid organ rejection is lifelong and uses combination drug therapy. Antirejection drugs suppress the cells and factors of the immune system that are responsible for rejection of transplanted tissues and organs by the patient's body. The dosages must be adjusted to the immune response of each patient because these drugs do cause some degree of general immunosuppression. In addition to corticosteroids and some DMARDs, the selective immunosuppressant drugs for this purpose are antiproliferative drugs and calcineurin inhibitors.

### Action

**Antiproliferative drugs** slow the growth of the lymphocytes most responsible for autoimmune diseases and transplant rejection. A less selective drug in this class is azathioprine. It inhibits the metabolism of purines, which are important in DNA synthesis and cell division. Inhibition suppresses the actions of T lymphocytes that can attack transplanted organs and are responsible for causing tissue damage in some autoimmune diseases. The names, adult dosages, and nursing implications of the antiproliferative drugs are listed in Table 15.1.

Mycophenolate is more selective in suppressing T- and B-lymphocyte activity because it inhibits an enzyme needed for lymphocyte reproduction. It also prevents T-cell activation. As a result, the immune responses most associated with autoimmune tissue destruction and transplant rejection are selectively suppressed.

Sirolimus selectively inhibits T-cell activation and reproduction by blocking the mammalian target of rapamycin (mTOR) signal pathways that promote completion of cell division for T cells. Fewer T cells produce less tumor necrosis factor (TNF) and other substances that can attack normal tissues and transplanted organs. Sirolimus also suppresses the growth and maturation of B cells, thereby reducing antibody production and attacks on normal tissues and transplanted organs.

### Table **15.1**  Examples of Selective Immunosuppressants for Transplant Rejection

*Antiproliferative drugs* reduce transplant rejection by slowing the growth of immune system cells that are responsible for transplant rejection.

*Calcineurin inhibitors* block the action of calcineurin, an enzyme that activates T cells. These drugs exert immunosuppressive effects by limiting T-cell function, which increases the likelihood of transplant survival.

| DRUG/ADULT DOSAGE | NURSING IMPLICATIONS |
|---|---|
| **Antiproliferative Drugs** | |
| azathioprine (Azasan, Imuran) 1–5 mg/kg orally once daily or 1–1.5 g IV<br>mycophenolate (CellCept, Myfortic) 1.5 g orally twice daily or 1.5 g IV twice daily<br>sirolimus (Rapamune) 6 mg orally loading dose, followed by 2 mg orally once daily for maintenance<br>everolimus (Zortress) 0.75 mg orally every 12 hours initially; dosages adjusted according to patient response | • Teach patients to look for signs of bleeding, such as bleeding gums, easy bruising, and nosebleeds, because these drugs can decrease platelet counts and WBC counts.<br>• All patients should have BUN and creatinine levels checked as ordered. Notify the healthcare provider about signs of renal failure such as decreased urine output, fatigue, swelling, or shortness of breath.<br>• Antiproliferative drugs commonly cause nausea and vomiting. Warn patients that they should notify the healthcare provider if these symptoms are accompanied by fever and diarrhea.<br>• Teach patients not to take these drugs with grapefruit juice because it can increase toxicity.<br>• Allopurinol use with azathioprine can increase toxicity of the drug, leading to an extreme decrease in WBCs and bone marrow suppression, which can be life-threatening.<br>• Mycophenolate is associated with congenital abnormalities if used during pregnancy. Remind female patients who are sexually active to use two forms of birth control while taking this or any antiproliferative drug.<br>• Mycophenolate can cause hyperglycemia. Caution diabetic patients that it may be difficult to control sugar levels.<br>• Doses of sirolimus and cyclosporine must be separated by at least 4 hours to ensure the best effect.<br>• Oral solutions of sirolimus must be mixed in a glass container with milk, orange juice, or apple juice and *not* water. |
| **Calcineurin Inhibitors** | |
| cyclosporine (Neoral, Gengraf, Sandimmune) 4–8 mg/kg orally twice daily initially<br>tacrolimus (Astagraf XL, Hecoria, Prograf)<br>Immediate-release capsules: 0.1 mg/kg orally every 12 hours<br>Extended-release capsules: 0.2 mg/kg orally once daily | • Both cyclosporine and tacrolimus can cause significant kidney and liver toxicity. Monitor serum electrolyte, BUN, and creatinine levels closely along with liver enzymes.<br>• All patients should have BUN and creatinine levels checked as ordered. Notify the healthcare provider for signs of renal failure, such as decreased urine output, fatigue, swelling, or shortness of breath.<br>• Teach patients who are taking cyclosporine to monitor their blood pressure daily because this drug causes hypertension.<br>• Teach patients who are taking cyclosporine to practice good oral hygiene because this drug can cause gingival hyperplasia.<br>• Neoral and Gengraf cannot be used interchangeably with Sandimmune because the absorption is different.<br>• These drugs should not be given with grapefruit juice because it can lead to toxicity.<br>• Many drug interactions can occur, most commonly with St. John's wort and NSAIDs. Remind the patient to never take any OTC drugs without checking first with the pharmacist or healthcare provider.<br>• Do not crush or split the tablets or capsules because they are an extended-release form and release of too much drug at once could cause toxicity.<br>• Oral solutions of cyclosporine must be mixed in a glass container with milk, orange juice, or apple juice and *not* water. |

*BUN*, blood urea nitrogen; *NSAIDs*, nonsteroidal anti-inflammatory drugs; *OTC*, over-the-counter; *WBC*, white blood cell.

Everolimus is a drug that acts similar to sirolimus. It also inhibits the mTOR pathway, reducing lymphocyte cell division and growth. It is more specific than the general antiproliferative drugs against the immune system cells that attack normal self-cells and transplanted organs.

Calcineurin inhibitors work by forming a complex with calcineurin in T lymphocytes, preventing calcineurin from activating those cells and reducing their ability to attack transplanted tissues and organs.

The two main calcineurin inhibitors are cyclosporine and tacrolimus. The names, usual adult dosages, and nursing implications of the antiproliferatives are listed in Table 15.1.

## Expected Side Effects

All selective immunosuppressants reduce immunity to some extent and thereby increase the risk of infection. For this reason, these drugs should not be used when a patient has a systemic infection. Reduced immunity and inflammation may obscure the symptoms of even a significant infection.

The side effects of selective immunosuppressants vary depending on the mechanism of action. All of these drugs cause GI problems and rashes. Tacrolimus can cause diabetes mellitus. Sirolimus and everolimus increase blood cholesterol levels.

The calcineurin inhibitors that increase blood cholesterol levels can lead to salt-sensitive hypertension. Those that increase blood glucose levels (hyperglycemia) make diabetes more difficult to control. Many patients who are taking cyclosporine develop gingival (gum) hyperplasia.

## Adverse Effects

All selective immunosuppressants increase the risk of cancer development, especially skin cancers, because they reduce immunity. This problem is thought to be related to reduced immunosurveillance, which leads to loss of early recognition by the immune system when normal cells transform into cancer cells. The risk is higher for the drugs that are taken for long periods, including the antiproliferatives and calcineurin inhibitors.

Antiproliferative drugs given intravenously can cause phlebitis and thrombosis at the administration site. Liver toxicity and liver failure have occurred with all of the antiproliferative drugs and calcineurin inhibitors. The risk is increased if the patient has other liver problems or is exposed to other substances that are toxic to the liver, such as alcohol and acetaminophen.

Other adverse effects vary by the drug's mechanism of action. Most of these drugs can cause imbalances of potassium, phosphorus, and magnesium. Patients who are taking selective immunosuppressant drugs are advised to avoid vaccinations with live vaccines because their reduced immunity increases their risk of getting the disease that the vaccine is designed to prevent.

## Drug Interactions

All selective immunosuppressants interact with numerous other drugs. Transplant recipients usually need other drugs in addition to lifetime immunosuppressant therapy, which increases the risk of drug interactions. To be safe when giving antiproliferative drugs and calcineurin inhibitors, it is important to take a detailed drug history and check with the pharmacist or a drug reference book for more information about specific drug interactions. For example, cyclosporine has 57 serious interactions and 36 moderate interactions with other drugs.

## ❖ Nursing Implications and Patient Teaching

◆ *Assessment.* The healthcare provider completes a detailed history and physical assessment for each patient who is to receive a transplant. Transplantation is a multifaceted medical and ethical issue, and the many transplant team members include specialty healthcare providers, nurses, nurse practitioners, social service workers, psychologists, and a variety of other professionals involved in the care of a transplant patient and the patient's family. Your continuing assessment after transplantation will be guided by the individual medical needs of the patient and is discussed next.

◆ *Planning and implementation.* The antiproliferative drugs can be absorbed through skin and mucous membranes, and they exert effects on whoever prepares them. Use of personal protective equipment (PPE), including gowns, gloves, and masks, is critical when preparing and giving these drugs to prevent accidental exposure.

Obtain a list of all other prescribed and over-the-counter (OTC) drugs that the patient takes because most selective immunosuppressant drugs interact with many other agents. Consult a drug reference book or pharmacist for more information about specific drug interactions. If needed, consult with the prescriber about dosage or changing the patient's other drugs.

All patients who are taking or receiving a selective immunosuppressant have baseline laboratory tests that include complete blood cell counts, electrolyte studies, platelet counts, kidney function tests, liver function tests, bilirubin levels, and electrocardiograms. These tests, as well as assessments and documentation of signs and symptoms of infection and bleeding, are repeated at regular intervals throughout the patient's lifetime to prevent drug toxicities. Review the results of laboratory tests, and notify the healthcare provider about any abnormal results.

For best effects, intravenous (IV) formulations of these drugs *must* be mixed with the manufacturer-recommended diluent. Do not mix or give selective immunosuppressants with other IV drugs, and do not give other drugs through the same IV line used for immunosuppressant therapy.

Assess the site for irritation, phlebitis, and thrombosis. Monitor patients closely during infusions of any immunosuppressant drugs for signs of allergic (hypersensitivity) reactions and anaphylaxis. If these occur, stop the infusion immediately, and follow your institution's protocol for an emergency situation. If you are in a clinic, make sure the crash cart or emergency drug box is close by. Document the reaction to the drug, flag the chart, and alert the patient that the drug should not be taken again.

Assess the functioning of all organ systems of the patient. Assess vital signs and report abnormalities. Ask the patient about fever, chills, fatigue, lethargy, cough, or difficult breathing that may indicate infection. Look in the mouth for signs of gum hyperplasia (which can be caused by cyclosporine) or evidence of fungal infection. Assess the patient for yellowing of the skin or whites of the eyes that may indicate liver dysfunction. Kidney function can be affected, especially with tacrolimus; weigh the patient to assess for changes in fluid balance. A weight gain of 1 kg is equal to 1 L of fluid. Check the blood urea nitrogen (BUN), creatinine, and electrolyte levels, and ask the patient about color, amount, and consistency of urine. Small amounts of dark yellow, concentrated urine can indicate dehydration, infection, or a problem with the kidneys caused by drug toxicity.

◆ *Patient and family teaching.* Tell the patient and family:
- Take your temperature daily, and watch for the common signs and symptoms of infection because these drugs reduce your ability to fight infection. Common indications of infection include fever, foul-smelling drainage, pain or burning on urination, sore throat, and cough.
- Immediately report any indication of infection to your healthcare provider.
- Check with your healthcare provider for what types of vaccinations you should have while receiving immunosuppressive therapy.
- Keep all appointments for monitoring of blood counts and other laboratory tests.

- Take your drugs exactly as prescribed to maintain their effectiveness in preventing transplant rejection. Even a few missed doses can lead to tissue-damaging responses and transplant rejection episodes.
- Notify your healthcare provider if you develop yellowing of the skin or eyes, darkening of the urine, or lightening of the stools. These problems are signs of liver toxicity, a serious adverse effect of these drugs.
- Avoid drinking alcohol or using acetaminophen while taking these drugs because they also can cause liver damage.
- If you are taking the oral suspensions of sirolimus or cyclosporine, mix the drug exactly as directed, using the recommended solution (i.e., milk, orange juice, or apple juice); *do not mix with water*. After drinking the suspension, rinse the container with the same solution and drink the rinse for better drug effectiveness. Remember that cyclosporine must be mixed in a glass container, not a plastic one.
- If you are taking both sirolimus and cyclosporine, separate the drug dosages by at least 4 hours to ensure the best effect.
- Do not take sirolimus or tacrolimus with grapefruit juice because it decreases the effectiveness of the enzyme that metabolizes these drugs, and the blood levels could become dangerously high, leading to toxic side effects.
- Do not take other drugs or supplements without checking with your healthcare provider because the antiproliferatives and calcineurin inhibitors interact with many other drugs.

 **Lifespan Considerations**

**Pregnancy and Selective Immunosuppressants**

Pregnancy is an absolute contraindication to the use of antiproliferative drugs because these drugs are associated with birth defects and other severe problems. Tell sexually active women of childbearing age to use two reliable methods of contraception during therapy and for at least 12 weeks after therapy is discontinued. These drugs also enter breast milk and can have an adverse effect on the infant.

# Get Ready for the Next-Generation NCLEX® Examination!

## Key Points

- Innate immunity helps protect a person from infection but does not provide true immunity to a specific infectious microorganism.
- The immune system cannot make an antibody against a specific antigen unless it is exposed to that antigen.
- Antibodies made by one person or animal can be transferred to another person for short-term passive immunity.
- The six types of vaccines currently available are inactivated (killed) vaccines, attenuated (live) vaccines, toxoids, biosynthetic vaccines, mRNA vaccines, and vector virus vaccines.

- Vaccinations usually require more than one dose and often must be boosted for best long-term immunity to a specific organism.
- For some infectious microorganisms (e.g., seasonal influenza viruses), there are many different strains, each of which requires vaccination for immunity.
- Pregnant women should receive seasonal influenza vaccination and the Tdap vaccination during every pregnancy. Most other vaccinations are avoided during pregnancy.
- Vaccinations are used to help people develop immunity to a dangerous disease without the risk of becoming sick first.

- Immunizing the majority of a community produces herd immunity, which prevents disease transmission to those who are unable to become vaccinated.
- The immune system of a patient who receives a transplanted organ (unless from an identical sibling) can attack and reject the new organ. These patients need to take immunosuppressive drugs daily to prevent transplant rejection.
- All patients who are taking immunosuppressive drugs are at increased risk for infection and cancer.
- Ask patients about all other drugs or supplements they take before giving any selective immunosuppressant drug because these drugs have many interactions.
- Use PPE when preparing or giving selective immunosuppressants to prevent accidental exposure to the drug.
- The antiproliferative drugs are associated with poor pregnancy outcomes. Teach sexually active women of childbearing age who are taking these drugs to use two reliable methods of contraception during therapy and for 12 weeks after antiproliferative drugs are discontinued.

## Clinical Judgment and Next-Generation NCLEX® Examination-Style Questions

### Case Study

The urgent care LPN/VN is caring for a 10-year-old girl who recently immigrated from Haiti. She has cold symptoms, swollen pink eyelids, small white spots inside her cheek, a fever of 102°F (38.8°C), and a flat, red rash on her forehead. She has never been immunized and has no allergies.

1. **Which actions by the nurse are important to carry out with this patient? Select all or any that apply.**

   1. Transfer the patient to the pediatric intensive care unit.
   2. Transfer the patient to the public health department.
   3. Admit the patient to a reverse isolation room.
   4. Don an N95 respirator.
   5. Administer an MMR vaccine to the patient.
   6. Administer intramuscular immune globulin.
   7. Administer 20,000 IU of vitamin A by mouth.
   8. Increase the patient's fluid intake.
   9. Administer acyclovir 200 mg by mouth.
   10. Administer aspirin by mouth for pain and fever.
   11. Contact the infection control nurse.

2. **The mother, who only speaks Spanish, is visibly stressed and shaking her head no—she does not understand as the nurse talks to her. What is the nurse's best action? Select all or any that apply.**

   1. Ask a Spanish-speaking coworker on another unit to translate information.
   2. Ask the patient's older brother, who does speak English, to translate.
   3. Use the hospital over-the-phone interpreting service.
   4. Use the iTranslate medical app on the nurse's iPhone.
   5. Direct the brother and mother to the cafeteria while taking care of the child.
   6. Give the mother a handout about measles written in Spanish.

3. **The nurse assistant reports the patient's vital signs and condition to the nurse: Temperature 100° F (37.7°), Pulse 88, Respirations 30, Oxygen Saturation level 93% on room air. She tells the nurse that morning care was completed and that the patient is drinking fluids, eating Jell-o, and coughing a little. What is the first action of the nurse?**

   1. Notify the healthcare provider.
   2. Apply oxygen by nasal cannula at 2L.
   3. Observe and perform a focused assessment on the patient's lungs.
   4. Ask the nurse assistant to take another set of vital signs in an hour.

4. **Instructions: For each vaccine listed below, drag the letter for the vaccination to the type of vaccination it is. Vaccinations can be used more than once.**

| VACCINATION | TYPE OF VACCINATION |
|---|---|
| a. Influenza | 1. _____ Inactivated |
| b. Hepatitis A | 2. _____ Attenuated |
| c. Ebola | 3. _____ Toxoid |
| d. COVID-19 | 4. _____ Biosynthetic |
| e. Tetanus | 5. _____ Vector Virus |
| f. Measles, mumps, rubella | 6. _____ mRNA |
| g. Hepatitis B | |

5. **A 34-year-old patient has just begun work as a produce inspector and quality control clerk. One of the mandates of the job is to be current on all immunizations. He states he has been immunized but does not have proof. Which nursing actions are appropriate? Select all or any that apply.**

   1. Tell the patient to contact his primary care provider to obtain copies of his vaccination.
   2. Tell the patient to contact the public health department for copies of his vaccination.
   3. Tell the patient he will need to take a leave of absence until all vaccines can be given.
   4. Send antibody titer levels for MMR, varicella, shingles, and hepatitis A, B, and C.
   5. Administer all the necessary vaccines to the patient at once.

6. **Which drug combination can be given together?**

   1. ibuprofen and cyclosporine
   2. prednisone and tacrolimus
   3. azathioprine and cyclosporine
   4. tacrolimus and atorvastatin

7. **A patient with a history of diabetes and chronic obstructive pulmonary disease declines getting the seasonal flu shot because he is allergic to eggs. What is the best action of the nurse?**

   1. Advise the patient to wear a well-fitting mask and wash his hands frequently.
   2. Ask the patient what kind of symptoms he gets if he eats eggs.
   3. Document the patient's allergy to the seasonal influenza vaccine.
   4. Ask the patient if he would accept an egg-free seasonal flu vaccine.

8. A patient tells the nurse that he broke out in a rash and hives when he started the prep for his colonoscopy. Which vaccination is contraindicated in this patient?

   1. Measles, mumps, and rubella
   2. Hepatitis B
   3. Meningococcal B
   4. Pneumococcal
   5. COVID mRNA
   6. Polio
   7. Varicella

9. A 45-year-old female patient is receiving cyclosporine after receiving a kidney transplant. The patient has a sore throat, fatigue, and a fever of 99.0°F (37.2°C). What should the nurse suspect at this time?

   1. The patient's kidney has begun to fail.
   2. The patient is rejecting the kidney.
   3. The patient may have an infection.
   4. The patient is beginning to have an adverse reaction to the cyclosporine.

10. A patient taking long-term immunosuppressants should adhere to which of the following instructions? **Select all or any that apply.**

    1. Stay away from persons who are sick.
    2. Wash your hands frequently.
    3. Routinely have a healthcare professional check for skin lesions.
    4. Receive only inactivated or dead vaccines.
    5. Wash fruits and vegetables well before eating.
    6. Notify your healthcare provider if you develop yellowing of the eyes and skin.

## Next-Generation NCLEX® (NGN) Examination–Style Question

**Nurse's Notes**
**1 Week Ago, 1200**

An 18-year-old female client presents to the outpatient primary care provider's office to establish care. The client states, "I'm just getting away from my parents. They never let me see a doctor growing up due to religious reasons, but I don't feel the same." The client states she has had no routine medical care and no childhood immunizations "that I can remember." The client says, "Obviously, I can't remember when I was two, but I don't think I was vaccinated." The client further states, "I think I had chickenpox though."

**Today, 1300**

The client returns for her follow-up visit as scheduled. She reports that she has been having morning nausea. She reports her last menstrual cycle was 6 weeks ago and states, "I'm ready to get my vaccination status updated."

**Laboratory Results**
**1 Week Ago, 1200**

| TEST/PANEL | RESULT | INTERPRETATION |
|---|---|---|
| Rubella IgG | < 7 international units/mL | No immunity to rubella |
| Measles IgG | Negative | No immunity to measles |
| Varicella IgG | Positive | Previous varicella infection |
| Polio IgG | Negative | No immunity to polio |
| Diphtheria | Negative | No immunity to diphtheria |
| Pertussis | Negative | No immunity to pertussis |

**Today, 1300**

| TEST/PANEL | RESULT |
|---|---|
| Urine HCG | positive |

**Flow Sheet**
**1 Week Ago, 1200**

Blood Pressure: 118/78 mm Hg
Heart Rate: 80/min
Respiratory Rate: 18/min
Temperature: 98.6°F (37°C)

**Today, 1300**

Blood Pressure: 122/78 mm Hg
Heart Rate: 78/min
Respiratory Rate: 18/min
Temperature: 98.6°F (37°C)

**Orders**
**1 Week Ago, 1200**

Check titers and return in 1 week for vaccinations.

A nurse is caring for a client in the outpatient primary care provider's office.

Which of the following immunizations does the nurse anticipate administering today?

*Select all or any that apply.*

- Tdap (tetanus, diphtheria, and acellular pertussis)
- MMR (measles, mumps, rubella)
- Influenza
- Rabies
- Polio
- Varicella

See answer on Evolve at http://evolve.elsevier.com/Visovsky/LPNpharmacology/.

# 16

# Drugs Affecting the Hematologic System

http://evolve.elsevier.com/Visovsky/LPNpharmacology

## Learning Outcomes

1. Describe the clotting mechanism in the human body.
2. Explain the difference between anticoagulant drugs and fibrinolytic drugs.
3. List the names, actions, possible side effects, and adverse effects of common platelet inhibitors.
4. Explain what to teach patients and families about platelet inhibitors.
5. List the names, actions, possible side effects, and adverse effects of common direct thrombin inhibitors.
6. Explain what to teach patients and families about direct thrombin inhibitors.
7. List the names, actions, possible side effects, and adverse effects of common indirect thrombin inhibitors.
8. Explain what to teach patients and families about indirect thrombin inhibitors.
9. List the names, actions, possible side effects, and adverse effects of vitamin K antagonists.
10. Explain what to teach patients and families about vitamin K antagonists.
11. List the names, actions, possible side effects, and adverse effects of fibrinolytic drugs.
12. Explain what to teach patients and families about fibrinolytic drugs.
13. List the names, actions, possible side effects, and adverse effects of erythropoiesis-stimulating agents.
14. Explain what to teach patients and families about erythropoiesis-stimulating agents.
15. List the names, actions, possible side effects, and adverse effects of various iron preparations.
16. Explain what to teach patients and families about drugs for iron replacement.

## Key Terms

**anticoagulant** Drug that interferes with one or more steps in the blood clotting process to reduce or prevent new clots from forming or prevent existing clots from getting larger.

**clot** A semisolid amount of coagulated (thickened) blood that blocks blood flow in a blood vessel; also referred to as a *thrombus*.

**deep vein thrombosis (DVT)** A clot lying in a deep vein, usually in a leg.

**direct thrombin inhibitors (DTIs)** Anticoagulants that delay blood clotting by directly inhibiting the enzyme thrombin.

**embolism** A blockage in an artery caused by a blood clot or air bubble.

**erythropoiesis-stimulating agent (ESA)** A synthetic form of the hormone erythropoietin, which stimulates the bone marrow to make more red blood cells at a faster rate.

**fibrin** A protein formed from fibrinogen during the clotting process; its netlike structure traps blood cells and platelets, building up a spongy mass that gradually hardens and contracts to form a blood clot.

**fibrinogen** A protein found in blood plasma that is converted to fibrin to help form a blood clot.

**fibrinolytic drug** A drug that uses enzymes to dissolve the fibrin in a clot; also known as a *thrombolytic drug* or *clot buster*.

**indirect thrombin inhibitors (ITIs)** Anticoagulant drugs that reduce clot formation by increasing the amount and action of the protein antithrombin III.

**platelet inhibitors** Drugs that interfere with blood clotting in arteries by preventing platelets from sticking and clumping together (aggregating).

**thrombin** An enzyme that acts on fibrinogen (a protein found in the blood plasma) to convert it to fibrin to help clots form.

**vitamin K antagonist** Anticoagulant drug that interferes with blood clotting by reducing the amount of vitamin K available to help the liver form clotting factors.

## BLOOD CLOTTING

Drugs that affect the hematologic system work by interfering with blood clotting, reducing existing blood clots, or stimulating the production of red blood cells (RBCs). Many such drugs are taken by patients on a daily basis, whereas others are given only in hospital settings. To understand the action of these drugs, it is important to review normal clotting mechanisms.

When blood flows freely through blood vessels, the cells of the body are provided with oxygen and

314

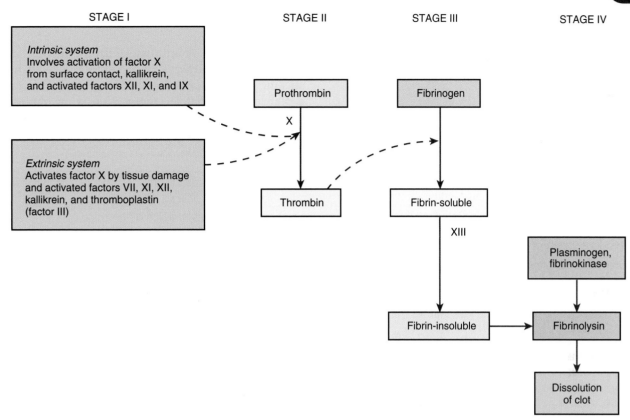

**Fig. 16.1** Blood coagulation and clot lysis.

nutrients, and waste products are removed from tissues and organs. When blood vessels become damaged, clot formation is needed to prevent blood from leaving the circulatory system and causing excessive bleeding. A clot is a semisolid amount of coagulated (thickened) blood that blocks blood flow in a blood vessel. At all times, the body functions that keep circulation going are balanced with blood functions that can start the formation of blood clots in areas of injury. In health, blood circulates to all tissues and organs continuously and forms clots only when and where they are needed.

Tissue damage starts a series of reactions to protect the body and repair the tissue injury (Fig. 16.1). In response to bleeding, various clotting factors made by the liver are released into the blood, and they act quickly in an organized series of events called a *cascade* that results in the formation of a blood clot. Tissue and blood vessel damage releases the enzyme thromboplastin, which acts on prothrombin in the bloodstream to form the clotting factor thrombin. **Thrombin** is an enzyme that then acts on **fibrinogen**, a protein found in blood plasma, to convert it to **fibrin** and form a netlike substance in the blood that traps blood cells and platelets to form the matrix, or frame, of a blood clot.

Vitamin K must be present to produce prothrombin and other clotting factors that are made in the liver. In addition to calcium, clotting factors, and RBCs, platelets and magnesium are needed for clot formation.

In the circulatory system, arterial vessels carry oxygenated blood throughout the body. If these small arteries become plugged with thrombi (clots made of fibrin, platelets, and cholesterol), oxygen cannot get to the tissues, and death may result. Abnormal blood clotting may produce a thrombus (a single clot) in one of the coronary arteries that nourish the heart muscle. Emboli (small pieces of a blood clot) may break off from the site of a thrombus or thrombophlebitis (inflammation of a vein wall and associated blood clot) in the lower extremities and travel through the bloodstream to block vessels in the brain or lungs. An **embolism** is a blockage in an artery caused by a blood clot or air bubble. In the brain, the blockage can cause stroke or death. In the lungs, the blockage can interfere with oxygenation of the blood.

## ANTICOAGULANTS

An **anticoagulant** is a drug that interferes with one or more steps in the blood clotting process. These drugs can reduce or prevent new **clots** from forming and help to prevent existing clots from getting larger (extending). They cannot dissolve formed clots. Anticoagulants are mistakenly called *blood thinners*, but they do not actually thin the blood. Drugs that act as anticoagulants are classified as platelet inhibitors, direct thrombin inhibitors (DTIs), indirect thrombin inhibitors (ITIs), or vitamin K antagonists. A summary of anticoagulants is provided in Table 16.1.

**Memory Jogger**

There are four classes of anticoagulant drugs:
- Platelet inhibitors
- Direct thrombin inhibitors
- Indirect thrombin inhibitors
- Vitamin K antagonists

## PLATELET INHIBITORS

### Action

Platelet inhibitors, or antiplatelet drugs, interfere with blood clotting in arteries by preventing platelets from sticking and clumping together (aggregating) to form a platelet plug. Platelet aggregation is an important

### Table 16.1    Anticoagulants

*Platelet inhibitors* use a variety of mechanisms to prevent platelets from sticking together (aggregating) to form a plug that starts the blood clotting cascade.

*Direct thrombin inhibitors (DTIs)* bind to prothrombin and prevent its conversion to thrombin, which is needed to convert fibrinogen to fibrin. With less thrombin, less fibrin is available to form the mesh network that traps red blood cells and provides the framework for a clot.

*Indirect thrombin inhibitors (ITIs)* indirectly prevent the conversion of prothrombin to thrombin by increasing the amount of active antithrombin III, a substance that interferes with that conversion.

*Vitamin K antagonists* reduce or prevent the formation of vitamin K in the intestinal tract. Vitamin K is required for the production of many clotting factors in the liver. With less vitamin K available, fewer clotting factors are made.

| DRUGS/ADULT DOSAGE | NURSING IMPLICATIONS |
|---|---|
| **Platelet Inhibitors** | |
| aspirin (Ecotrin, low-dose aspirin, Asaphen ♣, Entrophen ♣) 81–325 mg orally once daily<br>cilostazol (Pletal) 100 mg orally twice daily<br>clopidogrel (Plavix) 75 mg once daily<br>ticagrelor (Brilinta) 180 mg orally once as a loading dose, then 90 mg orally twice daily<br>ticlopidine (Ticlid) 250 mg orally twice daily | • Avoid taking OTC drugs, especially those that contain NSAIDs, because they increase the risk of bleeding. Fish oil is a natural anticoagulant, so taking fish oil may increase the risk of bleeding.<br>• Antacids interfere with antiplatelet drugs. Teach patients to take antiplatelet drugs 1 hour before or 2 hours after taking antacids.<br>• Most oral antiplatelet drugs are better tolerated when given with food to prevent nausea.<br>• Teach patients the symptoms of bleeding and to report any signs of abnormal bleeding to the healthcare provider.<br>• Teach patients to avoid the foods, herbs, and supplements that can interfere with antiplatelet drugs.<br>• Teach patients not to stop taking these drugs without talking to their provider. Antiplatelet drugs sometimes need to be withheld for certain surgical or dental procedures. Discuss all drugs with each healthcare provider.<br>• Antiplatelet drugs should be avoided during the last trimester of pregnancy and should not be taken while breast-feeding. Check labs and notify the healthcare provider for platelet levels below 100,000 per microliter. |
| **Direct Thrombin Inhibitors** | |
| apixaban (Eliquis) 2.5–5 mg orally twice daily<br>desirudin (Iprivask) 15 mg subcutaneously every 12 hours or 0.1 mg/kg/h as a continuous IV<br>dabigatran (Pradaxa) 150 mg orally twice daily<br>rivaroxaban (Xarelto) 20 mg orally daily or 15 mg orally twice daily<br>edoxaban (Savaysa) 60 mg orally once daily | • Watch for signs of abnormal bleeding, and teach patients to report abnormal bleeding, including heavy menses, to the healthcare provider.<br>• Monitor patients for signs of allergy or hypersensitivity to these drugs, such as wheezing, shortness of breath, chest tightness, facial swelling, rash, or hives.<br>• Teach patients to avoid aspirin and NSAIDs while taking thrombin inhibitors because serious hemorrhage or death could occur.<br>• Keep the drugs in their original containers; do not place them in plastic pill containers because they are sensitive to light. |
| **Indirect Thrombin Inhibitors** | |
| heparin, heparin sodium (Calcilean ♣, Hepalean ♣)<br>IV: adult dose for bolus is based on patient weight; usually 5000–10,000 units as an IV bolus, followed by continuous IV infusion<br>Subcutaneous injection: 8000–10,000 units every 8 hours or 5000–20,000 units every 12 hours | • The IV flow rate for continuous heparin infusion is ordered by the prescriber and based on aPTT test results. Monitor aPTT results and report them to the healthcare provider.<br>• Watch for signs of abnormal bleeding and teach patients to report abnormal bleeding, including heavy menses, to the healthcare provider, because these may indicate overdosage.<br>• Monitor patients who are receiving heparin for wheezing, shortness of breath, chest tightness, facial swelling, rash, or hives, because these are indications of allergy or hypersensitivity to the drug. |

| Table 16.1 | Anticoagulants—cont'd |
|---|---|
| **DRUGS/ADULT DOSAGE** | **NURSING IMPLICATIONS** |
| **Low-Molecular-Weight Heparins**<br>enoxaparin (Lovenox) 1 mg/kg every 12 hours or 1.5 mg/kg once daily subcutaneously<br>dalteparin (Fragmin) 100–200 U/kg once daily subcutaneously<br>tinzaparin (Innohep) 175 U/kg once daily subcutaneously<br>fondaparinux sodium (Arixtra) available in single-dose, prefilled syringe of 2.5–10 mg once daily subcutaneously | • Teach patients to avoid aspirin and NSAIDs while taking heparin preparations because the risk of excessive bleeding is greatly increased.<br>• Assess patients who are receiving heparin for low platelet counts and indications of clot extension because these are signs of heparin-induced thrombocytopenia, a life-threatening reaction to heparin.<br>• Ensure that the heparin antidote, protamine sulfate, is available so that it can be given quickly in case of overdose.<br>• LMWHs are given by deep subcutaneous injection. Do not expel air bubble or aspirate before giving the injection. Do not rub the injection site. All of these actions can cause excessive bleeding, bruising, and tissue damage at the injection site.<br>• Ask patients who are prescribed prefilled syringes of fondaparinux sodium (Arixtra) whether they have a latex allergy because these products contain latex rubber–tipped needle covers. |
| **Vitamin K Antagonists** | |
| warfarin (Coumadin, Jantoven, Warfilone) 2–10 mg orally daily for 2–4 days; then dose is adjusted based on INR laboratory test results | • Teach patients to limit the amount of green, leafy vegetables they eat because these vegetables are a natural source of vitamin K that can reduce the effect of warfarin.<br>• Monitor patients' INR test results to determine effectiveness.<br>• Remind patients to keep all appointments for INR laboratory tests because the dosage is adjusted based on the test results.<br>• Stress the importance of not taking aspirin or NSAIDs with this drug because it can lead to excessive bleeding.<br>• Teach patients the signs of abnormal bleeding to report to the healthcare provider.<br>• Ensure that the warfarin antidote, vitamin K, is available so it can be given quickly in case of an overdose.<br>• Caution women of childbearing age who are taking warfarin to avoid pregnancy because this drug can cause birth defects and bleeding.<br>• Many drugs and herbal supplements interfere with the action of warfarin and should be avoided. |

*aPTT*, activated partial thromboplastin time; *INR*, international normalization ratio; *LMWHs*, low-molecular-weight heparins; *NSAIDs*, nonsteroidal anti-inflammatory drugs; *INR*, international normalized ratio; *OTC*, over-the-counter.

defense mechanism when the body is injured; it seals the entry into the vascular system and prevents blood from going into body tissues. Platelet inhibitors work in the cardiovascular system to prevent clotting events in a patient who may have reduced blood circulation to the heart before a myocardial infarction (MI). Common platelet inhibitors are aspirin, clopidogrel, dipyridamole, eptifibatide, prasugrel, ticlopidine, tirofiban, and cilostazol.

## Uses

**Platelet inhibitors** are often the first drugs used to prevent clots in blood vessels (the vascular system). These drugs are often given prophylactically (for prevention) when a patient has a condition that may produce blood clots to prevent further extension of the clot or to prevent further development of blood clots. Although they can prevent some clotting, they can do nothing to dissolve clots that have already developed.

Some of these drugs are used to keep venous and arterial grafts open and to prevent strokes when blood vessels become blocked. They may be given as additional drugs (adjuncts) to thrombolytic therapy to patients who have had a heart attack to prevent them from having another one.

Acetylsalicylic acid (ASA), or aspirin, is the most commonly used antiplatelet drug. ASA reduces the risk of major blood vessel blockage that can lead to acute MI (heart attack), ischemic stroke, angina, and peripheral arterial disease (PAD). Although ASA use is helpful, it also carries the risk of gastrointestinal (GI) bleeding in older patients, in those with a history of peptic ulcer disease, and in patients using other nonsteroidal anti-inflammatory drugs (NSAIDs) or more than one antiplatelet therapy. Chapter 12 provides information on the actions and nursing implications for aspirin.

Clopidogrel (Plavix) is given to patients who have had an MI caused by a clot (thrombus) formed in a coronary artery. In patients who have had a stent placed into the coronary artery as a result of severe narrowing or blockage of the artery, clopidogrel prevents platelets from sticking to the stent mesh. For these patients, clopidogrel must be taken daily for a year or longer to prevent clots from developing and plugging the stent. It is also used in patients with PAD to prevent blood clots in the legs, for prevention of an MI, and as additional therapy along with thrombolytic drugs to prevent additional strokes after a recent ischemic stroke.

## Expected Side Effects

Most drugs that affect the blood clotting system have the potential to cause bleeding, especially when used in combination with other antiplatelet drugs. Easy bruising is common—for example, bleeding of the gums can occur when the patient brushes his or her teeth. GI effects such as diarrhea, nausea, dyspepsia (stomach discomfort after eating), vomiting, flatulence, and anorexia (lack of appetite) have been experienced. Skin effects such as rash, pruritus (itching), and purpura (bruising) have been reported.

## Adverse Reactions

Excessive bleeding, including acute hemorrhage, is the most common adverse effect. Allergic reactions to aspirin and NSAIDs typically occur within a few hours after taking the drug. Symptoms of allergic reactions include itching, hives, and runny nose, with more severe reactions causing swelling of the lips, tongue, or face. New acute cardiovascular events can occur when these drugs are stopped abruptly, and they should never be discontinued without the advice of the patient's healthcare provider. Some of these drugs, including clopidogrel, can decrease the platelet count (thrombocytopenia) and the white blood cell count (neutropenia).

---

**! Safety Alert!**

Patients who are taking anticoagulants should watch for early signs of bleeding:
- Easy bruising of knuckles, elbows, or any body part that experiences pressure (e.g., under watchband)
- New or excessive bleeding of gums when brushing teeth
- Blood in the urine or stool or tarry-colored stool
- Tachycardia
- Hypotension
- Shortness of breath
- GI pain

---

## Drug and Food Interactions

Anticoagulants have many interactions with other drugs and foods that can increase the risk of bleeding or decrease effectiveness of the drug. Platelet inhibitors such as aspirin and NSAIDs, if taken with other drugs that reduce coagulation, can cause excessive bleeding. Drinking alcoholic beverages can increase the risk of bleeding because of their effect on the liver, where some clotting factors are formed. Other drugs, such as vitamin K and oral contraceptives, decrease the effects of anticoagulants. Antibiotics can affect blood clotting when taken with anticoagulants.

Some drugs that protect the GI system, such as proton-pump inhibitors (PPIs), can interact with

---

**Box 16.1** Foods, Herbs, and Supplements That Affect the Clotting System

**FOODS THAT MAY INTERFERE WITH ANTICOAGULANTS**
- Tomatoes
- Onions
- Dark leafy greens
- Broccoli
- Garlic
- Bananas

**HERBS AND SUPPLEMENTS THAT INCREASE THE RISK OF BLEEDING IN ANTICOAGULATED PATIENTS**
- Angelica
- Cat's claw
- Chamomile
- Chondroitin
- Feverfew
- Fish oil
- Vitamin E
- Ginkgo
- Goldenseal
- Grape seed extract
- Green leaf tea
- Horse chestnut seed
- Psyllium
- Turmeric

---

clopidogrel and decrease its effectiveness. Green, leafy vegetables contain vitamin K and can decrease the effectiveness of anticoagulants. Many herbal products, vitamins, and supplements can interfere with anticoagulants. For example, St. John's wort further increases the risk of bleeding if it is used by someone who is taking an anticoagulant. Multivitamins often contain vitamin K, which reduces the effectiveness of warfarin (Box 16.1). Chapter 20 describes many herbal, vitamin, and supplemental products and some of their interactions with drugs.

### ❖ Nursing Implications and Patient Teaching

◆ *Assessment.* Before giving the first dose of any platelet inhibitor, it is important to ask the patient what other drugs he or she has taken in the past week, including over-the-counter (OTC) drugs, vitamins, minerals, and herbal products. Many of these drugs and products can interact with platelet inhibitors and greatly increase the risk of bleeding. Ask whether the patient currently has bruising or bleeding, especially from the gums, nose, or mouth, which is a sign of a low platelet count and increased bleeding risk.

Assess for signs of internal bleeding:
- Severe abdominal pain and tenderness
- Vomiting or diarrhea that contains frank red blood or is coffee colored
- Cold, clammy skin

Examine the mouth and skin for any signs of bleeding, such as pale mucous membranes, bruising, or petechiae (tiny red-purple spots on the skin, caused by a minor bleed into the skin) (Fig. 16.2).

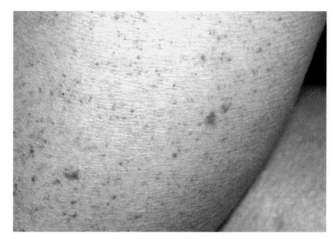

**Fig. 16.2** Petechiae. (Modified from Marks, J., & Miller, J. (2013). *Lookingbill and Marks' principles of dermatology* (5th ed.). Saunders.)

◆ *Planning and implementation.* Give platelet inhibitors, and record the doses given and the patient's response. Monitoring the patient's vital signs can alert you to possible adverse reactions. Tachycardia and hypotension can occur with bleeding, so monitor pulse and blood pressure at least once per shift.

Report the location and amount of any bruising or petechiae that occur. Assist with the collection of blood for ordered tests that are required to monitor therapy.

◆ *Evaluation.* Changes in vital signs and levels of consciousness provide important feedback about the possible risk of bleeding that can occur with these drugs. Watch for skin-related signs of bleeding, such as bruising or petechiae. Watch for signs of overdose and internal bleeding as therapy progresses. This includes bleeding gums when brushing the teeth, blood in the urine, and coughing up blood.

Determine whether the patient understands why he or she is taking the drug and the symptoms of overdose. Have the patient report any signs of bruising or easy bleeding.

### DIRECT THROMBIN INHIBITORS

### Action

All **direct thrombin inhibitors (DTIs)** prevent the formation of blood clots, or thrombi, by interfering with the activity of the enzyme thrombin (factor II). This action increases the time it takes for blood to clot, preventing new clots from forming. These drugs do not dissolve clots that have already occurred. Dabigatran (Pradaxa), rivaroxaban (Xarelto), apixaban (Eliquis), and edoxaban (Savaysa) are examples of DTIs (see Table 16.1). All of these drugs stop the coagulation cascade by binding to free thrombin in the blood and to thrombin that is bound to fibrin.

### Uses

DTIs are used to prevent clots in arteries and veins. They can also be used to prevent and treat **deep vein thrombosis (DVT)** or pulmonary embolism (PE) or to prevent clotting from atrial fibrillation, an abnormal heart rhythm in which the upper chambers of the heart (the atria) quiver instead of beating normally to move blood out of the atria and into the ventricles. The advantage of DTIs is that they do not require frequent laboratory blood testing as part of the monitoring process that is required for warfarin.

DTIs are used much like warfarin and other anticoagulants. They are prescribed for patients who are at risk for systemic embolism and stroke and especially for patients who have atrial fibrillation that is not caused by a heart valve problem. They are also used for prevention of blood clots after some types of surgery.

### Expected Side Effects

DTIs can cause bleeding. Easy bruising is common, including bleeding gums when the patient brushes his or her teeth. Another common side effect of DTIs is gastric upset when the drug is taken on an empty stomach.

### Adverse Reaction

By far, the most common adverse reactions from DTIs are excessive bleeding and thrombocytopenia. Early signs of overdose or internal bleeding include bleeding from the gums while brushing the teeth, excessive bleeding or oozing from cuts, unexplained bruising or nosebleeds, and unusually heavy or unexpected menses in women. These "must know" signs and symptoms indicate that the patient needs prompt attention.

### Drug Interactions

DTIs can interact with many commonly prescribed drugs and some supplements, including atorvastatin, azithromycin, carvedilol, clarithromycin, cyclosporine, diltiazem, and St. John's wort. When they are taken together, the concentration of DTIs increases, which greatly increases the risk of excessive bleeding. When taken with carbamazepine, dexamethasone, phenobarbital, phenytoin, or rifampin, the concentrations and actions of DTIs are reduced, decreasing their effectiveness. Antacids may also reduce the actions of DTIs.

 **Drug Interaction Alert**

- Common drugs that increase the activity and bleeding risks of DTIs are atorvastatin, azithromycin, carvedilol, clarithromycin, cyclosporine, and diltiazem.
- Drugs that decrease the effectiveness of DTIs are carbamazepine, dexamethasone, phenobarbital, phenytoin, rifampin, and antacids.

❖ **Nursing Implications and Patient Teaching**

◆ *Assessment.* Assess patients for any of the following, which may be a sign or symptom of serious bleeding:
- Unusual bruising
- Blood in the urine, stool, or vomitus

- Coughing up blood
- Headaches, dizziness, or weakness
- Recurring nosebleeds
- Unusual bleeding from gums
- Menstrual bleeding that is heavier than normal

◆ *Planning and implementation.* Teach the patient and family members to take DTIs on time. When a dose is missed, the scheduled dose should be taken as soon as possible on the same day, but if there will be less than 6 hours between scheduled doses, the missed dose should not be taken.

Accidental overdose may lead to excessive bleeding. If needed, the reversal agent (idarucizumab) can be prescribed by the healthcare provider.

Teach patients and family members not to discontinue DTIs without talking to the healthcare provider who prescribed it because the risk for serious clotting events increases.

Instruct patients to keep DTIs in the original bottle to protect the drug from moisture and light. Teach them not to put DTIs in pillboxes or pill organizers.

Teach patients not to chew or break the capsules before swallowing them because the drug may be absorbed too rapidly or destroyed by stomach acid. Instruct patients to take DTIs with a full glass of water to prevent stomach irritation and improve absorption.

◆ *Evaluation.* Watch for signs of overdose and internal bleeding. These include bleeding gums when brushing the teeth, blood in the urine, and coughing up or vomiting blood.

Have the patient or family explain to you the purpose of taking this drug and the symptoms of overdose. Note any signs of bruising or easy bleeding, and document your findings according to agency policy.

◆ *Patient and family teaching.* Tell the patient and family:
- Take DTIs on time.
- When a dose is missed, take it as soon as possible on the same day, but if there will be less than 6 hours before the next scheduled dose, the missed dose should not be taken.
- Accidental overdose can lead to excessive bleeding. If needed, the reversal agent (idarucizumab) can be prescribed by the healthcare provider.
- Do not discontinue a DTI without talking to the healthcare provider who prescribed it because the risk of serious clotting events increases.
- Keep DTIs in their original bottle to protect the drug from moisture and light. Do not put DTIs in pillboxes or pill organizers.
- Do not to chew or break the capsules before swallowing them because the drug may be absorbed too rapidly or destroyed by stomach acid.

- Take DTIs with a full glass of water to prevent stomach irritation and improve absorption.

## INDIRECT THROMBIN INHIBITORS

### Actions

Indirect thrombin inhibitors (ITIs) are anticoagulant drugs that reduce clot formation by increasing the amount and action of the protein antithrombin III. This protein inhibits thrombin from converting fibrinogen to fibrin in the blood clotting cascade, reducing clot formation.

Commonly used ITIs include heparin sodium (Calcilean, Hepalean) and the low-molecular-weight heparins (LMWHs) dalteparin (Fragmin), enoxaparin (Lovenox), tinzaparin (Innohep), and fondaparinux (Arixtra). Heparin is given only by injection because it cannot be absorbed orally.

LMWH is a special formulation of heparin that has a steady anticoagulation effect compared with unfractionated heparin sodium. LMWH works by binding to antithrombin and inhibiting factor Xa, which disrupts part of the clotting cascade. The half-life of LMWH is longer than that of heparin sodium, ranging from 2 to 4 hours after intravenous (IV) injection to 3 to 6 hours after subcutaneous injection.

Therapy with heparin sodium must be monitored for its anticoagulation effect by a blood test known as the *activated partial thromboplastin time (aPTT).* The prescriber maintains or adjusts dosages according to this test result. The LMWH formulation does not require testing.

### Uses

Heparin is used to prevent formation of new clots or to stop existing clots from growing in size. Heparin therapy is used prophylactically (as a preventive measure) during and after many types of surgery, especially surgery involving the heart or circulatory system. It is also used in patients with heart valve disease, in patients with certain dysrhythmias (irregular heartbeats), and in patients receiving hemodialysis. Any patient who is on bed rest for a long time is at risk for blood clots, especially patients with a history of clotting problems or recent orthopedic, thoracic, or abdominal surgery. LMWH is used especially in the prevention of venous thromboembolism and may often be used when pulmonary embolism is present.

### Expected Side Effects

Heparin sodium can cause easy bleeding and bruising, pain, redness, warmth, irritation, or skin changes where the drug was injected. Other side effects may include foot itching and bluish-colored skin.

### Adverse Reactions

Adverse reactions include hemorrhage, thrombocytopenia, shortness of breath, wheezing, chills, fever, alopecia, and hypersensitivity (allergic) reaction. In cases of heparin overdose, protamine sulfate is given to counteract the effect of heparin.

Serious adverse reactions include heparin-induced thrombocytopenia (HIT) and heparin-induced thrombocytopenia and thrombosis (HITT). In HIT, antibodies against heparin are formed and activate platelets, which then clump together and cause small clots in the bloodstream; the platelet count falls. If major clots develop and block vessels, the condition is even more serious and is called *HITT*.

### Drug Interactions

Heparin can interact with aspirin, NSAIDs, glucocorticoids, and other anticoagulants (warfarin) to increase the risk for GI bleeding. Antihistamines, digoxin, nicotine, and tetracycline decrease the anticoagulant effect of heparin.

### ❖ Nursing Implications and Patient Teaching

◆ *Assessment.* Heparin is derived from animal tissue and is more likely to cause an allergic reaction than other anticoagulants. When giving it to patients who have a history of allergy, observe them closely.

This drug should be used cautiously in patients with liver or kidney disease or hypertension, during menses, after delivery, and in patients with indwelling catheters. A higher incidence of bleeding may be seen among older patients.

◆ *Planning and implementation.* Dosages for heparin are given in units. Heparin is given only by IV injection, IV infusion, or subcutaneous injection. Heparin is not given by intramuscular (IM) injection because these injections produce hematomas, irritation, and pain at the injection site.

Do not shake the bottle containing the heparin; only roll it carefully between your hands before inserting the needle. If the heparin solution is discolored or contains a precipitate or particles at the bottom of the bottle, do not use it. Heparin is strongly acidic and is incompatible with many other drugs in solution, and it must not be piggybacked with other drugs into an infusion line. Never mix any drug with heparin in a syringe when bolus therapy is given.

> **⚠ Drug Alert**
>
> **ADMINISTRATION ALERT**
> Roll the heparin bottle between your hands rather than shaking it. Do not give heparin in the same IV line or the same syringe with any other drug.

Use a small (25-gauge) needle and a tuberculin syringe for the subcutaneous injection, which is often given in the abdomen around the umbilicus. Subcutaneous heparin is usually given every 12 hours. There are several things to remember about heparin injection. First, after the needle has been inserted into the patient, do not

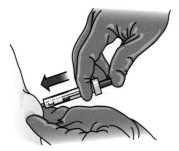

**Fig. 16.3** Deep subcutaneous injection for low-molecular-weight heparin. (From Workman, M. L., & LaCharity, L. A. (2016). *Understanding pharmacology: Essentials for Medication Safety* (2nd ed.). Elsevier.)

attempt to pull back on the plunger or aspirate blood before injection. Second, do not move the needle while the heparin is being injected. Third, do not massage the injection site before or after injection. Doing any of these things increases tissue damage from the heparin. Avoid giving IM injections of other drugs while the patient is receiving heparin because hematomas and bleeding into nearby areas may occur. LMWH preparations are given by deep subcutaneous injection (Fig. 16.3).

> **⊖ Top Tip for Safety**
>
> When injecting subcutaneous heparin, do not pull back on the syringe to aspirate for blood or move the needle in the tissue during the injection. Do not massage the injection site. All of these actions increase the risk of bleeding, bruising, and tissue damage at the injection site.

Rotate the sites of subcutaneous injections of heparin to avoid formation of hematomas (see Chapter 4 and Fig. 4.14 for recommended rotation sites). In the hospital setting, after the heparin is drawn into the syringe, double-check the dose drawn up with another nurse before giving it because of the adverse effects if an inaccurate dose is given.

If intermittent IV therapy is prescribed, draw blood for partial thromboplastin time (PTT) determination 1 hour before the next scheduled heparin dose. Blood for PTT can be drawn at any time after 8 hours of continuous IV heparin therapy. However, blood should not be drawn from the tubing of the heparin infusion line or from the vein being used for infusion. Blood should always be drawn from the arm not being used for heparin infusion.

Continuous intravenous therapy with heparin is first started by a bolus of heparin that is based on the weight of the patient (usually 5000–10,000 units). Obtaining an accurate weight is important before initiating heparin therapy. Check intravenous heparin infusions frequently, even if pumps are in good working order, to ensure that the proper dose is being given.

If heparin is being given at the same time as warfarin, blood should not be drawn for PTT within 5 hours after IV heparin administration or within 24 hours if heparin is given subcutaneously.

Patients who require rapid anticoagulation are commonly hospitalized. Heparin is usually started for an immediate effect and gradually replaced by oral anticoagulants.

The most commonly used blood test for determining the therapeutic range for heparin is the aPTT. The dosage of heparin is considered adequate when the aPTT is about 1.5 to 2.5 times the laboratory control value. PTT and international normalized ratio (INR) tests are ordered when the patient is started on oral anticoagulants and at regular intervals thereafter. The normal range for the INR is 0.8 to 1.2, with a therapeutic target range of 2.0 to 3.0. For patients with mechanical heart valves, this therapeutic range is slightly higher—2.5 to 3.5—because of the high risk of clot formation within the valve. When the oral anticoagulant shows proper effect and the prothrombin activity is in the therapeutic range, heparin therapy may be stopped and the oral anticoagulant therapy continued.

Be sure that the heparin antidote, protamine sulfate, is available for use when patients are given heparin therapy while hospitalized in case of accidental overdosage or an acute bleeding event. You need to urgently contact the appropriate healthcare provider for an order before giving protamine sulfate.

◆ *Evaluation.* If heparin is given by continuous IV infusion, the coagulation time should usually be determined every 4 hours in the early stages of treatment. Many medical centers have adopted protocols that indicate heparin dosing based on previous aPTT results and determine when the next aPTT level should be measured.

Watch for signs of allergy, such as difficulty breathing, wheezing, swelling around the eyes, itching, rash, or hives. Watch for signs of overdose and internal bleeding as therapy progresses. Check with the patient and/or family to ensure that they understand the dosage schedule, side effects, adverse effects, and which signs of adverse effects to report to the healthcare provider. These signs include bleeding gums when brushing the teeth, blood in the urine, and coughing up blood. Teach patients to report all drugs and supplements taken.

---

### 🔊 Top Tip for Safety

- Teach women of childbearing age to notify the healthcare provider if they are pregnant or plan to become pregnant while using heparin. There are risks of birth defects and bleeding in the last trimester that are associated with heparin use in pregnancy.
- If anticoagulation is needed for an expectant mother, heparin is the anticoagulant that will be used.
- Breast-feeding is safe during heparin therapy because the drug is not found in breast milk.
- The heparin antidote protamine sulfate should be available in the event of accidental overdose or hemorrhage.
- Monitor the patient's platelet counts for declines that can be associated with HIT or HITT.

---

## VITAMIN K ANTAGONISTS

Vitamin K is necessary for the production of specific proteins that are needed for the clotting process. A vitamin K antagonist is an anticoagulant drug that interferes with blood clotting by reducing the amount of vitamin K available to help the liver form clotting factors. These drugs are from the coumarin category of drugs. The most common drug in this class is warfarin (Coumadin).

### Actions

Vitamin K antagonists inhibit the enzyme needed for final activation of vitamin K. Without adequate amounts of vitamin K, the liver cannot make blood coagulation factors II, VII, IX, and X. Blood clotting requires the actions of all of the clotting factors, and limiting any clotting factor reduces blood clot formation.

### Uses

For long-term therapy in chronic conditions that may involve problems with clot formation (e.g., coronary artery disease, atrial fibrillation, knee and hip replacement surgery, immobility), warfarin is the drug of choice. Warfarin is given orally for the prevention of blood clots and emboli. Patients typically begin warfarin while taking heparin. Heparin is then discontinued after the INR result for blood clotting time reaches the therapeutic range.

### Expected Side Effects

Easy bruising and bleeding with warfarin are common. For example, bleeding gums may occur when the patient brushes his or her teeth; blood in the stool or urine is also common. Warfarin may produce GI upset (e.g., diarrhea, nausea), headache, and rash.

### Adverse Reactions

Adverse reactions of warfarin include excessive bleeding and hemorrhage that can occur with very heavy menstrual bleeding; frank blood or dark, tarry stools; or coffee-colored vomitus with excessive dosage. Warfarin can cause skin necrosis (death), which can occur within the first 10 days of therapy and is associated with larger doses (Fig. 16.4). Obese, menopausal women are at greatest risk for this rare adverse reaction. Warfarin is not given during pregnancy because it can cause birth defects or death of the fetus.

In response to some bleeding disorders or warfarin overdosage, a synthetic (human-made) form of vitamin K—phytonadione (AquaMephyton)—may be given orally or parenterally to help stimulate the liver to resume manufacture of prothrombin and to serve as an anticoagulant antagonist. However, clotting activity may not return for 48 to 72 hours. Blood products that contain clotting factors may have to be given to stop severe bleeding. Even in urgent situations, giving phytonadione requires an order from the healthcare provider.

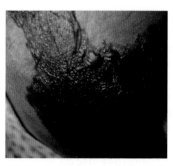

Fig. 16.4 Warfarin-induced skin necrosis. (From Hoffman, R., Benz, E. J., Jr., Shattil, S. J., Furie, B., Silberstein, L. E., McGlave, P., & Heslop, H. (2008). *Hematology: Basic principles and practice* (5th ed.). Churchill Livingstone.)

---

### ⌂ Top Tip for Safety

Several signs suggest internal bleeding:
- Abdominal pain or swelling, back pain, or constipation (resulting from paralytic ileus or intestinal obstruction)
- Bloody or tarry stools, bloody or dark-colored urine, coughing up or vomiting blood or a "coffee-ground" substance
- Dizziness or cold, clammy skin
- Severe or continuous headache
- Tachycardia (fast pulse), hypotension (low blood pressure), and tachypnea (rapid breathing)

---

## Drug and Food Interactions

Vitamin K antagonists (e.g., warfarin) interact with many other drugs. Use a drug reference or consult with the healthcare provider or pharmacist as needed for patient care or teaching because the list of drugs that interact with vitamin K antagonists is very long. In general, many antibiotics, anti-inflammatory drugs, antidysrhythmics, GI drugs, statins, and steroids can lengthen the bleeding time due to warfarin, whereas antacids, antihistamines, barbiturates, large doses of vitamin C, and oral contraceptives can shorten it. Lengthening the bleeding time greatly increases the risk of hemorrhage and death.

It is critically important for the patient and family to accurately report all current drugs before beginning therapy with warfarin. Vitamin K antagonists also interact with many herbal preparations and supplements, and patients should consult with the healthcare provider before beginning any of them while taking these drugs.

Anticoagulant effects may be increased with acute alcohol intoxication but are decreased with chronic alcohol abuse. Some antidiabetic drugs taken with anticoagulants may increase the effect of the diabetes drug or the anticoagulant, and close patient monitoring is needed. Green, leafy vegetables (e.g., spinach, broccoli) are a natural source of vitamin K and can decrease the effect of anticoagulants. Patients should avoid eating excessive amounts of these vegetables and eat a consistent amount each day.

## ❖ Nursing Implications and Patient Teaching

◆ *Assessment.* Obtain a complete health history from the patient, including the current health problem, medical and surgical histories, and any drug and food allergies or hypersensitivity reactions. Ask the patient for a current, accurate list of all drugs being taken, including herbal products, supplements, and OTC drugs.

Ask about conditions that would prevent the use of some anticoagulants, such as alcoholism, blood diseases and conditions associated with bleeding, and uncontrolled hypertension. Patients with heart failure may be more sensitive to vitamin K antagonists.

Make absolutely sure that female patients who are taking a vitamin K antagonist are not pregnant or breast-feeding. A pregnancy test may be performed for women of childbearing age before beginning these drugs. Teach sexually active women who are taking warfarin to use two reliable methods of birth control.

◆ *Planning and implementation.* Warfarin can have an unpredictable effect in some patients, especially in adults over age 65 and in patients of Asian descent. Warfarin has a very narrow range (therapeutic index) that produces the anticoagulant effects without also causing bleeding in the patient. Frequent blood tests are done to monitor bleeding risk while still providing the anticoagulation needed. To avoid variation in testing methods, the INR is used to standardize PTT reporting. In a person who is not receiving anticoagulation therapy, the normal INR is 0.9 to 1.1. The typical INR goal for a patient who needs anticoagulation therapy is 2 to 3, except in cases of mechanical cardiac valve replacement, in which case a higher INR is necessary to prevent clot formation. The INR goal may be different for specific disorders that require anticoagulation.

Initially, the prothrombin time test and INR (PT/INR) may be measured daily, but after stabilization, tests are performed at 1- to 4-week intervals, depending on patient response. For hospitalized patients and those in long-term care facilities, be sure to obtain the blood tests on time, and report abnormal findings to the healthcare provider as soon as they are received. The antidote for warfarin overdosage (vitamin K) should be available at all times.

◆ *Evaluation.* Warfarin takes up to 72 hours to reach an effective level for anticoagulation. Heparin is given when an immediate anticoagulant effect is required. For this reason, hospitalized patients often receive heparin and warfarin at the same time. Monitoring of the PT/INR is especially critical during this period.

Watch for signs of overdose and internal bleeding as therapy progresses. Indications include bleeding gums when brushing the teeth, blood in the urine or stool, and coughing up or vomiting blood.

Assess whether the patient understands why he or she is taking the drug and the symptoms of overdose. Have the patient explain the actions he or she would take if signs of bruising or easy bleeding were noted.

Remind patients to always consult their healthcare provider before starting any new drug (including OTC drugs and vitamins), changing a drug dose, or discontinuing any drug. Many drugs can change the effects of an anticoagulant in the body.

Determine whether the patient and family members understand the dietary instructions regarding the intake of green, leafy vegetables (e.g., broccoli, cabbage, collard greens, lettuce, spinach). Box 16.1 lists herbs that increase the risk of bleeding or interfere with anticoagulant action.

---

### Lifespan Considerations
**Older Adults**

Older adults may be more sensitive to the effects of anticoagulants, and a lower maintenance dose is usually recommended for older adult patients, along with very close supervision and monitoring. This is particularly true for patients who receive warfarin and may be deficient in vitamin K because of low intake of green, leafy vegetables.

---

### Memory Jogger

Heparin and warfarin can be taken at the same time, but most other anticoagulants cannot.

---

◆ *Patient and family teaching.* Tell the patient and family:
- Wear a medical alert bracelet or carry an identification card indicating the use of an anticoagulant.
- Teach patients and family members about warfarin, and tell them to immediately report expected side effects and adverse reactions to warfarin to the healthcare provider.
- Avoid adding any drugs, herbs, and/or supplements without the express permission of the healthcare provider because these agents can interfere with the actions of warfarin.
- Swallow the tablets whole, without cutting, crushing, or chewing them, to ensure proper drug absorption.
- Protect the drug from humidity and light exposure (they are dispensed in an opaque plastic container or a dark-colored glass container) because the drug's activity is reduced by exposure to light and moisture. Do not transfer the drug to another storage container.
- Avoid increasing the intake of green, leafy vegetables because they contain vitamin K and can decrease the effectiveness of warfarin.
- Avoid alcohol while taking warfarin because alcohol ingestion changes the drug's activity.
- Keep all appointments for laboratory tests and visits to the healthcare provider because blood clotting

ability can change, and dosage changes may be needed based on test results.
- Use caution when brushing teeth, trimming nails, and shaving. An electric shaver should be used whenever possible.
- Apply pressure to stop bleeding from accidental cuts or scrapes. If bleeding persists after 10 minutes, contact your healthcare provider.
- Do not suddenly stop taking any oral anticoagulant because this may trigger severe cardiovascular problems and clotting.
- Avoid contact sports or other activities that could lead to injuries.
- At least 2 days are usually required to recover blood clotting ability after anticoagulation is stopped.

---

### Top Tip for Clinical Care
- Teach patients to tell their dentist and all healthcare providers that they are taking anticoagulants.
- Patients who are taking anticoagulants and who require dental or surgical procedures may need to discontinue the drug before surgery to avoid bleeding problems. Procedures may pose a particular risk if patients have a traumatic injury or require emergency surgery.
- Drugs such as clopidogrel (Plavix), which is used after stent placement, should never be abruptly stopped without consultation with a cardiologist. Abruptly stopping clopidogrel in this case could lead to the stent becoming blocked with a clot.

---

## FIBRINOLYTIC DRUGS
### Action
**Fibrinolytic drugs** (formerly called *thrombolytic drugs*) actually do dissolve and break down existing blood clots. For this reason they are sometimes called *clot busters*. Fibrinolytic drugs work by converting plasminogen to the enzyme plasmin, which degrades or breaks down fibrin clots, fibrinogen, and other plasma proteins. These products are used especially for dissolving or lysis of thrombi and are used only in a critical care setting. Fibrinolytics are summarized in Table 16.2.

### Uses
Fibrinolytic drugs are used in acute care settings such as emergency departments and intensive care units. The drugs are given for a variety of reasons, including acute MI, acute pulmonary embolus, acute ischemic stroke, and acute arterial occlusion. These drugs dissolve clots and emboli, ultimately reducing the extent of cellular damage from arterial blockage.

Timing is a critical factor for use of these drugs. If fibrinolytics are begun within 12 hours after a heart attack or 3 hours after the onset of a stroke, the blood clot blocking the artery can be dissolved and blood flow restored. The most commonly used fibrinolytic drugs are alteplase (Activase, tPA), reteplase (Retavase), and tenecteplase (TNKase). Be careful not to confuse tPA and TNKase. Although both are fibrinolytics, the dosages and administrations are different. These drugs are high-alert drugs and are given through an IV line.

 Memory Jogger

All fibrinolytic drugs are given IV and are high-alert drugs.

### Expected Side Effects

Bleeding is the most obvious side effect of fibrinolytic drugs. Bleeding of the gums or bleeding at injection or IV sites can occur. Low blood pressure (hypotension) can also occur.

### Adverse Reactions

Allergic reactions and hypersensitivity can occur with symptoms of shortness of breath, wheezing, chest tightness, facial swelling, rash, or hives. Hemorrhage is the most critical adverse reaction that can occur, and because these drugs break up clots, there is a risk of stroke, especially in older adult patients with hypertension. Contraindications for giving fibrinolytic drugs include known bleeding disorders, pregnancy or recent delivery (< 24 hours), stroke within the past 2 months, hypertension with blood pressure greater than 200/120 mm Hg, head trauma, and aortic dissection.

### Drug Interactions

Giving fibrinolytic drugs together with other anticoagulants increases the potential for bleeding and hemorrhage.

### ❖ Nursing Implications and Patient Teaching

◆ *Assessment.* Fibrinolytic drugs are given by the healthcare provider or advanced practitioner in the life-threatening situations of MI or stroke. They are most helpful when given within the first hour after the onset of symptoms from thrombosis. Ask the patient or family when the chest pain (due to MI) or stroke symptoms began to determine the exact time sequence of events and what happened before the patient was brought to the hospital. Ask whether the patient has a history of a prior stroke or bleeding disorder.

Ask whether other drugs, such as aspirin, have been taken. Aspirin helps reduce platelet adhesion, and for patients with suspected MI, the standard protocol is to have the patient chew a 325-mg aspirin (ASA) tablet. The aspirin may have been taken at home or given by paramedics before arrival at the hospital.

Ask the patient or family whether the patient has had surgery or given birth within the past 48 hours.

◆ *Planning and implementation.* Fibrinolytic drugs come as a powder that requires reconstitution. Have all of the equipment and materials assembled and ready for infusion.

Carefully monitor and record the vital signs of the patient who is receiving fibrinolytic therapy. Report these findings to the healthcare provider. After the fibrinolytic drug has been given, do not remove IV lines or give IM injections because of increased risk of severe bleeding. If an IV line must be removed, apply pressure to the area for 30 minutes.

◆ *Evaluation.* Monitor the patient carefully for bleeding. Bleeding may be superficial, coming from the infusion site. Other, more significant bleeding indicates overdose and is shown by hematuria (blood in the urine), hematemesis (blood in the vomitus), abdominal pain and swelling, tachycardia, tachypnea, and hypotension, all of which can indicate internal bleeding.

| Table 16.2 | **Fibrinolytic Drugs** |
|---|---|
| *Fibrinolytic drugs* dissolve clots by activating plasminogen to form plasmin, which is an enzyme that breaks down the fibrin fiber network (mesh) holding a clot together. | |
| **DRUGS/ADULT DOSAGE** | **NURSING IMPLICATIONS** |
| alteplase (Activase, tPA; Activase, rtPA ♣): adult dose is based on the condition being treated<br>Myocardial infarction: 15 mg intravenous (IV) bolus, then 50 mg IV over 30 minutes, then 35 mg IV over 60 minutes; followed by heparin therapy<br>Pulmonary embolism: 100 mg IV over 2 hours; followed by heparin therapy<br>Stroke: 0.9 mg/kg IV over 1 hour (limit total dose to 90 mg, with 10% of the dose given as a bolus)<br>reteplase (Retavase) adult dose: 10 units IV bolus, then another 10 units IV bolus 30 min later<br>tenecteplase (TNKase) adult dose is based on weight: 30–50 mg IV push[a] | • Before therapy, ensure that the patient has no history of active internal bleeding, recent stroke, spinal surgery, blood pressure > 200/120 mm Hg, bleeding disorders, pregnancy or delivery, head trauma, prolonged cardiopulmonary resuscitation, or pending aortic dissection, because these conditions are absolute contraindications for fibrinolytic therapy.<br>• Watch for signs of hemorrhage, especially bleeding into the brain, because these drugs greatly increase the risk of bleeding anywhere.<br>• Monitor patients for symptoms of allergic reactions such as rash, facial swelling, hives, low blood pressure, or difficulty breathing.<br>• Monitor coagulation laboratory tests after initial dose is given because additional drugs or dosages are based on the results of these tests.<br>• Monitor for severe headache or changes in alertness because these may signal stroke from bleeding in the brain.<br>• Avoid giving intramuscular drugs because of the risk of bleeding. If the IV line is removed, apply pressure for 30 minutes. |

[a]Not given by LPN/VN.

◆ *Patient and family teaching.* Tell the patient and family:
- Ensure that the patient and family understand the purpose, risks, and benefits of fibrinolytic therapy.
- Teach the patient to report to the healthcare provider any unusual symptoms, signs of allergic reaction to the drug, or unusual bleeding that occurs.

## ERYTHROPOIESIS-STIMULATING AGENTS

### Action

An **erythropoiesis-stimulating agent (ESA)** is a synthetic form of the hormone erythropoietin, which stimulates the bone marrow to make more red blood cells (RBCs) at a faster rate. Erythropoietin is naturally produced by the kidneys when the RBC count declines because of anemia.

The hemoglobin in RBCs carries oxygen to the body organs and tissues, and decreases in RBCs result in poor tissue oxygenation. Anemia signals the kidneys to secrete erythropoietin, which then travels to the bone marrow, stimulating the marrow to increase production of RBCs. This process is known as *erythropoiesis.*

The synthetic forms of erythropoietin work just like the natural hormone. ESAs come in vials or in prefilled syringes, and they are given by IV or subcutaneous routes. A summary of ESAs is provided in Table 16.3.

### Uses

ESAs are usually given to patients who have a condition that causes anemia and need to increase the production of RBCs. Patients with chronic kidney disease cannot make enough erythropoietin to stimulate RBC production and provide adequate oxygen to tissues. Patients who are anemic from the effects of chemotherapy on the bone marrow or who may be anemic before surgery are often prescribed ESAs. These drugs reduce the need for transfusions and reduce the complications of transfusions, such as fluid overload.

### Expected Side Effects

Pain at the injection site is the most common side effect of ESAs. Generalized body aches and pain, rash, redness, or warmth at the injection site can occur.

### Adverse Reactions

The use of ESAs can pose significant risks. As RBC production increases, the blood becomes thicker. This can increase the risk of hypertension, blood clots, stroke, and MI. In some cases of advanced cancer, tumor growth increased when ESAs were given. There is a risk of severe allergic reactions to ESAs.

### ❖ Nursing Implications and Patient Teaching

◆ *Assessment.* Assess the patient's vital signs and weight. Report the finding of hypertension, which may need to be controlled before ESAs are started.

Obtain a complete health history, especially for a history of stroke, blood clots, MI, other blood clotting disorders, or sickle cell disease. Ask about symptoms of allergic reactions if the patient received ESAs in the past. Ask about the presence of latex allergy because the covers of prefilled syringes contain latex.

Assess the result of the patient's complete blood count (CBC). Notify the healthcare provider if the hemoglobin concentration is 12 g/dL or higher before giving ESAs. Monitor the patient's iron status (i.e., transferrin, serum ferritin) levels, and notify the healthcare provider of the results before beginning ESAs.

◆ *Planning and implementation.* Give supplemental iron as ordered by the healthcare provider. Do not give IV ESAs with any other drugs.

Do not expose the ESA vial to light, and do not shake the vial. Give subcutaneous injections in the outer area of the upper arm, the abdomen (except for a 2-inch area around the umbilicus), the front middle of the thighs, or the outer area of the buttocks. After giving the drug, discard any unused or leftover drug in the vial or in the prefilled syringes.

| Table 16.3 | Erythropoiesis-Stimulating Agents |
|---|---|

*Erythropoiesis-stimulating agents (ESAs)* induce bone marrow to increase the production of red blood cells and mobilize some other blood cells.

| DRUGS/ADULT DOSAGE | NURSING IMPLICATIONS |
|---|---|
| darbepoetin alfa (Aranesp) 0.45 mcg/kg intravenous (IV) or subcutaneously each week; can be given in divided doses<br>epoetin alfa (Epogen, Procrit, Eprex ♣) 50–100 U/kg IV or subcutaneously three times weekly to maintain hemoglobin level at prescribed range | • Monitor for increased blood pressure due to increased blood viscosity (thickness), headaches, body aches, fever, or chills.<br>• Monitor blood counts, especially hemoglobin levels, to help determine drug effectiveness.<br>• Follow directions for drug mixing and preparation because these vary by product and drug effectiveness depends on correct administration.<br>• Check for signs or symptoms of allergic reactions, which are possible adverse effects of these drugs.<br>• Teach patients to immediately report chest pain or shortness of breath, drooping face, or numbness in face or extremities and to call an ambulance for transport to the emergency department; these are signs of heart attack or stroke, and ESAs increase the risk of these health problems. |

◆ *Evaluation.* Report signs of an allergic reaction, such as rash, wheezing, facial swelling, difficulty breathing, or hypotension. Report signs of stroke, chest pain or shortness of breath, and increases in the patient's blood pressure.

◆ *Patient and family teaching.* Tell the patient and family:
- Weigh yourself daily, and report to your healthcare provider a weight gain of 2 pounds in 24 hours or 4 pounds in a week, because these drugs can cause water retention.
- Go immediately to the nearest hospital if you have chest pain because these drugs increase blood thickness and raise blood pressure, which can increase the risk of heart attack.
- Inform your healthcare provider if you are pregnant, breast-feeding, or plan to become pregnant.

## DRUGS FOR IRON DEFICIENCY ANEMIA

Erythropoietin is a hormone that is made in the kidney in response to low levels of oxygen in the tissue (hypoxia) and regulates the production of RBCs. Iron, folate, and vitamin $B_{12}$ (cobalamin) are needed for RBC production. Iron is a key component of hemoglobin in RBCs. Most iron is incorporated into hemoglobin, and the rest is stored as ferritin or myoglobin.

To maintain adequate numbers of RBCs, immature red blood cells known as *reticulocytes* are continually released into the circulation in small amounts by the bone marrow. To ensure adequate tissue oxygenation, a feedback loop involving erythropoietin helps to regulate erythropoiesis so that the rate of RBC production is equal to the removal of older, defective RBCs from the body. Iron deficiency anemia develops when there is not enough iron available for maintaining tissue oxygenation and the body's supply of stored iron gets used up.

Signs of iron deficiency anemia include weakness, shortness of breath, palpitations, tachycardia, and pale skin and mucous membranes. There are many causes of iron deficiency anemia, including bleeding, inability to absorb iron, and pregnancy.

Iron products are used to provide additional iron that is needed for producing hemoglobin and restoring body stores of iron. Oral iron supplements are the most common treatment for iron deficiency anemia because of their established safety profile, ease of administration, and low cost of therapy. Parenteral iron is typically given to patients who cannot tolerate oral iron, who have not responded to oral iron preparations, or who require a rapid increase in iron stores. Iron preparations are reviewed in Table 16.4.

### FERROUS SULFATE

Ferrous sulfate is an iron supplement that is given orally for the treatment of iron deficiency anemia.

#### Action
When given orally, ferrous sulfate is absorbed in the small intestine.

#### Uses
Ferrous sulfate is used to replace iron stores in patients with iron deficiency anemia.

#### Expected Side Effects
The most common side effects of ferrous sulfate are constipation, dark stool color, GI irritation, and nausea.

Table **16.4**   **Drugs for Iron Deficiency Anemia**

*Iron preparations* are used to treat iron deficiency anemia, which develops when there is not enough iron available for producing hemoglobin and maintaining tissue oxygenation.

| DRUGS/ADULT DOSAGE | NURSING IMPLICATIONS |
|---|---|
| Ferrous sulfate 325-mg tablet three times daily<br>Iron dextran<br>Intramuscular: 1 mL (100 mg iron) as a single dose; can be repeated in 10 days<br>Intravenous (IV): 2 mL or less IV once daily until desired level is reached (as determined by healthcare provider); administered by registered nurse | • Assess for signs and symptoms of bleeding, history of illnesses that can cause problems with iron absorption, or history of disease that can cause iron overload.<br>• Assess for a history of allergic reactions to other drugs.<br>• Monitor for signs of anaphylaxis.<br>• Assess the patient's vital signs.<br>• Assess skin and mucous membrane color.<br>• Assess the result of the patient's complete blood count, transferrin level, and serum ferritin level.<br>• Assess for signs and symptoms of bleeding.<br>• Assess for a history of allergic reactions to other drugs.<br>• Ensure that a test dose is administered before the total dose is given.<br>• Ensure that emergency resuscitation equipment is ready nearby.<br>• Monitor for signs of anaphylaxis.<br>• Assess the patient's vital signs.<br>• Assess the result of the patient's complete blood count, transferrin level, and serum ferritin level.<br>• Monitor skin for adverse effects at injection sites, such as abscess, changes in skin pigmentation, cellulitis, or inflammation. |

If an oral solution is given, temporary discoloration of the teeth can occur.

### Adverse Reactions

Hypersensitivity reactions to ferrous sulfate can occur. Iron overdose can lead to fatal poisoning in children younger than 6 years of age.

### ❖ Nursing Implications and Patient Teaching

◆ *Assessment.* Obtain a complete health history, including signs and symptoms of bleeding, history of illnesses that may cause problems with iron absorption, and history of any disease that can cause iron overload. Assess the patient's vital signs for tachycardia and increased respirations associated with anemia.

Assess for pale color of the skin and mucous membranes and for cold temperature of the hands and feet. Assess the result of the patient's CBC, especially hemoglobin level, and notify the healthcare provider of the results. Monitor the patient's iron status (transferrin and serum ferritin levels), and notify the healthcare provider of the results.

◆ *Planning and implementation.* You can expect a rise in hemoglobin levels after about 3 weeks of treatment. Give ferrous sulfate on an empty stomach, or 2 hours after a meal, for best absorption of the drug. Avoid giving ferrous sulfate with antacids because antacids decrease the effectiveness of the drug. When giving ferrous sulfate drops to an infant, use the dropper provided to carefully measure the dose, placing it in the back of the mouth.

◆ *Evaluation.* Report signs of hypersensitivity (allergic reaction), such as rash, wheezing, facial swelling, difficulty breathing, or hypotension. Report signs of severe anemia, such as tachycardia, chest pain, or shortness of breath.

◆ *Patient and family teaching.* Tell the patient and family:
- Take the oral tablet with a full glass of water.
- Avoid lying down for at least 10 minutes after taking the tablet.
- If using the enteric-coated, extended release form of ferrous sulfate, do not crush, chew, or split the tablet. Instead, swallow the tablet whole to prevent releasing all of the drug at once.
- If you are taking the oral solution (liquid) form of ferrous sulfate, shake the bottle well before each dose given. Take the solution through a straw to prevent staining of the teeth.

### IRON DEXTRAN

Iron dextran is another form of the iron mineral that is essential for many body functions, especially transportation of oxygen in the blood. Iron dextran is given by slow IV infusion or by IM injection. It is available in a

solution of 50 mg/mL (2 mL), and it is diluted with 250 to 1000 mL of normal saline for IV infusion. IM injections are given using the Z-track technique in the upper outer quadrant of the buttock.

### Action

The iron that is released into the bloodstream is deposited in the bone marrow, where it is incorporated into hemoglobin. Response to iron dextran can be expected within 3 to 10 days, with an increase in hemoglobin at 2 to 4 weeks.

### Uses

Iron dextran is used to treat iron deficiency anemia in patients for whom oral iron is not effective or not feasible.

### Expected Side Effects

Pain and brown-colored pigmentation at the injection site can be experienced. Use alternate sites on each buttock with each IM injection. Constipation is often a side effect of iron deficiency therapy.

### Adverse Reactions

 **Black Box Warning: Iron Dextran**

Iron dextran contains a black box warning because it can cause severe and sometimes fatal allergic reactions or severe low blood pressure in some patients. A test dose (prescribed by the healthcare provider) should be given before the first infusion. Give the test dose over 30 seconds, and observe the patient for hypersensitivity (allergic) reactions for the next hour. Always have resuscitation equipment and trained personnel ready. Other adverse reactions include GI effects such as diarrhea or vomiting and a sterile abscess at the IM injection site.

### ❖ Nursing Implications and Patient Teaching

◆ *Assessment.* Obtain a complete health history, including signs and symptoms of bleeding, history of illnesses that may cause problems with iron absorption, or history of disease that can cause iron overload. Assess for a history of allergic reactions to other drugs because patients with such a history are at higher risk for severe allergic reactions to iron dextran.

Monitor for signs of anaphylaxis (e.g., swelling of the face, throat, or lips; difficulty breathing; chest pain; rash). Assess the patient's vital signs for tachycardia and increased respirations associated with anemia. Assess for pale color of the skin and mucous membranes and for cold temperature of the hands and feet.

Assess the result of the patient's CBC, especially hemoglobin level, and notify the healthcare provider of the results. Monitor the patient's iron status (transferrin and serum ferritin levels) and notify the healthcare provider of the results. Monitor the skin for adverse effects at injection sites, such as abscess, changes in skin pigmentation, cellulitis, or inflammation.

Patients should avoid taking antacids, dairy products, tea, or coffee within 2 hours before or after this medication because they will decrease its effectiveness.

◆ *Planning and implementation.* You can expect a rise in hemoglobin levels after 2 to 4 weeks of treatment. Rotate injection sites in the buttocks for each injection.

◆ *Evaluation.* Report signs of hypersensitivity (allergic reaction), such as rash, wheezing, facial swelling, difficulty breathing, or hypotension. Report signs of severe anemia, such as tachycardia, chest pain, or shortness of breath.

◆ *Patient and family teaching.* Tell the patient and family:
* Report any signs or symptoms associated with allergic reactions to the drug.
* Take antihistamines as ordered during the treatment period.
* If using the enteric-coated, extended-release form of ferrous sulfate, do not crush, chew, or split the tablet. Instead, swallow the tablet whole to prevent releasing all the drug at once.
* Prevent constipation by increasing water and fiber intake and taking a stool softener daily during treatment.

## Get Ready for the Next-Generation NCLEX® Examination!

### Key Points

* Anticoagulants are used to prevent new clots from forming and existing clots from getting larger.
* Fibrinolytic drugs dissolve existing clots and reduce the formation of new clots.
* All anticoagulants and fibrinolytic drugs greatly increase the risk of excessive bleeding.
* Before starting anticoagulation therapy, ask the patient which other drugs (prescribed or OTC), vitamins, and herbal supplements he or she takes, and check with the pharmacist to determine whether any of them affect blood clotting.
* When injecting subcutaneous heparin, do not pull back on the syringe to aspirate blood or move the needle in the tissue during the injection.
* Do not massage the subcutaneous heparin injection site.
* The antidote for a heparin overdose is protamine sulfate.
* The risk of allergic reactions is higher with heparin than with other anticoagulants because heparin is made from animal products.
* Warfarin is teratogenic (causes birth defects) and should never be used during pregnancy.
* The antidote for warfarin overdose is vitamin K injection (AquaMephyton).
* DTIs are light sensitive and must be stored in their original opaque bottles, not in daily pill organizers.
* A patient may receive warfarin at the same time he or she receives heparin.
* The anticoagulation effect for patients who are taking warfarin daily is usually measured weekly by the INR.
* The "must know" signs that require prompt attention for patients who are taking anticoagulant drugs are excessive gum bleeding, continuous bleeding or oozing from cuts, unexplained nosebleeds, and unusually heavy menstrual flow.
* All fibrinolytic drugs are given intravenously and are high-alert drugs.
* ESAs are used to increase hemoglobin levels to improve oxygen transport to vital organs and tissues.
* Patient and family teaching is especially important for the patient who is undergoing long-term therapy.
* Severe, fatal allergic reactions can occur with iron preparations, especially when given IV.
* Iron dextran is a high-alert drug that carries a black box warning.
* Give a test dose of iron dextran before the full dose is administered.
* Assess the patient for signs and symptoms of allergic reactions, and have resuscitation equipment ready during iron dextran treatment.
* Monitor the CBC and iron, transferrin, and ferritin levels for patients being treated for iron deficiency anemia.

### Clinical Judgment and Next-Generation NCLEX® Examination-Style Questions

1. A 75-year-old male patient is hospitalized for new-onset atrial fibrillation. During his hospitalization, he received IV heparin. He will be discharged tomorrow after being started on warfarin 5 mg daily. He has been following a vegetarian diet for the past 30 years and states that he has a health regimen that includes his vegetarian diet and several supplements and herbal products.

Place an X next to the actions the nurse will emphasize for this client to prevent harm from warfarin.

| | |
|---|---|
| Report signs of abnormal bleeding. | |
| Increase your intake of green, leafy vegetables. | |
| You may continue all herbal supplements that you are currently taking. | |
| Avoid drinking alcohol. | |
| Keep all appointments for INR testing. | |
| Continue warfarin when you have dental or surgical procedures to prevent clots. | |
| Use a soft toothbrush. | |
| Avoid using electric razors. | |

## Get Ready for the Next-Generation NCLEX® Examination!—cont'd

2. A patient with a clotting disorder is prescribed an anticoagulant and asks you to explain the purpose of anticoagulant therapy. What is your best response?

   1. Anticoagulants are used to lyse existing clots.
   2. Anticoagulants are used to increase the flow of blood.
   3. Anticoagulants are used to prevent new clot formation.
   4. Anticoagulants are used to thin the viscosity of the blood.

3. You are caring for a patient who is taking an NSAID for treatment of arthritis and will also be treated with heparin. What should you expect the patient to experience?

   1. A decrease in arthritis pain
   2. An increase in arthritis pain
   3. A decreased effect of the heparin
   4. An increased effect of the heparin

4. Which of the following menu selections demonstrates understanding of the dietary teaching for a patient treated with an anticoagulant?

   1. Bacon, lettuce, and tomato sandwich and iced tea
   2. Chef salad, whole grain crackers, and orange juice
   3. Baked chicken, macaroni and cheese, and low-fat milk
   4. Pork chops, broccoli and cheese, and iced tea

5. Place an X next to the drugs belonging to the direct thrombin inhibitor class of anticoagulants.

| | |
|---|---|
| Acetylsalicylic acid | |
| Apixaban | |
| Clopidogrel | |
| Dabigatran | |
| Heparin | |
| Protamine sulfate | |
| Rivaroxaban | |
| Warfarin | |

6. You are caring for a patient who will be receiving warfarin sodium (Coumadin) 10 mg by mouth daily. You have warfarin 5-mg tablets available to give. What is your best action?

   1. Give the patient two (2) tablets.
   2. Skip this dose until you obtain 10 mg tablets.
   3. Break the tablet in half and give ½ tablet.
   4. Give 2½ tablets.

7. A patient is prescribed 2000 U/mL of heparin subcutaneously. The drug on hand is heparin 5000 U/mL. How many milliliters is the correct dose? _____ mL

8. You are caring for a patient who is to begin iron dextran for the treatment of iron deficiency anemia. What priority step should be taken before beginning the iron dextran?

   1. You should begin hydrating the patient with normal saline 30 minutes before the infusion.
   2. You should place the patient on oxygen by nasal cannula before the infusion.
   3. You should have resuscitation equipment and trained personnel ready before the infusion.
   4. You should place the patient in a supine position before the infusion begins.

# Drugs for Cancer Treatment

## Learning Outcomes

1. Understand the difference between normal cells and cancer cells.
2. Understand the different categories of cancer drugs.
3. Describe the common side effects of traditional cancer chemotherapy.

5. Understand the basis for hormone therapy for cancer, and common side effects.
6. Explain the basis of biologics/targeted therapy for cancer and common side effects.

## Key Terms

**alkylating agents** Cytotoxic drugs that cross-link DNA, making the two DNA strands bind tightly together, which prevents proper DNA and RNA synthesis and inhibits cell division.

**antimetabolites** Cytotoxic drugs similar to normal metabolites needed for vital cell processes that act as counterfeit metabolites and impair cell division.

**antitumor antibiotics** Cytotoxic drugs that damage the DNA of the cell and interrupt DNA or RNA synthesis.

**cancer** Abnormal cell growth that serves no useful purpose, is invasive, and without intervention would lead to death. Also known as *malignancy*.

**carcinogen** Any substance or event that can damage the DNA of a normal cell and cause cancer development.

**cytotoxic** Actions that are cell damaging and cell killing.

**ecchymosis** Skin discoloration from damaged, leaking blood vessels underneath the skin that appears as a bruise.

**extravasation** Leakage of an irritating chemotherapy drug into the tissues surrounding the vein used to infuse the drug, leading to tissue damage.

**gene expression** Information from a gene that is used to make RNA and gene products such as proteins.

**mitosis** The process by which a single parent cell divides to make two new daughter cells.

**mitotic inhibitors** Class of drugs that interfere with the formation of tubules so cells cannot separate during cell division. Also called *antimitotics*.

**petechiae** Red, brown, or purple, pinpoint and round, spots on the skin that result from bleeding under the skin.

**topoisomerase inhibitors** Cytotoxic drugs that disrupt an enzyme (topoisomerase) needed for DNA synthesis and cell division, which causes breakage of DNA (the genetic material in cells) and cell death.

## CANCER

### OVERVIEW OF CANCER

**Cancer** is a disease that results from abnormal cell growth. All cancer cells come from normal cells that have undergone changes to the normal DNA that result in damage or changes in **gene expression** and the loss of normal cell growth controls. As compared to normal cells, cancer cells grow uncontrollably, spreading to the bone and other organs.

 Memory Jogger

- Cancer cells arise from normal cells that, through DNA damage, have lost the strict control processes for normal growth and function.
- This loss of function now makes cancer cells grow and spread uncontrollably.

Growth of cells and tissues is expected during infancy and childhood, and many body cells continue to grow to replace damaged or dead cells long after maturation is complete. This growth is well controlled, ensuring that the right number of cells is always present in any tissue or organ.

Cell division (**mitosis**) occurs in the well-recognized pattern described by the cell cycle. Normal cells divide for only two reasons: to develop normal tissue or to replace lost or damaged tissue (Fig. 17.1). The steps of the cell cycle are tightly controlled. Normal cell division represents a balance between the proteins that promote cell division (known as *cyclins*) and those that limit cell division (known as *suppressor gene products*).

> **Memory Jogger**
>
> Cancer is a disease that results from abnormal cell growth.
>
> Normal cell division occurs with a balance between the cyclins that promote cell division and the suppressor gene products that limit cell division.

## CANCER CELL BIOLOGY

When new or continued abnormal cell growth occurs that is not needed for normal development or tissue replacement, it is known as *neoplasia*. Whether the abnormal cells form tumors that are *benign* (grow by expansion rather than invasion and do not spread) or cancerous, it is important to know that neoplastic cells develop from normal cells. Thus cancer cells were once normal cells but changed to no longer look, grow, or function normally; strict gene expression processes controlling normal cell growth and function have been lost. This occurs because the cells of the body have been exposed to conditions that can damage DNA and change gene expression for how the cells grow or function. When either cell growth or cell function is changed, the cells are abnormal (Table 17.1).

Cancer cells undergo continuous cell division, reentering the cell cycle for division almost as soon as they leave it. Cancer cells tend to divide more quickly than normal cells and do not respond to signals for normal cell death. As a result, cancer cells have an unlimited lifespan, overgrow, and spread *(metastasize)* by invasion into other body areas. This invasion can damage vital organs, often leading to death. Cancer cells can invade tissues both near and far away from the original tumor. This invasion and persistent growth make untreated cancer deadly (Fig. 17.2).

## CANCER DEVELOPMENT

The multistep process of changing a normal cell into a cancer cell is known as *malignant transformation* or *carcinogenesis*. The first step is DNA damage to genes that control cell division, which then allows other genes (oncogenes) that promote cell growth to be activated. Carcinogens are substances or events, such as chemicals, physical agents, or viruses, that can damage normal cell DNA and cause cancer development.

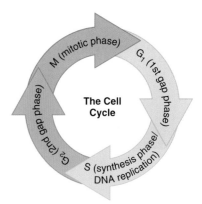

**Fig. 17.1** The cell cycle. **G₁:** In this phase, the cell prepares for division by taking in nutrients, making more energy, increasing fluid, and growing a larger membrane. **S:** Making one cell into two cells requires twice as much of everything, including DNA in the nucleus. So, in the S phase the cell must double its DNA content through DNA synthesis. **G₂:** The cell makes proteins that will be used in cell division and for normal cell functions to be done after cell division is complete. **M:** The single cell splits apart into two cells (mitosis) that are identical to each other. (From Guilbault, J., & Petersen, D. (2023). Oncological and hematological medications. In: Silvestri, A. E., & Silvestri, L. A. (Eds.), *Saunders comprehensive review for the NCLEX-RN® Examination* (9th ed.). Elsevier.)

The original site where a cancerous tumor occurs is known as the *primary tumor*. It is identified by where the tumor began, such as breast or lung cancer. When primary tumors are located in vital organs such as the brain or lungs, they grow quickly and damage the organ so it cannot perform its necessary functions. *Metastasis* occurs when cancer cells move from the primary tumor location through hematologic or lymphatic spread and establish new tumors in other areas, such as the liver, bone, or brain.

## CAUSES OF CANCER

Cancer development takes years and depends on several tumor and patient factors. Three interacting factors influence cancer development: exposure to carcinogens, genetic predisposition, and immune function. Personal and environmental factors increase the risk for cancer development. Environmental factors, including exposure to carcinogens, are responsible for about 80% of cancer development. Environmental carcinogens can be:
- Chemicals (including those in tobacco)
- Physical agents (radiation and chronic irritation of tissues from inflammatory diseases)
- Certain viruses known as *oncoviruses* (human papilloma virus, Epstein-Barr virus (EBV), hepatitis B virus (HBV), and hepatitis C virus (HCV))

Personal factors, including immune function, age, and genetic risk, also affect a person's risk for cancer development. These factors interact with external factors to affect cancer risk. Cancer is more likely to occur in older people, those whose immune systems are not functioning at optimal levels, and those who have inherited a mutated suppressor gene that increases cancer risk.

## Table **17.1**   Characteristics of Normal and Cancer Cells

| CHARACTERISTIC | NORMAL CELLS | CANCER CELLS |
|---|---|---|
| Cell division | No or slow cell division to replace lost or damaged cells. | Cell division is rapid, and continuous. |
| Appearance | Normal human cells come in many shapes and sizes depending upon the cell and function. Normal cells have a larger amount of cytoplasm and smaller nucleus. | Cancer cells are irregular in shape and contain a smaller amount of cytoplasm and larger nucleus. |
| Differentiated functions | Normal cells perform many different functions. | Retains some normal function or has complete loss of function. |
| Cell adherence | Normal cells are tightly adhered to each other. | Cancer cells are loosely adherent and easily break off to spread through the blood and lymph systems. |
| Cell migration | With the exception of some blood cells (leukocytes, erythrocytes), normal cells are not migratory. | Cancer cells migrate through the basement cell membrane and invade other tissues and vital organs. |
| Cell Growth | Normal cell growth is well regulated. These cells respond to signals for cell death (apoptosis). | Cancer cell growth is unregulated, invasive, and does not respond to signals for cell death. |

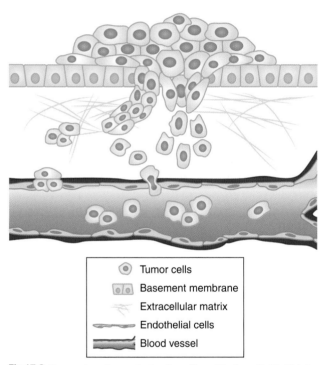

- Tumor cells
- Basement membrane
- Extracellular matrix
- Endothelial cells
- Blood vessel

Fig 17.2 Cancer invasion and migration. (From Novikov, N. M., Zolotaryova, S. F., Gautreau, A.M., & Denisov, E. V. (2021). Mutational drivers of cancer cell migration and invasion. *British Journal of Cancer, 124*(1), 102–114.)

 **Memory Jogger**

Aging is the most common and important risk factor for cancer. Exposure to carcinogens adds up over a lifetime, and immune protection decreases with age.

## CANCER TREATMENT APPROACHES

Cancer treatment options include surgery, radiation, traditional chemotherapy, hormone manipulation, and biologic or targeted agents. Some treatment approaches, such as surgery or radiation, treat the actual cancer cells in one body area. Traditional chemotherapy and hormonal therapy are systemic and are delivered throughout the body. Hormonal therapy slows or stops the growth of cancer that relies on certain hormones (such as estrogen) to grow. Hormone therapy is also called *hormonal therapy* or *endocrine therapy*.

 **Memory Jogger**

Common cancer therapies include these options:
- Surgery
- Radiation
- Traditional chemotherapy
- Hormone manipulation
- Biologic or targeted agents

The purpose of systemic therapies is to reach cancer cells that may have escaped from local tumors and spread (*metastasized*) to other areas but are too small to be seen using current imaging methods. Because systemic therapies are very widely distributed throughout the body, these drugs have more negative effects on normal tissues as compared to local treatments.

When given by intravenous (IV) line chemotherapy drugs can cause severe tissue damage if the IV access moves from the vein and leaks chemotherapy into the surrounding tissues, a process known as **extravasation**.

Typically, the therapies noted above are used in combination to kill cancer cells. Treatment regimens (known as *protocols*) have been established from clinical trials for most types of cancer.

 **Memory Jogger**

Surgery and radiation therapy are local treatments that are most effective for tumors and cancer cells confined to a limited, localized body area.

Traditional chemotherapy, hormone therapy, and biologics or targeted therapies are systemic therapies that can have a cancer-killing effect wherever cancer cells are present in the body.

## TRADITIONAL CHEMOTHERAPY

Traditional chemotherapy is the use of cytotoxic drugs to kill cancer cells. These killing effects are due to the ability of the drugs to damage cancer cell DNA and interfere with cell division. There are different categories of traditional chemotherapy drugs, each having different effects on cancer cell DNA for cytotoxic purposes, but the outcome is the same: limitation of cancer cell division leading to cancer cell death. Traditional chemotherapy drugs damage both normal cells and cancer cells. Normal cells that divide rapidly are most affected, including the skin, hair, cells of the gastrointestinal (GI) system, and blood-forming cells. Traditional chemotherapy drugs are classified by the types of action they exert in the cancer cell.

 **Memory Jogger**

All traditional chemotherapy drugs affect both normal cells and cancer cells.

Normal cells that rapidly divide (skin, hair, cells of the gastrointestinal [GI] system, and blood-forming cells) are most affected by systemic traditional chemotherapy.

### TRADITIONAL CHEMOTHERAPY DRUG TYPES

There are six categories of cancer chemotherapy drugs: alkylating agents, antimetabolites, antitumor antibiotics, topoisomerase inhibitors, and mitotic inhibitors (also known as *antimitotic agents*). Chemotherapy drugs can be cell-cycle specific (killing cancer cells only in a specific phase of the cell cycle) or cell-cycle nonspecific. Traditional chemotherapy is dosed based on the patient's body surface area (BSA) with an equation that takes the patient's height and weight into consideration. For this reason, drug dosages will be noted throughout this chapter only as appropriate.

There are many drug interactions with chemotherapy agents. Check with the pharmacist for any drug–drug interactions once a medication history is taken from the patient.

When patients receive chemotherapy, the absolute neutrophil count (ANC) is monitored closely as this test measures neutrophils, the most important infection fighting white blood cell. The ANC total white blood cell (WBC) X percent neutrophils/100. A healthy person has an ANC between 2,500 and 6,000.

All chemotherapy drugs are high-alert drugs that can cause serious harm if given at a dose that is too high or too low, if given to a patient for whom it was not prescribed, or if not given to a patient for whom it was prescribed. Only registered nurses who are chemotherapy certified may give traditional chemotherapy drugs.

 **Top Tip for Safety**

- Chemotherapy drugs are toxic to the patient and the nurse.
- Personal protective equipment (PPE: special gloves, eye protection, face shields, and gowns) are worn to protect healthcare providers when preparing and administering the drugs or when discontinuing or changing an IV after chemotherapy has been infused.
- Accurate dosing is critical, as dosing errors can have dire consequences.
- Although LPNs/VNs are not administering these drugs, it is a nursing responsibility to monitor the patient's IV for possible damaging infiltration and any adverse reactions during administration.

 **Memory Jogger**

The six major chemotherapy drug categories are:
- Alkylating agents
- Antimetabolites
- Antitumor antibiotics
- Topoisomerase inhibitors
- Mitotic inhibitors
- Miscellaneous agents

### ALKYLATING AGENTS

Alkylating agents were one of the first drugs to be used effectively in the treatment of cancer. Alkylating agents are cell-cycle nonspecific, as they work in all phases of the cell cycle.

#### Action

Alkylating agents work to prevent cancer cells from dividing by damaging its DNA. Alkylating agents make the two DNA strands stay bound tightly together, thereby preventing the DNA from separating into single strands and, by doing so, preventing cell division.

#### Uses

Alkylating agents are used to treat cancers of the lung, breast, and ovary as well as leukemia, lymphoma, Hodgkin disease, multiple myeloma, and sarcoma.

#### Expected Side Effects

Nausea and vomiting are frequent, common side effects of alkylating agents. Alopecia (hair loss) is also expected.

#### Adverse Reactions

There are several serious adverse effects that occur with alkylating agents, including bone marrow toxicity, particularly suppression of granulocytes and platelets, thereby increasing the risk for infection and bleeding. Gastrointestinal toxicities, including mucositis, stomatitis, esophagitis, and diarrhea, occur with high doses of alkylating agents. Pulmonary damage and pulmonary fibrosis are associated with almost all of the alkylating agents. Renal toxicity in the form of hemorrhagic cystitis can occur and is caused by the metabolites of these drugs, which are then excreted into the urine.

### Lifespan Considerations

**Childbearing Age**

Alkylating agents can be harmful to the developing fetus, causing birth defects.
Alkylating agents can cause gonadal damage in men, causing loss of active sperm.
Breast-feeding is contraindicated for patients taking alkylating agents.

### ❖ Nursing Implications and Patient Teaching

◆ *Assessment.* Understand the type of cancer the patient is being treated for. Review all chemotherapy drugs to be given for expected side effects and adverse effects that may occur during or after chemotherapy infusion (Table 17.2).

Routinely assess the patient's vital signs, especially for hypotension or fever. Assess the patient for symptoms of expected side effects or signs of allergic reactions such as flushing, swelling of the oral cavity or face, and itching or rash. Assess the patient's laboratory values for signs of low platelet or low granulocyte counts that can signal hematologic toxicity. Assess the IV infusion site continuously for pain, redness or swelling, which can indicate extravasation. Assess the patient's skin for bruising, petechiae, or ecchymosis related to low platelet counts. Assess the patient's urine for the presence of blood (hematuria). Assess for the presence of cough or shortness of breath.

*Planning and implementation.* Ensure that the patient receives adequate hydration through prescribed IV orders. Encourage oral fluid intake to prevent renal damage. Instruct the patient to take antiemetics as ordered to prevent nausea and vomiting. Report abnormal laboratory values to the supervising RN or the healthcare provider as appropriate. Report the presence of bruising, petechiae, or ecchymosis related to low platelet counts. Report the presence of frank bleeding in the urine to the supervising RN or healthcare provider. Report any signs or symptoms of allergic reaction immediately so emergency action can be taken. Report any signs of extravasation immediately to prevent tissue damage from infiltration of chemotherapy. Prepare for extravasation care per the institutional policy. Dispose of all IV equipment per institutional policy related to chemotherapy safety.

*Evaluation.* Evaluate the patient for expected side effects and any adverse effects. Monitor the patient's

| Table **17.2**   Alkylating Agents | |
|---|---|
| altretamine | ifosfamide |
| bendamustine | lomustine |
| busulfan | mechlorethamine |
| carboplatin | melphalan |
| carmustine | oxaliplatin |
| chlorambucil | temozolomide |
| cisplatin | thiotepa |
| cyclophosphamide | trabectedin |
| dacarbazine | |

laboratory reports and report abnormal findings or trends in hematologic or renal function tests. Following IV discontinuation, evaluate the area for signs of extravasation. Evaluate for the presence of nausea or vomiting. Evaluate the results of any patient and family teaching to ensure understanding of care following chemotherapy. Evaluate respiratory rate and breath sounds.

*Patient and family teaching.* Tell the patient and family:

- Avoid activities that can result in bruising or bleeding when platelet counts are low.
- Teach infection control measure such as frequent, thorough handwashing and avoidance of crowds or anyone who is sick.
- Take antiemetics as ordered around the clock. Waiting until the patient feels nauseated can result in vomiting, dehydration, and potentially, a visit to the urgent care or emergency room for IV antiemetics and fluids.
- Report unresolved nausea and vomiting that may occur despite antiemetic treatment.
- Teach the patient to eat small, frequent meals to avoid nausea.
- Teach the patient and family all side effects and adverse effects that can occur with their chemotherapy regimen, and when to call the oncology provider.
- Teach the patient to take their temperature several times a day when the white blood cell count may be at its lowest (known as the nadir) between 7-10 days following chemotherapy. A temperature of ≥37°C should be reported to the oncology provider.
- Drink plenty of fluids as alkylating agents can cause renal and bladder toxicity.
- Maintain good oral hygiene to prevent infection. Use mouthwashes that do not contain alcohol to avoid drying out the oral mucosa. Use a soft toothbrush to prevent bleeding of the gums.
- Teach patients and families to report the onset of shortness of breath or cough.

| Table **17.3** | Antimetabolites |
|---|---|
| azacitidine | gemcitabine |
| capecitabine | hydroxyurea |
| cladribine | 6-mercaptopurine |
| clofarabine | methotrexate |
| cytarabine | nelarabine |
| decitabine | pemetrexed |
| 5-fluorouracil | pentostatin |
| floxuridine | pralatrexate |
| fludarabine | thioguanine |

## ANTIMETABOLITES

Antimetabolites are considered cell-cycle-specific drugs as they exert their effect by interfering with DNA synthesis (Table 17.3).

### Action

The action of antimetabolite drugs is similar to the functions of normal metabolites needed for vital cell processes. Antimetabolite chemotherapy drugs act like "counterfeit" metabolites that fool cancer cells into using the antimetabolite in cellular reactions instead of the real metabolite. Because these drugs do not function as proper metabolites, their presence impairs cell division.

### Uses

Antimetabolites are commonly used to treat leukemias and cancers of the breast, ovary, head and neck, and GI system.

### Expected Side Effects

Common side effects of antimetabolites include nausea, vomiting, or loss of appetite, diarrhea, or constipation. Fatigue and headaches have also been reported. Patients can expect alopecia with antimetabolites.

### Adverse Reactions

Antimetabolites can result in liver damage (hepatotoxicity) and to bone marrow suppression leading to severe low blood cell counts, especially at higher doses. Severe GI effects such as stomatitis and diarrhea can also result. High doses of 5-fluorouracil can result in hemorrhagic colitis.

### Top Tip for Safety

For 48 hours after some antimetabolites are given, the patient's body fluids can contain the active drug. During this 48-hour period, nurses and caregivers should wear gloves when handling the patient's body fluids (vomitus, stool, urine, blood).

### ❖ Nursing Implications and Patient Teaching

◆ *Assessment.* Assess vital signs, especially temperature. Assess for symptoms of infection (fever, sore throat).

Check laboratory test results, especially liver function tests, complete blood count (CBC), and ANC. Assess the oral cavity for stomatitis and check the patient's ability to swallow, eat, and drink fluids. Assess the patient for diarrhea, as well as number and consistency of stools. Assess the patient for symptoms of dehydration. Assess for the presence of painful urination and hematuria.

◆ *Planning and implementation.* Monitor vital signs, especially temperature routinely according to institution policy. Report temperature of >37°F to the supervising RN or healthcare provider. Report abnormal liver function tests, CBC, and ANC results to the supervising RN or healthcare provider. Ensure the patient receives adequate hydration through prescribed IV orders and oral fluid intake to prevent renal damage. Instruct the patient to take antiemetics as ordered to prevent nausea and vomiting. Report the presence of painful urination or frank bleeding in the urine to the supervising RN or healthcare provider. Report diarrhea that does not resolve after 24 hours.

◆ *Evaluation.* Evaluate the patient for expected side effects and any adverse effects. Monitor the patient's laboratory reports and report abnormal findings or decreased trends in hematologic or renal function tests. Evaluate for the presence of nausea or vomiting. Evaluate the condition of the oral cavity and ability to swallow, eat, and drink fluids. Evaluate the results of any patient and family teaching to ensure understanding of care following chemotherapy.

###  Lifespan Considerations

**Pregnancy and Lactation**

Antimetabolites should not be used during pregnancy and breast-feeding because they are teratogens, meaning that they disrupt fetal development and can lead to birth defects.

◆ *Patient and family teaching.* Tell the patient and family:
- Limit alcohol intake to prevent liver damage.
- Avoid nonsteroidal anti-inflammatories (NSAIDs) as they can contribute to bleeding and other adverse renal effects.
- Teach patients to report temperature ≥ 98.6°F (37°C) immediately as this may signal febrile neutropenia.
- Teach infection control measures, including thorough handwashing.
- Teach the importance of oral hygiene measures including the use of alcohol-free mouthwash and soft toothbrushes.
- Take antiemetics as ordered around the clock.
- Report unresolved nausea and vomiting that may occur despite antiemetic treatment.
- Teach the patient to eat small, frequent meals to avoid nausea.

- Teach the patient and family all side effects and adverse effects that can occur with the chemotherapy regimen, and when to call the oncology provider.
- Drink plenty of fluids to avoid renal and bladder toxicity.

## ANTITUMOR ANTIBIOTICS

**Antitumor antibiotics** are cell-cycle nonspecific and act by binding with DNA to prevent the RNA (ribonucleic acid) synthesis that is needed to make critical proteins necessary for cell survival. There are two different subcategories of these agents: the anthracycline antibiotics and the nonanthracycline antibiotics.

Antitumor antibiotics are not like general antibiotics for infections. An important *adverse effect* (an undesired effect of a drug that can be serious) of the anthracycline antibiotics is potentially permanent damage to the cells of the heart muscle. Because of this adverse effect, there is a lifetime limit on how much of the anthracycline antitumor antibiotics any one person can receive. The nonanthracycline antitumor antibiotics do not have this lifetime dose limitation (Table 17.4).

### Action

Antitumor antibiotics block cell growth and spread by interfering with DNA, the genetic material in cells. Antitumor antibiotics are cell cycle non-specific, except for bleomycin, which acts in the G2 phase of the cell cycle.

### Uses

Antitumor antibiotics are used to treat many cancers. Doxorubicin is used in the treatment of sarcoma (tumors of the bones and fat or muscle tissue), breast cancer, ovarian cancer, lung cancer, Wilms tumor, and neuroblastoma. Daunorubicin is used for acute myeloid leukemia and acute lymphocytic leukemia, and idarubicin is indicated in the treatment of chronic myeloid leukemia. Epirubicin is used in the treatment of breast cancer and gastroesophageal cancer. Mitoxantrone is used for prostate cancer that fails to respond to hormone therapy.

### Expected Side Effects

Antitumor antibiotics are known to cause hair loss (alopecia), fatigue, nausea, and vomiting. Mouth sores, anemia, bruising, and bleeding can also occur.

### Adverse Reactions

Adverse reactions to antitumor antibiotics include heart failure due to heart muscle damage from anthracyclines. Bleomycin can result in severe irreversible lung damage, known as *pulmonary fibrosis*. Bone marrow suppression resulting in anemia and low platelet and white blood cell counts can lead to abnormal bleeding and high risk for infection.

Table 17.4   **Antitumor Antibiotics**

| ANTHRACYCLINE ANTIBIOTIC AGENTS | NONANTHRACYCLINE ANTIBIOTIC AGENTS |
|---|---|
| daunorubicin | bleomycin |
| doxorubicin | dactinomycin |
| epirubicin | mitomycin-C |
| idarubicin | mitoxantrone |
| valrubicin | |

❖ **Nursing Implications and Patient Teaching**

◆ *Assessment.* Ask the patient about a history of preexisting cardiac or lung disease that can increase their risk for pulmonary or cardiac toxicity from antitumor antibiotics. Assess vital signs, especially temperature. Ask the patient if symptoms of infection (fever, sore throat) are present. Check laboratory test results especially CBC and ANC. Assess the oral cavity for mouth sores and check the patient's ability to swallow, eat, and drink. Assess for signs of abnormal bleeding of the gums and the presence of petechiae or ecchymosis. Assess for difficulty breathing, rapid pulse or respiratory rate, dyspnea on exertion, rapid and unexplained weight gain, and edema that can signal pulmonary or cardiac complications. Assess the patient's pulse oximetry for abnormal oxygenation.

◆ *Planning and implementation.* Report the presence of abnormal cardiac or respiratory symptoms or low pulse oximetry findings to the supervising RN or healthcare provider. Monitor temperature and signs of infection routinely according to institution policy. Report temperature of ≥ 98.6°F (37°C) to the supervising RN or healthcare provider. Report abnormal CBC and ANC results to the supervising RN or healthcare provider. Instruct the patient to avoid crowds, or anyone who is ill in the 7- to 10-day period after chemotherapy, as this is when blood counts are expected to be lowest. Instruct the patient to take antiemetics as ordered to prevent nausea and vomiting. Report the presence of abnormal bleeding to the supervising RN or healthcare provider. Prepare the patient for hair loss that will occur by the second chemotherapy cycle. Assess the oral cavity for the presence of irritation or mouth sores that can occur 5 to 14 days after chemotherapy. Encourage good oral hygiene, as well as the use of prescribed mouthwashes or saliva substitutes as ordered. Instruct the patient to avoid any over-the-counter (OTC) mouthwashes that contain alcohol, which can dry and irritate the oral cavity.

◆ *Evaluation.* Evaluate the patient for expected side effects and any adverse effects. Monitor the patient's laboratory reports, and report abnormal findings or decreased trends in the CBC. Evaluate for the presence of nausea or vomiting despite antiemetic treatment.

Evaluate the condition of the oral cavity and ability to swallow, eat, and drink fluids. Evaluate the results of any patient and family teaching to ensure understanding of care following chemotherapy.

◆ *Patient and family teaching.*
- Instruct patients with long hair to cut their hair to a very short length prior to chemotherapy to lessen the disturbance of hair loss. Educate patient son choices of head coverings or wigs.
- Recommend a thorough dental care assessment before beginning chemotherapy to reduce the risk of mucositis.
- Instruct the patient in good oral hygiene practices to prevent mucositis.
- In accordance with institution policy: instruct the patient to swish ice chips in the mouth for 30 minutes at the time of chemotherapy infusion, sometimes referred to as "oral cryotherapy." This action may prevent or minimize mucositis.
- Teach the patient to take antiemetics around the clock as ordered after chemotherapy, even if nausea is not immediately present.
- Report unresolved nausea and vomiting that may occur despite antiemetic treatment.
- Teach the patient to eat small, frequent meals to avoid nausea.
- Teach the patient/family to report signs and symptoms of cardiac or pulmonary impairment immediately to the healthcare provider.
- Teach the patient to monitor temperature and to report a temperature of > 37°C.
- Teach the patient to use strict, frequent handwashing to minimize infection.

## TOPOISOMERASE INHIBITORS

Topoisomerase inhibitors inhibit are considered cell-cycle-specific drugs and are most active during the S and early G2 phases of the cell cycle. Topoisomerase inhibitors work by interfering with cell division and growth and DNA synthesis by disrupting the work of two different topoisomerase enzymes needed for these functions. Topoisomerase inhibitor drugs prevent the actions needed for maintaining DNA function, causing the DNA to break and leading to cell death.

The two subcategories of these drugs are based on which of the two types of topoisomerases they inhibit. Topoisomerase I inhibitors and topoisomerase II inhibitors. Both subcategories are derived from plants and are also known as *plant alkaloids* (Table 17.5).

### Action

Topoisomerase inhibitors can inhibit cell division and growth by preventing DNA replication, causing DNA damage, and preventing cells from going through the cell cycle. Topoisomerase inhibitors block the enzymes (topoisomerases) that break and reconnect DNA strands that are needed for cell division and growth.

### Uses

Topoisomerase inhibitors are used in the treatment of colorectal, lung, pancreatic, ovarian, breast, cervical, and hematological cancers.

### Expected Side Effects

Common side effects of topoisomerase inhibitors include alopecia, nausea, vomiting, fatigue, mouth sores, diarrhea, loss of appetite, and loss of taste sensation.

### Adverse Reactions

The most concerning adverse reactions of topoisomerase inhibitors include bone marrow suppression that results in low WBC, red blood cell, and low platelet counts, placing the patient at risk for infection and bleeding. Gastrointestinal issues such as severe diarrhea and nausea can also occur. Hypersensitivity (allergic) reactions have occurred during infusion. Impairment of the liver and kidney can also occur. Interstitial lung disease can develop and be fatal. Long-term survivors are at risk of cardiac toxicity and the development of other cancers, such as a secondary leukemia.

❖ **Nursing Implications and Patient Teaching**
◆ *Assessment.* Ask the patient about any history of severe allergic reactions, and report these to the healthcare provider. Assess vital signs, especially temperature for elevation. Ask the patient if symptoms of infection (fever, sore throat) are present. Check laboratory test results especially complete blood count (CBC) and ANC to determine if anemia, neutropenia, or thrombocytopenia are present. Assess for signs of abnormal bleeding. Assess results of kidney or liver function tests. Inspect the oral cavity for the presence of mouth sores. Check the patient's weight and skin turgor for signs of weight loss and dehydration. Ask the patient about the presence of nausea and diarrhea, and if present, the number and consistency of daily stools. Check respiratory rate and report the presence of shortness of breath or low oxygen saturation rate. Assess for complaints of hypersensitivity reactions during infusion such as itching, rash or swelling of the face or lips, or feelings of throat tightness.

◆ *Planning and implementation.* Immediately report any signs or symptoms of hypersensitivity reactions to the supervising RN or healthcare provider. Report

| Table **17.5** Topoisomerase Inhibitors | |
|---|---|
| **TOPOISOMERASE I INHIBITORS** | **TOPOISOMERASE II INHIBITORS** |
| irinotecan | etoposide |
| topotecan | mitoxantrone |
| | teniposide |

symptoms of difficulty breathing or shortness of breath and/or low pulse oximetry findings. Monitor temperature and signs of infection routinely according to institution policy. Report temperature of ≥ 98.6°F (37°C) to the supervising RN or healthcare provider. Instruct the patient to avoid crowds and anyone who is ill in the 7- to 10-day period after chemotherapy, as this is when blood counts are expected to be lowest. Report abnormal laboratory results to the supervising RN or healthcare provider. Instruct the patient to take antiemetics as ordered to prevent nausea and vomiting. Report the presence of abnormal bleeding to the supervising RN or healthcare provider. Prepare the patient for hair loss (alopecia) that will occur by the second chemotherapy cycle. Assess the oral cavity for the presence of irritation or mouth sores that can occur 5 to 14 days after chemotherapy. Encourage good oral hygiene, as well as use as ordered of prescribed mouthwashes or saliva substitutes. Instruct the patient to avoid any OTC mouthwashes that contain alcohol, which can dry and irritate the oral cavity.

◆ *Evaluation.* Determine if the chemotherapy infusion was tolerated without signs of hypersensitivity reaction. Evaluate the vital signs and laboratory reports for any abnormal findings. Evaluate the patient for expected side effects such as nausea, as well as for the effectiveness of antiemetics in controlling nausea. Evaluate the condition of the oral cavity and ability to swallow, eat, and drink fluids. Evaluate the skin, stools, urine, and oral cavity for signs of abnormal bleeding. Evaluate the results of any patient and family teaching to ensure understanding of care following chemotherapy.

◆ *Patient and family teaching.* Tell the patient and family:
- Report any signs/symptoms of hypersensitivity reactions during the chemotherapy infusion.
- Limit alcohol intake to prevent liver damage.
- Drink plenty of fluids to maintain hydration.
- Avoid NSAIDs as they can contribute to bleeding and adverse renal effects.
- Teach patients to report a temperature of ≥ 98.6°F (37°C) immediately as this may signal febrile neutropenia.
- Teach infection control measures, including thorough handwashing.
- Teach the importance of oral hygiene measures including the use of alcohol-free mouthwash and soft toothbrushes.
- Teach patients to report shortness of breath or difficulty breathing.
- Take antiemetics as ordered around the clock.
- Report unresolved nausea and vomiting that may occur despite antiemetic treatment.
- Teach the patient to eat small, frequent meals to avoid nausea.

- Instruct patients about hair loss and encourage patients to cut their hair short before chemotherapy begins.
- Instruct the patient about hair coverings and wigs as needed.
- Teach the patient and family all side effects and adverse effects that can occur with the chemotherapy regimen, and when to call the oncology provider.

## MITOTIC INHIBITORS

Mitotic inhibitors (also known as *antimitotic agents*) are cell-cycle-specific drugs and are considered a type of plant alkaloid that acts on the cell's *microtubules*. Microtubules are the hollow tubelike structures found in the cytoplasm (the fluid inside a cell). Microtubules help support the shape of a cell. They also help chromosomes move during cell division. There are two different subcategories of antimitotic agents, the *taxanes* and the *vinca alkaloids*. These drugs are somewhat different from other traditional chemotherapy drugs and cause peripheral nerve damage, known as *peripheral neuropathy*, that may be permanent (Table 17.6).

### Actions
Mitotic inhibitors interfere with the formation of the microtubules so cells cannot separate during cell division, and thereby cell division is prevented. They also cause cellular damage throughout the cell cycle, so the proteins needed for cell division are not produced.

### Uses
Mitotic inhibitors are used in the treatment of cancers of the breast, lung, and ovary, as well as lymphoma and leukemia.

### Expected Side Effects
Common side effects of mitotic inhibitors include nausea and vomiting, joint pain or stiffness, and skin reactions such as flushing and rashes.

### Adverse Reactions
Severe peripheral neuropathy (numbness, tingling, difficulty with walking and balance) are common with mitotic inhibitors and develop in the lower and upper extremities. Cardiovascular effects include slow heart rate (bradycardia). Bone marrow suppression can also be severe, predisposing patients to neutropenia, anemia, and low platelet counts (thrombocytopenia). Severe constipation can also occur due to autonomic

| Table **17.6** Antimitotic Agents | |
|---|---|
| **TAXANES** | **VINCA ALKALOIDS** |
| cabazitaxel | vinblastine |
| docetaxel | vincristine |
| Paclitaxel | vinorelbine |

neuropathy. Hearing loss from neuropathy involving the cranial nerves can also occur.

### ❖ Nursing Implications and Patient Teaching

◆ *Assessment.* Ask the patient about expected side effects such as nausea and vomiting, joint pain or stiffness, and any facial flushing or rashes. Check laboratory test results, especially liver and kidney function tests, CBC and ANC to determine if anemia, neutropenia, or thrombocytopenia are present. Assess for signs of abnormal bleeding. Assess vital signs, especially temperature, for infection and heart rate to assess for bradycardia. Assess for symptoms of infection (fever, sore throat). Ask the patient about the presence of nausea unrelieved by antiemetics.

Assess the ability of the patient to walk, and balance. Ask the patient about symptoms of numbness, tingling, pain, and loss of sensation in the feet and hands. Ask the patient about daily stools and assess for the presence of constipation. Ask the patient about hearing loss, and report to the healthcare provider for possible referral for a hearing specialist.

---

### 🔹 Top Tip for Safety

Children and adults with a hereditary neuropathy known as *Charcot–Marie–Tooth disease* are more predisposed to peripheral neuropathy from vincristine.

Ask patients and family about any hereditary forms of neuropathy that may be present before chemotherapy is planned.

---

◆ *Planning and implementation.* Report symptoms of severe fatigue, shortness of breath, dizziness, or activity intolerance that may signal low heart rate (bradycardia). Monitor temperature and signs of infection routinely. Report temperature of ≥ 98.6°F (37°C) to the supervising RN or healthcare provider. Instruct the patient to avoid crowds and anyone who is ill in the 7- to 10-day period after chemotherapy as this is when blood counts are expected to be lowest. Report abnormal laboratory results to the supervising RN or healthcare provider. Instruct the patient to take antiemetics as ordered to prevent nausea and vomiting and to report any unresolved nausea. Report the presence of abnormal bleeding to the supervising RN or healthcare provider. Report symptoms of peripheral neuropathy to the RN or healthcare provider for potential workup or referral. Report the presence of constipation as stool softeners or laxatives may be needed. Report any symptoms of hearing loss or tinnitus for possible evaluation and referral.

◆ *Evaluation.* Evaluate the patient for signs and symptoms of hypersensitivity during infusion. Evaluate the ability of the patient to walk with normal gait and balance. Evaluate the patient for expected side effects such as nausea, as well as the effectiveness of antiemetics for controlling nausea.

Evaluate vital signs, especially temperature and heart rate, and laboratory reports for any abnormal findings. Evaluate the patient's skin, mucous membranes, stools, and urine for signs of abnormal bleeding. Evaluate the bowel pattern for constipation. Evaluate the patient for self-report of hearing loss. Evaluate the results of any patient and family teaching to ensure understanding of care following chemotherapy.

---

### 🔹 Lifespan Considerations

**Children**

Younger children may be at greater risk of peripheral neuropathy from vincristine, due to the immaturity of the peripheral nervous system.

---

◆ *Patient and family teaching.* Tell the patient and family:

- Teach the patient and family to report signs and symptoms of potential hypersensitivity reaction during infusion.
- Teach the patient to report any difficulty walking or maintaining balance.
- Teach infection control measure such as frequent, thorough handwashing and avoidance of crowds or anyone who is sick. Maintain good oral hygiene to prevent infection.
- Teach the patient to take their temperature several times a day when the white blood cell count may be at its lowest (known as the nadir) between 7 to 10 days following chemotherapy. A temperature of ≥ 98.6°F (37°C) should be reported to the oncology provider.
- Take antiemetics as ordered around the clock. Waiting until the patient feels nauseated can result in vomiting, dehydration, and potentially, a visit to the urgent care or emergency room for IV antiemetics and fluids.
- Teach the patient to eat small, frequent meals to avoid nausea.
- Report unresolved nausea and vomiting that may occur despite antiemetic treatment.
- Teach the patient and family measures to prevent constipation. Eat high fiber foods, drink plenty of water, and use stool softeners and laxatives as needed.
- Avoid activities that can result in bruising or bleeding when platelet counts are low.
- Teach the patient to report signs of abnormal bleeding to the healthcare provider.
- Teach the patient to report symptoms of tinnitus or hearing loss.
- Teach the patient and family all side effects and adverse effects that can occur with their chemotherapy regimen, and when to call the oncology provider.

## COMBINATION CHEMOTHERAPY

Chemotherapy treatment for cancer typically involves *combination chemotherapy*. Combination chemotherapy refers to the combining of two or more chemotherapy drugs that are given at a specified time schedule, such as every 3 weeks. Using a combination of chemotherapy drugs that are cell-cycle specific and cell-cycle nonspecific kills cancer cells throughout the cell cycle. However, the side effects and damage caused to normal tissues also increase with combination chemotherapy.

 **Memory Jogger**

Combination chemotherapy uses a combination of chemotherapy drugs to kill cancer cells throughout the cell cycle.

## HORMONE THERAPY FOR CANCER TREATMENT

Some hormones make hormone-sensitive cancers grow and divide more rapidly (e.g., prostate cancer, breast cancer). So, decreasing the amounts of hormones to hormone-sensitive tumors can slow cancer growth for many years. Hormone therapy does not typically lead to a cure. For example, prostate cancer is a hormone-sensitive cancer that grows faster when the hormone testosterone binds to the testosterone receptors, preventing the patient's testosterone from binding to those sites. The blocking of testosterone slows the growth of prostate cancer increasing survival time.

### HORMONE THERAPY FOR BREAST CANCER

Estrogen is the hormone that increases the growth of some breast cancers. For breast cancer cells to be sensitive to estrogen, they must express significant numbers of estrogen receptors (ERs). Such tumors are termed *ER positive* (ER+). Hormone therapy involves either reducing the amount of estrogen present or preventing existing estrogen from binding to cancer cell estrogen receptors. The drug categories used for hormone manipulation of breast cancer cells are *aromatase inhibitors (AIs)*, *selective estrogen receptor modulators (SERMs)*, *estrogen receptor antagonists (ERAs)*, and *luteinizing hormone-releasing hormone (LHRH) agonists*. The duration of therapy is long term, usually for at least 5 years or until disease progression occurs (Table 17.7).

*Aromatase inhibitors (AIs)* work by inhibiting the enzyme aromatase that works to convert androgens into estrogens that continue to promote breast cancer cell growth. The aromatase inhibitors (AIs) prevent this conversion and reduce the amounts of estrogens in the blood.

*Selective estrogen receptor modulators (SERMs)* are drugs that block the estrogen receptors on breast cancer cells. This action interferes with breast cancer growth.

*Estrogen receptor antagonists* bind as tightly to estrogen receptors, and by doing so, it blocks estrogen from binding to the receptor and reduces the growth-promoting effects of estrogen on breast cancer cells.

*Luteinizing hormone releasing hormone (LHRH) agonists* are synthetic gonadotrophin-releasing hormones (GnRHs) that increases the production and release of follicle-stimulating hormone (FSH), which over the course of 4 weeks causes ovarian shrinkage with decreased estrogen production, especially in premenopausal women.

 **Memory Jogger**

Hormone therapy for breast cancer works by reducing the availability of estrogen to breast cancer cells, which inhibits or slows their growth.

**Table 17.7**   **Hormone Therapy for Breast Cancer**

| DRUG CATEGORY | DRUG NAME | USUAL DOSE |
|---|---|---|
| Aromatase inhibitors (AIs) | anastrozole (Arimidex) | 1 mg orally daily |
| | exemestane (Aromasin) | 25 mg orally once daily |
| | letrozole (Femara) | 2.5 mg orally once daily |
| Selective estrogen receptor modulators (SERMs) | tamoxifen (Nolvadex, Soltamox) | 20–40 mg orally once daily |
| | raloxifene (Evista) | 60 mg orally once daily |
| Estrogen receptor antagonists | fulvestrant (Faslodex) | Initially: two 250 mg intramuscular (IM) injections (one in each buttock) on days 1, 15, 29<br>Maintenance: Same dose once monthly |
| | toremifene (Fareston) | 60 mg orally once daily |
| Luteinizing hormone-releasing hormone (LHRH) agonists | goserelin (Zoladex) | 3.6 mg subcutaneously into the abdomen below the navel line every 28 days |
| | leuprolide (Fensolvi, Lupron, Viadur) | 11.25 mg subcutaneous once every 3 months for 2 years |
| | triptorelin (Trelstar, Triptodur) | 3.75 mg IM once monthly |

## Common Side Effects of Hormone Therapy for Breast Cancer

All hormone therapy drugs for breast cancer cause a return of perimenopausal symptoms that include vaginal dryness and hot flashes. For women who have not yet undergone menopause, menses become irregular and heavy. Other common side effects of AIs include bone, muscle, and joint pain.

Other hormone levels and have unique side effects. Breast atrophy is common, as are the *estrogen receptor antagonists* often induce headaches and nausea. These drugs are administered by IM injection, and injection side reactions are common.

*LHRH agonists* affect gastrointestinal problems of abdominal pain, flatulence, and diarrhea. Patients also report increased emotional ups and downs and more depression.

> **Memory Jogger**
>
> The most common side effects of all drugs for hormone therapy for breast cancer are hot flashes, vaginal dryness, and menstrual cycle irregularities with heavier menses.

## Adverse Effects of Hormone Therapy for Breast Cancer

All of the drugs used for hormone therapy with breast cancer can increase serum cholesterol levels, cause fluid retention with peripheral edema, increase blood pressure, and increase the risk for blood clots that can cause stroke and heart attack. They also are associated with a risk for elevated liver enzymes.

Specific additional possible adverse effects of *aromatase inhibitors* include the development of osteoporosis with bone fractures. Specific additional possible

adverse effects of *SERMs* include an increased risk for endometrial cancer and for cataract development.

Specific additional possible adverse effects of *LHRH agonists* include hyperglycemia and an uncommon but serious increase in the risk for seizures.

## HORMONE THERAPY FOR PROSTATE CANCER

Prostate cancer cells have receptors for and are sensitive to the presence of androgens, especially testosterone. Although prostate cancer cells are often slow growing, their growth rate is increased when androgen receptors are bound with testosterone. As a result of this sensitivity, drugs that suppress androgen production or function are used to slow the growth of prostate cancer cells. These drug categories include *androgen receptor antagonists*, *luteinizing hormone releasing hormone (LHRH) agonists*, and *luteinizing hormone releasing hormone (LHRH) antagonists* (Table 17.8).

*Androgen receptor antagonists* bind tightly to androgen receptors, preventing androgens from binding to and increasing the growth of prostate cancer cells.

*Luteinizing hormone releasing hormone (LHRH) agonists* are synthetic gonadotrophin-releasing hormones (GnRHs). In men, within 2 to 4 weeks of daily dosing, FSH and LH levels decrease causing blood testosterone levels to fall.

*Luteinizing hormone releasing hormone (LHRH) antagonists* bind tightly to GrRH receptors on the anterior pituitary gland. As a result, production of both FSH and LH is reduced or completely inhibited.

## Common Side Effects and Possible Adverse Effects of Hormone Therapy for Prostate Cancer

All hormone therapy for prostate cancer results in symptoms related to reduced testosterone levels or functions. These include the enlargement of breast tissue in males

### Table 17.8   Hormone Therapy for Prostate Cancer

| DRUG CATEGORY | DRUG NAME | USUAL MAINTENANCE DOSAGES |
|---|---|---|
| Androgen receptor antagonists | apalutamide (Erleada) | 200 mg orally once daily |
| | bicalutamide (Casodex) | 50 mg orally once daily |
| | darolutamide (Nubeqa) | 600 mg orally twice daily with food |
| | enzalutamide (Xtandi) | 160 mg orally once daily |
| | flutamide (Eulexin) | 250 mg orally every 8 hours |
| | nilutamide (Nilandron) | 150–300 mg orally once daily |
| Luteinizing hormone-releasing hormone (LHRH) agonists | goserelin (Zoladex) | 3.6 mg subcutaneously into the abdomen below the navel line every 28 days |
| | leuprolide (Lupron, Eligard) | 1 mg subcutaneously once daily |
| | triptorelin (Camcevi) | 3.75 mg IM once every 4 weeks into the buttocks |
| Luteinizing hormone-releasing hormone (LHRH) antagonists | degarelix (Firmagon) | Initially: two separate 120 mg subcutaneous injections once, followed by 80 mg subcutaneously every 28 days |
| | relugolix (Orgovyx) | First dose of 360 mg orally, followed by 120 mg orally once daily |

*known as (gynecomastia)*, reduced sexual desire or sexual dysfunction, and some degree of testicular atrophy. Other common hormone-related changes include hot flashes, fluid retention, and peripheral edema. Additional common side effects include fatigue and general body aches.

 **Memory Jogger**

Reduced androgen influence of hormone therapy for prostate cancer causes feminizing responses. Facial hair thins, breast tissue enlarges, facial skin becomes smoother, and body fat redistributes. Testicular and penile size decrease. Although sexual function may continue, achieving an erection is more difficult.

All classes of these drugs are associated with possible adverse effects: elevated liver enzymes and an increased risk for liver impairment, hypertension, osteoporosis with increased risk for bone fractures, and increased risk for blood clots, including heart attack and stroke. Those drugs that are given by injection often have injection site reactions, especially for those given intramuscularly. Additional side effects and adverse effects for androgen receptor antagonists include hyperglycemia and a very rare possibility of triggering seizure activity. The LHRH agonists have a slightly increased risk for triggering seizure activity or pituitary infarction.

# GET READY FOR THE NCLEX® EXAMINATION!

## Key Points

- Cancer cells were once normal cells that through DNA damage, lost the strict control over normal growth and function.
- Older age is the most common and important risk factor for cancer. Exposure to carcinogens increases over a lifetime, and immune function decreases with age.
- Traditional chemotherapy and hormone therapy are systemic therapies that are effective anywhere in the body where cancer is present.
- All chemotherapy drugs are high-alert drugs that can cause serious harm if given at a dose that is too high or too low, if given to a patient for whom it was not prescribed, or if not given to a patient for whom it was prescribed.
- Combination chemotherapy uses multiple drugs from different traditional chemotherapy categories to kill cancer cells in all phases of the cell cycle.
- Schedules for chemotherapy administration are timed to maximize the number of cancer cells killed, as well as to minimize damage to normal cells.
- The normal cells most affected by these drugs are those that divide rapidly, including skin, hair, cells of the gastrointestinal (GI) system, sperm, and blood-forming cells.
- Administration of chemotherapy must be performed only by chemotherapy-certified registered nurses. Monitoring the patient during chemotherapy administration is a responsibility of all LPN/VNs and registered nurses.
- Chemotherapy drugs are dangerous and can be absorbed through skin and mucous membranes of anyone who comes into contact with the drugs, always use PPE when mixing, handling, and giving these drugs and when handling the wastes and excretions of patients receiving them.
- Oral anticancer drugs are just as toxic to the person taking the drug and the person handling the drug as are traditional IV chemotherapy drugs. Nurses need to be

knowledgeable about handling precautions for these oral agents and ensure patients also are aware of them.
- Monitor the access site of any infusing chemotherapy at least every 30 minutes to prevent extravasation or limit damage by preventing leakage of larger volumes.
- Compare all patient assessment findings after chemotherapy with those obtained before administration. Report abnormal findings.
- Bone marrow suppression can result in febrile neutropenia and can be life threatening.
- Hormone therapy can help control the growth of hormone-sensitive cancers if those cancers express the receptor for the hormone.
- All of the drugs used for hormone therapy with breast cancer and prostate cancer can increase serum cholesterol levels, cause fluid retention with peripheral edema and increased blood pressure, and increase the risk for blood clots that result in stroke and heart attack.
- Men taking hormone therapy for prostate cancer usually develop the feminizing side effects of gynecomastia, thinning facial hair, and decreased libido because of either lower circulating levels of androgens (especially testosterone) or reduced function of androgens.

## Clinical Judgment and Next-Generation NCLEX® Examination-Style Questions

1. **Which statements are true concerning traditional chemotherapy? Select all or any that apply.**
   1. Chemotherapy affects only cancer cells.
   2. Chemotherapy mostly affects fast-growing normal cells.
   3. Chemotherapy is considered a local treatment for cancer.
   4. Chemotherapy drugs are toxic to the patient and the nurse.
   5. All chemotherapy drugs are high-alert drugs.
   6. Combination chemotherapy uses multiple drugs from different traditional chemotherapy.

2. Which precaution is **most important** for the nurse to teach a patient who received traditional chemotherapy 1 week ago?

   1. Avoiding crowds and people who are ill
   2. Using a soft-bristled toothbrush and not flossing
   3. Taking several naps or rest periods during the day
   4. Wearing a hat, protective clothing, and using sunscreen when outdoors

3. A patient is starting chemotherapy with the alkylating agent cyclophosphamide. The chemotherapy infusion is now in process.

   Use an X for the nursing action below that is <u>Indicated</u> (appropriate or necessary), <u>Contraindicated</u> (could be harmful), or is <u>Nonessential</u> (makes no difference or is not necessary) for the client's care with regard to administering this drug.

| NURSING ACTION | INDICATED | CONTRA-INDICATED | NON-ESSENTIAL |
|---|---|---|---|
| Check the patient for signs of hypersensitivity reaction. | | | |
| Explain to the patient that a fluid restriction is needed for patients taking this drug. | | | |
| Provide small snacks throughout the infusion period. | | | |
| Check the patient's vital signs before, during, and after the infusion. | | | |

| NURSING ACTION | INDICATED | CONTRA-INDICATED | NON-ESSENTIAL |
|---|---|---|---|
| Assess the patient's IV site. | | | |
| Instruct the patient to take antiemetics as soon as nausea begins. | | | |
| Teach the patient that the urine color will be dark pink or red after the infusion. | | | |

4. Which assessments should the nurse to perform with a patient who has received an antimitotic agent as chemotherapy? **Select all or any that apply.**

   1. 24-hour fluid intake and urine output
   2. Rate, rhythm, and quality of the pulse
   3. Color of the skin and sclera
   4. Rate, depth, and ease of respiration
   5. Complete blood count
   6. Sensation in the hands and feet

5. A 67-year-old patient with breast cancer taking an aromatase inhibitor tells the nurse that she now has hot flashes and night sweats again, years after her menopause. What is the nurse's best action?

   1. Documenting the patient's symptoms as the only action
   2. Asking the patient whether she has been taking the drug daily as prescribed
   3. Reassuring the patient that this is an expected and normal response to the therapy
   4. Instructing the patient to stop taking the drug immediately and notifying the prescriber

# Drugs for Reproductive Health

## Learning Outcomes

1. Explain the role of the reproductive system in general health and reproductive problems.
2. List the names, actions, possible side effects, and adverse effects of drugs for female reproductive problems.
3. Explain what to teach patients and families about drugs for female reproductive problems.
4. List the names, actions, possible side effects, and adverse effects of drugs for male reproductive problems.
5. Explain what to teach patients and families about drugs for male reproductive problems.

## Key Terms

**anabolic steroids** Synthetic drugs with the same use and actions as androgens.

**androgens** Synthetic or natural hormones that help to develop and maintain the male sex organs at puberty and develop secondary sex characteristics in men (e.g., facial hair, deep voice, body hair, body fat distribution, muscle development).

**estrogen** A hormone made by the body that helps develop and maintain female sex characteristics and the development and regulation of the female reproductive system.

**hormonal contraception** The use of hormones to suppress ovulation for the intentional prevention of pregnancy.

**hormone** A protein secreted by an endocrine gland that changes the action of another gland or tissue, known as its *target tissue*.

**hormone replacement therapy (HRT)** Temporary or permanent therapy with drugs that perform the function of natural endocrine hormones.

**menstruation** The regular discharge of blood and mucosal tissue from the inner lining of the uterus through the vagina. The menstrual cycle is triggered by falling progesterone levels and is a sign that pregnancy has not occurred.

**testosterone** A hormone made mainly in the testes (part of the male reproductive system). It is needed to develop and maintain male sex characteristics, such as facial hair, deep voice, and muscle growth.

## FEMALE SEX HORMONES

### OVERVIEW

**Hormones** secreted throughout a woman's menstruating years promote conception and pregnancy. The beginning of **menstruation**, also called *menarche*, occurs during adolescence. Menstruation depends on secretion of *gonadotropin-releasing hormone* (GnRH) in the brain, which begins at the start of puberty in females and males. GnRH initiates sex hormone secretion and starts the physical changes leading to interest in sexual activity (libido) and the ability to perform sexual intercourse. Shedding of the uterine lining occurs during menstruation and results from changes in hormone levels in females during their menstrual cycles. **Estrogen** is the main female sex hormone secreted by the ovaries and adrenal glands.

Secretion of GnRH from the hypothalamus in females stimulates the release of two hormones from the pituitary gland: *follicle-stimulating hormone* (FSH) and *luteinizing hormone* (LH) (Fig. 18.1). FSH triggers the

ovary to make and secrete estrogen and to bring one ovum (egg) to maturity each month. Rising estrogen levels allow the uterine lining to grow and thicken (see Fig. 18.1). After about 14 days (midcycle), the uterine lining is thick enough to allow a fertilized egg to implant. GnRH then triggers the release of LH, which causes secretion of progesterone by the ovary and allows the release of the mature ovum or egg *(ovulation)*.

When the ovulated egg is fertilized by a sperm, the egg's outer covering grows and secretes estrogen and progesterone. These two hormones keep the uterine lining intact and are able to support a pregnancy until the placenta forms and maintains the pregnancy. Therefore functional pregnancy resulting in birth requires conception, continued secretion of estrogen and progesterone, successful implantation 5 to 8 days after conception, and placental development.

If conception and pregnancy do not occur after ovulation, the outer covering from the released ovum degenerates, and circulating levels of estrogen and progesterone decline in about 12 days. Low levels of these hormones cause the uterine lining to shed as menstruation. Fig. 18.2 shows the feedback loops controlling the secretion of estrogen and progesterone.

## MENOPAUSE

*Menopause* is the period in a woman's life when menstruation and ovulation no longer occur. This happens because of age-related changes that make the ovary stop functioning. Estrogen secretion and ovulation stop. *Perimenopause* is defined as the transition from having regular menstrual periods based on hormone cycles to having no menstrual periods for at least a full year as a result of reduced hormone levels. The reduction in hormone levels causes a variety of uncomfortable symptoms.

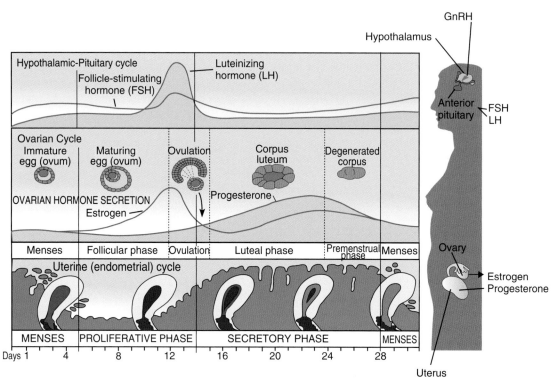

Fig. 18.1 Hormone interactions for ovulation and menstruation. *GnRH,* gonadotropin-releasing hormone. (From Workman, M. L., & LaCharity, L. A. (2016). *Understanding pharmacology: Essentials for Medication Safety* (2nd ed.). Elsevier.)

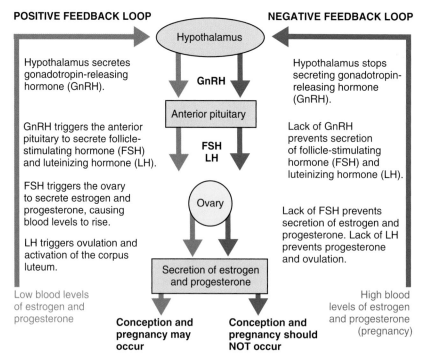

Fig. 18.2 Positive and negative feedback control over estrogen and progesterone secretion. (From Workman, M. L., & LaCharity, L. A. (2016). *Understanding pharmacology: Essentials for Medication Safety* (2nd ed.). Elsevier.)

As a result of negative feedback, decreased blood levels of estrogen trigger the brain to secrete GnRH, which then forces the pituitary gland to oversecrete FSH (see Fig. 18.2). However, the FSH no longer has an effect on the ovary because its cells are no longer functional, and blood levels of estrogen remain low. Continuing low blood estrogen levels constantly stimulate the brain to secrete GnRH in large amounts for a time, resulting in the secretion of even more FSH (Fig. 18.3). This extra FSH does not have any effect on the ovary but does cause responses in other body tissues. Box 18.1 lists the symptoms associated with decreased estrogen levels and increased FSH levels.

> ### Memory Jogger
> - Symptoms of menopause are caused by low levels of estrogen and high levels of FSH.
> - Hot flashes with facial redness and feelings of overheating are caused by high levels of FSH acting on blood vessels to make them dilate suddenly.
> - At night, hot flashes may be followed by excessive sweating that leaves nightclothes and bedding wet.

## DRUGS FOR MENOPAUSE RELIEF

### Action and Uses

Menopausal **hormone replacement therapy (HRT)** during the perimenopausal period consists of replacement of naturally secreted estrogen and progesterone with hormones given in the form of a drug. When a woman is given low doses of estrogen, blood estrogen levels are mildly increased, reducing perimenopausal symptoms (see Box 18.1) and suppressing the feedback system to lower the FSH levels. This action reduces hot flashes, night sweats, and difficulty sleeping.

Table 18.1 lists the names, dosages, and nursing implications for common drugs used for relief of menopausal symptoms. Consult a drug handbook or drug reference source for information about additional drugs for relief of menopausal symptoms.

### Expected Side Effects

The most common side effects of perimenopausal HRT are breast tenderness, breakthrough bleeding, fluid retention, weight gain, and acne. These occur with estrogen alone and when estrogen is combined with progesterone.

| Box 18.1 | Symptoms Associated with the Low Estrogen Levels and High Follicle-Stimulating Hormone Levels of Menopause |
|---|---|
| Symptoms caused by reduced estrogen levels:<br>• Irregular and absent menses<br>• Dry skin and vaginal mucous membranes<br>• Painful intercourse<br>• Increased rate of osteoporosis | Symptoms caused by increased follicle-stimulating hormone levels:<br>• Hot flashes<br>• Night sweats<br>• Sleep difficulty<br>• Difficulty concentrating on cognitive tasks |

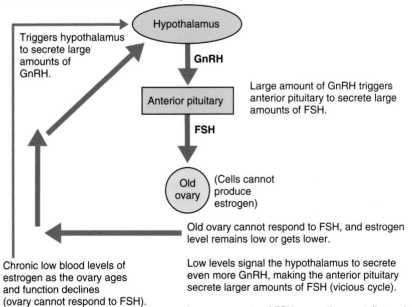

**Positive but ineffective feedback loop**

Triggers hypothalamus to secrete large amounts of GnRH.

Hypothalamus

GnRH

Large amount of GnRH triggers anterior pituitary to secrete large amounts of FSH.

Anterior pituitary

FSH

Old ovary (Cells cannot produce estrogen)

Old ovary cannot respond to FSH, and estrogen level remains low or gets lower.

Chronic low blood levels of estrogen as the ovary ages and function declines (ovary cannot respond to FSH).

Low levels signal the hypothalamus to secrete even more GnRH, making the anterior pituitary secrete larger amounts of FSH (vicious cycle).

Larger amounts of FSH cause the most distressing effects of menopause.

Fig. 18.3 Mechanism for hot flashes and night sweats associated with menopause. *FSH*, follicle-stimulating hormone; *GnRH*, gonadotropin-releasing hormone. (From Workman, M. L., & LaCharity, L. A. (2016). *Understanding pharmacology: Essentials for Medication Safety* (2nd ed.). Elsevier.)

| Table 18.1   Examples of Common Drugs for Relief of Menopausal Symptoms | |
|---|---|
| *Conjugated female sex hormones* reduce menopausal symptoms by providing enough estrogen or estrogen plus progesterone to disrupt the feedback loop and lower follicle-stimulating hormone levels. | |
| **DRUG/ADULT DOSAGE** | **NURSING IMPLICATIONS** |
| **Conjugated Female Sex Hormones** | |
| Conjugated estrogens (Cenestin, C.E.S. ♣, Enjuvia, Premarin) 0.3, 0.45, or 0.625 mg orally once daily, given cyclically or continuously, alone in women without a uterus or in combination with a progestin in women with a uterus<br>Conjugated estrogens plus progestin:<br>medroxyprogesterone (Premphase) 0.625 mg conjugated estrogens orally once daily on days 1–14, then one light blue tablet (0.625 mg conjugated estrogens plus 5 mg medroxyprogesterone acetate) orally once daily on days 15–28<br>medroxyprogesterone (Prempro) 0.3 or 0.45 mg conjugated estrogens along with medroxyprogesterone acetate 1.5 mg/day, *or* 0.625 mg conjugated estrogens along with medroxyprogesterone acetate 2.5 mg and then 0.625 mg along with 5 mg medroxyprogesterone acetate | • Teach the patient to take drugs for perimenopausal HRT exactly as prescribed to reduce the risk of excessive uterine bleeding.<br>• Advise the patient to quit or reduce smoking to reduce the risk of blood clots, heart attacks, and strokes.<br>• Teach the patient to assess the color of the roof of the mouth and the sclerae of the eyes weekly for jaundice.<br>• Instruct the patient to call 911 immediately for chest pain, difficulty breathing, swelling in one leg, or symptoms of stroke.<br>• Teach the patient that taking HRT for long periods increases the risk of cancers of the cervix, breast, ovary, and uterus. |

*HRT,* hormone replacement therapy.

## Adverse Effects

Women who are taking estrogen-based HRT have a slightly higher incidence of myocardial infarction (heart attack). For this reason, perimenopausal HRT is not recommended for long-term therapy.

Estrogen and progesterone drugs increase the risks of blood clotting and inappropriate development of thrombi and emboli. These risks increase with age and are greatly increased with cigarette smoking. Potential health problems associated with increased clot formation include heart attack, stroke, pulmonary embolism, and deep vein thrombosis.

The uterine lining in women who have a uterus and take perimenopausal HRT can become very thick and bleed excessively. Perimenopausal HRT promotes the growth of hormone-sensitive cancers of the cervix, uterus, ovary, and breast, and these hormones should not be used by women who have a history of or are at high risk for these types of cancer. Perimenopausal HRT also is associated with liver impairment, gallbladder disease, and pancreatitis.

❖ **Nursing Implications and Patient Teaching**
◆ *Patient and family teaching.* Tell the patient and family:
• Take drugs for perimenopausal HRT exactly as prescribed with regard to dosage and timing. Taking perimenopausal HRT drugs more often than prescribed or not following instructions for timing increases the risk for excessive uterine bleeding.
• Quit or reduce smoking while you are taking these drugs to reduce your risk for blood clots, heart attacks, and strokes.
• Check the color of the roof of your mouth and the whites of your eyes weekly for a yellow tinge because these drugs can impair the liver. If you see

yellowing, report it to your healthcare provider as soon as possible.
• Go to the emergency department or call 911 immediately if you have chest pain or difficulty breathing, swelling in one leg, or symptoms of stroke.
• Taking HRT for long periods increases the risk of cancers of the cervix, breast, ovary, and uterus. Discuss the optimal length of time for taking these drugs with your healthcare provider.

## DRUGS FOR HORMONAL CONTRACEPTION

Hormonal contraception is the use of hormones to suppress ovulation for the intentional prevention of pregnancy. When used correctly, hormonal contraception is highly effective. These hormones can be taken orally; used as topical applications in the form of transdermal patches, vaginal rings, or intrauterine devices; implanted under the skin; or injected parenterally as a slow-absorbing drug form (Table 18.2). *Oral contraceptives* (OCs; often called *birth control pills* or *BCPs*) are the most commonly used form of hormonal contraceptive. The mechanism of action and side effects of hormonal contraception are the same for all forms.

## Action and Uses

Natural secretion of estrogen and progesterone is controlled through an endocrine feedback system involving the hypothalamus, the pituitary gland, and the ovary (see Fig. 18.2). In a manner similar to perimenopausal HRT, OCs provide enough estrogen and/or progesterone to signal the hypothalamus that further secretion of these hormones is not needed. Just as in pregnancy, GnRH, FSH, and LH secretion are stopped, and the ovary has no stimulation to produce estrogen

Table 18.2 Common Hormonal Contraceptives

| GENERIC NAMES | TRADE NAMES |
|---|---|
| **Combination Oral Contraceptives** | |
| drospirenone, ethinyl estradiol | Yasmin |
| ethinyl estradiol, desogestrel | Apri, Azurette, Caziant, Cyclessa, Desogen, Kariva, Mircette, Ortho-Cept, Pimtrea, Reclipsen, Solia, Velivet |
| ethinyl estradiol, ethynodiol diacetate | Demulen, Kelnor, Zovia |
| ethinyl estradiol, levonorgestrel | Aviane, Enpresse, Jolessa, Lessina, Levlen, Levlite, Levora, Lutera, Portia, Quasense, Seasonale, Seasonique, Sronyx, Tri-Levlen, Triphasil, Trivora |
| ethinyl estradiol, norethindrone | Aranelle, Balziva, Brevicon, Femcon, Genora, Jenest, Leena, Modicon, Necon, Norinyl, Nortrel, Ortho-Novum, Ovcon, Tri-Norinyl, Zenchent |
| ethinyl estradiol, norethindrone acetate | Estrostep, Femhrt, Junel, Loestrin, Microgestin, Pirmella, Tilia, Tri-Legest |
| ethinyl estradiol, norgestimate | MonoNessa, Ortho Tri-Cyclen, Previfem, Sprintec-28, Tri-Previfem, Tri-Sprintec, TriNessa |
| ethinyl estradiol, norgestrel | Cryselle, Low-Ogestrel, Ogestrel, Ovral |
| mestranol, norethindrone | Genora, Necon, Necon, Norinyl, Ortho-Novum |
| **Combination Topical Contraceptives** | |
| **Vaginal Rings** | |
| ethinyl estradiol, etonogestrel | NuvaRing |
| **Patches** | |
| ethinyl estradiol, norelgestromin | Ortho Evra |
| **Progestin-Only Oral Contraceptives** | |
| norethindrone | Aygestin, Camila, Errin, Jolivette, Nor-QD, Nora-BE, Ortho Micronor |
| norgestrel | Ovrette |
| **Intrauterine Contraceptives (Progestin Only)** | |
| levonorgestrel | Mirena |
| **Subcutaneous Implants (Progestin Only)** | |
| etonogestrel | Implanon |
| levonorgestrel | Norplant |

or progesterone. Ovulation does not occur; the cervical mucus thickens, making fertilization difficult; and the lining of the uterus becomes too thin to support pregnancy.

The most effective OCs contain a synthetic estrogen and progestin, a synthetic progesterone. The specific drugs in combination and their dosages vary, as does the dosing schedule. Consult a drug handbook for specific dosages and scheduling.

*Mini-pills* are OCs that contain only progestin rather than a combination of estrogen and progestin. They increase blood levels of progesterone, turning off the hormone pathway with positive feedback, which prevents ovulation. Mini-pills are not as effective as combination OCs, and most must be taken daily continuously.

### Expected Side Effects

The most common side effects of OCs are breast enlargement and tenderness, nausea, fluid retention, and weight gain. Depending on the dosage and whether the OC contains estrogen and progestin or only progestin, breakthrough vaginal bleeding can occur. Acne can become worse for some women or clear up for others while taking OCs.

### Adverse Effects

Like other types of sex hormones, OCs increase the risk of blood clot formation. This problem can lead to deep vein thrombosis, pulmonary embolism, myocardial infection, and stroke. The risk increases among women who smoke and in those older than age 35.

Most hormonal contraceptives cause fluid and sodium retention, which can lead to hypertension. Hormonal contraception is not recommended for women with moderate to severe hypertension.

The estrogen and progestin in OCs can cause liver toxicity. Indications of liver toxicity include elevated liver enzyme levels, yellowing of the skin and the whites of the eyes, tiredness, coffee-colored urine, clay-colored stools, and nausea. Hormonal contraceptives are not recommended for women with known liver problems.

The estrogen and/or progestin of OCs promote the growth of hormone-sensitive cancers of the cervix, uterus, ovary, and breast. Hormonal contraceptives should not be used by women who have a history of or are at high risk for these types of cancer.

OCs that use drospirenone (Ocella, Yasmin, YAZ28) as the progestin can increase the serum potassium level, which can lead to heart block and other irregular heart rhythms. Contraceptives that contain drospirenone are not recommended for women who have kidney, liver, or adrenal disease and those who are taking other drugs that increase potassium levels (e.g., angiotensin-converting enzyme inhibitors for hypertension, potassium-sparing diuretics).

### Drug Interactions

Many drugs and herbal supplements interact with OCs. Ask women who are prescribed OCs about all other drugs and supplements they are taking. Check with the pharmacist to avoid a possible drug interaction.

❖ **Nursing Implications and Patient Teaching**

◆ *Patient and family teaching.* Tell the patient and family:
- Use an additional method of contraception during the first cycle because OCs require a full cycle before they are effective.
- Take the drug as prescribed; otherwise an unplanned pregnancy may result because scheduling is important for best effectiveness.
- Remember that OCs are effective at preventing pregnancy only when taken *exactly* as prescribed.
- Take the OC with food once daily and at the same time each day for best effect.
- Do not smoke or use nicotine in any form to reduce the risk of blood clots, heart attacks, and strokes.
- If you miss one dose during your monthly cycle, the drug should still be effective in preventing pregnancy. However, if you miss more than one dose in a cycle, especially two doses in a row, continue to use it but also use another method of contraception for the rest of that cycle.
- Because of the potential for drug interactions, tell other healthcare providers that you are taking this drug.
- To prevent possible interactions, do not take any over-the-counter drug without checking with the healthcare provider who prescribed the contraceptive.
- Notify your healthcare provider if you develop yellowing of the skin or eyes, darkening of the urine, or lightening of the stools. These problems are signs of liver toxicity, a serious adverse effect of hormonal contraceptives.

 **Lifespan Considerations**

**Pregnancy and Lactation**

- Hormonal contraceptives should not be used during pregnancy because they can interrupt the pregnancy and can cause birth defects. Women should know for certain that they are not pregnant before starting hormonal contraceptives. Instruct women to immediately notify their healthcare provider if a pregnancy is suspected.
- Hormonal contraceptives interfere with lactation. They are also present in breast milk and may harm the infant. These drugs should not be used by lactating women.

## MALE SEX HORMONES

### OVERVIEW

Male sex hormones are produced under the influence of the anterior pituitary gland. The male hormone testosterone and its related hormones are called *androgens*. Androgens are synthetic or natural hormones that help to develop and maintain the male sex organs at puberty and to develop secondary sex characteristics in men (e.g., facial hair, deep voice, body hair, body fat distribution, muscle development). They promote the anabolic or tissue-building processes in the body.

Anabolic steroids are synthetic drugs with the same uses and actions as androgens. These drugs may be given as replacement therapy for testosterone deficiency.

### ANDROGENS

#### Action and Uses

Androgens are steroid hormones that are synthesized from cholesterol in the adrenal gland; they stimulate or control the development and maintenance of male characteristics, including the activity of the male sex organs and the development of male secondary sex characteristics. Androgens and anabolic steroids are primarily used in the treatment of hypogonadism, hypopituitarism, *eunuchism* (absence of testes or undeveloped gonads in a male), *cryptorchidism* (undescended testes), *oligospermia* (lack of sperm in the semen), and general androgen deficiency in males. The most commonly used androgen is testosterone. Androgens also help in the development of skeletal muscle cells by exerting action on several cell types in skeletal muscle tissue.

#### Expected Side Effects

Common side effects of androgens include edema caused by sodium retention (usually with larger doses), acne, *hirsutism* (excessive body hair), male pattern baldness, mouth irritation, diarrhea, nausea, and vomiting.

#### Adverse Reactions

Administration of some testosterone injections that contain oils have been associated with cases of pulmonary oil embolisms and serious allergic reactions. These allergic reactions can occur anytime during the course of therapy, including after the first dose. Observe patients in the healthcare setting for 30 minutes after an injection in order to provide appropriate medical treatment in the event of serious hypersensitivity reactions or anaphylaxis.

Tumors of the liver, liver cancer, and hepatitis have occurred with long-term, high-dose androgen therapy. Adverse reactions to androgens also include jaundice, a decreased sperm count, *gynecomastia* (enlargement of the breasts), impotence, and urinary retention. In

Table 18.3   Androgen Drugs

| DRUGS/ADULT DOSES | NURSING IMPLICATIONS |
|---|---|
| testosterone (Andriol)<br>50–400 mg IM every 2 to 4 weeks | Inject deep into the gluteal muscle. Take care to avoid intravascular injection.<br>For subsequent injections, alternate injection site.<br>Monitor patient for 30 minutes following each injection in order to provide appropriate medical treatment in the event of serious pulmonary oil microembolism reaction or anaphylaxis. |
| testosterone enanthate subcutaneous injection (Xyosted) | Do not remove the cap until ready to inject.<br>Wash hands with soap and water.<br>Wipe the abdomen injection site with an alcohol swab. Allow the site to dry on its own. Only use the left or right side of the abdomen for injection sites. Do not use the area within 2 inches around the navel. Do not use in areas where the skin is tender, bruised, red, scaly, or hard. Avoid areas with scars, tattoos, or stretch marks. |
| testosterone gel (AndroGel) 50 mg daily | Wash hands with soap and water before and after applying the gel.<br>Apply to the skin of the abdomen, shoulders, or upper arms that will be covered by a shirt.<br>Do not apply to the penis or scrotum.<br>Allow the medicine to dry for at least 5 minutes before dressing.<br>Avoid showering, swimming, or bathing for at least 2 hours after the application. |
| testosterone transdermal patch (Androderm)<br>4 mg daily | Apply transdermal patch to the to the arm or upper body once daily.<br>Remove all old patches before applying a new patch. |
| testosterone mouth patch (Striant) 30 mg every 12 hours | Apply to the upper gums close to the two front teeth. Remove all old patches before applying a new patch. |
| testosterone pellets (Testopel) 150 to 450 mg every 3 to 6 months | Testopel pellets are inserted with a minor surgical procedure in the office or clinic.<br>The pellets are placed under the skin on the back side of the hip area, usually once every 3 to 6 months.<br>The implants slowly release testosterone and are absorbed over time. |

children, use of androgens may result in early puberty and short stature because of premature closing of the bone growth plates. Testosterone is contraindicated in patients with a history of breast or prostate cancer, uncontrolled heart failure, or those with a myocardial infarction or cerebrovascular accident within the past 6 months.

### Lifespan Considerations

**Pregnancy and Lactation**

Testosterone may cause birth defects if a pregnant woman comes in contact with the medicine.

### Drug Interactions

Androgens and anabolic steroids may increase the effects of anticoagulants, antidiabetic agents, and other drugs. Corticosteroids given at the same time as androgens increase the possibility of edema. Barbiturates decrease the therapeutic effects of androgens because of increased breakdown in the liver (Table 18.3).

 **Top Tip for Safety**

- When giving testosterone observe and exercise appropriate precautions for handling, preparation, administration, and disposal.
  - *INJECTIONS:* Use double chemotherapy gloves and a protective gown. Eye/face and respiratory protection may be needed during preparation and administration.
  - *TOPICAL or TRANSDERMAL:* Use double chemotherapy gloves and protective gown. Eye/face and respiratory protection may be needed during preparation and administration.

❖ **Nursing Implications and Patient Teaching**
◆ *Patient and family teaching.* Tell the patient and family:
- Take androgens only as instructed by your healthcare provider.
- Do not increase the dose without consulting your healthcare provider, even if you do not see the expected effects within the first 1 to 2 months, because response to the drug may take several months.
- Report any new or troublesome symptoms that may develop, including fluid retention (especially in

the feet and hands), breast enlargement, shortness of breath, excessive physical or sexual stimulation, prolonged or painful erection of the penis, impotence, urinary retention, and jaundice.

- If you are using a topical gel form of the drug, do not let women or children come into contact with the areas where you have applied it to prevent them from absorbing the drug.

## Get Ready for the Next-Generation NCLEX® Examination!

### Key Points

- Use of HRT to relieve menopausal symptoms increases the risks of blood clot formation, heart attack, stroke, pulmonary embolism, and deep vein thrombosis.
- Teach patients using the topical gel form of testosterone to avoid letting women or children come into contact with the areas where the drug has been applied to prevent them from accidentally absorbing the drug.

### Clinical Judgment and Next-Generation NCLEX® Examination-Style Questions

1. **What should a woman who takes a combination oral contraceptive do if she misses two consecutive doses?**

   1. Finish the package as prescribed for the rest of the cycle and start the next cycle's package without taking any time off.
   2. Finish the package as prescribed for the rest of the cycle and use an additional method of contraception.
   3. Take two tablets daily for the next 2 consecutive days and then finish the package as prescribed.
   4. Take two tablets daily for the rest of the current cycle.

2. **A patient experiencing symptoms related to menopause asks you to explain the cause of her symptoms. What is your best response?**

   1. "Symptoms of menopause are caused by low levels of estrogen and high levels of FSH."
   2. "Symptoms of menopause are caused by high levels of estrogen and low levels of FSH."
   3. "Symptoms of menopause are caused by low levels of estrogen and low levels of FSH."
   4. "Symptoms of menopause are caused by high levels of estrogen and high levels of FSH."

3. **A 72-year-old man has been prescribed testosterone as androgen therapy for hypogonadism.**

   **Highlight or place a check mark next to the statements that should be included when teaching your patient about testosterone.**

   - ___ You may increase the dose of testosterone after 2 weeks if no effect is seen.
   - ___ You should report signs of fluid retention to your healthcare provider.
   - ___ You should avoid crowds because this drug decreases your immunity.
   - ___ You may experience enlargement of the breasts with this drug.
   - ___ Testosterone can increase the effects of the drugs you take for your diabetes.
   - ___ To enhance absorption, drink a warm fluid when taking the buccal form of this drug.
   - ___ The expected response to testosterone may not be seen for several months.
   - ___ Notify your healthcare provider if you experience a painful or prolonged erection.
   - ___ This drug can only be given by injection.
   - ___ You should report the presence of jaundice to your healthcare provider.

4. **A 26-year-old woman has begun an initial course of oral contraceptives (OCs). Which of the following is a serious side effect of OCs?**

   1. Blood clots
   2. Risk for infection
   3. Fracture of the jaw
   4. Bone marrow suppression

5. **You are teaching the patient about safe administration of testosterone gel by _____1_____ and _____2_____.**

| OPTIONS FOR 1 | OPTIONS FOR 2 |
|---|---|
| Placing the gel only on the penis and scrotum | Allowing the gel to dry for 5 minutes before dressing |
| Applying the gel to the covered skin of the abdomen, shoulders, or upper arms | Using a sterile tongue blade to apply the gel |
| Applying the gel only before sexual intercourse | Covering the gel once applied with a sterile bandage |

## Next-Generation NCLEX® (NGN) Examination–Style Question

### History and Physical
### 6 Months Ago, 1000

A 53-year-old female client presents to the outpatient OB/GYN office for their routine physical. The client reports having hot flashes and excessive sweating at nighttime over the last 4 months. The client also reports their last menstrual cycle was 5 months ago and states, "Do you think I'm in menopause?"

Physical Exam:

General: flushed, red face

Respiratory: breath sounds clear bilaterally

Breast Exam: nontender breasts

Cardiovascular: no edema

Skin: warm and dry

### Today, 1300

"My hot flashes are so much better, but I just haven't felt well the last week or so." The client also reports occasional breakthrough bleeding over the last month and complains of urinary frequency.

Physical Exam:

General: no acute distress, white sclerae

Respiratory: breath sounds clear bilaterally

Breast Exam: tender breasts

Cardiovascular: trace bilateral edema

Skin: warm and dry, facial acne noted

### Flow Sheet
### 6 Months Ago, 1000

Blood Pressure: 138/78 mm Hg

Heart Rate: 80/min

Respiratory Rate: 18/min

Temperature: 98.6°F (37°C)

Weight: 155 pounds (70.5 kg)

### Today, 1300

Blood Pressure: 158/82 mm Hg

Heart Rate: 84/min

Respiratory Rate: 18/min

Temperature: 99.8°F (37.7°C)

Weight: 161 pounds (73.2 kg)

### Orders
### 6 Months Ago, 1000

Medroxyprogesterone 0.625 mg conjugated estrogens orally once daily on days 1–14, then 0.625 mg conjugated estrogens plus 5 mg medroxyprogesterone acetate orally once daily on days 15–28

### Imaging Studies
### Today, 1300

Mammogram: mass noted to left upper quadrant of the left breast, concern for cancerous lesion

A nurse is caring for the client in the outpatient OB/GYN office.

**Click to highlight the findings that are considered side effects or complications of the client's hormone replacement therapy.**

### Today, 1300

"My hot flashes are so much better, but I just haven't felt well the last week or so." The client also reports occasional breakthrough bleeding over the last month and complains of urinary frequency.

Physical Exam:

General: no acute distress, white sclerae

Respiratory: breath sounds clear bilaterally

Breast Exam: tender breasts

Cardiovascular: trace bilateral edema

Skin: warm and dry, facial acne noted

### Today, 1300

Blood Pressure: 158/82 mm Hg

Heart Rate: 84/min

Respiratory Rate: 18/min

Temperature: 99.8°F (37.7°C)

Weight: 161 pounds (73.2 kg)

### Today, 1300

Mammogram: mass noted to left upper quadrant of the left breast, concern for cancerous lesion

See answer on Evolve at http://evolve.elsevier.com/Visovsky/LPNpharmacology/.

# Drugs for Thyroid and Adrenal Problems

## Learning Outcomes

1. Explain the role of the endocrine system in general health and thyroid and adrenal problems.
2. List the names, actions, possible side effects, and adverse effects of drugs for thyroid problems.
3. Explain what to teach patients and families about drugs for thyroid problems.

4. List the names, actions, possible side effects, and adverse effects of drugs for adrenal gland problems.
5. Explain what to teach patients and families about drugs for adrenal gland problems.

## Key Terms

**antithyroid drug** A drug that works directly in the thyroid gland to stop production of new hormones by preventing an enzyme from connecting iodine (iodide) with tyrosine to make active thyroid hormones.

**thyroid hormone agonist** Drug that mimics the effect of the thyroid hormones $T_3$ and $T_4$, helping to regulate metabolism.

## OVERVIEW OF THE ENDOCRINE SYSTEM

The endocrine system involves many glands that secrete hormones (Fig. 19.1). A hormone is a protein secreted by an endocrine gland that changes the action of another gland or tissue, known as its *target tissue*. Unlike some glandular secretions (e.g., from the salivary glands) that move through a duct directly to their site of action, hormones do not require a duct to reach their target tissues. For this reason, endocrine glands are known as *ductless glands*. The hormones are released into the bloodstream, in which they circulate throughout the body. When a specific hormone, such as insulin, reaches a tissue or organ that has insulin receptors, the hormone recognizes its target tissue and binds to its receptors, causing a change in the activity of the target tissue. Endocrine glands sometimes develop problems and are no longer able to produce adequate amounts of specific hormones. In other cases, an endocrine gland may be surgically removed for a specific problem, making the person deficient in that hormone.

### THYROID AND ADRENAL HORMONES

The thyroid gland releases triiodothyronine ($T_3$) and thyroxine ($T_4$). These hormones work to regulate weight, energy levels, body temperature, skin, hair, nail growth, and metabolism. Having too much $T_3$ in the bloodstream results from overactivity of the thyroid gland, or *hyperthyroidism*. Hyperthyroidism

occurs in conditions such as Graves' disease, a disorder of the immune system that results in an overproduction of thyroid hormones (hyperthyroidism). Hypothyroidism occurs if the thyroid gland does not produce enough of the thyroid hormone due to autoimmune conditions, such as Hashimoto's thyroiditis, certain medications, or pituitary issues.

The adrenal glands are located at the top of both kidneys. Adrenal glands produce hormones that regulate the immune system, blood pressure, metabolism, and the stress response. Adrenal hormones include aldosterone, adrenaline, cortisol, norepinephrine, and dehydroepiandrosterone (DHEA).

The regulation of hormones works on a negative feedback loop. For example, when the level of thyroid hormones is high enough to meet bodily needs, the hormone feedback loop stops the hypothalamus from secreting thyrotropin-releasing hormone (TRH) and the pituitary from secreting thyroid-stimulating hormone (TSH). As a result, the thyroid stops secreting its hormones. If the negative feedback loop fails, the result is undesirable consequences, as many hormones are necessary for life.

Depending on how important the function of the hormone is to a patient's health and well-being, *hormone replacement therapy (HRT)*—temporary or permanent therapy with drugs that perform the function of natural endocrine hormones—may be needed. HRT may be used for a short time, such as for relief of menopausal symptoms, or permanently, such as for replacement of thyroid hormones after removal of the thyroid gland. HRT is commonly used for thyroid problems, adrenal gland problems, sex hormone replacement, contraception, and diabetes. The issues for diabetes management are complex and are discussed separately in Chapter 20.

> 💡 **Memory Jogger**
> - The thyroid gland releases triiodothyronine (T₃) and thyroxine (T₄).
> - Adrenal hormones include aldosterone, adrenaline, cortisol, norepinephrine, and dehydroepiandrosterone (DHEA).

## DRUGS FOR THYROID PROBLEMS

As mentioned, the thyroid gland is located in the neck (see Fig. 19.1) and produces two thyroid hormones that are critical for life: triiodothyronine (T₃) and thyroxine (T₄). These hormones enter all cells in the body, where they bind to receptors inside the cell and activate various genes for metabolism. T₃ and T₄ increase the rate of metabolism, which is the energy use and work performed in the body. These hormones are critical for the following body actions:

- Brain development and function, including the ability to think, remember, and learn
- Heart and skeletal muscle contraction and strength
- Endocrine system production of other hormones
- Breathing and oxygen use in all cells

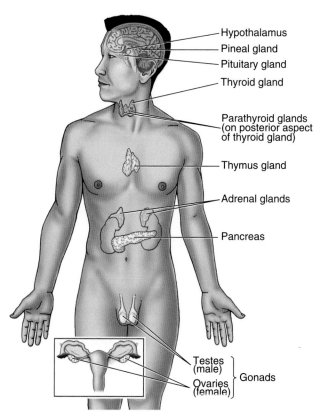

Fig. 19.1 The endocrine system. (Modified from Herlihy, B. (2014). *The human body in health and illness* (5th ed.). Elsevier.)

## HYPOTHYROIDISM

*Hypothyroidism*, also known as *underactive thyroid*, is a common problem in which the thyroid gland produces little or no thyroid hormones, slowing all aspects of metabolism. Other symptoms, such as weakness, fatigue, weight gain, or depression, also occur. If hypothyroidism is left untreated, serious problems of the cardiovascular, pulmonary, and nervous systems and brain result. Children may have such poor brain development that they are cognitively impaired. Adult metabolism can slow to the point that death from cardiac or respiratory failure can occur.

These problems can be prevented by HRT with drugs known as *thyroid hormone agonists*. Therapy with thyroid hormone replacement is usually needed for the rest of the person's life. Box 19.1 lists the symptoms associated with hypothyroidism.

## THYROID HORMONE AGONISTS

### Action and Uses

A **thyroid hormone agonist** is a drug that mimics the effect of the thyroid hormones T₃ and T₄, helping to regulate metabolism. These drugs work like natural thyroid hormones by moving through the blood and entering all cells. The drugs then enter the nucleus

| Box 19.1 | Symptoms Associated with Thyroid Problems |
|---|---|

**HYPOTHYROIDISM**
- Feeling tired, no energy, sleeps a lot
- Gaining weight while eating minimal amounts
- Lower heart rate, blood pressure, and respiratory rate for the person's age and size
- Always feeling cold when others are comfortable
- A body temperature below normal
- Constipation
- Increased facial and body hair, with decreased scalp hair
- Decreased interest in surroundings and appearing to think more slowly
- The tongue seems thicker, making speech more difficult
- Skin that is dry and flaky
- Decreased sex drive
- Decreased or absent menstruation
- Erectile dysfunction

**HYPERTHYROIDISM**
- Having lots of energy with difficulty sleeping
- Experiencing weight loss even when appetite and eating are increased
- Increased heart rate and blood pressure
- Always feeling too warm when others are comfortable
- A body temperature above normal
- Having multiple bowel movements daily, diarrhea
- Thinning of the scalp hair
- Skin that is moist or sweaty
- Difficulty concentrating, being irritable
- Hand tremors

and bind to receptors on the DNA, which activates the genes for metabolism. As a result of turning on these genes, thyroid hormone agonists increase the cells' rate of metabolism, which speeds up the energy use and work of each cell.

Table 19.1 lists the names, dosages, and nursing implications for the most commonly prescribed thyroid hormone agonists. Consult a drug reference or pharmacist for information about other thyroid hormone agonists.

## Expected Side Effects

Thyroid hormone agonist drugs have few side effects because they mimic normal hormones. As cell metabolism increases, the patient may experience symptoms of hyperthyroidism. The symptoms most easily noticed are diarrhea, rapid pulse, high blood pressure (hypertension), difficulty sleeping (insomnia), excessive sweating, and heat intolerance.

## Adverse Effects

The most serious adverse effects of thyroid hormone agonists occur in the cardiac and nervous systems. The activities of both systems increase, sometimes to

dangerous levels. Increased cardiac activity can lead to angina (chest pain), myocardial infarction (heart attack), or heart failure. Increased nervous system activity can lead to seizures, although this is more likely to occur in patients who already have a seizure disorder.

## Drug Interactions

When thyroid hormone agonists are taken with drugs that reduce blood clotting (anticoagulants), especially warfarin (Coumadin), their actions are increased. This response can cause excessive bleeding and bruising.

### ❖ Nursing Implications and Patient Teaching

◆ *Assessment.* Before giving the first dose of a thyroid hormone agonist drug, check the patient's heart rate and blood pressure because these drugs can increase metabolic rate and cardiac activity. Check the patient's entire drug list—including prescription drugs, vitamins, minerals, and supplements—for potential interactions with thyroid hormone agonist drugs. Report the use of anticoagulants or NSAIDs to the healthcare provider because these drugs can interact with thyroid

| Table **19.1** | Examples of Common Drugs for Thyroid Problems |
|---|---|

*Thyroid hormone agonists* have the same structure as thyroid hormones and work in the same way to activate genes for metabolism, speeding up the energy use and work output of each cell.

*Antithyroid drugs* reduce thyroid hormone levels by entering the thyroid gland and combining with the enzyme responsible for connecting iodine (iodide) with tyrosine. Without this iodide–tyrosine connection, thyroid hormone production is suppressed.

| DRUG/ADULT DOSAGE | NURSING IMPLICATIONS |
|---|---|
| **Thyroid Hormone Agonists** | |
| levothyroxine sodium [synthetic] (Estre, Eltroxin ♣, Levo-T, Levothroid, Levoxyl, Synthroid, Unithroid) Oral: 25–250 mcg once daily IV: 12.5–150 mcg once daily liothyronine sodium [synthetic] (Cytomel, Triostat) 25–100 mcg orally once daily | • Check the patient's heart rate and blood pressure before giving this drug because increased heart rate and blood pressure can result. <br>• Check the patient's entire prescription and OTC drug list for potential interactions with thyroid hormone agonist drugs. <br>• Report the use of anticoagulants or NSAIDs because these drugs can interact with levothyroxine and cause excessive bruising and bleeding. <br>• Pregnant women may need a higher dose, and women who are taking thyroid hormone agonists are advised not to breast-feed because the drug can be found in breast milk. <br>• Check the dose and the specific drug name carefully. Thyroid hormone agonists are *not* interchangeable because the strengths of these drugs vary. <br>• Levothyroxine may affect the blood sugar of diabetic patients. Check blood sugar levels closely. |
| **Antithyroid Drugs** | |
| methimazole (Northyx, Tapazole) maintenance 5–30 mg orally every 8 hours propylthiouracil (Propacil, Propyl-Thyracil ♣, PTU) maintenance 100–150 mg orally every 8 hours | • Check the patient's CBC for signs of bone marrow suppression such as a low WBC count, anemia, or thrombocytopenia. <br>• Assess the patient for signs of infection. <br>• Assess the patient's skin for signs of bruising or bleeding, such as ecchymosis or petechiae. <br>• Check the patient's drug list for drugs that have antiplatelet actions, such as warfarin. <br>• Check the patient's liver function test results before giving these drugs. Both thyroid-suppressing drugs (methimazole and propylthiouracil) are hepatotoxic. Check the patient daily for yellowing of the skin or sclera that indicates jaundice. <br>• Check the dose and the specific drug name and prescribed dosage carefully. These drugs are not interchangeable because the strength of each drug varies. <br>• Notify the healthcare provider if adverse effects, such as bone marrow suppression or altered liver function, occur. |

*CBC,* complete blood cell count; *NSAIDs,* nonsteroidal anti-inflammatory drugs; *OTC,* over-the-counter; *WBC,* white blood cell.

hormone agonists and cause excessive bruising and bleeding.

Assess women of childbearing age for possible pregnancy before beginning thyroid hormone agonists. Pregnant women may need a higher dose, and women who are taking thyroid hormone agonists are advised not to breast-feed because the drug can be found in breast milk.

Carefully check the drug name and dose because thyroid hormone agonist drugs are *not* interchangeable. Although the actions are similar, the strength of each drug varies.

### Top Tip for Safety

Do not give one brand of thyroid hormone in place of another. The strength of different brands and types varies, and so can patient responses. For example, liothyronine is four times as potent as levothyroxine.

◆ *Planning and implementation.* When hypothyroidism is first diagnosed, the thyroid hormone drug dose is kept low for the first several weeks. The drug dose is then increased slowly every 2 to 3 weeks until the patient has normal blood levels of thyroid hormone and signs of normal metabolism.

The absorption of thyroid hormone agonists in the gastrointestinal (GI) tract is greatly reduced by food and fiber. Give the drug 2 hours before a meal or fiber supplement or at least 3 hours after a meal or a fiber supplement has been taken.

◆ *Evaluation.* The effects of the drug may not be apparent for several weeks. Check the patient's heart rate and blood pressure to determine whether the drug is working and to check for side effects because hypothyroid symptoms may be most notable in the cardiac system. The following changes indicate that the drug is effective, and that the dose is appropriate:
- The patient's vital signs (i.e., body temperature, heart rate, blood pressure, and respiratory rate) are within normal limits.
- The patient's activity level and mental status are normal for him or her.
- The patient's body weight is consistent with the number of calories consumed and his or her activity level.
- The patient's bowel habits are what they were before the thyroid problem occurred.

Assess the patient for indications of adverse effects on the cardiac system. The first indications may be chest pain or discomfort and hypertension.

For patients who are also taking drugs that affect blood clotting, especially warfarin, assess the patient at least once per shift for any sign of increased bleeding. Indications are bleeding from the gums, unusual or excessive bruising anywhere on the skin, bleeding around intravenous (IV) sites, bleeding for more than 5 minutes after an intramuscular (IM) injection

or discontinuation of an IV, and visible blood in urine, stool, or vomit.

◆ *Patient and family teaching.* Teach the patient and family:
- Take only the dose that is prescribed because increasing the drug too quickly can lead to adverse effects such as a heart attack or seizures.
- Do not skip doses, and you must take the drug daily to maintain normal body function.
- Take a missed dose as soon as you remember it. However, if it is almost time for the next dose, skip the missed dose and continue your regular dosing schedule. Do not take a double dose to make up for a missed one.
- To prevent underdosing or overdosing, do not stop the drug suddenly or change the dose (up or down) without contacting your healthcare provider.
- Because food and fiber greatly decrease absorption of the drug, take the drug 2 to 3 hours before a meal or fiber supplement or at least 3 hours after a meal or fiber supplement.
- Check your pulse each morning before taking the drug and again each evening before going to bed. If the pulse rate becomes 20 beats higher than the normal rate for 1 week or it becomes consistently irregular, notify your healthcare provider.
- Go to the emergency department immediately if you start to have chest pain.
- If you are ill and cannot take the drug orally, contact your healthcare provider to get an injection dose of the drug.
- If you also take warfarin, keep all follow-up appointments and appointments for blood-clotting tests because these drugs increase the effectiveness of warfarin.
- Avoid situations that can lead to bleeding and other drugs that can make bleeding worse (e.g., aspirin).

 **Lifespan Considerations**

**Pediatric Patients**

Thyroid hormone agonist drugs are safe to take during pregnancy and are needed to maintain the pregnancy and prevent problems with the fetus. These drugs do enter breast milk and can cause problems for the nursing infant. Therefore a mother being treated with thyroid hormone agonists should not breast-feed.

 **Lifespan Considerations**

**Pediatric Patients**

Hypothyroidism can occur in children, and some are born with it. Any child with the disorder must take thyroid hormone replacement drugs for his or her entire life. Infants and children going through periods of rapid growth need higher dosages of thyroid agonist drugs.

**Lifespan Considerations**

**Older Adults**

Adults older than 65 years are usually prescribed a lower initial dose of thyroid hormone agonists because they are more likely to experience serious adverse cardiac and nervous system effects. For this reason, doses are increased more slowly in older adults than in younger adults until an appropriate maintenance dose is reached.

## HYPERTHYROIDISM

*Hyperthyroidism,* also called an *overactive thyroid* or *thyrotoxicosis,* is a condition in which the thyroid gland secretes excessive amounts of thyroid hormones ($T_3$ and $T_4$). This hormone excess causes general body metabolism to be greatly increased. Although there are different causes of hyperthyroidism, the most common is Graves' disease. Box 19.1 lists the symptoms associated with hyperthyroidism. Some types of hyperthyroidism cause the patient to have a *goiter,* which is a swelling in the neck caused by an enlarged thyroid gland. Continued excessive amounts of thyroid hormones can cause toxic side effects in some organs, especially the heart and nervous system. When hyperthyroidism is caused by Graves' disease, bulging or protruding eyes (exophthalmos) (Fig. 19.2) and blurred vision may occur.

Severe hyperthyroidism that causes life-threatening hypertension, heart failure, and seizures is called a *thyroid crisis* or *thyroid storm.* A fever is often the first indication of a problem. This condition is an emergency and can lead to death if the thyroid hormone levels are not decreased immediately.

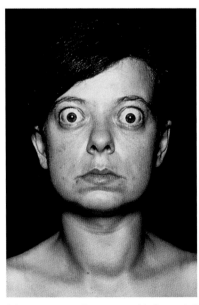

Fig. 19.2 Facial appearance of a woman with Graves' disease. (From Ignatavicius, D. D., & Workman, M. L. (2016). *Medical-surgical nursing: Patient-centered collaborative care* (8th ed.). Saunders.)

## ANTITHYROID DRUGS

### Actions and Uses

Without treatment, hyperthyroidism has serious consequences. For some people, treatment consists of surgical removal of all or part of the thyroid gland. Radiation therapy with radioactive iodine can also reduce thyroid gland function and production of thyroid hormones. Therapy with antithyroid drugs can be used short term before surgery or long term to prevent thyroid hormone production and control the disease. Methimazole and propylthiouracil are common antithyroid drugs and belong to the thionamide class of drugs.

Table 19.1 lists the names, dosages, and nursing implications for the common antithyroid drugs. These drugs are not interchangeable because methimazole is 10 times stronger than propylthiouracil.

 **Top Tip for Safety**

Do not substitute methimazole for propylthiouracil because methimazole is 10 times stronger than propylthiouracil.

**Antithyroid drugs** work directly in the thyroid gland to stop production of new hormones by preventing an enzyme from connecting iodine (iodide) with tyrosine to make active thyroid hormones. The drug serves as a decoy for the enzyme so that it works on the drug instead of connecting these two substances. As a result, new hormones are not made, but the ones already made and stored in the thyroid gland are not affected by the drug. The drugs do not affect stored hormones, so it may take several weeks before the effects of all the stored thyroid hormones are gone.

 **Top Tip for Safety**

Teach patients that thyroid-suppressing drugs must be taken for 3 to 4 weeks to start being effective because they have no effect on thyroid hormones already stored in the thyroid gland.

### Expected Side Effects

Most common side effects of antithyroid drugs are minor and include taste changes, headache, itchiness, rash, muscle and joint aches, drowsiness, nausea, vomiting, enlarged lymph nodes, and swelling of the lower extremities.

### Adverse Effects

Bone marrow suppression can occur, causing anemia and increasing the risk of infection. These drugs often induce hypothyroidism in patients who take them. Propylthiouracil can be hepatotoxic (causing liver damage). Methimazole is preferred over propylthiouracil. In some patients, these drugs can also damage the kidneys.

## Drug Interactions

Both methimazole and propylthiouracil increase the effectiveness of anticlotting drugs, especially warfarin. Patients who are taking antithyroid drugs with any anticlotting drug are at greater risk for excessive bleeding and bruising.

### ❖ Nursing Implications and Patient Teaching

◆ *Assessment.* Assess the patient's vital signs, especially for elevated temperature that may be associated with infection. Check the patient's blood counts for signs of bone marrow suppression, such as a low white blood cell count, anemia, or thrombocytopenia.

Check the patient's drug list for drugs that have antiplatelet actions, such as warfarin. Assess the patient's skin for signs of bruising or bleeding, such as ecchymosis or petechiae. Notify the healthcare provider if these appear.

Before giving these drugs, check the patient's liver function tests because both methimazole and propylthiouracil are toxic to the liver *(hepatotoxic)*, especially propylthiouracil. For patients who already have liver problems, the effects of antithyroid drugs on the liver are more severe and occur at lower doses.

◆ *Planning and implementation.* Carefully check the dose and the specific drug name and prescribed dosage. These drugs are not interchangeable because methimazole is 10 times stronger than propylthiouracil. Notify the healthcare provider if adverse effects such as bone marrow suppression or altered liver function occur.

◆ *Evaluation.* Check the patient's complete blood cell count whenever it is determined because these drugs cause some degree of bone marrow suppression. When WBCs are reduced, the patient's risk for infection increases. Report changes in blood cell counts to the healthcare provider.

Bone marrow suppression can increase the risk of bleeding. These drugs increase the action of anticlotting drugs. For patients who also take anticlotting drugs, look for bleeding from the gums, unusual or excessive bruising anywhere on the skin, bleeding around IV sites or bleeding that lasts longer than 5 minutes after discontinuation of an IV, and the presence of blood in urine, stool, or vomit.

Both of these drugs are hepatotoxic, especially propylthiouracil. Check the patient daily for yellowing of the skin or sclerae (jaundice), coffee-colored urine, and clay-colored stools. These are all symptoms of liver problems.

◆ *Patient and family teaching.* Tell the patient and family:
- Even if you do not notice a reduction of your symptoms in the first 1 to 2 weeks, do not increase the dosage on your own. These drugs take several weeks to become effective.
- Keep all follow-up appointments and appointments for blood-clotting tests because these drugs increase the effectiveness of warfarin.
- Avoid situations that can lead to bleeding and other drugs that can make bleeding worse.
- Avoid crowds and people who are ill because these drugs can reduce your immunity and resistance to infection.
- Check the color of the roof of the mouth and the whites of your eyes daily for a yellow tinge that may indicate a liver problem. If this appears, notify your healthcare provider as soon as possible.

### Lifespan Considerations
**Pregnancy and Breast-Feeding**

- Antithyroid drugs increase the risk of birth defects, fetal damage, and miscarriages. They should not be taken during pregnancy unless the benefits of treatment outweigh the risks. Women who are taking antithyroid drugs should not breast-feed because these drugs enter breast milk and can suppress the infant's thyroid function.
- Methimazole is the treatment of choice in the second or third trimester of pregnancy, whereas propylthiopuracil is the treatment of choice in the first trimester.

### Lifespan Considerations
**Older Adults**

Older adults who are taking antithyroid drugs are more likely to have more severe adverse effects. The older patient's immune system function is already lower than that of a younger person, which increases the older person's risk of infection. Bone marrow suppression from these drugs increases the risk of severe infection. For older adults who take warfarin (Coumadin), the risks of bleeding are even greater while taking an antithyroid drug.

## DRUGS FOR ADRENAL GLAND PROBLEMS

### ADRENAL GLAND HYPOFUNCTION

The adrenal glands are a pair of small endocrine glands located on top of the kidneys, although they are not part of kidney function (Fig. 19.3). They have an outer layer known as the *cortex* and an inner layer known as the *medulla*. In addition to sex hormones (discussed later), the adrenal cortex secretes aldosterone and cortisol. Both are steroid hormones, also called *corticosteroids*, which means their main structure is composed of the steroid cholesterol. *Aldosterone* controls sodium and water balance. It is also known as a *mineralocorticoid* because it regulates sodium. *Cortisol*, of which there are many types, has many functions that are essential for life. Cortisol helps maintain critical blood glucose levels, the stress response, excitability of cardiac muscle, immunity, and blood sodium levels. Cortisol is called a *glucocorticoid* because it was first discovered to affect blood glucose levels.

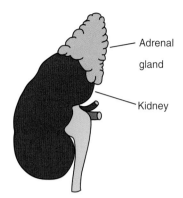

Adrenal gland

Kidney

Fig. 19.3 Location of the adrenal gland on top of the kidney. (From Workman, M. L., & LaCharity, L. A. (2016). *Understanding pharmacology: Essentials for Medication Safety* (2nd ed.). Elsevier.)

Adrenal gland hypofunction is a disorder in which the adrenal gland produces little or no cortisol and aldosterone. Conditions that cause reduced adrenal gland function include an autoimmune disease that attacks and destroys the adrenal glands, adrenalectomy, abdominal radiation therapy, and reduced function of the anterior pituitary gland. Major problems resulting from adrenal gland hypofunction are *hypoglycemia* (low blood glucose levels), salt wasting, hypotension, weakness, and high blood potassium levels.

## Memory Jogger

**GLUCOCORTICOIDS**

Without replacement of cortisol and aldosterone, adrenal gland hypofunction eventually leads to death. Corticosteroid replacement therapy involves the glucocorticoids, especially prednisone. If further help is needed to replace aldosterone action, fludrocortisone (Florinef) may be used.

## Action and Uses

Although glucocorticoids (corticosteroids) are used for HRT, their most common use is as powerful anti-inflammatory drugs. Chapter 13 discusses corticosteroid drug therapy, including specific drugs, side effects, adverse effects, and nursing implications.

Glucocorticoid drugs act like natural cortisol. Because glucocorticoids also have some mineralocorticoid action, many people with adrenal gland hypofunction only need HRT with glucocorticoids. When this replacement is not enough to manage blood sodium levels, fludrocortisone may be added to correct the deficiency.

Fludrocortisone is a synthetic drug that acts like natural aldosterone. With the use of this drug, more sodium is retained and more potassium is excreted to prevent dangerously high blood potassium levels. Fludrocortisone helps prevent hyponatremia, hyperkalemia, and hypotension. The usual adult dosage is 0.1 to 0.2 mg orally once daily.

## Expected Side Effects

Side effects of fludrocortisone therapy include hypertension, edema formation, low blood potassium levels, and high blood sodium levels. The cause of these problems is the drug's action on fluid and electrolyte balance.

## Adverse Effects

Heart failure is a serious adverse effect of fludrocortisone. If heart failure develops, the drug dose is reduced or stopped.

## ❖ Nursing Implications and Patient Teaching

◆ *Patient and family teaching.* Tell the patient and family:
- Take fludrocortisone at the same time daily with food to prevent GI problems.
- Weigh yourself daily and keep a record because the drug can cause fluid retention with weight gain, edema, and heart failure.
- Report edema of the lower extremities because this may be a sign of heart failure.
- Report immediately to the healthcare provider a weight gain of 2 lb in a day or 3 lb in a week. Rapid weight gain can signal fluid retention due to heart failure.

## ADRENAL GLAND HYPERFUNCTION

Most of the time when adrenal gland hyperfunction occurs, only one hormone is oversecreted. Excessive secretion of cortisol is known as *hypercortisolism* or *Cushing disease or Cushing syndrome*. With Cushing syndrome, the excess cortisol can come from issues inside the body or from external sources, such as certain drugs (e.g., prednisone). Excessive secretion of aldosterone is called *hyperaldosteronism*. The most common cause of adrenal gland hyperfunction is an adrenal gland tumor. Sometimes, a problem in the pituitary gland produces excessive amounts of hormones that stimulate the adrenal gland to produce adrenal hormones in excess.

## Action and Uses

Surgery is the most common treatment for adrenal gland hyperfunction that is caused by a problem in the adrenal gland. Drug therapy can help manage the problems caused by adrenal gland hyperfunction before surgery and in patients who are unable to have surgery.

Table 19.2 lists the names, dosages, and nursing implications of the most common drugs used to manage adrenal gland hyperfunction. Some of these drugs reduce cortisol production, whereas others help control the problems caused by hyperaldosteronism.

Mitotane (Lysodren) is a steroid production inhibitor that works by directly preventing adrenal gland production of cortisol and other adrenal cortex hormones. Mifepristone (Korlym), a specialized drug for hypercortisolism, works by blocking corticosteroid receptors. Although this does not reduce cortisol levels, it does inhibit cortisol responses in different tissues. It is approved for use *only* in people who have diabetes type 2 and hypercortisolism.

| Table 19.2 | Examples of Common Drugs to Treat Adrenal Gland Hyperfunction |
|---|---|

*Corticosteroid receptor blockers* reduce symptoms and problems of hypercortisolism by interfering with the binding of cortisol with its receptor, acting as an antagonist.

*Steroid production inhibitors* reduce the symptoms and problems of hypercortisolism by preventing the adrenal cortex from producing cortisol and other adrenal cortex hormones.

| DRUG/ADULT DOSAGE | NURSING IMPLICATIONS |
|---|---|
| **Corticosteroid Receptor Blocker** | |
| mifepristone (Korlym) 300 mg orally once daily; can be increased to 1200 mg orally daily | • This drug is used *only* for people who have diabetes type 2 and hyperglycemia along with hypercortisolism.<br>• Instruct sexually active women of childbearing age to use two reliable forms of birth control while taking mifepristone because this drug can cause a pregnancy loss. |
| **Steroid Production Inhibitors** | |
| mitotane (Lysodren) 1–2 g orally every 6–8 hours | • Teach patients the signs and symptoms of adrenal insufficiency: hypoglycemia, salt craving, muscle weakness, hypotension, and fatigue.<br>• Teach patients the importance of laboratory blood work because these drugs affect levels of sodium and potassium.<br>• Teach patients to take these drugs with food because they can cause nausea, vomiting, and other gastrointestinal upsets. |

Drug therapy for hyperaldosteronism focuses on reducing potassium levels and relies on spironolactone (Aldactone, Spironol, Novo-Spiroton), a potassium-sparing diuretic. Chapter 9 provides more information on spironolactone therapy.

### Expected Side Effects

Common side effects for drugs that suppress adrenal hormone production are likely to cause nausea, vomiting, rashes, and dizziness. Mitotane can also cause bloody urine (hematuria). Mifepristone has many side effects, including menstrual irregularities.

### Adverse Effects

Any drug that suppresses adrenal production of cortisol can lead to problems of adrenal insufficiency. Allergic reaction to mifepristone can occur, and emergency help is needed for hives, difficult breathing, and swelling of the face, lips, tongue, or throat. Mifepristone is also used to induce abortion and can cause pregnancy loss.

### ❖ Nursing Implications and Patient Teaching

Teach the signs and symptoms of adrenal insufficiency to patients who are taking any drug that suppresses

adrenal hormone production. Common indicators are salt craving, muscle weakness, hypotension, hypoglycemia (with headache, difficulty concentrating, shakiness), and fatigue.

◆ *Patient and family teaching.* Tell the patient and family:
- Keep all appointments for laboratory blood work because these drugs alter blood levels of sodium and potassium.
- Report symptoms of adrenal insufficiency to your healthcare provider immediately.
- Take these drugs with food because they can cause nausea, vomiting, and other GI upsets.
- If you are a sexually active woman in your childbearing years, use two reliable forms of birth control while taking mifepristone because this drug can cause a pregnancy loss.

 **Lifespan Considerations**

**Pregnant and Pediatric Patients**

The drugs used for suppressing adrenal hormone production are not approved for use in children or in women who are pregnant or breast-feeding.

## Get Ready for the Next-Generation NCLEX® Examination!

### Key Points

- Hormones exert their actions only on target tissues that have receptors for the specific hormone.
- HRT is commonly used for thyroid and adrenal gland problems.
- Overdoses of thyroid replacement hormones cause the same symptoms as hyperthyroidism.
- Older adults with hypothyroidism are very sensitive to the drugs and are started on lower initial doses than are younger adults.
- Thyroid crisis (or thyroid storm) is an emergency that can lead to death without prompt treatment.
- The effects of antithyroid drugs usually are not felt until 2 to 4 weeks after therapy has started because these drugs do not affect the levels of stored thyroid hormones.

### Clinical Judgment and Next-Generation NCLEX® Examination-Style Questions

1. Which drug therapy for an endocrine problem drug can cause pregnancy loss?

   1. liothyronine sodium (Cytomel)
   2. spironolactone (Aldactone)
   3. mifepristone (Korlym)
   4. mitotane (Lysodren)

2. Which precaution is most important to teach a patient who is taking hormone replacement therapy for hypothyroidism?

   1. Take the drug at least 3 hours before or 3 hours after taking an oral fiber supplement.
   2. Avoid aspirin and aspirin-containing products while on this therapy.
   3. Stop taking the drug as soon as you feel normal again.
   4. Use reliable birth control methods during this therapy.

3. You are preparing to give instructions to an older adult patient who is starting treatment with thyroid hormone. Which symptom reported by the patient indicates an adverse effect of the drug?

   1. Difficulty swallowing
   2. Sleep apnea
   3. Chest pain
   4. Increased temperature

4. Which food or beverage will you advise a patient who is taking methimazole to avoid?

   1. Alcohol
   2. Aged cheese
   3. Dairy products
   4. Leafy green vegetables

5. A patient is prescribed levothyroxine 30 mcg by IV push. The drug on hand is levothyroxine sodium 100 mcg/mL. How many mL should be given?

   1. 30 mL
   2. 0.3 mL
   3. 5 mL
   4. 0.5 mL

6. A patient is prescribed Synthroid 100 mcg orally daily. The drug on hand is Synthroid 25 mcg per tablet. How many tablets should be given?

   1. 2 tablets
   2. 2½ tablets
   3. 4 tablets
   4. ¼ tablet

7. A patient is diagnosed with adrenal gland hyperfunction. The patient asks you to explain how the adrenal glands work.

   Place an X next to the following statements that are true.

   | | |
   |---|---|
   | "Adrenal hormones differ by age and gender." | |
   | "Aldosterone controls sodium and water balance." | |
   | "Glucocorticoid hormones are necessary for life." | |
   | "The most common cause of adrenal gland hyperfunction is an adrenal gland tumor." | |
   | "Low levels of adrenal hormones can lead to stroke." | |
   | "The adrenal cortex secretes aldosterone and cortisol." | |
   | "When adrenal hormones are overproduced, cancer can result." | |

8. Which drugs belong to the bisphosphonate class of drug? **Select all or any that apply.**

   A. alendronate (Fosamax)
   B. denosumab (Prolia)
   C. estrogen/bazedoxifene (Duavee)
   D. ibandronate (Boniva)
   E. raloxifene (Evista)
   F. risedronate (Actonel)
   G. zoledronic acid (Reclast)

## Next-Generation NCLEX® (NGN) Examination–Style Question

### History and Physical
### 6 Weeks Ago, 1000

A 48-year-old female client presents to the outpatient primary care provider's office and reports fatigue, a decreased sex drive, and feeling cold "all the time."
Physical Exam:
General: appears fatigued
Respiratory: breath sounds clear
Heart Rate: regular rate and rhythm
Skin: dry, flaky

### Today, 0900

The client returns to the office for a follow-up from the previous visit. The client reports feeling "like a new person." The client reports sleeping much better and no longer being cold.
Physical Exam:
General: no acute distress, no exophthalmos noted
Respiratory: breath sounds clear
Heart Rate: regular rate and rhythm
Skin: warm, dry

### Laboratory Results
### 6 Weeks Ago, 1000

| TEST/PANEL | RESULT | NORMAL |
|---|---|---|
| TSH | 17.2 µU/mL (17.2 mU/L) | 0.3–5 µU/mL or 0.3–5 mU/L |
| Free T$_4$ | 0.1 ng/dL (1.2872 pmol/L) | 0.8–2.8 ng/dL or 10–36 pmol/L |
| Hemoglobin | 11.5 (7.1369 mmol/L) | 12–16 g/dL or 7.4–9.9 mmol/L |
| Aldosterone | 21 ng/dL (0.78 nmol/L) | 5–30 ng/dL or 0.14–0.8 nmol/L |

### Flow Sheet
### 6 Weeks Ago, 1000

Blood Pressure: 98/58 mm Hg
Heart Rate: 62/min
Respiratory Rate: 12/min
Temperature: 96.8°F (36°C)
Weight: 150 pounds (68.2 kg)

### Orders
### 6 Weeks Ago, 1000

Levothyroxine 100 mcg PO every morning.
The nurse is preparing to check the client's vital signs and repeat the lab work from the client's previous visit.

**The nurse anticipates that the assessment findings will have increased, decreased, or show no change anticipated from the client's previous visit.**

*Each row must have only one response option selected.*

| ASSESSMENT FINDING | INCREASED | DECREASED | NO CHANGE ANTICIPATED |
|---|---|---|---|
| Body Temperature | | | |
| Heart Rate | | | |
| TSH | | | |
| Body Weight | | | |
| Hemoglobin | | | |
| Blood Pressure | | | |
| Aldosterone | | | |

See answer on Evolve at http://evolve.elsevier.com/Visovsky/LPNpharmacology/.

## Learning Outcomes

1. Describe the differences between diabetes mellitus type 1 and type 2 and explain why most drugs used for type 2 are not useful for type 1.
2. List the names, actions, possible side effects, and adverse effects of insulin stimulators and biguanides.
3. Explain what to teach patients and families about insulin stimulators and biguanides.
4. List the names, actions, possible side effects, and adverse effects of insulin sensitizers and alpha-glucosidase inhibitors.
5. Explain what to teach patients and families about insulin sensitizers and alpha-glucosidase inhibitors.
6. List the names, actions, possible side effects, and adverse effects of incretin mimetics and amylin analogs.
7. Explain what to teach patients and families about incretin mimetics and amylin analogs.
8. List the names, actions, possible side effects, and adverse effects of DPP-4 inhibitors and sodium-glucose cotransport inhibitors.
9. Explain what to teach patients and families about DPP-4 inhibitors and sodium-glucose cotransport inhibitors.
10. List the names, actions, possible side effects, and adverse effects of insulin preparations.
11. Explain what to teach patients and families about insulin preparations.

## Key Terms

**alpha-glucosidase inhibitor** A category of oral non-insulin antidiabetic drugs that lower blood glucose levels by preventing enzymes in the intestinal tract from breaking down starches and more complex sugars into glucose.

**amylin analogs** A category of injectable non-insulin antidiabetic drugs similar to natural amylin, which is a hormone produced by pancreatic beta cells that works with and is co-secreted with insulin in response to blood glucose elevation. It prevents hyperglycemia by delaying gastric emptying and making the patient feel full so he or she eats less.

**biguanides** A category of oral non-insulin antidiabetic drugs that lower blood glucose levels by reducing the amount of glucose the liver releases and by reducing how much and how quickly the intestines absorb the glucose from food.

**diabetes mellitus (DM)** A common chronic endocrine condition in which the lack of insulin or poor function of insulin impairs glucose metabolism, leading to problems in the metabolism of fat and protein.

**DPP-4 inhibitors** A category of non-insulin antidiabetic drugs that help prevent hyperglycemia by reducing the amount of the enzyme dipeptidyl peptidase-4 (DPP-4), which inactivates the normal incretins glucagon-like peptide (GLP) and gastric inhibitory polypeptide (GIP). This action allows the naturally produced incretins to work with insulin to control blood glucose levels.

**glucagon** A hormone produced by alpha cells of the pancreas that raises the concentration of glucose and fat in the bloodstream.

**glucose** A simple sugar that is critically important for energy production in cells and organs.

**hyperglycemia** A condition of higher-than-normal blood glucose levels.

**hypoglycemia** A condition of lower-than-normal blood glucose levels.

**incretin mimetics** A category of non-insulin antidiabetic drugs that act like the natural gut hormones (e.g., glucagon-like peptide 1) that are secreted in response to food in the stomach. They work with insulin to prevent blood glucose levels from becoming too high after meals, resulting in an increase in insulin secretion, a decrease in glucagon secretion, and a slower rate of gastric emptying.

**insulin** A protein hormone produced by the pancreas or injected as a drug that binds to insulin receptors on many cells, which then promotes the movement of glucose from the blood into cells. Sulfonylureas and meglitinides are the two classes of drugs in this category.

**insulin sensitizers** A category of oral non-insulin antidiabetic drugs that lower blood glucose levels by making insulin receptors more sensitive to insulin, which increases cellular uptake and use of glucose.

**insulin stimulators** A category of oral non-insulin antidiabetic drugs that lower blood glucose levels by triggering the release of insulin stored in the beta cells of the pancreas. Sulfonylureas and meglitinides are the two classes of drugs in this category.

**non-insulin antidiabetic drugs** Oral and injectable drugs that use a variety of mechanisms other than binding to insulin receptors to help lower blood glucose levels.

**sodium-glucose cotransport inhibitors** A category of non-insulin antidiabetic drugs that lower blood glucose levels by preventing the kidney from reabsorbing glucose

that was filtered from the blood into the urine. The glucose remains in the urine and is excreted rather than being moved back into the blood.

## DIABETES

### BLOOD GLUCOSE CONTROL

**Diabetes mellitus (DM)** is a chronic, metabolic disease characterized by elevated levels of blood glucose (or blood sugar), which leads over time to serious damage to the heart, blood vessels, eyes, kidneys, and nerves. Diabetes results in the inability of the body to regulate glucose, increasing the patient's risk of acute and chronic health problems and early death. **Glucose** is a simple sugar important for energy production in cells and organs. Glucose is also a part of many carbohydrates. DM type 1 is a chronic condition in which the pancreas produces little or no insulin by itself. In DM Type 2, the body becomes resistant to insulin or does not make enough insulin to support the body's needs.

**Insulin** is a hormone produced by the area of the pancreas known as the *islets of Langerhans* and works to regulate the amount of glucose in the blood. Like other hormones, insulin is a "key" that binds to its cellular receptors, which act as "locks." When insulin binds to its receptors, "doors" on cell membranes open, allowing glucose to enter cells, which lowers the blood glucose level. Glucose in the cells is metabolized to generate the cellular energy needed to maintain maximum cellular and organ function.

When blood glucose levels are lower than normal (**hypoglycemia**), cells and organs cannot metabolize it to provide energy, and cellular function can be greatly reduced. However, too much blood glucose (**hyperglycemia**) leads to severe complications over time, including cardiovascular disease, peripheral nerve damage (neuropathy), kidney failure, and damage to the blood vessels of the retina (diabetic retinopathy) that causes blindness.

Good glucose control, sometimes called *glycemic control*, requires balancing blood glucose so that levels are constantly in the normal range. Table 20.1 lists the desired laboratory values that indicate good blood glucose control for the two most common tests: fasting blood glucose levels and hemoglobin A1c.

#### Table 20.1  Goals for Blood Glucose Control

| LABORATORY TEST | INDICATORS OF GOOD BLOOD GLUCOSE CONTROL |
|---|---|
| Fasting blood glucose (FBG) | Less than 100 mg/dL or 5.6 mmol/L Controlled levels for older adults usually increase by about 1.0 mg/dL (or 0.05 mmol/L) for every decade of life. |
| Glycosylated hemoglobin (hemoglobin A1c) | 4%–6% |

The healthy pancreas controls blood glucose levels through the actions of insulin and another hormone, glucagon. Insulin prevents hyperglycemia by allowing body cells to take up, use, and store carbohydrate, fat, and protein. It is called the *hormone of plenty* because its release is triggered by a high blood glucose level. The actions of **glucagon** are the opposite of those of insulin. It prevents low blood glucose levels by triggering the release of glucose from storage sites in the liver and skeletal muscle. Glucagon is called the *hormone of starvation* because its release is triggered by a lower-than-normal blood glucose level. When these two hormones are released appropriately, blood glucose levels remain in the normal range.

> **Memory Jogger**
> - Insulin is the *hormone of plenty*, which is released when blood glucose levels are above normal. Its function is to lower blood glucose levels and prevent hyperglycemia.
> - Glucagon is the *hormone of starvation*, which is released when blood glucose levels are lower than normal. Its function is to raise blood glucose levels and prevent hypoglycemia.

In addition to insulin and glucagon, other organs and hormones help maintain normal blood glucose levels by balancing glucose uptake by cells and glucose production by the liver. Blood glucose levels after a meal are controlled by the emptying rate of the stomach and the delivery of nutrients to the small intestine, where they are absorbed into circulation. Incretins are metabolic hormones that stimulate a decrease in blood glucose levels. Incretins are released after eating and support the secretion of insulin. Incretin hormones (e.g., glucagon-like peptide 1 [GLP-1]), secreted in response to the presence of food in the stomach, work with insulin to prevent blood glucose levels from becoming too high after meals.

The brain and other parts of the nervous system require a continuous supply of glucose from the blood because they cannot store it. Other organs can use fats as well as glucose to generate energy. In the liver and muscles, glucose is stored as glycogen. Fats are stored as triglycerides in fat cells. During a prolonged fast or after illness, proteins are broken down, and some of their amino acids are converted into glucose. Insulin keeps blood glucose levels from becoming too high, helps maintain blood lipid levels in the normal range, and prevents muscle protein breakdown.

### LOSS OF GLUCOSE CONTROL

Recall that in DM, the *lack of insulin* or *poor function of insulin* impairs glucose metabolism. When glucose metabolism is poor, problems in fat metabolism and protein metabolism also occur. When there is not enough insulin or when insulin does not bind well to its receptor, glucose does not enter cells and instead circulates unused and at high levels in the blood. For this reason, the main feature of DM is chronic hyperglycemia.

 **Memory Jogger**

The main feature of DM is chronic high blood glucose levels (hyperglycemia) because glucose movement from the blood into cells and organs is impaired.

About 34.2 million people in the United States and 5.7 million people in Canada are living with DM. Almost one-third of people with DM have not been diagnosed and are not being treated. Another 96 million have *prediabetes*, which is abnormal glucose metabolism that carries a high risk for developing into actual DM.

Poorly controlled DM can reduce the function of all organs and tissues. The most serious complications of uncontrolled or poorly controlled DM are hypertension, high blood lipid levels, early-onset cardiovascular disease, kidney failure, strokes, and blindness. The complications of DM can be delayed or reduced by maintaining good glycemic control and keeping blood pressure and blood cholesterol levels as close to normal as possible. The classic symptoms of DM are *polydipsia* (increased fluid intake), *polyuria* (excessive urination), and *polyphagia* (hunger with excessive eating). The person with untreated DM remains in a condition of metabolic starvation until insulin is available to move glucose into the cells.

If insulin is not produced by the pancreas or there is a problem with insulin binding to its receptor, cells cannot use glucose for energy. To make up for this problem, the body breaks down fat and protein to provide energy and increase the production of glucose from other sources. Muscle protein is reduced, and the body also moves fatty acids into the blood to use instead of glucose for cellular energy. When this stored fat is used for energy, ketoacids are formed and collect in the blood, resulting in a dangerous and potentially fatal condition known as *ketoacidosis*.

 **Memory Jogger**

**HYPERGLYCEMIA**
**Early Signs**
- Frequent urination
- Increased thirst
- Increased hunger
- Blurred vision
- Fatigue
- Headache

**Late Signs**
- Fruity-smelling breath
- Abdominal pain
- Nausea and vomiting
- Shortness of breath
- Weakness
- Confusion
- Coma

## CLASSIFICATION OF DIABETES MELLITUS

In addition to the diabetes that can occur with pregnancy (*gestational diabetes*), there are two main types of DM. DM type 1 is an autoimmune disorder in which the beta cells of the pancreas that store and release insulin are destroyed. When this occurs, the immune system takes destructive actions and produces antibodies against them. DM type 1 can occur as a result of a genetic predisposition or as a response to infection by certain viruses, such as rotavirus or coxsackievirus. DM type 1 is often diagnosed in childhood, sometimes even before the child is 1 year old. Older names for DM type 1 are *insulin-dependent diabetes mellitus (IDDM)* and *juvenile diabetes*. With DM type 1, the pancreas produces no insulin. The patient must take insulin daily for life unless a pancreas transplant is received.

DM type 2 is a disorder in which the person continues to make some insulin, but it does not bind well to its receptors, and there is a reduced response of the body to insulin, called *insulin resistance*. Eventually, the pancreas makes less and less insulin. Insulin resistance is a complex condition in which the body does not respond as it should to insulin. Several genetic and lifestyle factors can contribute to insulin resistance, such as genetic predisposition, obesity, and decreased physical activity. Usually, DM type 2 develops in adulthood, although with childhood obesity on the rise, some children are being diagnosed with this form of diabetes. Older names for DM type 2 are *non–insulin-dependent diabetes mellitus (NIDDM)* and *adult-onset diabetes*.

About 90% of people with diabetes have DM type 2. Because the pancreas still makes some insulin, their symptoms slowly progress, and many are not aware that they have the disease until long-term complications begin. Although far fewer people have DM type 1, it is usually diagnosed more quickly because the initial symptoms are sudden and severe. It is important to remember that whether a person has DM type 1 or type 2, the long-term complications are the same and often shorten the lifespan.

 **Bookmark This!**

The American Diabetes Association: http://www.diabetes.org

## DRUG MANAGEMENT FOR DIABETES MELLITUS

### NON-INSULIN ANTIDIABETIC DRUGS

Patients with diabetes type 2 usually have a pancreas that functions a little and can be stimulated by drugs to produce more insulin. Although insulin may be necessary for some people with DM type 2, diet, weight reduction, and non-insulin antidiabetic drugs are often effective in maintaining good glycemic control.

**Non-insulin antidiabetic drugs** are oral and injectable drugs that use a variety of mechanisms other than binding to insulin receptors to help lower blood glucose levels. The goal of drug therapy for DM type 2 is to help keep blood glucose levels within the normal target range for each person—not to make the person hypoglycemic. Hypoglycemia is a serious adverse effect of some of these drugs, not the desired effect.

Non-insulin antidiabetic drugs are prescribed when diet and exercise alone are not enough for a patient with DM type 2 to maintain the blood glucose target range identified for that patient. These drugs are not a substitute for diet and exercise for blood glucose control but are used in addition to achieve glucose control. Usually, one drug is started at the lowest effective dose and increased every 1 to 2 weeks until the patient reaches his or her target blood glucose levels or the maximum drug dose is reached without the desired blood glucose control. If the first drug does not adequately control blood glucose levels, a second non-insulin antidiabetic drug that works differently may be added to the first or used alone. Insulin therapy is used only when blood glucose target ranges cannot be met with the use of two or three different types of non-insulin antidiabetic agents.

The non-insulin antidiabetic drugs are divided into eight categories: *insulin stimulators, biguanides, insulin sensitizers, alpha-glucosidase inhibitors, incretin mimetics, DPP-4 inhibitors, amylin analogs,* and *sodium-glucose cotransport inhibitors*. Non-insulin antidiabetic drugs can be in oral or subcutaneous form. Table 20.2 lists the common drugs for each class, their mechanisms of action, usual adult dosages, and nursing implications.

> **Memory Jogger**
>
> There are eight categories of non-insulin antidiabetic drugs:
> - Insulin stimulators
> - Biguanides
> - Insulin sensitizers
> - Alpha-glucosidase inhibitors
> - Incretin mimetics
> - Amylin analogs
> - DPP-4 inhibitors
> - Sodium-glucose cotransport inhibitors

## INSULIN STIMULATORS

### Action and Uses
**Insulin stimulators** are oral non-insulin antidiabetic drugs that lower blood glucose levels by stimulating the release

### Table 20.2  Examples of Insulin Stimulators and Biguanides

*Insulin stimulators* lower blood glucose levels by triggering the release of preformed insulin from beta cells.

*Biguanides* lower blood glucose levels by reducing the amount of glucose the liver releases and by reducing how much and how quickly the intestines absorb the glucose in food.

| DRUG/ADULT DOSAGE | NURSING IMPLICATIONS |
|---|---|
| **Insulin Stimulators** | |
| **Second-Generation Sulfonylurea Agents**<br>glimepiride (Amaryl, Apo-Glimepiride ♣) 1–4 mg orally once daily with breakfast<br>glipizide (Glucotrol) 10–20 mg orally once daily before breakfast<br>glyburide (Diabeta, Micronase) 1.25–20 mg orally daily<br><br><br>**Meglitinide Analogs**<br>nateglinide (Starlix) 120 mg orally three times daily with meals<br>repaglinide (Prandin) 0.5–4 mg orally with meals up to four times daily | • To prevent hypoglycemia, assess patients for indications of hypoglycemia before giving the drug.<br>• If a patient is NPO (nothing by mouth) or is not eating a meal, do not give that dose of the drug.<br>• Teach patients the indications of hypoglycemia: hunger, headache, tremors, sweating, and confusion.<br>• Instruct patients to take these drugs with or just before a meal to prevent hypoglycemia.<br>• Instruct patients taking a sulfonylurea to check with their healthcare provider or a pharmacist before taking any supplements or over-the-counter drugs because sulfonylureas interact with many other drugs.<br>• Instruct patients about the expected common side effects of sulfonylureas.<br>  • Administer within 30 minutes before a meal.<br>  • Teach patients common side effects, including nausea and diarrhea.<br>  • For patients who skip meals, instruct patients to skip a scheduled dose prior to the skipped meal to reduce the risk of hypoglycemia. |
| **Biguanides**<br>metformin<br>Immediate release: 500–850 mg orally twice daily with meals<br>Extended release: 500–2000 mg orally once daily with evening meal | • To reduce the risk of kidney damage, stop metformin for 24 hours before and for 48 hours after a test that uses a radioactive dye.<br>• Tell patients not to cut, crush, or chew the extended-release capsule to prevent rapid absorption of the drug that could lead to adverse effects.<br>• Teach the patient to take metformin with food to avoid gastrointestinal upset.<br>• Inform the patient that metformin may cause diarrhea. |

of insulin stored in the beta cells of the pancreas. The patient must have some functioning beta cells for these drugs to work. They improve the movement of glucose into cells by *increasing the number* of insulin receptors on the cells or *enhancing the actions* of activated insulin receptors. They are used only for DM type 2 and are often used with other non-insulin antidiabetic drugs for best blood glucose control. They also can be used with insulin.

Sulfonylureas and meglitinides are the two classes of drugs in this category. Names, usual adult dosages, and nursing implications of the insulin stimulators are listed in Table 20.2. Consult a drug reference book for more information about specific insulin stimulators.

The sulfonylureas were the first type of non-insulin antidiabetic drugs available to help manage DM type 2. These early drugs, known as *first-generation* sulfonylureas, are rarely used today because of the extensive number of drug interactions. The second-generation sulfonylureas are much more potent than the first-generation drugs and have fewer interactions with other drugs.

The meglitinide analogs are newer insulin stimulators. They work in the same way as sulfonylureas but are more likely to increase insulin release just after a meal, when it is most needed.

### Expected Side Effects

Some common side effects of sulfonylureas are heartburn, nausea, vomiting, abdominal pain, and diarrhea caused by increased gastric acid secretion. They also increase sun sensitivity, which increases the risk of severe sunburns. Common side effects of meglitinides are upper respiratory infections, back and joint pain, and dizziness.

### Adverse Reactions

All insulin stimulators can cause hypoglycemia because they force the pancreas to secrete insulin even when blood glucose levels are normal or low. Hypoglycemia is more pronounced and prevalent in the elderly. A serious problem with insulin stimulators is that over long periods they eventually cause the beta cells of the pancreas to stop producing insulin, a condition known as *secondary beta cell failure*. All of these drugs can affect the liver and increase liver enzyme levels.

 **Memory Jogger**

**INDICATIONS OF HYPOGLYCEMIA**
- Headache
- Hunger sensation
- Difficulty concentrating
- Nervousness
- Tremors
- Increased sweating
- Pale, clammy skin
- Rapid heart rate
- Anxiety, confusion

### Drug Interactions

Sulfonylureas and meglitinides interact with many other drugs. Some drugs or drug groups enhance the hypoglycemic effect of insulin stimulators. They include aspirin and other nonsteroidal anti-inflammatory drugs (NSAIDs), angiotensin II receptor blockers (ARBs), angiotensin-converting enzyme inhibitors (ACEIs), beta-blockers, warfarin, azole antifungal drugs, and many antibiotics. Other common drugs increase the risk of hyperglycemia by reducing the effectiveness of insulin stimulators. These include corticosteroids, furosemide, isoniazid, pseudoephedrine, antiretroviral protease inhibitors, and thiazide diuretics. Always consult a drug reference book or pharmacist for more information about specific drug interactions with sulfonylureas and the meglitinides.

 **Top Tip for Safety**

**DRUG INTERACTIONS**
Sulfonylureas may decrease the effectiveness of certain contraceptive drugs. Women of childbearing years who are taking this antidiabetic drug need an alternative contraceptive method to avoid pregnancy.

### ❖ Nursing Implications and Patient Teaching

◆ *Planning and implementation.* To avoid making hypoglycemia worse, assess patients for signs or symptoms of hypoglycemia before giving an insulin stimulator. Signs of hypoglycemia include tremors, sweating, confusion, rapid heart rate, hunger, headache, nervousness, and inability to concentrate. If any indications are present, check the patient's blood glucose level.

Do not give an insulin stimulator at the same time as other drugs known to increase the hypoglycemic effect. When in doubt, consult a drug reference book or pharmacist about which other drugs increase hypoglycemic effects.

Ensure that these drugs are given with a meal or no more than 15 minutes before a meal to prevent hypoglycemia. It is a good idea to wait until the patient's tray is in the room before giving the drug. If the patient is NPO (nothing by mouth) or is not eating a meal for some other reason, do not give the drug.

 **Top Tip for Safety**

Do not give an insulin stimulator drug to a patient who is NPO or who is skipping a meal.

◆ *Patient and family teaching.* Tell the patient and family:
- Take these drugs with or just before meals to prevent hypoglycemia. If you must skip a meal, also skip the drug dose.
- For signs and symptoms of hypoglycemia, including hunger, nervousness, confusion, sweating, and

tremors, consume some sugar, such as glucose tablets or gel, ½ cup of juice or regular soda, or 1 tablespoon of honey or sugar.
- Check with your healthcare provider or a pharmacist before taking any supplements, over-the-counter drugs, or other prescribed drugs because they interact with many other drugs that can change your blood glucose levels.
- Common but expected side effects of these drugs are nausea, headache, and weight gain.

## BIGUANIDES

### Action and Uses
**Biguanides** are oral, non-insulin antidiabetic drugs that lower blood glucose levels by reducing the amount of glucose the liver releases and by reducing how much and how quickly the intestines absorb the glucose from food. Biguanides improve insulin binding to its cellular receptor site. Unlike the insulin stimulators, biguanides do not force the pancreas to release insulin from beta cells.

The only drug in this class is metformin. The dosages and nursing implications for this drug are presented in Table 20.2.

### Expected Side Effects
The most common side effects of metformin are related to the gastrointestinal system. These include nausea, diarrhea, flatulence, and weight loss. These side effects usually decrease over time.

### Adverse Reactions
Metformin use is associated with a risk of lactic acidosis, an unusually high concentration of lactate in the body. Signs of lactic acidosis include nausea, vomiting, rapid and deep breathing, and weakness. When used without other antidiabetic drugs, metformin alone does not cause hypoglycemia.

### Drug Interactions
Metformin interacts with the radioactive dye (contrast medium) used in some diagnostic tests, which can lead to kidney failure. For this reason, metformin is stopped at least 24 hours before a radioactive dye is used and is not started again until 48 hours after the test is completed.

**Memory Jogger**

**SIGNS OF LACTIC ACIDOSIS**
- Nausea
- Vomiting
- Rapid, deep breathing
- Weakness

### ❖ Nursing Implications and Patient Teaching
◆ *Planning and implementation.* Assess the patient's kidney function. Metformin should not be given to patients with kidney disease because it can cause kidney failure. Assess the patient for signs of lactic acidosis, and report any concerning findings to the healthcare provider.

Check the patient's blood glucose level as ordered, and assess the patient for signs of hypoglycemia. Metformin is safe in pregnancy for the treatment of gestational diabetes.

◆ *Patient and family teaching.* Tell the patient and family:
- Avoid drinking alcohol while taking metformin because this can increase the chance of developing lactic acidosis.
- The common side effects of metformin are mostly forms of GI upset. Nausea, vomiting, and diarrhea may occur, especially when the drug is first started or the dose is increased.
- Metformin should be stopped at least 24 hours before any test that uses radioactive dye and not started again until 48 hours after the test is completed.
- Long-term use of metformin is associated with increased homocysteine levels (a risk factor for cardiovascular disease) and vitamin $B_{12}$ (cobalamin) deficiency. Laboratory tests can be done to check homocysteine and $B_{12}$ levels for prevention and treatment strategies.

 **Top Tip for Safety**
- Metformin should be stopped 24 hours before any diagnostic test that uses radioactive dye.
- Metformin should not be restarted until 48 hours after the test is completed.

## INSULIN SENSITIZERS

### Action and Uses
**Insulin sensitizers** are oral non-insulin antidiabetic drugs that lower blood glucose levels by making insulin receptors more sensitive to insulin, which increases cellular uptake and use of glucose. The drugs in this class are the thiazolidinediones (TZDs), also called *glitazones*. They are used only for DM type 2 and are often used together with other non-insulin antidiabetic drugs for best glycemic control. They also can be used with insulin.

The U.S. Food and Drug Administration (FDA) has issued a black box warning indicating that these drugs are not to be used by patients who have symptomatic heart failure or other specific types of cardiovascular disease. A *black box warning* is a government designation indicating that a drug has a serious side effect and must be used with caution.

The names, usual adult dosages, and nursing implications of the thiazolidinediones are listed in Table 20.3.

### Expected Side Effects
Hypoglycemia is a potential side effect of rosiglitazone (and all agents used to treat diabetes). It can be more

## Table 20.3  Examples of Insulin Sensitizers and Alpha-Glucosidase Inhibitors

*Insulin sensitizers* (thiazolidinediones) lower blood glucose levels by making insulin receptors more sensitive to insulin, which increases cellular uptake and use of glucose.

*Alpha-glucosidase inhibitors* are non-insulin antidiabetic drugs that lower blood glucose levels by preventing enzymes in the intestinal tract from breaking down starches and more complex sugars into glucose.

| DRUG/ADULT DOSAGE | NURSING IMPLICATIONS |
|---|---|
| **Insulin Sensitizers: Thiazolidinediones** | |
| pioglitazone (Actos) initial dose: 15–30 mg orally daily with meal; may increase dose by 15 mg with careful monitoring to 45 mg daily maximum<br>rosiglitazone (Avandia) initial dose: 4 mg orally once daily or in divided doses as 2 mg every 12 hours; dose may be increased to 8 mg orally once daily or in divided doses as 8 mg every 12 hours | • Tell patients to report immediately to the healthcare provider symptoms of allergic reactions (itching, hives, facial swelling).<br>• Monitor patients carefully for signs and symptoms of heart failure (e.g., excessive and rapid weight gain, dyspnea, edema).<br>• Monitor for symptoms of hypoglycemia. |
| **Alpha-Glucosidase Inhibitors** | |
| acarbose (Prandose, Precose) initial dose: 25 mg orally three times daily at the start (with first bite) of each main meal, with a maximum dose of 100 mg orally three times daily<br>miglitol (Glyset)<br>Initial dose: 25 mg orally every 8 hours at meals (with first bite); maintenance dose: 50 mg orally every 8 hours, with a maximum dose of 100 mg orally every 8 hours | • Assess the patient for signs of allergic reaction to the drug.<br>• Monitor the patient for hypoglycemia, especially when this drug is combined with insulin or other antidiabetic drugs.<br>• Monitor the patient for gastrointestinal discomfort or diarrhea, and report findings to the healthcare provider.<br>• Give these drugs at the start of a meal. |

frequent and severe if rosiglitazone is used in combination with insulin as part of the diabetes treatment plan. Headache, sneezing, and sore throat can also occur.

### Adverse Reactions

TZDs have been associated with severe cardiovascular side effects and must be used with care. Currently, rosiglitazone is available only to selected patients, but pioglitazone is still generally available, although closely monitored. Rosiglitazone can also cause fluid retention, liver problems, and macular edema. In addition, TZDs show an increased bone fracture risk in female patients.

### Drug Interactions

Many drugs interact with rosiglitazone. Gemfibrozil, rifampin, and drugs used to treat hypertension all interact with rosiglitazone. Check your drug reference guide or ask your pharmacist about specific drug interactions.

### ❖ Nursing Implications and Patient Teaching

◆ *Planning and implementation.* Assess the patient for signs of allergic reaction (e.g., hives, facial swelling, itching). Assess for signs of heart failure (e.g., weight gain, shortness of breath, tachycardia, edema) and for symptoms of hypoglycemia (e.g., hunger, sweating, pale skin, irritability, dizziness, feeling shaky, trouble concentrating).

◆ *Patient and family teaching.* Tell the patient and family:
• Take the drug as prescribed. If you miss a dose, take it as soon as possible. If you miss a dose and it is almost time for the next one, skip the dose. Do not double up on the drug to make up for missed doses.

• Immediately report to your healthcare provider itching, hives, or swelling of the face or hands if any of these symptoms of allergic reaction occur.
• Report any changes in vision or blurred vision to your healthcare provider.
• Report swelling of the feet or ankles or any rapid weight gain to your healthcare provider.
• Avoid alcohol while taking this drug, because alcohol can affect blood glucose levels, causing hypoglycemia or hyperglycemia, depending on how much alcohol is ingested.
• When signs and symptoms of hypoglycemia are present (e.g., hunger, sweating, pale skin, irritability, dizziness, feeling shaky, or trouble concentrating), eat or drink something that contains real sugar, as directed by your healthcare provider.
• When signs or symptoms of hyperglycemia are present and persist (e.g., headache, increased thirst, dry mouth, blurred vision, fatigue, abdominal pain, or weakness), notify your healthcare provider.
• Check your blood sugar frequently, especially during times of stress or illness because such circumstances can affect blood glucose levels.

### ALPHA-GLUCOSIDASE INHIBITORS

### Action and Uses

An **alpha-glucosidase inhibitor** is an oral non-insulin antidiabetic drug that lowers blood glucose levels by preventing enzymes in the intestinal tract from breaking down starches and more complex sugars into glucose. This action slows glucose absorption. These drugs are primarily prescribed for patients who have high blood glucose levels after meals.

These drugs were first approved to help manage DM type 2 but can also be used for DM type 1 (along with insulin) because they work in the GI tract independently from insulin. Used alone, they cannot cause hypoglycemia. Alpha-glucosidase inhibitors can be used with sulfonylureas, insulin, or metformin. The names, usual adult dosages, and nursing implications of the alpha-glucosidase inhibitors are listed in Table 20.3.

### Expected Side Effects
The alpha-glucosidase inhibitors prevent the breakdown of complex carbohydrates (starches such as bread, cereals, corn, potatoes) into glucose. The carbohydrates remain in the intestine, causing the passing of gas (flatulence), bloating, and diarrhea. These signs and symptoms go away as the body adjusts to the drug and dose.

### Adverse Reactions
Alpha-glucosidase inhibitors can cause the worsening of conditions associated with inflammation of the bowel such as colitis, Crohn's disease, and intestinal obstruction. There is the potential for hypoglycemia when alpha-glucosidase inhibitors are taken with insulin or other drugs for the treatment of diabetes. They also can cause liver impairment, and liver enzymes should be monitored.

### Drug Interactions
There is a risk of hypoglycemia when alpha-glucosidase inhibitors are combined with other antidiabetes drugs such as sulfonylureas, insulin, and meglitinides.

 **Top Tip for Safety**

Alpha-glucosidase inhibitors can cause liver damage. Check liver enzymes as ordered, and report elevations to the healthcare provider.

### ❖ Nursing Implications and Patient Teaching
◆ *Planning and implementation.* Assess the patient for signs of allergic reaction to the drug (e.g., hives, itching, facial swelling). Monitor for signs or symptoms associated with hypoglycemia when this drug is combined with insulin or other antidiabetic drugs. Monitor the patient for GI discomfort or diarrhea, and report findings to the healthcare provider because a dose adjustment may be needed.

◆ *Patient and family teaching.* Tell the patient and family:
- These drugs work best when they are used in conjunction with a proper diet and exercise.
- These drugs are competitive inhibitors of the digestive enzymes, and they must be taken at the start of meals to get the most benefit.
- The drug effect on blood glucose levels after meals depends on the amount of complex carbohydrates in the meal.
- Avoid alcohol because of the potential for liver impairment.
- Report any signs of allergic reaction to the healthcare provider immediately.

## INCRETIN MIMETICS
### Action and Uses
Incretin mimetics are injectable drugs that act like the natural gut hormones (e.g., GLP-1) that are secreted in response to food in the stomach. Just like gut hormones, these drugs work with insulin to prevent blood glucose levels from becoming too high after meals by increasing insulin secretion, decreasing glucagon secretion, and slowing the rate of gastric emptying. The drugs provide satiety (feeling full), which may help the person to eat less.

The injected drugs work with naturally secreted insulin, and they are approved only for patients who have DM type 2 that has not been controlled with oral drugs. They are given by the subcutaneous route, and some (albiglutide, dulaglutide, and exenatide extended release) are long-acting drugs, requiring only weekly dosing. The names, usual adult dosages, and nursing implications of the incretin mimetics are listed in Table 20.4.

### Expected Side Effects
Common side effects of the incretin mimetics include nausea, vomiting, diarrhea, and upper respiratory tract symptoms. Many patients lose weight when taking this drug.

### Adverse Reactions
Incretin mimetics can cause allergic reactions (hives, facial swelling, trouble breathing). There are several long-term adverse effects. Pancreatitis can occur in obese patients with DM type 2, and there is an increased risk of thyroid cancer.

### Drug Interactions
Many herbal products and drugs interact with incretin mimetics. Ask the healthcare provider or pharmacist about potential interactions. Sulfonylureas increase the risk for hypoglycemia. Incretin mimetics slow the absorption of other drugs, including antibiotics and contraceptive drugs. Take other drugs 1 hour before taking an incretin mimetic.

### ❖ Nursing Implications and Patient Teaching
◆ *Planning and implementation.* Assess the patient for signs of allergic reaction to the drug. Check for signs of abdominal pain, bloating, and nausea. Monitor the patient's blood glucose level, especially after beginning this drug. Evaluate the patient for signs of thyroid cancer, such as a lump in the throat or difficulty swallowing.

## Table 20.4 Examples of the Incretin Mimetics and Amylin Analogs

*Incretin mimetics* are non-insulin antidiabetic drugs that act like the natural gut hormones (e.g., GLP-1) secreted in response to food in the stomach. They work with insulin to prevent blood glucose levels from becoming too high after meals. This results in an increase in insulin secretion, a decrease in glucagon secretion, and a slower the rate of gastric emptying.

*Amylin analogs* are injectable non-insulin antidiabetic drugs that are similar to natural amylin, which is a hormone produced by pancreatic beta cells that works with and is co-secreted with insulin in response to blood glucose elevation. They prevent hyperglycemia by delaying gastric emptying and making the patient feel full so that he or she eats less.

| DRUG/ADULT DOSAGE | NURSING IMPLICATIONS |
|---|---|
| **Incretin Mimetics** | |
| albiglutide (Tanzeum) 30–50 mg subcutaneously once weekly in a single-dose, prefilled pen<br>dulaglutide (Trulicity) 0.75–1.5 mg subcutaneously once weekly in a single-dose, prefilled pen or syringe<br>exenatide immediate release (Byetta) 5–10 mcg subcutaneously every 12 hours within 60 minutes before a meal using a single-dose, prefilled pen<br>exenatide extended release (Bydureon) 2 mg subcutaneously once every 7 days using a single-dose, prefilled pen<br>liraglutide (Victoza) 0.6 mg subcutaneously once daily for 7 days, then 1.2–1.8 mg once daily subcutaneously using a single-dose, prefilled pen | • Assess for signs of allergic reaction to the drug.<br>• Assess the patient for pancreatitis (abdominal pain, bloating, and nausea).<br>• Assess the patient's blood sugar level.<br>• Teach the patient and family the correct procedures for preparing the skin, injecting the drug with the pen injector, and disposing needles and syringes.<br>• Assess the patient for signs of thyroid cancer (lump in the throat or difficulty swallowing).<br>• Instruct the patient to avoid alcohol. |
| lixisenatide (Adlyxin) initial dose (green pen: 50 mcg/mL in 3 mL): 10 mcg subcutaneously before first meal of the day—pen provides 14 doses of 10 mcg/dose; maintenance dose (burgundy pen: 100 mcg/mL in 3 mL): 20 mcg subcutaneously 1 hour before first meal of the day—pen provides 14 doses of 20 mcg/dose<br>Semaglutide oral: 3 mg orally once daily for 30 days, then 7 mg orally once daily; may increase the dose to 14 mg orally once daily after at least 30 days; maximum dose: 14 mg/day<br>Semaglutide subcutaneous injection: 0.25 mg subcutaneously once weekly for 4 weeks, then 0.5 mg subcutaneously once weekly; may increase the dose to 1 mg subcutaneously once weekly after 4 weeks; maximum dose: 2 mg/week | • Administer oral drug at least 30 minutes before the first meal or medication to prevent decreasing semaglutide absorption.<br>• Take the oral drug with no more than 4 ounces of plain water.<br>• Swallow oral tablets whole. Do not split, crush, or chew tablets.<br>• Inspect injectable drug for particulate matter and discoloration prior to administration.<br>• Injection pens should never be shared among patients.<br>• Instruct patients/caregivers on proper injection technique.<br>• If a dose is missed, give as soon as possible within 5 days after the missed dose.<br>• Assess the patient for pancreatitis (abdominal pain, bloating, and nausea).<br>• Assess the patient's blood sugar and HA1c levels |
| Dual Glucose-Dependent Insulinotropic Polypeptide (GIP) Receptor and Glucagon-like Peptide-1 (GLP-1) Receptor Agonist<br>tirzepatide (Mounjaro) 2.5 mg subcutaneously once weekly for 4 weeks, then 5 mg subcutaneously once weekly; may increase dose by 2.5 mg/week after at least 4 weeks if needed; maximum dose: 15 mg/week | • Tirzepatide is subcutaneously administered once weekly.<br>• Inspect the drug for particulate matter and discoloration prior to administration.<br>• If particulate matter or discoloration is seen, contact the pharmacist.<br>• Injection pens should never be shared among patients.<br>• Instruct patients/caregivers on proper injection technique.<br>• If a dose is missed, give as soon as possible within 4 days of the missed dose.<br>• Teach patients that GI effects such as nausea, vomiting, and diarrhea can occur.<br>• Assess the patient for pancreatitis (abdominal pain, bloating, and nausea).<br>• Assess the patient's blood sugar and HA1c levels. |
| **Amylin Analogs** | |
| pramlintide (Symlin) by pen injector initial dose: 15 mcg subcutaneously immediately before each meal; maintenance dose: 30–60 mcg subcutaneously immediately before each meal | • Assess for signs of allergic reaction to pramlintide.<br>• Check the blood glucose level after each meal.<br>• Monitor the patient for symptoms of hypoglycemia.<br>• Monitor the patient for dizziness.<br>• Teach the patient and family proper skin preparation and how to correctly inject the drug using the pen injector.<br>• Do not mix pramlintide in the same syringe with any type of insulin.<br>• Teach the patient and family how to rotate the injection sites and properly dispose of the needles and syringes.<br>• Instruct the patient to avoid alcohol. |

Ensure that the patient and family members understand and can demonstrate how to cleanse the skin, inject the drug, rotate injection sites, and properly dispose of the needles and syringes.

◆ *Patient and family teaching.* Tell the patient and family:
- Report any signs or symptoms of allergic reaction to your healthcare provider.
- Avoid alcohol intake because the risk of pancreatic inflammation is already higher due to the way the drug works in your body.
- Monitor your blood glucose level regularly, especially if you are taking more than one drug for your diabetes.
- Seek immediate help for severe abdominal pain and nausea, which can signal pancreatitis.
- If a dose is accidentally missed, do not double up injections, but take the missed dose as soon as possible.
- Give the subcutaneous injection in the thigh, upper arm, or abdomen, rotating injection sites regularly.
- Give the drug 60 minutes before meals, not after meals.
- Refrigerate unused injectable pens until they are used or expired. Dispose of them in a regulation sharps container.

 **Memory Jogger**

**SIGNS AND SYMPTOMS OF ACUTE PANCREATITIS**
- Severe upper abdominal pain that radiates to the back
- Indigestion
- Nausea and vomiting
- Bloating with distended abdomen
- Rapid heart rate
- Elevated blood amylase and lipase levels

## AMYLIN ANALOGS

### Action and Uses
An **amylin analog** is an injectable non-insulin antidiabetic drug similar to natural amylin, which is a hormone produced by pancreatic beta cells that works with and is co-secreted with insulin in response to blood glucose elevation.

The only drug in this class is pramlintide, which prevents hyperglycemia by delaying gastric emptying and making the patient feel full so that he or she eats less. It is used for patients with DM type 1 or type 2. Patients with DM type 1 take this drug because people who do not secrete insulin are usually deficient in amylin. The usual adult dosages and nursing implications for pramlintide are listed in Table 20.4.

### Expected Side Effects
Nausea, vomiting, headache, abdominal pain, weight loss, and fatigue can occur with pramlintide.

### Adverse Reactions
Pramlintide can cause severe hypoglycemia, especially if it is used with insulin to treat diabetes. This effect usually develops within 3 hours after injection of the drug. This drug can cause dizziness.

### Drug Interactions
Some drugs can affect how pramlintide works, including aspirin, atropine, dysopyramide, fluoxetine, pentoxifylline, certain blood pressure and cholesterol drugs, and monoamine oxidase (MAO) inhibitors. Pramlintide can interfere with the actions of antibiotics and birth control pills, and those and other oral drugs should be taken 1 hour before pramlintide.

 **Top Tip for Safety**

Patients taking pramlintide can develop severe hypoglycemia. This occurs most often within 3 hours after injection of the drug, and it is important to monitor patients carefully for signs and symptoms of hypoglycemia during that period.

### ❖ Nursing Implications and Patient Teaching
◆ *Planning and implementation.* Assess for signs of allergic reaction to pramlintide. Check blood glucose levels after meals to assess the effectiveness of the drug and to screen for hypoglycemia. Monitor the patient for dizziness; if present, notify the healthcare provider because the dose may need adjustment.

Ensure that the patient and family understand and can demonstrate the procedures for drawing up the drug, cleansing the skin, injecting the drug, rotating injection sites, and properly disposing the needles and syringes.

◆ *Patient and family teaching.* Tell the patient and family:
- This drug is injected into the thigh or stomach area, and the injection sites are rotated regularly.
- Opened vials and injectable pens should be kept refrigerated. If not refrigerated, they must be used within 28 days and then discarded.
- Allow the drug to warm to room temperature before injecting it.
- Give this injectable drug just before your meal.
- Never mix pramlintide with insulin in the same syringe.
- Dispose of all used syringes and needles in a regulation sharps container.
- If you miss a dose and cannot take it within a reasonable time, skip the dose. Do not double up on doses to make up for a missed dose.
- Do not drink alcohol while taking pramlintide.
- Check your blood glucose level regularly. Do not take pramlintide if your blood sugar is too low.
- This drug can cause dizziness. Do not drive or operate machinery until you know how this drug affects you.

- Report signs and symptoms of hypoglycemia to your healthcare provider.

## DPP-4 INHIBITORS

### Action and Uses

DPP-4 inhibitors are a category of non-insulin antidiabetic drugs that help prevent hyperglycemia by reducing the amount of the enzyme dipeptidyl peptidase-4 (DPP-4), which inactivates the gut hormones (incretins) glucagon-like peptide (GLP) and gastric inhibitory polypeptide (GIP). This action allows the naturally produced incretins to work with insulin to control blood glucose levels. These drugs are approved only for patients who have DM type 2. The names, usual adult dosages, and nursing implications of the DPP-4 inhibitors are listed in Table 20.5.

### Expected Side Effects

Nasopharyngitis, with coldlike symptoms of sneezing, runny nose, cough, and swelling of the nasal passages, can occur. Diarrhea has also been reported with the use of DPP-4 inhibitors.

### Adverse Reactions

Hypoglycemia can occur when DDP-4 inhibitors are given in combination with insulin or a sulfonylurea. Allergic reactions with symptoms of hives, facial swelling, and itching can occur. Reports of acute or fatal pancreatitis have occurred with these drugs. It is unknown whether persons with a history of pancreatitis are at increased risk.

An increased risk of heart failure has been reported among patients receiving saxagliptin and alogliptin.

---

### Table 20.5   Examples of DPP-4 Inhibitors and Sodium-Glucose Cotransport Inhibitors

*DPP-4 inhibitors* are non-insulin antidiabetic drugs that help prevent hyperglycemia by reducing the amount of the enzyme DPP-4, which inactivates the normal incretins, GLP and GIP. This action allows the naturally produced incretins to be present and work with insulin to control blood glucose levels.

*Sodium-glucose cotransport inhibitors* are non-insulin antidiabetic drugs that lower blood glucose levels by preventing the kidney from reabsorbing glucose that was filtered from the blood into the urine. The glucose remains in the urine and is excreted rather than moved back into the blood.

| DRUG/ADULT DOSAGE | NURSING IMPLICATIONS |
|---|---|
| **DPP-4 Inhibitors** | |
| alogliptin (Nesina) 25 mg orally daily<br>linagliptin (Tradjenta) 5 mg orally daily<br>saxagliptin (Onglyza) 2.5–5 mg orally daily<br>sitagliptin (Januvia) 100 mg orally daily | • Assess for signs of allergic reaction or angioedema (swelling of the face, mouth, tongue, or larynx, often accompanied by hives).<br>• Assess patients taking alogliptin for signs and symptoms of heart failure.<br>• Check the patient's blood glucose level regularly.<br>• Monitor for signs and symptoms of hypoglycemia.<br>• Assess for signs and symptoms of pancreatitis. |
| **Sodium-Glucose Cotransport Inhibitors** | |
| canagliflozin (Invokana) initial dose: 100 mg orally daily taken before the first meal of the day; dose may be increased to 300 mg daily in specified patients<br>dapagliflozin (Farxiga) initial dose: 5 mg orally daily in the morning, with or without food; dose may be increased to 10 mg orally daily in specified patients<br>empagliflozin (Jardiance) 10 mg orally daily in the morning, taken with or without food; may increase to 25 mg orally daily<br>ertugliflozin (Steglatro) 5 mg orally daily; maximum dose 15 mg daily | • Assess the patient for signs of allergic reactions.<br>• Assess the patient's blood glucose level.<br>• Assess the patient for signs and symptoms of hypoglycemia.<br>• Assess the patient for unintended weight loss.<br>• Monitor the patient for symptoms of UTI (urgency, burning, painful urination, bloody or dark-colored urine, fever, chills, and back pain).<br>• Monitor female patients for symptoms of vaginal infection (vaginal discharge with itching, redness, burning, and soreness).<br>• Assess the patient for signs of dehydration (increased thirst, dry mouth, decreased urine output, dizziness, and headache).<br>• Monitor the patient's serum potassium level, and assess for symptoms of hyperkalemia (muscle twitching, numbness and tingling, and irregular heart rate).<br>• Teach patients the signs and symptoms of hyponatremia (muscle weakness, abdominal cramping, rapid heart rate, and orthostatic hypotension) because these drugs increase sodium loss. |

*GIP*, gastric inhibitory polypeptide; *GLP*, glucagon-like peptide; *UTI*, urinary tract infection.

Severe arthralgia (joint pain) has been reported in patients taking DPP-4 inhibitors. Bullous pemphigoid, a rare skin condition that results in large, fluid-filled blisters that most often occur on the lower abdomen, upper thighs, or armpits, has also been reported (Fig. 20.1).

### Drug Interactions
The effectiveness of DPP-4 inhibitors may be reduced when they are given in combination with a strong P-glycoprotein inducer (e.g., erythromycin) or a CYP3A4 inducer (e.g., ketoconazole).

### ❖ Nursing Implications and Patient Teaching
◆ *Planning and implementation.* Assess for signs of allergic reaction or angioedema (swelling of the face, mouth, tongue, or larynx, often accompanied by hives; Fig. 20.2). If present, notify the healthcare provider immediately.

Check the patient's blood glucose level to assess the effectiveness of the drug and to screen for hypoglycemia, especially if the patient is taking insulin or a sulfonylurea. Monitor for signs and symptoms of heart failure in patients receiving saxagliptin or alogliptin.

◆ *Patient and family teaching.* Tell the patient and family:
- Take the drug as ordered. If a dose is accidentally missed and cannot be taken within a reasonable time, do not double up on the drug dose. Take the next doses as scheduled.
- Check your blood glucose level regularly, and report any hypoglycemia incidents to your healthcare provider.
- If taking saxagliptin or alogliptin, check your weight daily. Report a weight gain of 2 or more pounds in a day or onset of shortness of breath.
- Report symptoms of allergic reaction or angioedema associated with the drug.
- Report symptoms of acute pancreatitis, such as upper abdominal pain radiating to the back, nausea and vomiting, fever, or rapid pulse.

- Inform your healthcare provider if you become pregnant because it is not known whether these drugs are safe for use in pregnancy or breast-feeding.
- Tell your healthcare provider all the drugs you are taking, including over-the-counter and herbal drugs and supplements, because many drugs can interfere with the effectiveness of DPP-4 inhibitors.

> **⚠ Safety Alert!**
> **DRUG INTERACTIONS**
> - Many drugs used to treat diabetes interact with other drugs the patient may be taking.
> - Obtain a complete list of all drugs and supplements the patient is taking.
> - Drugs for diabetes can interact with oral contraceptives and antibiotics, reducing their effectiveness.

## SODIUM-GLUCOSE COTRANSPORT INHIBITORS
### Action and Uses
Sodium-glucose cotransport inhibitors is a new category of non-insulin antidiabetic drugs that lower blood glucose levels by preventing the kidney from reabsorbing glucose that was filtered from the blood into the urine. The glucose remains in the urine and is excreted rather than being moved back into the blood. These drugs are approved only for patients who have DM type 2. The names, usual adult dosages, and nursing implications of sodium-glucose cotransport inhibitors are listed in Table 20.5.

### Expected Side Effects
An increased need to urinate has been reported by patients taking sodium-glucose cotransport inhibitors.

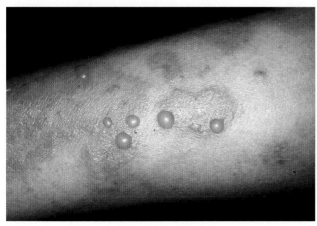
Fig. 20.1 Bullous pemphigoid.

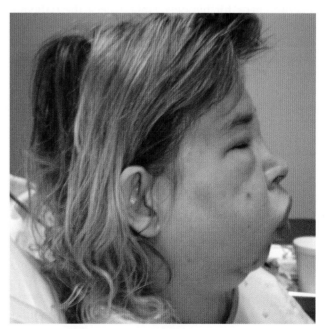
Fig. 20.2 Angioedema. (From Workman, M. L., & LaCharity, L. A. [2016]. *Understanding pharmacology: Essentials for Medication Safety* (2nd ed.). Elsevier.)

Because glucose is excreted in the urine, patients using glucose strips to check the urine see a positive result most of the time. Weight loss, initially through the loss of fluid, followed by loss of fat mass, can occur.

## Adverse Reactions

Vaginal yeast infections and urinary tract infections are the most commonly reported adverse effects, with the greatest risk occurring among female patients and uncircumcised men. Kidney failure, hyperkalemia (high level of potassium in the blood), ketoacidosis, increased risk of bladder cancer, and hypotension (low blood pressure) are other potential serious adverse effects. Allergic reactions, hypoglycemia, and dehydration can occur.

## Drug Interactions

Combining sodium-glucose cotransport inhibitors with insulin increases the likelihood of hypoglycemia. When these drugs are given with diuretics, the frequency of urination increases and dehydration can result. Some drugs, such as rifampin, phenytoin, ritonavir, and phenobarbital, decrease the efficacy of sodium-glucose cotransport inhibitors, requiring an increased dose.

### Memory Jogger

Sodium-glucose cotransport inhibitors can predispose patients to urinary tract and vaginal yeast infections.

### ❖ Nursing Implications and Patient Teaching

◆ *Planning and implementation.* Assess the patient for signs of allergic reaction to sodium-glucose cotransport inhibitors. Monitor the patient's blood glucose level to check for hypoglycemia. Check the patient's weight at the start of therapy and at regular intervals thereafter because these drugs can cause weight loss.

Monitor the patient for symptoms of urinary tract infection (UTI): urgency, burning, painful urination, bloody or dark-colored urine, fever, chills, and back pain. Monitor female patients for symptoms of vaginal infection (vaginal discharge with itching, redness, burning, and soreness).

Assess the patient for signs of dehydration (increased thirst, dry mouth, decreased urine output, dizziness, and headache). Monitor the patient's serum potassium level and for symptoms of hyperkalemia (muscle twitching, numbness and tingling, and irregular heart rate).

◆ *Patient and family teaching.* Tell the patient and family:
- Notify your healthcare provider if you have any symptoms of an allergic reaction to the drug.
- Check your blood glucose level at regular intervals.
- Weigh yourself at least once each week, and report any undue or unexpected weight loss.

- Report signs of a UTI or vaginal infection to your healthcare provider.
- Make sure you are drinking enough fluids throughout the day to prevent dehydration.
- You will see the presence of glucose in your urine if you test your urine with a glucose test strip. This is to be expected because the drug works by excreting glucose into the urine for elimination.

## INSULIN

### Action and Uses

The pancreas is responsible for making insulin and glucagon, both of which work to maintain blood glucose levels. Insulin is made by the beta cells of the pancreas. When blood sugar levels become elevated, insulin is released from the beta cells; this helps restore normal glucose levels by moving insulin into cells and allowing insulin to bind to insulin receptors on the cell membrane (Fig. 20.3). A fasting glucose level of 70 to 90 mg/dL is considered normal. As soon as insulin binds to its receptor, a series of reactions take place, making it easier for glucose to pass into the cell.

In addition to its role in glucose control, insulin is important in fat metabolism. Adequate amounts of insulin inhibit the release of fatty acids into the blood, preventing high blood lipid levels. Insulin is an *anabolic* hormone: one that converts simple substances into more complex compounds; it helps maintain stores of fatty acids, glycogen, and protein. Insulin is considered a *high-alert drug.*

### ⬆ Top Tip for Safety

**HIGH-ALERT DRUG**
- Insulin is a high-alert drug that can cause great harm when it is given at too high or too low a dose, is not given to a patient for whom it has been prescribed, or is given to someone who does not have diabetes.
- If insulin is given at too high a dose or is given to a patient without diabetes, the patient can become severely hypoglycemic, with a risk of death.
- If insulin is given at too low a dose, the patient's blood glucose level will be poorly controlled, increasing the risk of severe hyperglycemia, ketoacidosis, and death.
- Older patients with poor vision may benefit from prefilled insulin syringes, cartridges, or pens to prevent dosing errors.

For glucose control in DM type 1, multiple-dose insulin injections (three to four injections per day), known as *intensive insulin therapy,* or continuous subcutaneous insulin infusion by an insulin pump is recommended (Fig. 20.4). Insulin is destroyed by stomach acids and intestinal enzymes, so it must be given by the parenteral route. Most patients use dedicated insulin syringes with a small, thin needle designed specifically for insulin dosage (in units); they inject the insulin subcutaneously into the thigh, upper arm, or abdomen (Fig. 20.5).

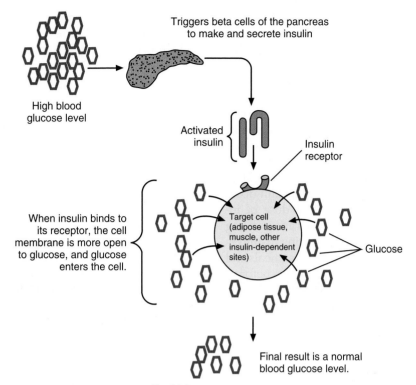

Triggers beta cells of the pancreas
to make and secrete insulin

High blood
glucose level

Activated
insulin

Insulin
receptor

When insulin binds to
its receptor, the cell
membrane is more open
to glucose, and glucose
enters the cell.

Target cell
(adipose tissue,
muscle, other
insulin-dependent
sites)

Glucose

Final result is a normal
blood glucose level.

Fig. 20.3  Action of insulin.

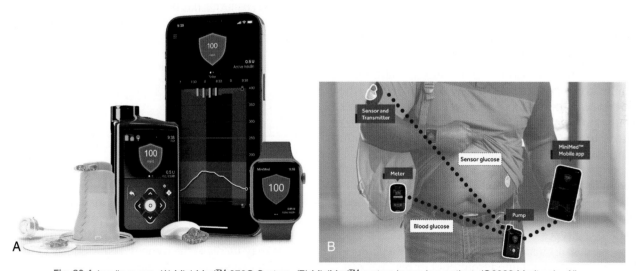

Fig. 20.4  Insulin pump. (A) Mini-Med™ 670G System. (B) MiniMed™ system in use in a patient. (©2023 Medtronic. All rights reserved. Used with the permission of Medtronic.)

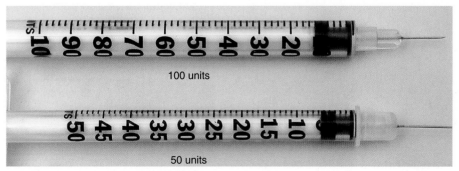

100 units

50 units

Fig. 20.5  U-100 and U-50 syringes. (From Workman, M. L., & LaCharity, L. A. (2016). *Understanding pharmacology: Essentials for Medication Safety* (2nd ed.). Elsevier.)

Various other injection devices have been developed to simplify insulin injection. Some of these devices are designed to look like a pen (Figs. 20.6 and 20.7). The patient sets the dial to the insulin dosage needed and touches the tip of the device to the skin, where the insulin is automatically injected (Box 20.1). These products do not need to be refrigerated, and they can easily be carried by the patient. Internal or external insulin pumps are computer driven and can be programmed to release small doses of insulin continuously, as needed, or hourly.

Each diabetic patient who needs insulin is prescribed an *insulin regimen*, which is a schedule of insulin doses aimed at preventing hyperglycemia. The dose of insulin and how often it should be given varies among patients. Typically, patients take a long-acting insulin in the morning and short-acting insulin to cover meals and snacks. Whenever short-acting insulin is given before a meal, the patient needs to eat the meal within 15 minutes of receiving the injection to prevent hypoglycemia.

The insulin regimen is determined by the patient's blood glucose levels, age, activity level, and eating habits. Some insulin regimens require the patient to self-inject two types of insulin once daily (Box 20.2). Patients need to be taught how to perform home glucose testing and maintain a written or electronic record of their test results. This information, along with hemoglobin A1c testing, is used by the healthcare provider to adjust the insulin regimen.

Patients with DM type 2 may require insulin because type 2 tends to worsen over time, and the pancreas no longer makes enough insulin. The addition of insulin also increases the glucose-lowering effect when oral drugs alone are not adequate. Insulin may also be used for patients with DM type 2 who have allergies to the oral drugs, have liver or renal dysfunction, or are pregnant or contemplating pregnancy.

### Types of Insulin

Many types of insulin are available, including rapid, short-acting, intermediate-acting, and long-acting formulas. The types differ mostly in their duration of action. Almost all insulin used today is synthetic. In the past, insulin was obtained from pork or beef pancreas,

but the development of antibodies to this type of insulin prompted development of human synthetic insulin, which is used today. All types of insulin are regarded as *high-alert drugs* because of the severity of effects that can occur if insulin is given in the wrong dose or to the wrong patient (Table 20.6).

### Expected Side Effects

Expected side effects include mild allergic reactions such as swelling, itching or redness around the injection site, and changes to the skin at injection sites (e.g., lipodystrophy). Lipodystrophy is abnormal fat distribution that resembles a small lump or nodule from repeated injections in the same spot.

### Adverse Reactions

The most important adverse reaction is hypoglycemia. Hypoglycemia can be dangerous because the brain is quite sensitive to low blood glucose levels, which can lead to loss of consciousness and death. Hypoglycemia may develop because of an insulin overdose, increased work or exercise, skipping a meal, or illness associated with vomiting or diarrhea.

> **Top Tip for Safety**
>
> **INSULIN SUBCUTANEOUS INJECTION**
> - Make sure you are preparing the right insulin concentration (U-50, U-100, or U-500) and using the correct syringe designed for that insulin concentration.
> - It is important to rotate injection sites regularly when giving insulin subcutaneously, or lipodystrophy may develop. You should document each site used when giving subcutaneous insulin, according to your institution's policy.

### Drug Interactions

A patient's insulin needs may be increased by other drugs that are considered to be insulin antagonists, such as oral contraceptives, corticosteroids, epinephrine, and thiazide diuretics. Alcohol and anabolic steroids may increase the hypoglycemic effects of insulin. Beta-blockers can mask the signs and symptoms of hypoglycemia.

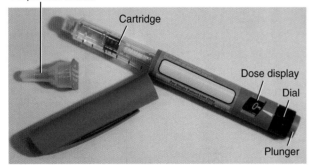

Disposable needle
Cartridge
Dose display
Dial
Plunger

Fig. 20.6 Insulin pen. (From Stein L.N.M. & Hollen C. J. (2024). Concept-based clinical nursing skills: fundamental to advanced competencies (2nd ed.). St. Louis, Elsevier.)

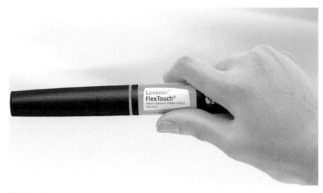

Fig. 20.7 Example of an insulin pen injector. (Courtesy Novo Nordisk Inc.)

## Box 20.1   Giving Insulin with a Pen Device

- Wash your hands.
- Check the order and the drug label.
- Remove the cap.
- If the insulin contains NPH, be sure it is evenly mixed.
- Wipe the tip of the pen with an alcohol swab where the needle will attach.
- Remove the protective pull tab from the needle and screw it onto the pen.
- Remove both the plastic outer cap and the inner needle cap.
- Check the dose window on the pen device, turning the device knob to the appropriate dose.
- Holding the pen with the needle pointing upward, press the button until at least a drop of insulin appears. This is called the *cold shot*, *air shot*, or *safety shot*. Repeat this step if needed until a drop appears.
- Dial the number of units needed,
- Hold the pen perpendicular to and press against the injection site with your thumb on the dosing knob.
- Press the dosing knob slowly all the way to dispense the dose.
- Hold the pen in place for 6 to 10 seconds, then withdraw it from the skin.
- Replace the outer needle cap; unscrew until the needle is removed, and dispose of the needle in a hard plastic or sharps container.
- Replace the cap on the insulin pen.

## Table 20.6   Timed Activity of Pharmaceutical Insulin

| PREPARATION | BRAND | ONSET (hr) | PEAK (hr) | DURATION (hr) |
|---|---|---|---|---|
| **Rapid-Acting Insulin Analogs** | | | | |
| Insulin aspart injection | NovoLog | 0.25 | 1–3 | 3–5 |
| Insulin glulisine injection | Apidra | 0.3 | 0.5–1.5 | 3–4 |
| Human lispro injection | Humalog | 0.25 | 0.5–1.5 | 5 |
| Human lispro injection U-200 | Humalog U-200 | 0.25 | 0.5–1.5 | 5 |
| Insulin human inhalation powder | Afrezza | 0.25 | 1–1.25 | 2.5 |
| **Short-Acting Insulin** | | | | |
| Regular human insulin injection | Humulin R | 0.5 | 2–4 | 5–7 |
| | Novolin R | 0.5 | 2.5–5 | 8 |
| | ReliOn R | 0.5 | 2.5–5 | 8–12 |
| Humulin R (concentrated U-500) | Humulin R (U-500) | 1.5 | 4–12 | 24 |
| **Intermediate-Acting Insulin** | | | | |
| Isophane insulin NPH injection | Humulin N | 1.5 | 4–12 | 16–24+ |
| | Novolin N | 1–4 | 4–14 | 10–24+ |
| | ReliOn N | 1–4 | 4–14 | 10–24+ |
| 70% human insulin isophane suspension/30% human insulin injection | Humulin 70/30 Novolin 70/30 ReliOn 70/30 | 0.5 | 2–12 | 24 |
| 70% insulin aspart protamine suspension/30% insulin as part injection | NovoLog Mix 70/30 | 0.25 | 1–4 | 24 |
| 75% insulin lispro protamine suspension/25% insulin lispro injection | Humalog Mix 75/25 | 0.25 | 1–2 | 24 |
| **Long-Acting Insulin Analogs** | | | | |
| Insulin glargine injection | Lantus | 2–4 | None | 24 |
| Insulin glargine injection U-300 | Toujeo | 2–4 | 12 | 24 |
| Insulin detemir injection | Levemir | 1 | 6–8 | 5.7–24 |
| Insulin degludec injection U-100, U-200 | Tresiba U-100/Tresiba U-200 | 11 | 99 | 4242 |

### ❖ Nursing Implications and Patient Teaching

◆ *Planning and implementation.* Test the patient's blood glucose level before every insulin injection. Carefully check the order for the time, type, and amount of insulin to be given.

Ensure that you are giving the right insulin concentration (U-50, U-100, or U-500) and using the correct syringe designed for the insulin concentration (Fig. 20.8). Check insulin vial for color and clarity. Some insulins are clear, including rapid-acting, short-acting, insulin glargine (Lantus), and insulin detemir (Levemir). All other types of insulin have a cloudy appearance.

If drawing up two different types of insulin, be sure the prescribed insulins are compatible for mixing. Insulin glargine (Lantus) and insulin detemir (Levemir) cannot be mixed with any other type of insulin. Draw up the shorter-acting insulin first, followed by the longer-acting insulin (Fig. 20.9). Be sure to gently roll the insulin vial or device between your hands to gently mix and warm the insulin.

Select the injection site (Fig. 20.10), and cleanse the site with alcohol. Grasp a skin fold with your nondominant hand, insert the needle at a 90-degree angle, and inject the insulin (without aspirating). Withdraw the

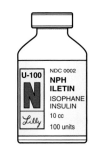

**Fig. 20.8** NPH insulin multidose vial.

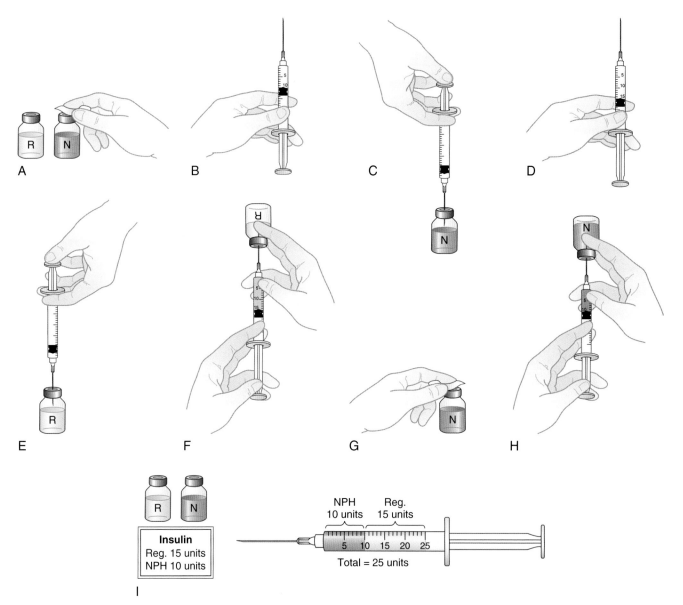

**Fig. 20.9** Mixing two types of insulin in one syringe. (From Clayton, B. D., & Willihnganz, M. L. (2017). *Basic pharmacology for nurses* (17th ed.). Elsevier.)

needle, and place mild pressure on the injection site without massaging it.

Make sure to document the injection site and rotation of sites to prevent lipodystrophy. Make sure the patient has a meal ready to eat before giving insulin. Check the patient at hourly intervals for signs and symptoms of hypoglycemia.

◆ *Patient and family teaching.* Tell the patient and family:
- Teach patients the signs and symptoms of hypoglycemia and hyperglycemia and the appropriate actions to take for each.
- Tell patients to seek emergency treatment for symptoms of ketoacidosis, which include nausea, vomiting, and changes in level of consciousness.
- Teach patients the correct procedure for testing blood glucose levels at home and how to maintain a chart of the results.
- Teach patients the correct procedure to store, draw up, and inject insulin; rotating injection sites; or the care and use of an insulin pump. Use a return demonstration to ensure the effectiveness of the teaching plan (Box 20.2).
- An insulin vial in use may be stored in the refrigerator or for 1 month at room temperature.
- Insulin should be warmed to room temperature for use because the injection of cold insulin may irritate the tissues.
- Check the expiration date of the insulin vial to ensure that the insulin is not out of date.

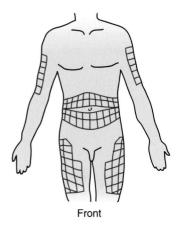

Front

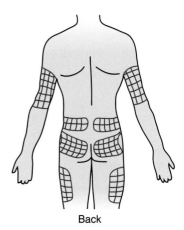

Back

**Fig. 20.10** Injection sites for insulin.

---

| Box 20.2 | **Patient Education Guide for Self-Injection of Insulin** |

- Wash your hands.
- Inspect the insulin container for the type of insulin and the expiration date.
- For rapid-acting insulin, short-acting insulin, insulin glargine, or insulin detemir, inspect the bottle for color and clarity. If particles are present or the insulin is cloudy, discard the bottle and open a new one.
- For other insulins, gently rotate the bottle or container between the palms of your hands to mix the insulin.
- Clean the bottle stopper with an alcohol sponge (leave out this step if you are using a prefilled pen or cartridge).
- Remove the cover from the needle and pull back the plunger to draw in the same amount of air into the syringe as the amount of insulin you will be withdrawing from the bottle.
- Push the needle through the rubber stopper, and inject the air into the insulin bottle with the bottle in the upright position (do not let the air bubble into the insulin).
- With the needle still in the bottle stopper, turn the bottle upside down and withdraw the same amount of insulin from the bottle as the air you put into the bottle.
- Make sure that the tip of the plunger is on the line of the syringe for your insulin dose.
- If air bubbles are present, tap the syringe while holding it upside down, letting the bubbles come to the top of the syringe where the needle is attached. Push out any air bubbles and recheck to ensure that the tip of the plunger is on the same line as your insulin dose.
- Remove the needle from the bottle stopper and recap the needle until you are ready to inject the insulin.
- Select an area within your usual injection site that has not been injected within the past 2 weeks.
- Cleanse the skin area with an alcohol swab.
- Remove the cap from the needle on the insulin syringe.
- Pinch a fold of skin in the area you cleaned and push the needle in at a 90-degree angle.
- Push the plunger all the way down to ensure that the entire insulin dose is injected.
- Release the fold of skin and remove the needle straight out quickly.
- Do not rub or massage the spot where you injected the insulin.
- Place the syringe with the needle (without recapping it) into a puncture-proof container.

From Workman, M. L., & LaCharity, L. A. (2016). *Understanding pharmacology: Essentials for Medication Safety* (2nd ed.). Elsevier.

- Gently roll the insulin vial before drawing up the insulin. Vigorous shaking may result in air bubbles and breaks down protein molecules in the insulin.
- Avoid drinking alcohol because it can intensify the hypoglycemia produced by insulin, causing blood glucose levels to fall too low.
- Insulin requirements increase when you are under stress or are ill with an infection. Check your blood glucose level frequently, and report abnormal results to your healthcare provider.
- Always carry a readily available source of sugar in case symptoms of hypoglycemia develop suddenly.

## Get Ready for the Next-Generation NCLEX® Examination!

### Key Points

- Insulin is the hormone of plenty, which is released when blood glucose levels are *above* normal. Its function is to lower blood glucose levels and prevent hyperglycemia.
- Glucagon is the hormone of starvation, which is released when blood glucose levels are *lower* than normal. Its function is to raise blood glucose levels and prevent hypoglycemia.
- Most patients with diabetes have DM type 2, and many have prediabetes but are not aware they have the disease.
- Patients diagnosed with DM type 1 or type 2 can develop serious long-term complications that shorten the lifespan.
- Good management of DM consists of keeping blood glucose levels within the normal range to delay or prevent serious complications.
- People who have DM type 1 must use insulin to control blood glucose levels for the rest of their lives because their bodies produce no insulin.
- All insulin stimulator drugs can cause hypoglycemia when taken alone.
- Do not give an insulin stimulator drug (sulfonylurea or meglitinide) to a patient who is NPO or who is skipping a meal.
- Insulin is a high-alert drug that can cause great harm when given at too high a dose, at too low a dose, or to someone who does not have diabetes.

### Clinical Judgment and Next-Generation NCLEX® Examination-Style Questions

1. Complete the following sentences by choosing the most probable option for the missing information that corresponds with the same numbered list of options provided.

   You are preparing an injection of insulin for a diabetic patient, and you note the fluid appears cloudy, so you _____1_____. As you prepare to give the patient insulin, the correct procedure includes _____2_____. After insulin is given, the patient should be instructed to _____3_____. The nurse should monitor the patient for the adverse effect of _____4_____ when giving insulin.

| OPTIONS FOR 1 | OPTIONS FOR 2 |
|---|---|
| notify the pharmacy | shaking the insulin vial vigorously before drawing the drug up into the syringe |
| shake the vial to disperse the drug | assessing and rotating the injection sites |
| administer the insulin as scheduled | giving the insulin at a 45-degree angle |
| administer a rapid-acting insulin instead as they are interchangeable | giving the insulin at a cold temperature, directly from the refrigerator |

| OPTIONS FOR 3 | OPTIONS FOR 4 |
|---|---|
| massage the injection site to prevent bleeding | hyperglycemia |
| eat a meal within 15 minutes of receiving the injection to prevent hypoglycemia | hypoglycemia |
| recap the syringe before disposing of it in a sharps container | hypertension |
| check their blood sugar 1 hour after the injection | respiratory distress |

2. Which statement made by a female patient would raise concern that she is experiencing an adverse effect of the prescribed sodium-glucose cotransport inhibitor?

   1. "I have a very bad headache."
   2. "I seem to be forgetting some things lately."
   3. "I have burning when I urinate."
   4. "I have had a bloody nose this morning."

3. A patient with DM type 2 has been prescribed sitagliptin 100 mg daily. You have 50-mg tablets available. How many tablets should you give this patient?

   1. Three tablets
   2. One and a half tablets
   3. Two tablets
   4. None. This drug is available only in an injectable form

4. An obese 72-year-old woman with DM type 2 has been prescribed the amylin analog pramlintide. In addition to diabetes, her medical history includes high cholesterol levels and hypertension.

   Place an X next to the information that should be included in her drug teaching plan.

| | |
|---|---|
| Take this drug daily with food. | |
| Weight loss and fatigue can occur when taking pramlintide. | |
| If a dose is missed, double the next dose to be taken. | |
| Warm this drug to room temperature before injecting it. | |
| Check your blood glucose level regularly. | |
| Avoid alcohol when taking this drug. | |
| Pramlintide can result in excessive blood clotting. | |
| You can add your insulin to the same syringe with pramlintide. | |
| Dizziness can occur with pramlintide. | |

5. A 35-year-old female patient with diabetes mellitus who is taking an oral antidiabetic drug comes in for a regularly scheduled clinic appointment. She tells you that she is currently taking an oral contraceptive agent for birth control. What is your best response?

   1. "Oral contraceptives are contraindicated for diabetics."
   2. "Oral contraceptives can be taken only if you are on insulin."
   3. "Oral contraceptives can be safely taken with oral antidiabetic agents."
   4. "Oral contraceptives reduce their effectiveness of oral antidiabetic agents."

6. What instructions should be included in the medication safety teaching for a patient taking metformin?

   1. "Wash your hands and prepare the skin before injecting this drug to prevent infection."
   2. "Stop metformin for 24 hours before and for 48 hours after a test that uses a radioactive dye."
   3. "Metformin can cause severe constipation, so use a stool softener daily."
   4. "Take metformin on an empty stomach to increase absorption."

## Next-Generation NCLEX® (NGN) Examination–Style Question

### History and Physical
#### 1300

A 67-year-old male client presents to the emergency department with complaints of shortness of breath and left-sided chest pain that "started suddenly."
Past Medical History: hypertension, diabetes mellitus type 2
Home Medications: metformin 1000 mg orally twice daily, insulin glargine 20 units subcutaneous every evening, lisinopril 20 mg orally daily
Social History: denies tobacco or alcohol use

### Nurse's Notes
#### 1500

The client is admitted to the medical-surgical unit for further care.

#### 1900

The nurse is called to the client's room. The client reports nausea, vomiting, and weakness.

### Flow Sheet
#### 1300

Blood Pressure: 138/88 mm Hg
Heart Rate: 88/min
Respiratory Rate: 18/min
Temperature: 101.2°F (38.4°C)

#### 1900

Blood Pressure: 132/84 mm Hg
Heart Rate: 84/min
Respiratory Rate: 26/min
Temperature: 100.6°F (38.1°C)

### Imaging Studies
#### 1300

EKG: normal sinus rhythm

#### 1330

Computed tomography chest with and without iodinated contrast: no pulmonary embolism detected. Findings consistent with left lower lobe pneumonia.
A nurse is caring for the client on a medical-surgical unit.

Choose the most likely options for the information missing from the statement(s) by selecting from the lists of options provided.

The nurse should first check the client's ____1____ in order to assess for the development of ____2____.

| OPTIONS FOR 1 | OPTIONS FOR 2 |
|---|---|
| Hemoglobin A1c | Hyperglycemia |
| Fasting glucose | Anemia |
| Serum lactate | Hypoglycemia |
| Hemoglobin | Lactic acidosis |
| Homocysteine levels | Cardiovascular disease |

See answer on Evolve at http://evolve.elsevier.com/Visovsky/LPNpharmacology/.

## Learning Outcomes

1. List the names, actions, possible side effects, and adverse effects of bisphosphonates to treat osteoporosis.
2. Explain what to teach patients and families about bisphosphonates to treat osteoporosis.
3. List the names, actions, possible side effects, and adverse effects of selective estrogen receptor modulators to treat osteoporosis.
4. Explain what to teach patients and families about selective estrogen receptor modulators.
5. List the names, actions, possible side effects, and adverse effects of calcitonin to treat osteoporosis.
6. Explain what to teach patients and families about calcitonin to treat osteoporosis.
7. List the names, actions, possible side effects, and adverse effects of parathyroid hormone analogs and

parathyroid hormone-related protein analogs to treat osteoporosis.
8. Explain what to teach patients and families about drugs about parathyroid hormone analogs and parathyroid hormone-related protein analogs to treat osteoporosis.
9. List the names, actions, possible side effects, and adverse effects of select monoclonal antibodies to treat osteoporosis.
10. Explain what to teach patients and families about select monoclonal antibodies to treat osteoporosis.
11. List the names, actions, possible side effects, and adverse effects of select sclerostin inhibitors.
12. Explain what to teach patients and families about select sclerostin inhibitors.

## Key Terms

**bisphosphonates** Bone-modifying drugs that prevent loss of calcium and increase bone density by moving blood calcium into the bone, binding to calcium in the bone, and preventing osteoclasts from destroying bone cells and resorbing calcium.

**bone remodeling** The continuous process in which old bone is resorbed and new bone is formed.

**bone resorption** The process in which osteoclasts breakdown old bone, releasing calcium and phosphate into the blood. It leads to a decrease in bone mass and bone density.

**calcitonin** A hormone, normally produced by specialized cells in the thyroid gland, that decreases bone resorption by the osteoclasts. The drug calcitonin is available to treat osteoporosis.

**osteoblast** Specialized cells that form bone and synthesize collagen and other substances that help create bone matrix.

**osteoclast** Specialized cells that break down old bone in the process of bone resorption.

**osteoclast monoclonal antibodies** Laboratory-made drugs that are designed to serve as substitute antibodies to target immature osteoclasts and decrease bone resorption.

**osteocyte** The most common cells in bone that help regulate bone remodeling and bone resorption.

**osteoporosis** The gradual loss of bone density and strength, which leads to spinal shortening and increased risk for bone fractures.

**parathyroid hormone analogs and parathyroid hormone-related protein analogs** These drugs can stimulate osteoblasts to build bone. This results in an increase in bone remodeling and bone strength. Reserved for patients with a high risk of fracture.

**sclerostin inhibitors** Drugs are used for patients at high risk for fracture. It helps increase activity of osteoblasts, resulting in formation of new bone.

**selective estrogen receptor modulators (SERMs)** Drugs for osteoporosis that target specific estrogen receptors. The SERMs are used to treat osteoporosis and act by activating estrogen effects on bone tissue (decreasing bone resorption and increasing bone density) while blocking estrogen effects on the breast and the uterine tissue.

## OVERVIEW OF OSTEOPOROSIS

**Osteoporosis** is metabolic bone disorder that causes the bones to become weak and brittle from the gradual loss of bone density (think *porous bone*). It affects about 10 million people in the United States over the age of 50, with an additional 43 million with low bone density *(osteopenia)*. It is not a normal part of aging but,

rather, a significant skeletal disease that causes the bone to be increasingly fragile and more likely to fracture. Patients with osteoporosis are more likely, even with minor falls, to have fractures of the hip, lumbar vertebrae, and forearms. They also have a greater risk for pain, disability, placement in long-term care, and premature death (Box 21.1).

| Box 21.1 | Examples of Risk Factors for Osteoporosis |

- Female
- Age 50 or older
- Decreased intake of calcium and/or vitamin D
- Smoking
- Rheumatoid arthritis
- Sedentary lifestyle
- White or Asian race
- Positive family history
- Increased alcohol intake
- Low testosterone
- History of any previous fracture
- Increased caffeine intake
- Low body weight/small body frame
- Hyperthyroidism
- Early menopause (e.g., surgical)
- Cushing syndrome

Adapted from Visovsky, C., Zamboroski, C., & Lutz, R. M. (2023). Osteoporosis medications. In *Edmunds pharmacology for the primary care provider* (5th ed.). Elsevier.

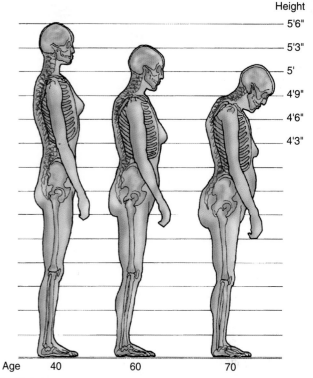

Height

— 5'6"
— 5'3"
— 5'
— 4'9"
— 4'6"
— 4'3"

Age      40            60            70

**Fig. 21.1** A normal spine at 40 years of age, and osteoporotic changes at 60 and 70 years of age. (From Ignatavicius, D. D., & Workman, M. L. (2016). *Medical-surgical nursing: Patient-centered collaborative care* (8th ed.). Saunders.)

Bone cells are continually in a process of building and breakdown (**bone remodeling**), responding to factors such as amount of weight bearing, repair from bone injury, influence of certain hormones, and nutritional intake. Normally, bone mass increases through childhood and adolescence, with peak bone mass reached between about 20 and 30 years of age. Bone density stabilizes until it begins a gradual decrease around age 40. As people age, the rate of bone loss occurs at a faster rate than bone remodeling, resulting in an overall loss of bone mass (Fig. 21.1). In other words, the process of breaking down bone (**bone resorption**) by cells called **osteoclasts** occurs at a faster rate than **osteocytes** and **osteoblasts** can rebuild bone. When excessive osteoclastic activity occurs, minerals (especially calcium) are lost from the bones, making them thinner and weaker, with an increased risk for bone fractures (Fig. 21.2).

 **Memory Jogger**

Bone density requires a constant supply of calcium, and dietary calcium requires activated vitamin D for absorption from the intestinal tract. Both are essential for healthy bones!

Osteoporosis can affect people of all genders and races. However, the rate and degree of bone density loss varies from person to person. For some people, osteoporosis occurs as early as age 40. For others, loss of bone density may not be obvious until age 75 or older. Bone loss accelerates in women at the age of menopause (typically in the late 40s or early 50s) and can lead to a significantly increased risk of fracture. Men can also be affected by osteoporosis, although it tends to occur at an older age (Fig. 21.3).

A variety of factors can contribute to the development of osteoporosis including age, lifestyle, family history, and race (Box 21.1). For example, prevalence of osteoporosis is higher in females who are of Asian and white heritage. While Asians and whites are more

likely to be diagnosed with osteoporosis, people of black heritage are still at risk for and more likely to die from fracture due to osteoporosis (see Box 21.2). Certain medications and medical conditions are associated with an increased risk of osteoporosis. For example, you may have a patient who has chronic lung disease who is taking long-term glucocorticoids or a patient with Barrett's esophagus who is taking long-term proton pump inhibitors and may develop osteoporosis (see Box 21.3).

Although osteoporosis cannot be fully prevented or cured, its progress can be slowed with drug therapy. Drugs and supplements that are used to manage the disorder include *bisphosphonates, selective estrogen receptor modulators (SERMS), calcitonin, parathyroid and parathyroid-hormone related protein analogs, osteoclast monoclonal antibodies, sclerostin inhibitors, calcium,* and *activated vitamin D*. The names, dosages, and nursing implications for common examples of these drugs are summarized in Table 21.1.

 **Bookmark This!**

**INTERNATIONAL OSTEOPOROSIS FOUNDATION CALCIUM CALCULATOR: https://www.iofbonehealth.org/calcium-calculator**
Dietary intake of calcium and vitamin D is important in the prevention and treatment of osteoporosis. This online calcium calculator is available for use in seven languages and for countries around the world. It can be used by nurses or patients to better understand their calcium needs.

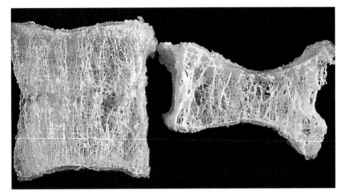

Fig. 21.2 Normal vertebral body (left) left compared to a vertebral body that has been shortened by compression fractures from osteoporosis (right). (From Kumar V, et al. (2021) *Robbins & Cotran pathologic basis of disease* (10th ed.). Elsevier.)

# DRUGS FOR OSTEOPOROSIS

Drugs used to treat osteoporosis generally act by either *decreasing resorption of bone* or by *increasing bone formation*. Bisphosphonates, SERMS, calcitonin, and osteoclast monoclonal antibodies decrease resorption of bone. The *parathyroid and parathyroid-hormone related protein analogs* help to build bone. Sclerostin inhibitors primarily increase bone formation but also can decrease bone resorption. Calcium and vitamin D are supplements essential for bone health and so will be discussed here.

## BISPHOSPHONATES

### Action and Uses

Bisphosphonates are the most commonly used drugs to treat osteoporosis. Bisphosphonates act by decreasing the ability of osteoclasts to break down bone cells. They can reduce the risk of hip, vertebral, and nonvertebral fractures in females diagnosed with osteoporosis. They also can decrease the risk of vertebral fracture in males diagnosed with osteoporosis. Additional uses are for prevention of skeletal fractures in patients with bone metastases or multiple myeloma, treatment of Paget disease, and treatment of cancer-induced hypercalcemia. Bisphosphonates are available in oral and intravenous (IV) forms and may be administered on a variety of schedules, including daily, weekly, monthly, even up to every 2 years depending on the individual drug.

### Expected Side Effects and Adverse Effects

Common side effects of the bisphosphonates are nausea, muscle and joint pain, nausea, and diarrhea. Other gastrointestinal (GI) effects include esophagitis, esophageal ulceration, and esophageal erosion that can lead to bleeding if not prevented. While relatively rare, jawbone necrosis *(osteonecrosis)* can develop with tooth extraction or other invasive dental procedures in which the jawbone is damaged (Fig. 21.4); this adverse reaction is more common in patients who are taking higher doses or the IV form of the drug.

### ❖ Nursing Implications and Patient Teaching

◆ *Assessment.* Because these drugs can cause esophageal erosion, it is imperative to consider the patient's

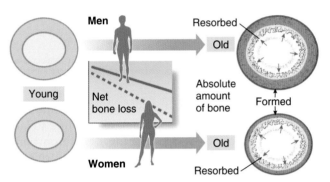

Fig. 21.3 Bone loss comparison in men and women. With aging, the absolute amount of bone resorbed on the inner bone surface and formed on the outer bone surface is greater in men than in women. (From Rogers, J. L. (2024). *McCance & Heuther's pathophysiology: The biologic basis for disease in adults and children* (9th ed.). Elsevier.)

ability to swallow if taking an oral bisphosphonate. They must be able to sit up or stand at least 30 minutes after taking the oral form. Remaining upright at least 30 minutes is the best way to help prevent GI complications. Report any use of aspirin or any nonsteroidal anti-inflammatories (NSAIDs) as these should be avoided while taking bisphosphonates. Assess for any dental concerns and report to the healthcare provider.

◆ *Planning and implementation.* Oral forms should be given first thing in the morning before any food, beverages, or other drugs have been taken. It should be given with *plain water only*, and the patient must be able to sit or stand for at least 30 minutes. If the patient misses a dose, they should not take it later in the day but should return to the usual schedule the next day.

◆ *Evaluation.* Report any jaw or esophageal pain to the healthcare provider as this may indicate adverse effects from bisphosphonates. Ensure that the patient also is maintaining adequate calcium and vitamin D intake.

◆ *Patient and family teaching.* Tell the patient and family:
  • Take oral bisphosphonates first thing in the morning with a full glass of plain water.

| Box 21.2 | Risk for Osteoporosis in Black Females |
|---|---|

While black females typically have a greater bone density than white females, they still have risk factors that may lead to diagnosis, including the following:

- More prone to lactose intolerance
- More likely to be diagnosed with sickle cell anemia or lupus both linked to higher risk
- Less likely to be screened for osteoporosis
- Less likely to receive an osteoporosis therapy when diagnosed
- Less awareness of osteoporosis risk
- More likely to have decreased calcium intake overall

From National Council on Aging. (2022). Osteoporosis: The risk factors for Black women. https://www.ncoa.org/article/osteoporosis-the-risk-factors-for-black-women

- Do not take any food, beverages, or drugs for at least 30 minutes after taking oral bisphosphonates. In certain oral bisphosphonates, it is best to wait at least 2 hours before a standard breakfast is eaten, so always check with the pharmacy.
- Remain in the upright position (sitting, standing, or walking) for at least 30 minutes after taking these drugs to prevent esophageal irritation.
- Inform your dentist or oral surgeon that you are taking a bisphosphonate before you have a tooth extraction or invasive dental procedure involving the jawbone.
- Report any swelling, pain, redness, or other signs of infection in the gums that may indicate osteonecrosis.

## SELECTIVE ESTROGEN RECEPTOR MODULATORS (SERMS)

### Action and Uses

Selective estrogen receptor modulators (SERMs) that are used in treating osteoporosis produce an estrogen-like effect on bone. They are "selective" because they are targeted to decrease bone breakdown by osteoclasts but do not have significant estrogen effects on the breast and endometrium. They do, however, increase estrogen effects on clotting and on lipid metabolism, so they can increase the risk of cardiovascular effects if improperly used. They are used in postmenopausal women at risk for vertebral fracture. SERMs are not used as often as other drugs for osteoporosis because of their cardiovascular effects. The main drug in this category is raloxifene.

### Expected Side Effects and Adverse Effects

The most common side effects are hot flashes, nausea, joint aches, and muscle cramps. Weight gain has been reported in about 9% of patients. Because these drugs can affect clotting, they can cause deep vein thrombosis, pulmonary embolism, and even stroke.

❖ **Nursing Implications and Patient Teaching**

◆ *Assessment.* Raloxifene should only be used in postmenopausal females, so it is important to verify that

| Box 21.3 | Examples of Medications and Medical Conditions That May Cause Loss of Bone Mass and Osteoporosis |
|---|---|

- Glucocorticoids
- Lithium
- Proton pump inhibitors
- Tamoxifen
- Anticonvulsants
- Medroxyprogesterone acetate
- Aromatase inhibitors
- Selective serotonin reuptake inhibitors
- Serotonin and norepinephrine reuptake inhibitors
- Thiazolidinediones
- Calcineurin inhibitors
- Certain chemotherapy agents
- Cushing disease
- Multiple myeloma
- Chronic obstructive pulmonary disease
- Diabetes
- Chronic kidney disease
- Chronic liver disease
- Hypogonadism
- Inflammatory bowel diseases (Crohn's disease and ulcerative colitis)
- Anorexia nervosa and/or bulimia nervosa
- Hyperparathyroidism

Adapted from Visovsky, C., Zamboroski, C., & Lutz, R. M. (2023). Osteoporosis medications. In *Edmunds pharmacology for the primary care provider* (5th ed.). Elsevier.

the patient meet this criterion. In addition, report if the patient has any history of deep vein thrombosis, pulmonary emboli, or cardiovascular events. Assess to determine whether the patient uses alcohol or tobacco products as these can increase the risk for adverse effects.

◆ *Planning and implementation.* It is important for patients taking raloxifene to report any symptoms of leg swelling, shortness of breath, or chest pain to the healthcare provider immediately. In addition, they should continue to maintain adequate intake of calcium and vitamin D.

As a nurse, it is important to avoid handling crushed or broken tablets and to wash hands after giving the drug

◆ *Evaluation.* Notify the healthcare provider if patients report any significant side effects or adverse effects of raloxifene.

◆ *Patient and family teaching.* Tell the patient and family:
- Raloxifene can be given without regard to meals.
- Because this drug can increase the risk of clotting, it is important to report any chest pain, confusion, shortness of breath, leg swelling, trouble speaking, severe headache, or any weakness of the face, arms, or legs (especially on one side of the body).
- Avoid smoking or using tobacco products as they may increase the risk for clotting.

Table **21.1**  **Examples of Common Drugs for Osteoporosis**

*Bisphosphonates* reduce the rate of osteoporosis by moving blood calcium into the bone, binding to calcium in the bone, and preventing osteoclasts from destroying bone cells and resorbing calcium.

*Selective estrogen receptor modulators* (SERMs) slow the rate of osteoporosis by activating estrogen receptors in the bone, which leads to reduced calcium resorption and increased bone density. They can be used in prevention and treatment of osteoporosis.

*Calcitonin* decreases breakdown of calcium in the bone by osteoclasts. It can be used in women who are at least 5 years past menopause.

*Parathyroid hormone analogs* and *parathyroid hormone-related protein analogs,* when given intermittently, can stimulate bone-building cells, resulting in new bone formation. They can be used to treat and prevent osteoporosis.

*Osteoclast monoclonal antibodies* bind receptors on immature osteoclasts and on certain white blood cells, preventing them from becoming mature and attacking bone tissue. The result is decreased bone loss and increased bone density and strength.

*Sclerostin inhibitors* are used for patients at high risk for fracture or for whom other therapies have failed. They consist of a glycoprotein from osteocytes that, when inhibited, stimulate osteoblast activity and formation of new bone.

| DRUG/ADULT DOSAGE | NURSING IMPLICATIONS |
|---|---|
| **Bisphosphonates** | |
| alendronate (Fosamax) 5–10 mg tablet orally daily or 35–70 mg once weekly (weekly tablets, oral solution or effervescent tablets for oral solution)<br><br>ibandronate (Boniva) 150 mg orally once per month, or 3 mg intravenous (IV) bolus once every 3 months<br><br>risedronate (Actonel, Atelvia) 5 mg orally daily (daily tablets), or 35 mg orally once weekly (weekly tablets), or 75 mg orally on 2 consecutive days once a month, or 150 mg orally once per month (monthly tablets)<br><br>zoledronic acid (Reclast) 5 mg IV infusion slowly over a minimum of 15 minutes once yearly or every other year | • Teach patients to take the drug first thing in the morning, at least 30 minutes before breakfast and before taking other drugs, for best absorption and to prevent drug interactions.<br>• Tell patients to remain upright (sitting or standing) for 30 minutes after taking the drug to help prevent esophageal irritation or reflux.<br>• Remind patients to have a dental examination every 6 months and to tell the dental professional about taking a bisphosphonate because it can cause jawbone osteonecrosis.<br>• Infuse the IV form of the drug slowly over a minimum of 15 minutes. These must be administered by healthcare professionals and are typically used in patients with esophageal abnormalities. |
| **Selective Estrogen Receptor Modulators** | |
| estrogen/bazedoxifene (Duavee) for prevention of osteoporosis in postmenopausal women, one tablet orally daily (contains 0.45 mg of conjugated estrogen and 20 mg of bazedoxifene)<br><br>raloxifene (Evista) 60 mg orally once daily | • Urge patients not to smoke while taking these drugs to reduce the risk of blood clots, heart attacks, and strokes. |
| **Calcitonin** | |
| **Calcitonin-salmon** 100 IU intramuscularly or subcutaneously once daily, or 200 IUs (1 spray) intranasally in one nostril once daily | • Consider periodic nasal examination for signs of nasal trauma for those using the nasal route.<br>• If using intranasally, rotate nostrils every other day.<br>• Ensure adequate calcium and vitamin D intake.<br>• Reserve use for patients more than 5 years past menopause in whom alternative treatments are not suitable.<br>• Read package instructions carefully for proper storage and administration. |
| **Parathyroid hormone analogs and parathyroid hormone-related protein analogs** | |
| teriparatide (Forteo) 20 mcg subcutaneously once daily<br>abaloparatide (Tymlos) 80 mcg subcutaneously once daily | • Available in a prefilled pen for injection.<br>• Administer as directed subcutaneously. Do not administer intramuscularly or IV.<br>• Generally used for no longer than 2 years due to the risk of complications.<br>• Watch for signs of hypercalcemia and hypercalciuria, such as nausea, vomiting, constipation, depression, and palpitations.<br>• Teach patient to stand slowly after sitting or lying down in case of orthostatic hypotension.<br>• Carefully follow package instructions for storage and administration. |

| Table 21.1 | Examples of Common Drugs for Osteoporosis—cont'd |
| --- | --- |
| **DRUG/ADULT DOSAGE** | **NURSING IMPLICATIONS** |
| **Osteoclast Monoclonal Antibodies** | |
| denosumab (Prolia) 60 mg subcutaneously once every 6 months | • Remind patients to have a dental examination every 6 months and to tell the dental professional about taking this drug, because it can cause jawbone osteonecrosis.<br>• Carefully follow package instructions for proper administration. This drug must be given by a healthcare professional. |
| **Sclerostin Inhibitor** | |
| romosozumab (Evenity) 210 mg subcutaneously monthly for 12 doses in two separate injections to receive the total dose | • Carefully follow package instructions for proper administration.<br>• Tell the patient to go to the emergency room if symptoms of myocardial infarction or stroke occur.<br>• Remind patients to have a dental examination every 6 months and to tell the dental professional about taking this drug because it can cause jawbone osteonecrosis. |

• Weight-bearing physical activity may decrease the rate of bone loss. Talk to your healthcare provider about physical activities you may enjoy.

• Avoid taking over-the-counter or herbal drugs while taking raloxifene.

• Make sure to get enough calcium and vitamin D in your diet.

• Wash your hands before and after taking this drug. Family members should avoid touching raloxifene. Keep out of the reach of children.

 Bookmark This!

The Office of Disease Prevention and Health Promotion and the Center for Nutrition Policy and Promotion are in partnership to provide Dietary Guidelines for Americans. Here is a link for food sources of calcium: https://www.dietaryg uidelines.gov/food-sources-calcium. Here is a link for food sources of vitamin D: https://www.dietaryguidelines.gov /resources/2020-2025-dietary-guidelines-online-materials/f ood-sources-select-nutrients/food-sources.

## CALCITONIN

### Action and Uses

Calcitonin is a hormone that is usually secreted by special cells in the thyroid gland to help regulate calcium levels in the blood. It acts by decreasing the breakdown of calcium in the bone by osteoclasts so that calcium levels in the blood are not too high. As a drug, calcitonin can be used to decrease breakdown of bone in patients with osteoporosis. It can be used in women who are at least 5 years past menopause. In addition, calcitonin can be used in the treatment of hypercalcemia or Paget's disease.

### Expected Side Effects and Adverse Effects

The most common side effects are mild nausea and vomiting, rhinitis, and a mild injection site reaction in some cases. Potential adverse effects include serious allergic reaction, hypertension, and heart dysrhythmias. Older adults are more likely to experience adverse effects.

❖ **Nursing Implications and Patient Teaching**

◆ *Planning and implementation.* Calcitonin is available in three main routes: intranasal spray, intramuscular or subcutaneous injection. For nasal spray, make sure that the drug is at room temperature. In addition, the patient should alternate the nostril used daily. The nasal spray should be used no longer than 30 days once opened. If using the injection route, make sure to rotate sites carefully. If giving intramuscularly (IM), make sure to inject into a large muscle. For subcutaneous injection, make sure to avoid intradermal injection.

◆ *Evaluation.* As with other drugs used to treat osteoporosis, it is important to encourage adequate dietary intake of calcium and vitamin D. In patients using nasal spray, make sure there are no signs of irritation of the nares. For patients receiving subcutaneous or IM injection, monitor the sites carefully for signs of irritation or any symptoms that would suggest allergic response, such as rash or itching. If these occur, make sure to report them to the healthcare provider.

◆ *Patient and family teaching.* Tell the patient and family:

• Be sure to use the proper techniques for drug administration.

• If you are using the intranasal spray, alternate nostrils daily.

• If you are using subcutaneous IM injections, rotate sites.

• Calcitonin as nasal spray and as injectable can only be kept at room temperature for 30 days.

### PARATHYROID HORMONE ANALOGS AND PARATHYROID HORMONE-RELATED PROTEIN ANALOGS

### Action and Uses

Normally parathyroid hormone increases bone resorption by osteoclasts to increase serum calcium. You may wonder, how does it help in osteoporosis?

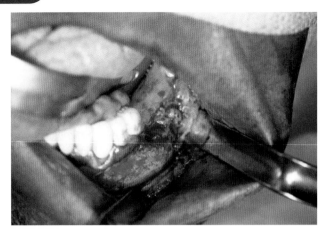
Fig. 21.4 Osteonecrosis of the jaw.

These parathyroid *hormone analogs and parathyroid hormone-related protein analogs* (PTH analogs and PTH hormone-related protein analogs), when given in intermittent doses, can stimulate osteoblasts to build bone. This results in an increase in bone remodeling and bone strength. These drugs are reserved for patients with a high risk of fracture and are usually given for a maximum of 2 years. These drugs can be used in patients with a high risk of fracture, including postmenopausal women, men with osteoporosis, and adults with osteoporosis from the use of glucocorticoid drugs.

### Expected Side Effects and Adverse Effects
Common side effects include nausea, weakness, fatigue, and mild injection-site reactions (pain, swelling, slight redness). Orthostatic hypotension occurs in about 5% of patients but can be relieved with positioning and lasts only a few days. Severe allergic reactions are rare. Hypercalcemia and hypercalciuria may occur. Increased blood uric acid levels may occur in patients taking the parathyroid hormone-related protein analogs.

### ❖ Nursing Implications and Patient Teaching
◆ *Assessment.* Determine if the patient has any history of orthostatic hypotension and report to the healthcare provider before giving these drugs. Parathyroid hormone analogs and parathyroid hormone-related protein analogs are not recommended for patients with severe kidney disease.

◆ *Planning and implementation.* These drugs are typically available in a prefilled pen. Carefully review the packaging for proper drug administration and storage. Follow safety protocols carefully to avoid falls in that these drugs may cause orthostatic hypotension, particularly early in treatment.

◆ *Evaluation.* Monitor patient tolerance to the drug, especially for signs of orthostatic hypotension. This may occur within 4 hours of administration.

◆ *Patient and family teaching.* Tell the patient and family:
- Make sure to rotate injection sites as directed,
- Stand up slowly in case you get dizzy. If the dizziness does not get better after a few doses, make sure to contact your healthcare provider.
- Make sure to maintain adequate calcium and vitamin D intake daily.
- You may need to have blood work drawn, such as blood calcium and serum uric acid levels. Make sure to follow up with your healthcare providers.

## OSTEOCLAST MONOCLONAL ANTIBODIES
### Action and Uses
Osteoclast monoclonal antibodies are drugs that are used in patients with high risk for osteoporosis. They are generally reserved for patients who are not able to take other drugs for treating osteoporosis, such as biphosphonates. They decrease the activity of the osteoclasts, resulting in a decrease in bone resorption. The main example is denosumab.

### Expected Side Effects and Adverse Effects
Side effects include fatigue, muscle ache, mild back pain, rash, constipation, and gastroesophageal reflux. Patients receiving denosumab may experience an acute reaction within the first 3 days, including chills, fever, flushing, and joint pain. In addition, they have an increased risk for infection. Patients taking denosumab are at increased risk for osteonecrosis. Patients may have an increased risk for hypocalcemia and cardiac dysrhythmias.

### ❖ Nursing Implications and Patient Teaching
◆ *Assessment.* Prior to beginning therapy, lab tests including serum calcium will be ordered to achieve a baseline. Assess adequacy of dietary intake of calcium and vitamin D. These drugs do not replace the need for good nutrition.

◆ *Planning and implementation.* Denosumab should only be administered by healthcare professionals and is not for home administration. Follow administration instructions very carefully to avoid adverse effects. It is designed for subcutaneous use.

◆ *Evaluation.* Patients will require regular lab tests to monitor serum calcium. Ensure that patients continue to maintain adequate dietary intake of calcium and vitamin D.

◆ *Patient and family teaching.* Tell the patient and family:
- Watch for and report any signs and symptoms of infection.
- Communicate to your dentist that you are taking these drugs, because there is an increased risk of osteonecrosis.

- Make sure to get adequate amounts of calcium and vitamin D daily.
- Notify your healthcare provider if you have any muscle cramping or spasms, tingling in the lips or fingers, or confusion as these may be signs of low blood calcium.

## SCLEROSTIN INHIBITORS
### Action and Uses
Sclerostin is a glycoprotein that is produced by osteocytes. When sclerostin is inhibited, osteoblast activity becomes stimulated and results in the formation of new bone. Sclerostin inhibitors are used for patients who are at high risk for fracture or for whom other therapies for osteoporosis have failed. The main example is romosozumab.

### Expected Side Effects and Adverse Effects
Sclerostin inhibitors are contraindicated for patients who have hypocalcemia (low serum calcium levels). Hypocalcemia must be corrected before these drugs can be given. Hypersensitivity reactions include swelling of the mouth and lips (angioedema) or rash. There is a risk of osteonecrosis of the jaw, which can occur without warning. The most serious adverse effect is the risk of cardiovascular events (e.g., myocardial infarction (MI), stroke).

### ❖ Nursing Implications and Patient Teaching
◆ *Assessment. Determine the patient's nutritional status including their dietary intake of calcium and vitamin D. Report to the healthcare provider if there is any history of MI or stroke. Check the patient's serum calcium prior to administration as this drug is contraindicated in hypocalcemia.*

◆ *Planning and implementation.* Romosozumab is only given by healthcare providers. Keep emergency equipment in the room with the patient while administering the drug. Assess the patient for an allergic reaction during and after subcutaneous injection of romosozumab. It is given at two injection sites. Recommended injection sites include the thigh, abdomen, or outer area of the upper arm. It is important to rotate sites with each injection. Avoid injecting in areas where the skin is tender, bruised, red, or hard. Do not administer in areas with scars or stretch marks.

◆ *Patient and family teaching.* Tell the patient and family:
- Inform your dentist or oral surgeon that you are taking romosozumab (Evenity) before you undergo a tooth extraction or invasive dental procedure involving the jawbone.
- This drug can cause allergic (hypersensitivity) reactions. Report any swelling of the lips or rash immediately. If you start having chest pain, shortness of breath, dizziness, or just do not feel right when you are receiving this drug, call for help immediately.

- Notify your healthcare provider immediately if you have any signs of a stroke, such as numbness or weakness of the face, arms, or legs; confusion; or difficulty speaking or understanding speech.
- Notify your healthcare provider immediately if you have any chest pain, shortness of breath, or jaw or neck pain, as these may be signs of a heart problem.
- Report any swelling, pain, redness, or other signs of infection in the gums that may be signs of osteonecrosis.

## CALCIUM AND VITAMIN D
### Action and Uses
Bones contain about 99% of the total calcium in the body. Calcium helps build and maintain bones, whereas vitamin D helps the body to absorb calcium. Standard recommendations for postmenopausal women with osteoporosis are to consume 1000 to 1200 mg of calcium (in the diet, as a supplement, or both). For males, the requirements increase at the age of 70 to 1200 mg per day of calcium. For vitamin D, recommendations typically range from 600 to 800 units per day. Dosages may be higher for patients with osteopenia or osteoporosis.

### Expected Side Effects and Adverse Effects
The side effects of calcium and vitamin D supplementation include nausea, vomiting, constipation, bone pain, muscle weakness, and increased thirst. High doses of calcium and vitamin D supplements may cause kidney stones, hypercalcemia, and impaired renal function.

### ❖ Nursing Implications and Patient Teaching
◆ *Assessment.* Carefully review your patient's dietary intake of calcium. If available, you may want to refer the patient to a dietician or nutritionist. Many times, the patient can meet calcium intake through their diet, but if not, they may require supplements.

◆ *Planning and implementation.* Calcium and vitamin D tablets should be given with food or within 1.5 hours after a meal to help the body absorb the calcium. Avoid taking the calcium with milk or other dairy products as they can actually decrease absorption of calcium. If the total calcium dose is greater than 600 mg, the dose may be divided and given at several times over the course of a day to prevent GI upset. If using the powder for oral solution, make sure to follow the package instructions carefully prior to administering. It is important to note that patients should discuss with their provider the use of supplements as high doses of supplemental calcium may be associated with cardiovascular risk.

◆ *Patient and family teaching.* Tell the patient and family:
- Calcium and vitamin D tablets come in different strengths. Be sure to obtain the correct strength recommended for you.
- Take calcium and vitamin D tablets with food.

- If using the liquid form of the supplement, carefully measure the dose using an accurate measuring container designed for drugs.
- If taking the chewable form, chew the drug carefully; do not swallow it whole.

- Do not crush extended-release forms of the drug.
- Eat a diet rich in foods that contain calcium and sources of vitamin D.

## GET READY FOR THE NEXT-GENERATION NCLEX EXAMINATION!

### Key Points

- **Osteoporosis** is a metabolic bone disorder that causes the bones to become weak and brittle from the gradual loss of bone density.
- Bone cells are continually in a process of building and breakdown, responding to factors such as amount of weight bearing, repair from bone injury, influence of certain hormones, and nutritional intake.
- As people age, the rate of bone loss occurs at a faster rate than bone remodeling, resulting in an overall loss of bone mass.
- Osteoporosis can affect people of all genders and races.
- Certain medications and medical conditions are associated with an increased risk of osteoporosis.
- Although osteoporosis cannot be fully prevented or cured, its progress can be slowed with drug therapy. Drugs used to treat osteoporosis generally act by either *decreasing resorption of bone* or by *increasing bone formation.*
- All patients who are at risk for osteoporosis or who have been diagnosed with osteoporosis should be evaluated for adequate calcium and vitamin D intake.
- **Bisphosphonates** are the most commonly used drugs to treat osteoporosis.
- Bisphosphonates act by decreasing the ability of osteoclasts to break down bone cells. Common side effects of the bisphosphonates are nausea, muscle and joint pain, and diarrhea.
- It is critical to consider the patient's ability to swallow and sit or stand for a minimum of 30 minutes in order to prevent esophageal erosion.
- Oral forms of bisphosphonates should be given first thing in the morning before any food, beverages, or other drugs have been taken. It should be given with *plain water only,* and the patient should be able to sit or stand for at least 30 minutes.
- Patients must remain in the upright position (sitting, standing, or walking) for at least 30 minutes after taking these drugs to prevent esophageal irritation.
- Report any use of aspirin or any NSAIDs as these should be avoided while taking bisphosphonates.
- Selective estrogen receptor modulators (SERMs) used in treating osteoporosis produce an estrogenlike effect on the bone. They help decrease bone breakdown but do not have significant estrogen effects on the breast and endometrium.
- SERMs increase estrogen in clotting and lipid metabolism, so they can increase the risk of cardiovascular effects. They are not used as often as other drugs for treating osteoporosis.
- Teach patients taking SERMs to report any chest pain, confusion, shortness of breath, leg swelling, trouble

speaking, severe headache, or any weakness of the face, arms, or legs (especially on one side of the body).
- Remind patient to avoid smoking or using tobacco products as they may increase the risk for clotting.
- Calcitonin is a hormone that is usually secreted by special cells in the thyroid gland to help regulate calcium levels in the blood. It acts by decreasing the breakdown of calcium in the bone by osteoclasts so that calcium levels in the blood are not too high.
- As a drug, calcitonin can be used to decrease breakdown of bone in patients with osteoporosis. It can be used in women who are at least 5 years postmenopause.
- The most common side effects of calcitonin are mild nausea and vomiting, rhinitis, and a mild injection-site reaction in some cases.
- Calcitonin is available via three main routes: intranasal spray, intramuscular injection, or subcutaneous injection.
- Parathyroid hormone analogs and parathyroid hormone-related protein analogs, when given in intermittent doses, can stimulate osteoblasts to build bone. These drugs are reserved for patients with a high risk of fracture and are usually given for a maximum of 2 years.
- Patients taking a parathyroid hormone analog and a parathyroid hormone-related protein analog are at risk for hypercalcemia.
- Monitor patients taking a parathyroid hormone analog and a parathyroid hormone-related protein analog for signs of orthostatic hypotension. This may occur within 4 hours of administration.
- Osteoclast monoclonal antibodies are used in patients with high risk for osteoporosis and who are not able to take other drugs for treating osteoporosis. Drugs in this category decrease bone resorption. The main example is denosumab.
- Patients receiving denosumab may experience an acute reaction within the first 3 days, including chills, fever, flushing, and joint pain, and they have an increased risk for hypocalcemia.
- Denosumab should only be administered by healthcare professionals and is not for home administration.
- Sclerostin inhibitors are used for patients who are at high risk for fracture or for whom other therapies for osteoporosis have failed. The main example is romosozumab.
- Sclerostin inhibitors are contraindicated for patients who have hypocalcemia. The most serious adverse effect is the risk of cardiovascular events (e.g., MI, stroke). Like denosumab, romosozumab must be given by a healthcare professional.
- Although relatively rare, jawbone necrosis is an adverse effect that can occur with many of the drugs used for

treating osteoporosis. Teach the patient to report any swelling, pain, redness, or other signs of infection in the gums and to notify their dentist they are taking drugs that might cause osteonecrosis.

- Calcium and vitamin D supplements may be recommended for patients to prevent or to help treat osteoporosis.
- Standard recommendations for postmenopausal women with osteoporosis are to consume 1000 to 1200 mg of calcium (in the diet, as a supplement, or both). For males age 70 and older, the requirements increase to 1200 mg per day of calcium.
- Doses of calcium and vitamin D supplements that are too high may cause kidney stones, hypercalcemia, and impaired renal function.

## Clinical Judgment and Next-Generation NCLEX® Examination-Style Questions

1. **Which assessment findings indicate a risk for osteoporosis? Select all or any that apply.**

   1. Postmenopausal female
   2. Nonsmoker
   3. Runs 30 miles per week
   4. Overweight
   5. Increased alcohol intake
   6. History of previous fracture
   7. Chronic kidney disease
   8. Takes an estrogen cream for symptoms of menopause

2. **Julia Parson is a 74-year-old who has been prescribed alendronate to treat osteoporosis. Which of the following statements by Ms. Parson indicates a need for more teaching?**

   1. "I should take this drug with food or milk so I don't irritate my stomach."
   2. "I should make sure to notify my dentist that I am taking this drug."
   3. "I need to sit or stand for at least 30 minutes after taking my medication."
   4. "It is best to take this drug first thing, at least 30 minutes before breakfast."

3. **A 62-year-old postmenopausal woman is prescribed raloxifene for prevention of osteoporosis. While doing your assessment, you discover the patient has a history of a deep vein thrombosis after a previous surgery. What is your best action?**

   1. Assess her calcium and vitamin D intake.
   2. Notify her healthcare provider before giving the drug.
   3. Administer the drug with food or milk to avoid GI upset.
   4. Teach the patient to report any hot flashes.

4. **A 72-year-old woman has been prescribed intranasal calcitonin for osteoporosis after being unable to take other more effective drugs. Which of the following actions should you include in caring for this patient? Select all or any that apply.**

   1. Assess both nostrils for any signs of irritation.
   2. Teach the patient to alternate nares with each dose.
   3. Assess the patient's dietary history for calcium and vitamin D intake.
   4. Teach the patient that the nasal spray can be left at room temperature for about 6 months.
   5. Teach the patient that they may experience a mild runny nose and congestion.
   6. Remind the patient to stand or sit for at least 30 minutes after taking calcitonin.

5. **Elizabeth Moore is newly diagnosed with osteopenia and is discussing meal planning. Which of the following menu selections would demonstrate a need for more teaching?**

   1. Two eggs, two slices of wheat toast, a cup of skim milk, and one orange
   2. Two waffles with syrup, cup of yogurt, and dried figs
   3. Omelet with cheese, two slices bacon, and wheat toast
   4. Two eggs, two slices of bacon, two slices white toast, and coffee with cream

6. **A 76-year-old female with a history of hip fracture has been on bisphosphonates for 5 years; however, she is no longer able to tolerate the drug, so her provider is beginning therapy with a sclerostin inhibitor (romosozumab). Complete the following sentence by choosing from the list of options.**

   The patient is at the highest risk for developing ____1____ associated with the patient's ____2____.

   | OPTIONS FOR 1 | OPTIONS FOR 2 |
   | --- | --- |
   | osteonecrosis of the jaw | low blood calcium |
   | hypercalcemia | history of hip fracture |
   | esophageal necrosis | intake of high calcium foods |
   | nausea and vomiting | history of dental problems |

7. **A 75-year-old male is admitted to the skilled nursing facility for rehabilitation after a stroke. The nurse is reviewing the patient's medical record. Complete the following sentence by choosing from the list of options.**

   The nurse should hold the ____1____ related to the patient ____2____.

   | OPTIONS FOR 1 | OPTIONS FOR 2 |
   | --- | --- |
   | alendronate 10 mg orally once daily | takes a 600 mg calcium vitamin D supplement daily |
   | raloxifene 60 mg once daily | having a history of occasional constipation |
   | calcitonin 100 IU subcutaneously daily | complains of difficulty swallowing |
   | romosozumab 210 mg subcutaneously once a month | recently had a fractured forearm from a fall |

8. Deborah Jackson has a long history of osteoporosis with a history of vertebral fracture and hip fracture. She has been treated with several drugs but is no longer able to tolerate them. Her healthcare provider has determined that she should begin denosumab therapy. Highlight or place a check mark next to the statements that should be included when teaching your patient about denosumab.

---

- ___ You will be able to give this drug at home every 6 months.
- ___ Make sure to let your dentist know you are on this drug.
- ___ Schedule a dental exam at least every 2 years.
- ___ This drug helps to build bone.
- ___ This drug may increase your risk for infection.
- ___ Make sure to eat plenty of fruits and vegetables as this drug can cause constipation.
- ___ Some patients experience a flulike syndrome about 3 days after administration of denosumab. Notify your healthcare provider if you have fever, chills, or muscle and joint ache.
- ___ This drug can be given intranasally as a spray.
- ___ Make sure you include enough calcium and vitamin D in your diet.
- ___ Notify your provider if you have signs of low blood calcium, such as fast heartbeat, muscle pain, or tingling or numbness in the hands or feet.

---

9. Roberta Thomas is a 68-year-old postmenopausal female who has been diagnosed with osteoporosis. Her primary care provider prescribed alendronate 70 mg orally once a week. The pharmacy has 35 mg weekly tablets available. How many tablets will the patient require with each dose?

**Case Study**

Jody Smith is a 57-year-old female with a long history of an eating disorder. Now in recovery from her eating disorder, she is now about 3 years since her last period. Her healthcare provider is concerned that she is now postmenopausal and may have had some bone loss relating to her history of an eating disorder. After a dual-energy x-ray absorptiometry (DEXA) scan, it is determined that she has osteopenia. Because of her history, her provider determines that she should be prescribed 150 mg orally once a month for prevention of osteoporosis.

1. What are the primary factors that should be considered when beginning therapy with an oral bisphosphonate?

2. What resources would you use to help evaluate Ms. Smith's nutritional status? What are some good sources of calcium that you might recommend?

3. Most people do not get enough vitamin D from the sun. What are some other sources of vitamin D?

4. Develop a teaching plan for a patient who has osteopenia.

## Next-Generation NCLEX® (NGN) Examination–Style Question

### History and Physical
### 3 Months Ago, 0900

CC: "I fell and hurt my wrist."

HPI: A postmenopausal, 68-year-old white female presents to the office with the complaint of wrist pain. The client reports yesterday she tripped over a rug a home, but states "I didn't land hard." Client reports she woke this morning with significant right wrist pain and swelling.

Physical Exam:

General: no acute distress, stooped posture

Respiratory: breath sounds clear bilaterally

Cardiovascular: S1, S2, no murmur

Musculoskeletal: right wrist with swelling and tenderness to palpation

### Today, 1100

CC: "I'm having terrible heartburn."

HPI: The client presents to the office for a follow-up visit. The client reports that the only issue she has been having since her previous visit is the development of heartburn. The client reports she has been taking TUMS daily, but states "I think I need something stronger." The client reports that she saw the orthopedist after her previous visit and "had a cast for 2 months."

Physical Exam:

General: no acute distress, stooped posture

Respiratory: breath sounds clear bilaterally

Cardiovascular: S1, S2, no murmur

Musculoskeletal: no swelling or tenderness to right wrist

### Flow Sheet
### 3 Months Ago, 0900

Blood Pressure: 142/88 mm Hg

Heart Rate: 98/min

Respiratory Rate: 18/min

Temperature: 98.6°F (37°C)

### Today, 1100

Blood Pressure: 138/84 mm Hg

Heart Rate: 93/min

Respiratory Rate: 16/min

Temperature: 98.6°F (37°C)

### Orders
### 3 Months Ago, 0900

Refer to orthopedics for wrist injury.

Alendronate 10 mg orally daily

### Imaging Studies
### 3 Months Ago, 0900

Right wrist x-ray: distal radius fracture

Dual-energy x-ray absorptiometry (DEXA):

>2.5 SD below normal, indicating osteoporosis

A nurse is caring for the client in the outpatient primary care provider's office.

**Which of the following nursing statements are indicated? Select all or any that apply.**

- "You must stay in a sitting or standing position for at least 30 minutes after taking your medication."
- "You should avoid taking acetaminophen for pain. Ibuprofen is a better choice."
- "You should report any gum or jaw pain or swelling immediately."
- "You should take your medication with orange juice to improve absorption."
- "You should avoid taking aspirin while on this medication."
- "You should take your medication first thing in the morning."
- "You should not eat for 10 minutes after taking your medication."
- "You should avoid exercise for 1 hour after taking your medication."

See answer on Evolve at http://evolve.elsevier.com/Visovsky/LPNpharmacology/.

# 22 Drugs for Eye and Ear Problems

## Learning Outcomes

1. Explain what types of drugs are used topically to manage ear problems.
2. Describe the proper technique to give drugs for the ear to adults or children.
3. List the names, actions, possible side effects, and adverse effects of cerumenolytics.
4. Explain what types of drugs are used topically to manage eye problems.
5. Describe the proper technique to give eye drops and eye ointments.
6. List the names, actions, possible side effects, and adverse effects of drugs for glaucoma.
7. Explain what to teach patients and families about the different drug categories used to manage glaucoma.
8. Describe lifespan considerations for drugs to manage glaucoma.

## Key Terms

**alpha-adrenergic agonists** Drugs that bind to receptor sites in the eye and reduce the amount of aqueous humor produced.

**beta-adrenergic antagonists** Drugs that inhibit adrenergic receptor sites in the eye and decrease production of aqueous humor; also called *beta-blockers*.

**carbonic anhydrase inhibitor (CAI)** A type of diuretic that also can lower intraocular pressure by decreasing production of aqueous humor by 50% to 60%.

**cerumenolytics** Drugs that soften earwax.

**cholinergic drugs** Drugs that increase the availability of acetylcholine to activate specific receptors. This leads to

decreased production and improved outflow of aqueous humor, reducing intraocular pressure.

**glaucoma** Glaucoma is a chronic condition in which increased IOP damages the optic nerve. If left untreated, glaucoma can cause loss of peripheral (side) vision and blindness.

**ophthalmic drugs** Liquid drops or ointments that are prepared to place on the eye or the conjunctiva.

**otic drugs** Drugs that are prepared for delivery into the external ear canal.

**prostaglandin agonists** Drugs that bind to specific prostaglandin receptor sites in the eye, causing increased outflow of aqueous humor.

## EAR PROBLEMS

### EAR STRUCTURE AND FUNCTION

The ear is the organ, along with the neural connections in the brain, that allows the sense of hearing to occur. The ear has three parts that are important to hearing: the external ear, the middle ear, and the inner ear.

The external ear is called the *pinna* (Fig. 22.1). It is made of cartilage covered by skin and is attached to the side of the head. The external ear extends from the pinna through the *ear canal* (auditory canal), ending at the *tympanic membrane* (eardrum) (Fig. 22.2). The *ear canal* is a slightly curved S-shaped tube open to the outside that ends at the eardrum. This canal is lined with hair cells and cells that produce *cerumen* (earwax) and oil. Cerumen helps protect and lubricate the canal. In adults, the ear canal tilts downward and is about 1 to 1.5 inches (2.5–3.75 cm) long. In children, the canal is shorter and straighter.

The middle ear is a small compartment that extends from the eardrum to the oval and round windows of

the wall separating it from the inner ear. It contains the top opening of the eustachian tube and three small bones known as the *bony ossicles*, which are the *malleus* (hammer), the *incus* (anvil), and the *stapes* (stirrup); the stapes is connected to the oval window (see Fig. 22.2).

The bony ossicles are joined loosely, which allows them to move slightly in response to the vibrations created when sound waves hit the eardrum. The *eustachian tube* extends from the floor of the middle ear to the back of the throat, allowing pressure on both sides of the eardrum to equalize. (You might have felt this as a popping sensation when you swallow or yawn, especially when traveling up or down steep hills or in an airplane.)

The eustachian tube normally allows secretions to drain from the middle ear into the throat. This opening from the throat to the middle ear also allows organisms in the throat to move upward (ascend) into the middle ear, which can cause *otitis media* (middle ear infection).

The inner ear lies on the other side of the *oval window*. It contains the semicircular canals, cochlea, vestibule, and end of the eighth cranial nerve (see Fig. 22.2). The *semicircular canals* are three tubes that contain fluid and hair cells that respond to rotational movements of the head. The *vestibule* contains organs that sense the position of the head with respect to gravity. Both send electrical signals to the eighth cranial nerve (CN VIII) to help maintain the sense of balance. The *cochlea* is a fluid-filled organ that also contains hair cells and sensory neurons; it detects vibrations produced by sound and sends electrical impulses to the eighth cranial nerve. CN VIII is called the *vestibulocochlear nerve* because it receives signals for balance and hearing.

Hearing (auditory perception) is the main function of the ear. Hearing begins when sound waves move through the air and into the external ear canal. These waves hit the movable eardrum, creating vibrations that are transferred to the ossicles of the middle ear. The movements of these bones transmit the vibrations from the middle ear to the cochlea of the inner ear, where the sensory neurons translate them into electrical signals that stimulate the nerve of hearing (CN VIII). The impulse is then carried to the areas of the brain that allow the nerve impulses to be interpreted as sounds.

## DRUGS TO MANAGE EAR PROBLEMS

The most common ear problems are infection and inflammation that occur in the external ear and in the middle ear. When these problems occur in the middle ear, antimicrobial and anti-inflammatory drugs are given systemically, most often by the oral route. The actions, side effects, and nursing implications of systemic antimicrobials are discussed in Chapters 5 and 7. The actions, side effects, and nursing implications of systemic anti-inflammatories are discussed in Chapter 13.

Infections and inflammation of the pinna and the ear canal are most often managed by topical drug application because the external ear can be reached from the outside. The actions of topical antimicrobial and anti-inflammatory drugs are the same as those given systemically and are discussed in Chapters 5 and 13. Drugs that are prepared for delivery into the external ear canal are **otic drugs**. Box 22.1 lists the techniques involved in placing *(instilling)* ear drops into the ear canal. Fig. 22.3 shows the correct techniques for instilling ear drops in adults and in children younger than 3 years of age (Fig. 22.3B).

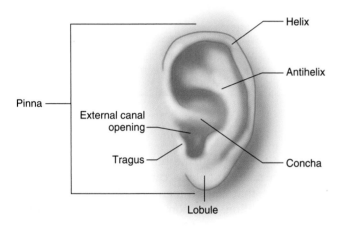

Fig. 22.1 Anatomy of the external ear (pinna). (From Ignatavicius, D., Workman, M. L., & Rebar, C. (2018). *Medical-surgical nursing* (9th ed.). Saunders.)

### Top Tip for Safety

Instill only drugs and liquids labeled "for otic use" into the ear canal.

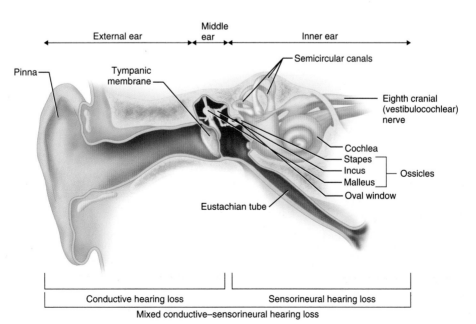

Fig. 22.2 Anatomy of the middle and inner ear. (From Ignatavicius, D., Workman, M. L., & Rebar, C. (2018). *Medical-surgical nursing* (9th ed.). Saunders.)

## Lifespan Considerations

The length and angle of ear canals are different in young children and adults. In adults, the ear canal tilts downward, is longer, and is slightly curved in an S-shape. In children, the canal is shorter and straighter. These differences require different techniques when instilling drugs into the ear canal.

- When instilling drops into an adult's ear, gently pull the external ear up and back (see Fig. 22.3A).
- When instilling drops into a young child's ear, gently pull the external ear down and back (see Fig. 22.3B).

| Box 22.1 | Technique for Instilling Ear Drops into a Patient's Ear |
|---|---|

- Make sure that the patient's eardrum is intact. This may require assessment by the registered nurse or other healthcare provider. Never give an ear drug if there is damage to the eardrum.
- Read the label of the drug carefully to ensure that it is "for otic use." Never put any solution in the ear that is not labeled specifically for use in ears.
- Verify the drug using the *9 Rights of Drug Administration* (Chapter 1).
- Wash your hands and don a pair of clean gloves.
- Warm the ear drops to room temperature.
- Ask the patient to lie down with the head turned so that the affected ear is turned upward; if the patient is sitting in a chair, tilt the patient's head so the affected ear is up.
- For a child younger than 3 years of age, gently pull the pinna down and back; for an older child or adult, pull the pinna up and back.
- Using the applicator, place only the prescribed number of drops into the patient's ear. Aim the drops onto the side of the ear canal, and let them run into the ear.
- Insert a cotton ball into the opening of the ear canal to keep the drops from rolling out of the ear.
- Remind the patient to keep his or her head in this position for 2 to 5 minutes as directed to allow the drops to flow.
- Remove your gloves and wash your hands.

Another problem in the external ear canal occurs when there is such an excessive buildup of cerumen that sound waves are blocked, hearing is reduced, and the patient has ear pain. For this problem, instillation of **cerumenolytics** (drugs that soften earwax) may be used, followed by irrigation of the ear. (Review ear irrigation in your fundamentals or medical-surgical nursing textbook.) These drugs are available over the counter and most often contain a carbamide peroxide (urea plus hydrogen peroxide) combination (Table 22.1). Teach patients to *never* use such a product in an ear that has drainage or discharge because the eardrum may not be intact and the solution could enter the middle ear, causing an infection.

Do not instill a cerumenolytic or irrigate the ear canal in a person who is dizzy, because these actions will increase the dizziness. Reports suggest that distilled water or saline may be just as effective as oil- or peroxide-based solutions. Carefully review the order, and do not hesitate to ask the healthcare provider if you have questions.

### Top Tip for Safety

Never place a drug into the ear canal or irrigate the ear canal if drainage is present because the fluid can enter the middle ear and cause an infection.

## EYE PROBLEMS

Together the eye and the brain allow sight (vision). Although many problems can affect the eye and vision, those that can be managed with drug therapy are inflammation, infection, and glaucoma. Drugs for these problems are **ophthalmic drugs**, which come in liquid drops or ointment form. Chapter 13 discusses various types of anti-inflammatory drugs, nearly all of which have an ophthalmic form. Chapters 5, 6, and 7 discuss antimicrobial drug therapies. Many antimicrobial and anti-inflammatory drugs have an ophthalmic form, and their actions are the same as the systemic forms. Follow directions carefully when giving the ophthalmic form to avoid underdosing or overdosing.

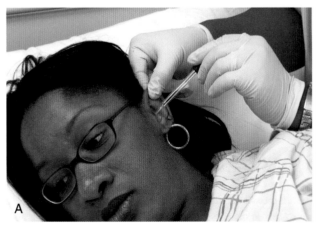
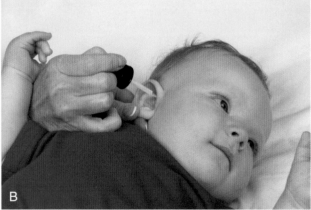

**Fig. 22.3** Correct techniques for giving ear drops to an adult (A) and to a child younger than 3 years of age (B). (From Perry, A., Potter, P., & Ostendorf, W. (2014). *Clinical nursing skills and techniques* (8th ed.). Mosby.)

| Table **22.1**  Example of Cerumenolytic Drugs | |
|---|---|
| *Cerumenolytics* are typically solvents used to break up or soften earwax so that it can be easily removed. | |
| **DRUG/ADULT DOSAGE** | **NURSING IMPLICATIONS** |
| carbamide peroxide (Debrox, Murine Ear Wax Removal) adults, adolescents, and children 12 years or older: instill 5–10 drops twice daily in the affected ear for up to 4 days; keep drops in ear for 5 minutes by keeping head tilted or placing cotton in the ear; do not use for longer than 4 days; kit comes with an ear syringe for flushing | • Teach patients that side effects are rare and may include redness, itching, or rash. <br> • Do not give the drug if the patient has any symptoms of ear infection or any discharge from the ear because this may cause damage to the middle or inner ear. <br> • To avoid dizziness, give the drug while the patient is lying down and the affected ear is turned upward. <br> • To avoid contamination of the tip or damage to the ear, do not insert the tip of the applicator into the ear canal. <br> • Remind the patient to remain lying down for at least 5 minutes after the drops are given for maximum effectiveness. <br> • Make sure that the drug is at room temperature. Drugs that are too cold or too warm can cause dizziness, nausea, and even burns to the ear. <br> • To avoid infection, do not share this drug with other patients. <br> • Gently flush the ear with warm water after application of the drug, using a bulb syringe or the syringe provided by the manufacturer. <br> • Remind the patient that a bubbling sound may be heard after the ear drops are instilled. |

This chapter focuses on drug therapy to manage the chronic eye disorder called *glaucoma*, which cannot be cured but can be controlled. Although the actions and uses for these drugs are different, some nursing implications are the same for all of them. Many of the points to teach patients and families about these drugs are the same. Box 22.2 describes the common nursing considerations for ophthalmic drugs, and Box 22.3 describes general patient teaching points. Nursing considerations and patient teaching issues specific to single drug types are listed in the individual drug categories.

Drug therapy for any eye problem requires that the drops or ointment be instilled using correct technique to ensure that the drug is in contact with the eye and that no harm or infection occurs (Figs. 22.4, 22.5, and 22.6). Box 22.4 describes the correct technique for giving ophthalmic drugs to a patient, and Box 22.5 describes the correct technique for patients to place drugs into their own eyes.

## EYE STRUCTURE AND FUNCTION

Vision results from light moving through the eye and meeting the optic nerve, which connects to the brain, where images are interpreted. Fig. 22.7 shows the basic anatomy of the eye, the *lacrimal gland* (tear gland), *lacrimal sac* (tear sac), and *nasolacrimal duct*. Fig. 22.8 shows the eye in much greater detail.

The eye is divided into the *anterior segment* and the *posterior segment*. The anterior segment divides into the *anterior chamber* and the *posterior chamber*. The space between the cornea and the lens is filled with a watery fluid called *aqueous humor*.

Aqueous humor is produced by the *ciliary body* and flows from the posterior chamber to the anterior chamber, where it drains through the trabecular meshwork and canal of Schlemm into the blood for reabsorption by the body. Normal circulation of the fluid through the anterior chamber is important in maintaining the *intraocular pressure* (IOP) at a normal level (10–20 mm Hg). Maintenance of a normal IOP keeps the eye healthy and helps prevent blindness. This will be important when you learn later in this chapter how drugs work to treat glaucoma.

The cornea covers the eye (see Fig. 22.8). The clarity of the cornea is important because the cornea allows light to enter the eye.

The iris is a flat, muscular ring located behind the cornea of the eye, and it has an adjustable circular opening in the center called a *pupil* (see Figs. 22.7 and 22.8). Pigments in the iris produce the color of your eyes (as determined by your genetic makeup). The smooth muscles in the iris control the size of the pupil to determine how much light enters the eye at any time.

Impulses from the autonomic nervous system cause the muscle to either constrict the pupil, reducing the amount of light that enters the eye, or dilate it, increasing the light let into the eye (Fig. 22.9). Constriction of the pupil is called *miosis*; dilation of the pupil is called *mydriasis*. There is an easy way to remember this: "miosis—small word, small pupil; mydriasis—large word, large pupil."

Constriction and dilation of the pupil occur continually as we adjust to varying levels of light in the environment. For example, when you walk from a dark room into the sunlight, your pupil constricts to reduce the amount of light that reaches the retina (too much

| Box 22.2 | General Nursing Considerations for Ophthalmic Drug Therapy |
|---|---|

- Always wash your hands before and after giving eye drops (use gloves if available).
- Assess the patient's eye(s) for redness, drainage, or open areas. In some cases, redness is a side effect of the eye drugs, but it also may be a sign of infection. If any new symptoms are present, notify the registered nurse or healthcare provider before giving the eye drugs.
- To avoid contamination and reduce the risk for infection, never touch the tip of the applicator/dropper or the inside of the cap.
- Always make sure that you are giving the correct concentration of the drug and the correct number of drops in the correct eye(s).
- Only use drugs that are specifically labeled for ophthalmic use.
- Remove the patient's contact lenses before giving eye drops, and read the drug inserts carefully to see whether the patient may use his or her contact lenses over the course of the therapy.
- If giving more than one type of eye drop, wait at least 5 minutes between instillations to avoid drug interaction.
- Teach the patient that his or her vision may be slightly blurry for a few minutes after eye drops are given and slightly longer for eye ointment.
- To reduce the risk for falls, teach the patient to avoid any significant activity until the blurred vision passes.
- Always report any sudden eye pain or sudden change in vision to the healthcare provider immediately because these symptoms may indicate potential for eye injury and even blindness.
- Follow the directions in Box 22.4 for instilling eye drops or ointments into a patient's eye.
- Fig. 22.4 shows the correct technique for applying eye drops.
- After giving eye drops, ask the patient to close his or her eyes for 2 minutes; this reduces the amount of drug absorbed systemically. A second option to reduce systemic absorption of the drug is to apply gentle pressure with the index finger over the tear duct in the inner corner of the eye for about 3 minutes after giving the eye drops (Fig. 22.5).
- Fig. 22.6 shows the correct technique for applying eye ointments.

light can be very uncomfortable). When you come from the daylight into a dark movie theater, your pupils dilate to let more light in so that you can get to your seat (see Fig. 22.9).

 **Memory Jogger**

Pupil constriction is *miosis* (small word, small pupil size). Pupil dilation is *mydriasis* (larger word, larger pupil size).

The *posterior segment* of the eye contains the retina and the optic nerve (see Fig. 22.8). The *retina* is the lining on the back of the eye. It contains special cells (rods and cones) that are sensitive to light energy and turn it into electrical impulses. The posterior segment is filled with a jellylike fluid called *vitreous humor*. The optic nerve in the back of the eye carries signals from the light-sensitive retinal cells to the brain, where they are interpreted as visual images. Any increase in pressure in the eye can injure blood vessels in the retina, which can damage the rods and cones and the optic nerve.

 **Memory Jogger**

Normal IOP is between 10 mm Hg and 20 mm Hg. Maintenance of a normal IOP keeps the eye healthy and helps prevent blindness in patients with glaucoma.

 **Bookmark This!**

The National Eye Institute (NEI) (https://nei.nih.gov) has fantastic resources for healthcare professionals, patients, and their families about a wide range of eye disorders. In particular, the NEI has an extensive bank of photographs and videos that help explain what happens in these disorders. Resources are available in English and in Spanish.

## GLAUCOMA

**Glaucoma** is a chronic condition in which increased IOP damages the optic nerve (Fig. 22.10). If left untreated, glaucoma can cause loss of *peripheral* (side) vision and blindness (Fig. 22.11). The disease is often described as a "silent thief of sight" because the patient typically has no symptoms other than a gradual loss of peripheral vision. By the time the patient realizes that vision is decreased, he or she has already experienced a degree of permanent vision loss. Those at greatest risk include blacks older than 40 years, patients with a family history of glaucoma, and patients older than 60 years of age, especially Mexican Americans. Although glaucoma typically occurs in adults, eye trauma can cause glaucoma in children.

Glaucoma is an eye disorder that results from too much aqueous humor. Aqueous humor is a fluid (similar to blood plasma) that is produced by the ciliary body in the eye (see Fig. 22.8). This fluid provides oxygen and nutrients to the cornea, the trabecular meshwork, and the lens of the eye. Normally, aqueous humor flows freely in the eye, providing nutrition and removing waste products. The most common type of glaucoma by far is *primary open-angle closure glaucoma*, in which aqueous humor does not drain through the normal pathways. It results in a buildup of fluid and increased IOP in the anterior chamber of the eye (see Fig. 22.10). The fluid increases pressure in the eye, leading to damage of the retina and the optic nerve.

In rare situations, a condition called *acute angle closure glaucoma* causes a sudden increase in IOP. This causes severe eye pain, nausea, and vomiting, and the patient may report seeing halos around lights. Acute angle closure glaucoma is a medical emergency. Any patient with symptoms of acute angle closure glaucoma should receive emergency treatment to avoid blindness.

### Box 22.3   General Teaching Points for Patients and Families During Topical Eye Drug Therapy

- Use only drugs that are labeled "for ophthalmic use only." Never place any solution in the eye that is not properly labeled.
- Eye drops are typically clear, thin, liquid drugs that are supplied in a bottle specifically labeled "for ophthalmic use only."
- Eye ointments are thick, often appear greasy, and come in a squeezable tube. Ointment remains in contact with the eye for a longer period than eye drops do.
- The concentration of the drug is on the label and must be carefully compared with the drug order.
- Use only the prescribed number of eye drops in the eye because too much of the drug can have adverse effects.
- To avoid eye injury and decrease risk for infection, never share eye drops or ointments with another person.
- Wash your hands thoroughly before giving eye drugs, and if available, put on clean gloves.
- Ask the patient to remove eyeglasses or contact lenses before giving eye drugs. Contact lenses must be removed because they can absorb eye drugs.
- Remove the cap of the eye drug container and place it upside down on the table to avoid contamination.
- Never touch the tip of the eye dropper/applicator with your finger or let it touch the patient's eye. The tip should remain sterile.

- Ask the patient to tilt his or her head back slightly and look at the ceiling. With a tissue, gently retract the lower lid to expose the conjunctival sac.
- Teach the patient (or family) the proper technique for giving eye drops. Over-the-counter saline drops can be used to practice the technique and avoid waste of the eye drugs.
- The patient should never drive or use heavy machinery if having blurred vision after taking the eye drugs.
- After giving eye drops, ask the patient to close his or her eyes for 2 minutes; this reduces the amount of drug absorbed systemically. A second option to reduce systemic absorption of the drug is to apply gentle pressure with the index finger over the tear duct in the inner corner of the eye for about 3 minutes after giving the eye drops.
- Always immediately report to the healthcare provider sudden eye pain or a sudden change in vision because these symptoms may indicate potential for eye injury and blindness.
- Teach patients to inform their healthcare provider immediately if there are any new symptoms while taking the drug (whether related to the eye or general symptoms).
- Teach the patient to go to the emergency department or call 911 if there is a sudden decrease or loss of vision.

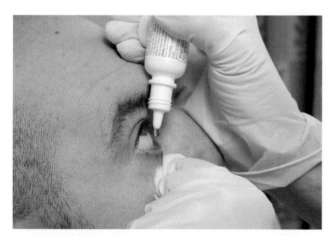

Fig. 22.4 Correct technique for instilling eye drops. (From Perry, A., Potter, P., & Ostendorf, W. (2017). *Clinical nursing skills and techniques* (9th ed.). Mosby.)

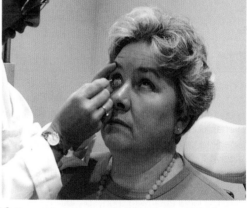

Fig. 22.6 Correct technique for instilling ointment into the eye. (From Ignatavicius, D., Workman, M. L., & Rebar, C. (2018). *Medical-surgical nursing* (9th ed.). Saunders.)

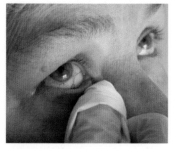

Fig. 22.5 Applying punctal occlusion (digital nasolacrimal occlusion) to prevent systemic absorption. (From Workman, M. L., & LaCharity, L. A. (2016). *Understanding pharmacology* (2nd ed.). St. Louis: Elsevier.)

 **Memory Jogger**

Glaucoma is a chronic disease with no cure. Drug therapy can prevent further damage and blindness and must continue for the rest of the patient's life.

Drug therapy for patients with glaucoma involves reducing the amount of aqueous humor produced by the ciliary body or improving drainage and reabsorption of the aqueous humor. Both treatments decrease fluid pressure in the eye (IOP) and relieve pressure on the retina and the optic nerve. Drugs for glaucoma are typically given as eye drops instilled into the affected eye. In emergency cases of

| Box **22.4**    Technique for Giving Eye Drops or Ointments to a Patient |
|---|

1. Check the name, strength, expiration date, color, and clarity of the eye drops to be instilled. If the drug is an ointment, be sure that it is an ophthalmic (eye) preparation and not a general topical ointment.
2. Check whether both eyes or only one eye is to receive the drug.
3. If both eyes are to receive the same drug and one eye is infected, use two separate bottles or tubes and carefully label each with "right" or "left" for the correct eye.
4. Wash your hands and put on gloves.
5. Explain the procedure to the patient.
6. Make sure the patient is not wearing contact lenses; if the patient is, ask him or her to remove them.
7. Have the patient sit in a chair while you stand behind the patient (or stand in front of the patient who is sitting in a chair, or over the patient who is lying in bed).
8. Ask the patient to tilt his or her head backward, with the back of the head resting against you or the back of the chair, and look up at the ceiling.
9. Gently pull the lower lid down against the patient's cheek, forming a small pocket.
10. Hold the container of eye drops or the ointment tube (with the cap off) like a pencil, with the tip pointing down.
    a. For ointment, squeeze a small amount out onto a tissue (without touching the applicator tip to the tissue), and discard it.
    b. For eye drops, gently squeeze the bottle and release the prescribed number of drops into the pocket that you have made with the patient's lower eyelid. Do not touch any part of the eye or the container lid with the tip of the bottle. For ointment, gently squeeze the tube and release a small amount of ointment into the pocket that you have made with the patient's lower eyelid. Do not touch any part of the eye or lid with the tip of the tube.
11. Gently release the lower eyelid.
12. Ask the patient to close his or her eye gently, without squeezing the lids tightly, and roll the eye under the lid for about 2 minutes to spread the drug across the eye.*
13. Without pressing on the eyelid, gently blot or wipe away any excess drug or tears with a tissue.
14. Remove your gloves.
15. Recap the tube or bottle.
16. Wash your hands again.
17. Replace contact lenses if appropriate.
18. Remind patients that their vision will be blurry and not to drive until their vision clears.

*An alternative to closing the eyes after giving eye drops: Using a gloved finger, gently press and hold the corner of the eye nearest the nose to close off the tear duct for about 3 minutes to prevent the drug from being absorbed systemically.
Adapted from Workman, M. L., & LaCharity, L. A. (2016). *Understanding pharmacology: Essentials for medication therapy* (2nd ed.). Elsevier.

| Box **22.5**    Technique for Self-Administration of Eye Drugs |
|---|

1. Check the name, strength, expiration date, color, and clarity of the eye drops to be instilled. If the drug is an ointment, be sure that it is an ophthalmic (eye) preparation and not a general topical ointment.
2. Check to see whether both eyes or only one eye is to receive the drug.
3. If both eyes are to receive the same drug and one eye is infected, use two separate bottles or tubes, and carefully label each with "right" or "left" for the correct eye.
4. Wash your hands.
5. Remove the cap from the bottle or tube, keeping the cap upright to avoid contaminating it.
6. Remove contact lenses if present.
7. Tilt your head backward, open your eyes, and look up at the ceiling.
8. Using your nondominant hand, gently pull the lower lid down against your cheek, forming a small pocket.
9. Hold the container of eye drops or the ointment tube (with the cap off) like a pencil, with the tip pointing down, with your dominant hand.
10. For ointment, squeeze a small amount out onto a tissue (without touching the applicator tip to the tissue), and discard it.
11. Rest the wrist that is holding the bottle or tube against your mouth or upper lip.
12. For eye drops, gently squeeze the bottle and release the prescribed number of drops into the pocket that you have made with your lower eyelid. Do not touch any part of the eye or the container lid with the tip of the bottle. For ointment, gently squeeze the tube and release a small amount of ointment into the pocket that you have made with your lower eyelid. Do not touch any part of the eye or lid with the tip of the tube.
13. Gently release your lower eyelid.
14. Close your eye gently (without squeezing the lids tight), and roll your eye under the eyelid to spread the drug across the eye.
15. Keep your eye closed for about 2 minutes.*
16. Without pressing on your eyelid, gently blot or wipe away any excess drug or tears with a tissue.
17. Recap the bottle or tube.
18. Replace contact lenses as appropriate.
19. Wash your hands again.
20. Do not drive or operate heavy machinery while your vision is blurry.

*An alternative to keeping your eye(s) closed for 2 minutes: Gently press and hold the corner of the eye nearest to your nose to close off the tear duct for about 3 minutes and prevent the drug from being absorbed systemically.
Adapted from Workman, M. L., & LaCharity, L. A. (2016). *Understanding pharmacology: Essentials for medication safety* (2nd ed.). Elsevier.

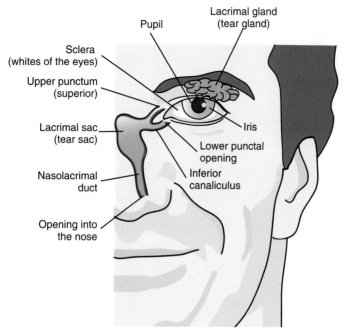

**Fig. 22.7** Features of the external eye (front view) along with the tear gland and duct system. (From Workman, M. L., & LaCharity, L. A. (2016). *Understanding pharmacology: Essentials of medication safety* (2nd ed.). Elsevier.)

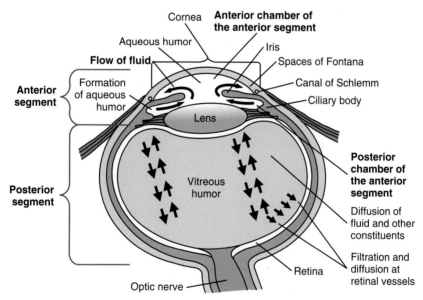

**Fig. 22.8** Side view (cutaway) of the internal features of the eye and the flow of aqueous humor. (From Workman, M. L., & LaCharity, L. A. (2016). *Understanding pharmacology: Essentials for medication safety* (2nd ed.). Elsevier.)

acute angle closure glaucoma, drugs may be given orally or intravenously to rapidly reduce IOP. To manage glaucoma, healthcare providers may recommend drugs from five classes: prostaglandin agonists (sometimes called *prostaglandin analogs*), beta-adrenergic antagonists (beta-blockers), alpha-adrenergic agonists, cholinergic drugs, and carbonic anhydrase inhibitors (CAIs).

### Memory Jogger

There are five classes of drugs to treat glaucoma:
- Prostaglandin agonists
- Beta-adrenergic antagonists
- Alpha-adrenergic agonists
- Cholinergic drugs
- Carbonic anhydrase inhibitors (CAIs)

## PROSTAGLANDIN AGONISTS

### Action and Uses

Prostaglandin agonists bind to prostaglandin receptor sites in the eye, increasing the outflow of aqueous humor. They help to control glaucoma by relaxing smooth muscles in the blood vessels of the eye, which allows these vessels to dilate and absorb aqueous humor. As a result, more aqueous fluid enters the blood and less is present in the eye, lowering the IOP. For many people, the prostaglandin agonists are very effective for controlling IOP. They are used only once a day and have fewer systemic side effects than other glaucoma drugs.

The names, usual adult dosages, and nursing implications of these drugs are listed in Table 22.2. Consult a drug reference book for more information about specific prostaglandin agonists.

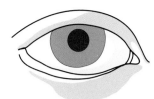

A Normal pupil slightly dilated for moderate light.

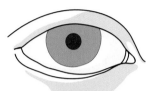

B Miosis–pupil constricted when exposed to increased light or for close work, such as reading.(Smaller word, smaller opening.)

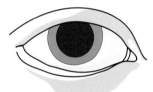

C Mydriasis–pupil dilated when exposed to reduced light or when looking at a distance. (Larger word, larger opening.)

Fig. 22.9 Comparison of pupil sizes: normal (A), miosis (B), and mydriasis (C). (From Workman, M. L., & LaCharity, L. A. (2016). *Understanding pharmacology: Essentials for medication safety* (2nd ed.). Elsevier.)

### Expected Side Effects

The most common side effects of prostaglandin agonists are eye itching and eye redness when the drugs are first applied. In some cases, patients have a foreign body sensation (i.e., feels like something is in their eye).

Over time, patients who take prostaglandin agonists may gradually but permanently develop changes in the color of the iris from lighter colors to brown (Fig. 22.12). This occurs because prostaglandins increase the production of the brown pigment *melanin*. The drug also causes thickening and lengthening of the eyelashes and darkening of the skin on the eyelids.

### Adverse Reactions

In rare cases, patients who are taking prostaglandin agonists can experience systemic effects, including infection, asthma, and corneal erosion (damage to the cornea).

### ❖ Nursing Implications and Patient Teaching

◆ *Assessment.* In addition to the general nursing considerations related to eye drug therapy listed in Box 22.2, assess the patient's understanding that glaucoma is a chronic disease that will require adherence to drug therapy to prevent decreased vision and blindness. For all patients who are taking prostaglandin agonists, it is important to check the affected eye for scratches (corneal

abrasions) or other signs of trauma. Never give these drugs if there is any damage to the eye surface.

 **Top Tip for Safety**

Never instill prostaglandin agonists into an eye that has been scratched or has an infection. Contact the healthcare provider for instructions about continuing glaucoma therapy and managing the corneal problem.

◆ *Patient and family teaching.* In addition to the general teaching points listed in Box 22.3, tell the patient and the family:
- Avoid using higher-than-prescribed doses because higher doses can reduce the effectiveness of the drug in controlling glaucoma.
- If you have lighter-colored eyes, your iris and eyelid color can change over time, and the lashes can become thicker and longer. If only one eye has glaucoma, the color and lash changes will occur only in that eye.
- If you have glaucoma only in one eye, do not place the drops in the unaffected eye even though the colors of your eyes may become different.

### BETA-ADRENERGIC ANTAGONISTS

#### Actions

Beta-adrenergic antagonists (also called *beta-blockers*) reduce the amount of aqueous humor produced from the ciliary body of the eye. They do this by binding to beta-adrenergic receptors in the ciliary body of the eye. Normally cells in the ciliary body produce aqueous humor, so blocking the action of these cells reduces the production of aqueous humor. Common beta-blockers for glaucoma, dosages, and nursing implications are listed in Table 22.2. Be sure to consult a drug reference book for more information about specific beta-blocking agents to control glaucoma.

#### Expected Side Effects

Expected side effects for beta-adrenergic antagonists often occur within a few minutes of instilling the drops in the eye. These include temporary blurring of vision, slight burning or stinging, and tearing of the eye. Later the patient may notice less tear production and dry, itchy, or red eyes. Beta-blockers constrict the pupil (i.e., cause miosis). It is important for patients to understand that the pupils will not dilate as easily when they go into a dark room.

 **Memory Jogger**

To determine whether a drug is a beta-blocker, look for the suffix (word ending) *-olol.*

#### Adverse Reactions

The greatest risk with ophthalmic use of beta-blockers occurs when the drops are unintentionally absorbed through the conjunctiva, the tear ducts, the nose, or other eye tissues. In fact, systemic absorption can cause the same effects seen with oral beta-blockers, as discussed in Chapter 10. Patients can experience decreased heart

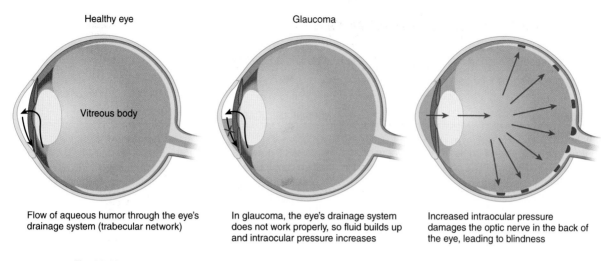

Fig. 22.10 In glaucoma, increased intraocular pressure from too much aqueous humor causes damage to the optic nerve.

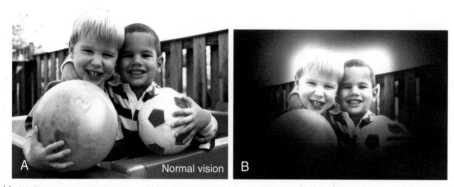

Fig. 22.11 (A) Scene as viewed by a person with normal vision. (B) The scene as viewed by a person with glaucoma. (Courtesy National Eye Institute, National Institutes of Health.)

rate, decreased blood pressure, and even heart failure. Systemic absorption of beta-blockers can also cause bronchoconstriction and asthma symptoms.

### ❖ Nursing Implications and Patient Teaching

◆ *Assessment.* In addition to the general nursing considerations related to eye drug therapy listed in Box 22.2, determine the patient's baseline vital signs. Watch for changes in heart rate and blood pressure. If the patient has respiratory problems such as asthma or chronic obstructive pulmonary disease (COPD), monitor for shortness of breath or changes in pulse oximetry. Determine whether the patient is also taking oral beta-blockers to control blood pressure or other heart dysrhythmia (see Chapter 9). If so, notify the healthcare provider to ensure that he or she is aware of the oral drug before giving the eye drops. Ophthalmic beta-blockers may increase the risk of expected side effects and adverse effects of the oral beta-blocker.

◆ *Planning and intervention.* Never touch the tip of the eye dropper to the patient's eye or with your finger to avoid contaminating the tip. To decrease systemic absorption of eye drops, use only the prescribed amount.

After giving the drops, ask the patient to close his or her eyes for 2 minutes. This reduces the amount of drug absorbed systemically.

Another option to reduce systemic absorption of the drug is *punctal occlusion* (also called *digital nasolacrimal occlusion*). This means putting gentle pressure with the index finger over the tear duct in the inner corner of the eye for about 3 minutes after instilling the eye drops. Caution is warranted because even with the techniques to decrease systemic absorption of the eye drops, you still must carefully monitor for adverse reactions to the drug.

> **⌂ Top Tip for Safety**
>
> To reduce systemic absorption of eye drops, give only the prescribed number of drops; then ask the patient to close his or her eyes for 2 minutes, or place a gloved finger over the tear duct and apply gentle pressure for about 3 minutes (punctal occlusion).

◆ *Evaluation.* Monitor the patient for expected side effects and adverse effects. Report significant changes in vital signs, particularly blood pressure lower than 90/60

| Table 22.2 | Examples of Prostaglandin Agonist and Beta-Adrenergic Antagonist Drugs |
|---|---|

*Prostaglandin agonists* help control glaucoma by binding to prostaglandin receptor sites in the eye and relaxing smooth muscles in blood vessels, which allows the vessels to dilate and absorb aqueous humor.

*Beta-adrenergic antagonists* reduce the amount of aqueous humor by binding to beta-adrenergic receptors in the ciliary body of the eye.

| DRUG/ADULT DOSAGE | NURSING IMPLICATIONS |
|---|---|
| **Prostaglandin Agonists** | |
| bimatoprost (Lumigan) adults and adolescents 16 years of age or older, 1 drop of 0.01% or 0.03% solution as prescribed in affected eye daily in the evening<br>latanoprost (Xalatan 0.005% solution and Xelpros 0.005% emulsion) adults, 1 drop (1.5 mcg) in affected eye daily in the evening<br>tafluprost (Zioptan 0.0015% ophthalmic solution) 1 drop in affected eye daily in the evening<br>travoprost (Travatan 0.004%, Travatan Z 0.004%) adults and adolescents 16 years of age and older, 1 drop in affected eye daily in the evening | • Check the eye carefully for any scratches or signs of trauma. If any are found, withhold the drug and contact the registered nurse or healthcare provider because these drugs should not be given if there are any breaks in the tissue.<br>• Ensure that you are administering the correct concentration of the solution to avoid medication error.<br>• Teach patients that they may notice changes in the color of the affected eye (usually it becomes darker). Patients may notice a slightly darker color on the eyelid. These color changes may be permanent.<br>• Eyelashes on the affected eye may grow longer and thicker. Do not attempt to use the drops in the unaffected eye to make the eyelashes match because the drug may be dangerous if used inappropriately. |
| **Beta-Adrenergic Antagonists** | |
| betaxolol hydrochloride (Betoptic) 1–2 drops (0.5% solution) in affected eye twice daily; 0.25% resin-formulated suspension 1 drop (0.25%) in the affected eye twice daily<br>carteolol 1 drop (1% solution) in affected eye twice daily<br>levobunolol (Betagan, Betagan with C Cap) 1–2 drops (0.25% solution) in affected eye twice daily; 1–2 drops (0.5% solution) in affected eye once daily<br>metipranolol (OptiPranolol) 1 drop (0.3% solution) in affected eye twice daily<br>timolol (Betimol, Istalol, Timoptic) 1 drop (0.25% solution or 0.5% solution) in affected eye once or twice daily<br>timolol GFS (gel-forming solution) (Timoptic-XE) 1 drop (0.25% solution or 0.5% solution) in affected eye once daily | • To reduce the risk of systemic absorption, perform punctal occlusion on the affected eye or remind the patient to keep the eye closed for 2–3 minutes.<br>• Check vital signs every 4–8 hours while the patient is receiving these drugs to assess for any decreases in heart rate or blood pressure; note any increased respiratory effects because these can be signs of systemic absorption.<br>• Recheck the blood glucose level in patients with diabetes regularly because beta-blockers can mask the symptoms of hypoglycemia.<br>• Ensure that you are administering the correct concentration of the solution to avoid medication error. |

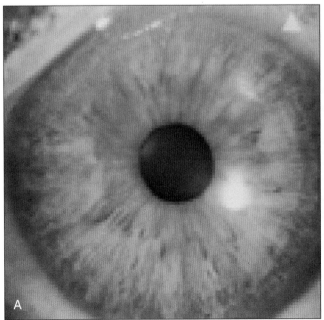 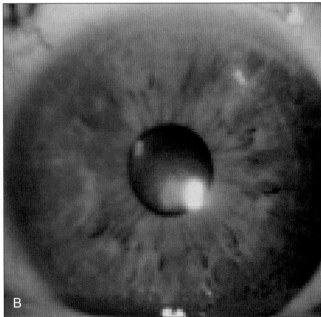

Fig. 22.12 Changes in iris color associated with prostaglandin agonist drug therapy for glaucoma. (A) Before treatment. (B) After treatment. (From Yanoff, M., & Duker, J. (2014). *Ophthalmology* (4th ed.). Mosby.)

Table 22.3    **Examples of Common Alpha-Adrenergic Agonists and Cholinergic Drugs for Glaucoma**

*Alpha-adrenergic agonists* reduce the amount of aqueous humor produced in the eye. They also improve the flow of aqueous humor out of the anterior chamber of the eye. These actions reduce intraocular pressure.

*Cholinergic drugs* increase availability of acetylcholine to activate specific receptors, which decreases production of aqueous humor and improves outflow of aqueous humor to decrease intraocular pressure.

| DRUG/ADULT DOSAGE | NURSING IMPLICATIONS |
|---|---|
| **Alpha-Adrenergic Agonists** | |
| apraclonidine (0.5% ophthalmic solution) 1–2 drops in affected eye every 8 hours three times daily<br>dipivefrin hydrochloride (0.1% ophthalmic solution) 1 drop in affected eye every 12 hours<br>brimonidine (0.1%, 0.15%, 0.2% ophthalmic solution) adults, adolescents, and children 2 years and older, 1 drop into the affected eye(s) 3 times daily about 8 hours apart | • Remind patients that, although these drops can sometimes make them feel they have something in their eye, they should not rub the eyelid.<br>• Monitor vital signs regularly because these drugs can cause increased or decreased blood pressure if absorbed systemically.<br>• Report upper respiratory symptoms such as cough, shortness of breath, sore throat, or runny nose because these can be adverse effects of the alpha-adrenergic agonists.<br>• These drugs may be used for short-term reduction of intraocular pressure or in addition to other types of drugs for patients who do not respond to other drugs.<br>• Wait at least 5 minutes after taking these drops before using other types of eye drops. |
| **Cholinergic Drugs** | |
| carbachol (Isopto Carbachol; 1.5% solution or 3% solution) 2 drops in affected eye up to three times daily<br>pilocarpine (Isopto Carpine; 1% solution or 2% solution) 1 drop in affected eye up to 4 times daily depending on the strength of solution and patient response to the drug; ophthalmic gel, apply ½-inch ribbon in the lower conjunctival sac of the affected eye once daily at bedtime; also available as an ocular insert—follow administration directions carefully | • Remind patients that vision may be decreased at night and that they may need to avoid night driving.<br>• Teach patients to wear protective sunglasses in bright lights because these drugs can cause photophobia.<br>• Report symptoms such as sweating, bradycardia, drop in blood pressure, diarrhea, nausea, and vomiting because they may indicate systemic absorption.<br>• Remind patient to follow appropriate eye drop administration techniques to reduce risk of systemic exposure. |

mm Hg or heart rate less than 60 beats/min. Watch for changes in respiratory status, including shortness of breath or wheezing, and for decreased oxygenation of the blood (pulse oximetry below 92%).

 **Top Tip for Safety**

To avoid contamination, never touch the tip of the applicator to the patient's eye or with your finger.

◆ *Patient and family teaching.* In addition to the general teaching points listed in Box 22.3, tell the patient and family:

• Do not increase the dose or use the drug more often than prescribed because excessive use increases the risk for heart and breathing problems, especially if you have asthma, COPD, or other respiratory problems.
• Use good lighting when reading. Use caution in darker rooms because the pupil will not dilate to let in more light, and it may be harder to see objects in dim light. This problem can increase the risk of falls.
• Avoid driving at night because your vision will be reduced.

• If you have diabetes, check your blood glucose more often because these drugs can mask the symptoms of hypoglycemia if the drug is absorbed systemically.

 **Lifespan Considerations**

**Older Adults**

Before giving beta-adrenergic blocker eye drops to older patients, make sure they are not taking any oral beta-blockers for a cardiac condition. If they are, notify the healthcare provider. Older adults are more likely to have cardiac and respiratory problems due to systemic absorption of eye drops.

## ALPHA-ADRENERGIC AGONISTS

### Action and Uses

In patients with glaucoma, alpha-adrenergic agonists bind to receptor sites in the eye and reduce the amount of aqueous humor produced. They also improve the flow of aqueous humor out of the anterior chamber, and both of these actions reduce the IOP. Common alpha-adrenergic agonists for glaucoma, their dosages, and nursing implications are listed in Table 22.3. Consult a drug reference book for more information about specific alpha-adrenergic agonists to control glaucoma.

### Expected Side Effects

Side effects commonly experienced by patients who are taking alpha-adrenergic agonists for their glaucoma include tearing, redness, blurring of vision, and burning or stinging after receiving the eye drops. Some patients may experience the sensation of a foreign body in the eye.

### Adverse Reactions

Adverse reactions to alpha-adrenergic agonists include bradycardia or tachycardia and a drop in blood pressure. These effects can result from giving too many drops of the drug, causing systemic absorption. Other adverse effects include allergic reaction, fatigue, and respiratory symptoms.

### ❖ Nursing Implications and Patient Teaching

◆ *Assessment.* In addition to the general nursing considerations related to eye drug therapy listed in Box 22.2, assess the patient's vital signs, especially heart rate, because the drug can cause tachycardia or bradycardia. Patients may also experience a drop in blood pressure and/or orthostatic hypotension. Let the prescriber know if the patient is taking antianxiety agents (particularly benzodiazepines), antidepressants, or sedatives, because these drugs may increase central nervous system (CNS) effects.

◆ *Planning and implementation.* Carefully monitor the patient's heart rate and blood pressure for changes after giving the eye drops. Read the label carefully to confirm that you are giving the correct concentration of the drug. To decrease the risk of adverse effects, give the exact number of eye drops prescribed by the healthcare provider to the patient. Ask the patient to close his or her eyes for 2 minutes, or place a gloved finger over the tear duct and apply gentle pressure for about 3 minutes. Always wipe off any excess drug that spills on the eyelid or face to avoid systemic absorption.

◆ *Patient and family teaching.* In addition to the general teaching points listed in Box 22.3, tell the patient and family:
- Read packaging carefully because some drugs may need to be stored in the refrigerator and protected from light to maintain potency.
- Wear dark glasses when you are in the sunlight or other bright light conditions because your pupil will be dilated and your eye will be sensitive to light.
- If you have been prescribed this drug for a limited time such as 1 week, do not continue taking it beyond that period. These drugs can continue to lower IOP below normal, which can cause additional problems with your vision.

## CHOLINERGIC DRUGS

### Action and Uses

Cholinergic drugs lead to decreased IOP by reducing the amount of aqueous humor produced and improving its flow. When the amount of acetylcholine is increased, the pupil becomes smaller (miosis). This increases the amount of space between the lens and the iris, allowing the aqueous fluid to flow freely and decreasing IOP.

Common cholinergic drugs for glaucoma, their dosages, and nursing implications are listed in Table 22.3. Be sure to consult a drug reference book for more information about specific cholinergic drugs to control glaucoma.

### Expected Side Effects

Expected side effects of cholinergic drugs include tearing, stinging, redness of the eye, and blurred vision. Cholinergic drugs cause miosis, and patients may experience difficulty with vision at night or have night blindness. As with other eye drugs discussed in this chapter, systemic side effects are possible; they include headache, increased saliva, increased urination, and sweating. Side effects are intensified if patients are prescribed an oral form of a cholinergic drug.

### Adverse Reactions

Adverse reactions are more common with systemic absorption of the drug. Examples include changes in blood pressure and abnormal heart rhythms. Other adverse effects include double vision and retinal detachment.

### ❖ Nursing Implications and Patient Teaching

◆ *Assessment.* In addition to the general nursing considerations related to eye drug therapy listed in Box 22.2, carefully monitor the patient's vital signs. Assess blood pressure, heart rate, and respiratory rate because they may be sensitive to changes caused by cholinergic drugs. Assess the patient for the side effects expected from any drug that increases acetylcholine, including increased saliva, increased urination, and sweating.

 **Memory Jogger**

Patients who are taking eye drugs for glaucoma may have unequal pupil sizes. If there is any question about neurologic status, contact the RN or healthcare provider for assessment.

Cholinergic drugs should be avoided by people who have breathing problems such as asthma or chronic bronchitis. These drugs should be avoided by patients with gallbladder or liver disease. Always use the correct dose, and wipe any excess drug off of the patient's skin because it can be absorbed and cause systemic effects. Use the punctal occlusion technique or ask the patient to close his or her eyes for at least 2 minutes after giving the drug.

**Top Tip for Safety**

To decrease the risk of side effects and adverse reactions, wipe off any excess drug from the skin rather than let it be absorbed. Never give more drops than are prescribed.

◆ *Evaluation.* Report significant changes in the patient's vital signs, including decreased heart rate (< 60 beats/min) or trouble breathing. Symptoms such as drooling, severe sweating, respiratory failure, and severe neuromuscular weakness indicate cholinergic toxicity.

**Top Tip for Safety**

A sudden change in blood pressure, change in heart rate, or difficulty breathing may be related to cholinergic eye drugs. Notify the healthcare provider immediately.

◆ *Patient and family teaching.* In addition to the general teaching points listed in Box 22.3, tell the patient and family:

- Your pupils will not dilate normally, and it may be difficult to see. Use caution in moving from light to dark rooms, and use good lighting for reading and other daily activities.
- To avoid absorption, remove any excess drug if it spills on your skin.
- Report immediately to your healthcare provider increased drooling or sweating or any difficulty breathing because those symptoms may indicate a toxic level of the drug.

## CARBONIC ANHYDRASE INHIBITORS

### Action and Uses

A **carbonic anhydrase inhibitor (CAI)** lowers IOP by reducing aqueous humor in the anterior chamber of the eye. CAIs are a type of diuretic and are available in oral forms, as eye drops, and intravenously (for patients who need a rapid decrease in IOP to prevent serious optic nerve damage). Common CAIs for glaucoma, their dosages, and nursing implications are listed in Table 22.4. Be sure to consult a drug reference book for more information about specific CAIs to control glaucoma.

### Expected Side Effects

Eye drops can cause slight burning or stinging with administration. Some patients may experience a bitter or sour taste in the mouth. In rare cases, redness of the conjunctiva can occur. CAIs can cause CNS effects and must be used with caution. Patients may experience drowsiness, fatigue, and headache with oral and intravenous forms. Blood glucose levels may fluctuate when the patient is taking oral CAIs.

### Adverse Reactions

Some CAIs are related to sulfonamide drugs and may cause an allergic reaction in patients who are allergic to any sulfa drug. The allergic response can happen even with eye drops, so notify the healthcare provider before giving a CAI to a patient with a sulfa allergy.

When CAIs are taken orally or intravenously, the patient can experience a wide range of adverse effects, including neurologic effects (e.g., confusion, dizziness, numbness of the hands and feet, paralysis), severe skin infections, severe electrolyte imbalances, and liver failure.

### ❖ Nursing Implications and Patient Teaching

◆ *Assessment.* In addition to the general nursing considerations related to eye drug therapy listed in Box 22.2, monitor the patient for side effects and adverse reactions, particularly CNS effects, which are more likely with the oral or intravenous drugs. Ask about and report sulfa allergy to the healthcare provider before giving any CAI.

**Top Tip for Safety**

Never give a CAI to a patient who has a sulfa allergy because some of these drugs are sulfonamides.

◆ *Evaluation.* Assess the patient's response to the drug. Report severe side effects or adverse reactions to the healthcare provider. One side effect, a bitter or sour

| Table 22.4 | Examples of Carbonic Anhydrase Inhibitors |

*Carbonic anhydrase inhibitors* lower intraocular pressure by reducing aqueous humor in the anterior chamber of the eye.

| DRUG/ADULT DOSAGE | NURSING IMPLICATIONS |
|---|---|
| acetazolamide (Diamox)<br>sustained-release capsules: 250 mg orally one to four times daily<br>extended-release capsules: 500 mg by mouth twice daily<br>brinzolamide (Azopt; 1% solution) 1 drop in affected eye three times daily<br>dorzolamide (Trusopt; 2% solution) 1 drop in affected eye three times daily<br>methazolamide 50–100 mg orally two to three times daily | • Double-check allergies before giving these drugs because some may have cross-sensitivity with sulfonamide antibiotics.<br>• Report any gastrointestinal problems to the healthcare provider because they may be side effects of these drugs.<br>• Monitor electrolytes (particularly sodium and potassium) because these drugs are also categorized as diuretics.<br>• Monitor for central nervous system side effects such as drowsiness, fatigue, depression, and irritability. These may require a change in drugs.<br>• Notify the healthcare provider if the patient has a history of gout because these drugs may increase the uric acid level. |

taste in the mouth, may affect the patient's dietary intake, and it should be monitored carefully. Shortness of breath, dizziness, hives, or itching may be symptoms of an allergic response.

### Lifespan Considerations

**Carbonic anhydrase inhibitors** (CAIs) should not be given to children because they can slow growth if used long term.

CAIs should be avoided during pregnancy and breast-feeding.

---

## Get Ready for the Next-Generation NCLEX® Examination!

### Key Points

- Apply only drugs and liquids labeled "for otic use" into the ear canal.
- When instilling ear drops into an adult's ear, gently pull the external ear up and back. When instilling ear drops into a young child's ear, gently pull the external ear down and back.
- Place ear drops or solutions only in the affected ear.
- Never instill a drug in the ear canal or irrigate the ear canal if drainage is present, to avoid causing a middle ear infection.
- Glaucoma is a chronic disease with no cure; drug therapy can prevent blindness and must continue for the patient's life.
- Pupil constriction is *miosis* (small word, small pupil size). Pupil dilation is *mydriasis* (larger word, larger pupil size).
- Normal intraocular pressure (IOP) is between 10 mm Hg and 20 mm Hg. Maintenance of a normal IOP keeps the eye healthy and helps prevent blindness in patients with glaucoma.
- Never instill prostaglandin agonists into an eye that has been scratched or has an infection. In these cases, contact the healthcare provider for instructions about continuing glaucoma therapy and managing the corneal problem.
- Prostaglandin agonists can change the color of the iris of the eye and increase the length of eyelashes.
- Before giving beta-adrenergic antagonist eye drops to a patient, make sure he or she is not also taking any oral beta-blocker for a cardiac condition. If he or she is, make sure to notify the prescriber prior to administration.
- Use punctal occlusion to reduce systemic absorption of eye drops. Give only the prescribed number of drops; then ask the patient to close his or her eyes for 2 minutes, or place a gloved finger over the tear duct and apply gentle pressure for about 3 minutes.
- All ophthalmic drugs must be labeled specifically "for ophthalmic use."
- Give eye drops or eye ointment in the affected eye only.
- To avoid contamination, never touch the tip of the bottle or tube to your finger or directly to the patient's eye.
- Gently pull the lower lid of the affected eye down so that you can place the eye drops or ointment into the conjunctival sac.
- Glaucoma drugs are typically available in various strengths. Read the label carefully, and give the correct strength prescribed for the patient.
- Adrenergic agonists cause mydriasis. The patient's pupils are dilated, and the eyes are more sensitive to bright lights.

Patients may need to wear protective sunglasses in bright conditions.
- Beta-blockers and cholinergic drugs cause miosis. Patients may have difficulty adjusting to dim lighting because their pupils are smaller. Patients need to use caution to avoid falls.
- Teach patients to report dizziness or shortness of breath to the healthcare provider because these symptoms indicate side effects of the glaucoma drugs.
- Advise patients with diabetes that beta-blockers can mask the symptoms of low blood sugar. Checking blood glucose levels regularly is very important.
- Symptoms of too much cholinergic drug include increased saliva, increased urination, and sweating.
- Patients who are taking eye drugs for glaucoma may have unequal pupil size. If there is any question about neurologic status, contact the registered nurse or healthcare provider for assessment.
- Cholinergic drugs should be avoided by people who have breathing problems such as asthma or chronic bronchitis.
- To decrease the risk of side effects and adverse reactions to spilled ophthalmic drug, wipe any excess drug from the skin rather than let it absorb.
- CAIs can cause severe neurologic or electrolyte imbalances and must be given with caution.
- CAIs are not approved for children because they can slow growth.
- CAIs are not used during pregnancy or breast-feeding because they are known to cause birth defects in animals.

### Clinical Judgment and Next-Generation NCLEX® Examination-Style Questions

1. A 78-year-old woman is prescribed 1 drop of 0.25% timolol ophthalmic solution (Timoptic) to her left eye every day for glaucoma. How does the licensed practical/vocational nurse (LPN/VN) teach the patient to perform punctal occlusion?

   1. Teach the patient to gently press her index finger against the inner corner of her eye over the tear duct for 3 minutes after putting in the eye drops.
   2. Teach the patient to press her index finger over the outer portion of her eye (between the eye and the cheek) for 3 minutes after putting in the eye drops.
   3. Teach the patient to press her index finger against the inner part of the eye over her tear duct for 10 to 20 seconds after putting in the eye drops.
   4. Teach the patient to press her index finger over the outer portion of her eye (between the eye and the cheek) for 10 to 20 seconds after putting in the eye drops.

2. The LPN/VN is assessing a patient who is taking cholinergic eye drops. Which symptoms should be reported to the healthcare provider? **Select all or any that apply.**

   1. Redness of the eyes
   2. Burning sensation in the eyes
   3. Diarrhea
   4. Hypotension
   5. Increased salivation
   6. Increased heart rate

3. A 74-year-old female with a long history of glaucoma has now been prescribed brimonidine 0.2%, an alpha-adrenergic agonist, that causes miosis. Which of the following statements indicates a need for more teaching?

   1. "This drug may make my eyelashes grow a little longer."
   2. "I will avoid touching the eye dropper to prevent eye infection."
   3. "I understand that this drug is usually needed for harder to treat glaucoma."
   4. "I will keep taking my eye drops, even if I feel well."

4. A patient is prescribed an ophthalmic beta-blocker for glaucoma. Which of the following adverse effects are possible if the drug is absorbed into the blood system? **Select all or any that apply.**

   1. Heart rate less than 60 beats/min
   2. Decreased blood pressure
   3. Increased tearing
   4. Dizziness
   5. Redness of the eyes

5. Which of the following are common side effects of prostaglandin agonists? **Select all or any that apply.**

   1. Changes in color of the affected eye
   2. Increased length of eyelashes
   3. Dilation of the pupil
   4. Foreign body sensation
   5. Increased heart rate

6. The nurse is instructing the patient about latanoprost (Xalatan) drops. Which statement indicates a need for further instruction?

   1. "I can stop the drops after my intraocular pressure goes down."
   2. "I need to notify the healthcare provider if I injure my eye."
   3. "My eyelashes may become thicker and longer."
   4. "The iris of my eyes may become darker."

7. The patient is taking metoprolol for high blood pressure. The healthcare provider orders timolol eye drops for the patient's glaucoma. Which of the following actions will the nurse do first?

   1. Monitor the patient's blood pressure four times a day while the patient is taking the drugs.
   2. Give the eye drops and apply punctal occlusion to prevent systemic absorption.
   3. Increase fluid intake to 2000 to 3000 mL/day to avoid dehydration.
   4. Contact the healthcare provider to clarify the order to avoid a potential adverse drug effect.

8. An elderly woman with cognitive impairment accidentally takes three times the prescribed number of pilocarpine eye drops for her glaucoma. Which of the following symptoms suggest cholinergic toxicity? **Select all or any that apply.**

   1. Increased sweating
   2. Constipation
   3. Drooling
   4. Diarrhea
   5. Dilated pupils

9. The patient is prescribed latanoprost (Xalatan) 0.005% ophthalmic solution as 1 drop (1.5 mcg) to the left eye every evening for glaucoma. The bottle holds 2.5 mL. In latanoprost, 1 mL is equal to 35 drops. How many days will the drug last if the patient uses the drug exactly as prescribed?

10. A patient is prescribed the carbonic anhydrase inhibitor acetazolamide 250 mg by mouth three times a day for glaucoma. How many milligrams will the patient take each day?

11. A 72-year-old diabetic patient is prescribed carteolol 1 drop in both eyes twice daily for glaucoma. Which of the following statements by the patient indicate a need for more teaching?

    1. "I will keep my eyes closed for 2 to 3 minutes after taking the eye drops to avoid getting the drug in my system."
    2. "I will notify my doctor if I have any dizziness or shortness of breath."
    3. "I will continue to check my blood sugar regularly because it may mask the symptoms if my blood sugar gets low.
    4. "This drug will dilate my pupil, so I will need to wear sunglasses in brightly lit rooms."

12. A patient comes to the outpatient clinic and states that hearing is decreased in the left ear. The nurse practitioner checks the patient's ear and notices a large amount of earwax obstructing the eardrum. The LPN/VN carefully reads the label of the drug to ensure that it is "for otic use." Place the nurse's next actions in the correct order.

    1. Ask the patient to lie down with the head turned so that the affected ear is turned upward; if the patient is sitting in a chair, tilt the patient's head so the affected ear is up.
    2. Using the applicator, place only the prescribed number of drops into the patient's ear. Aim the drops onto the side of the ear canal and let them run into the ear.
    3. Insert a cotton ball into the opening of the ear canal to keep the drops from rolling out of the ear.
    4. Wash your hands and don a pair of clean gloves.
    5. For an older child or adult, pull the pinna up and back.
    6. Remove your gloves and wash your hands.

**Case Study 1**

Ms. James is a 41-year-old black patient who was diagnosed with glaucoma after a screening event sponsored by her church. Her healthcare provider prescribed bimatoprost (Lumigan) 0.01% ophthalmic solution 1 drop in both eyes once daily.

1. What are the risk factors for glaucoma?

2. Bimatoprost belongs to which class of glaucoma drugs?

3. What are common side effects of bimatoprost?

4. Ms. James is having difficulty applying her eye drops. What teaching strategies would you use to assist her?

5. Ms. James enjoys wearing eye makeup daily. What additional teaching would you include in her plan of care?

6. As Ms. James is leaving the office, she mentions that she just could not believe she had glaucoma because "only old people get glaucoma." You are concerned that she may have difficulty adhering to her treatment plan. What information would you provide the patient to help increase her understanding of glaucoma?

7. What resources (e.g., Web site[s]) would help Ms. James?

**Case Study 2**

The nurse is working with a patient who was recently diagnosed with glaucoma. She has been prescribed latanoprost (Xalatan) 0.005% solution 1 drop in the right eye daily. **Choose the *most likely* options for the information missing from the statements below by selecting from the list of options provided.**

When administering the latanoprost, the nurse will _____ prior to administering, double check that he or she has selected the correct _____, and then administer 1 drop to the right eye. The nurse will teach the patient that ___ on the affected eye may become longer and thicker and that the _____ may become darker.

| OPTIONS |
|---|
| eyelid |
| cornea |
| solution concentration |
| eyelashes |
| right |
| left |
| check for any scratches or signs of trauma |

---

## Next-Generation NCLEX® (NGN) Examination–Style Question

**History and Physical**
**0700**

A 63-year-old male Mexican American client is admitted to the medical-surgical unit for evaluation and treatment of congestive heart failure exacerbation. The client is resting quietly with no complaints. The nurse administers the client's scheduled ophthalmic medication.

Past Medical History: glaucoma, congestive heart failure
Physical Exam:
General: no acute distress
HEENT: decreased peripheral vision, pupils 3 mm and reactive to light
Respiratory: faint bilateral crackles
Cardiovascular: S1, S2, no murmur, 2+ bilateral lower-extremity edema
Skin: warm dry

**Nurse's Notes**
**0900**

The nurse returns to reassess the client.

**Laboratory Results**
**0700**

| TEST/PANEL | RESULT | NORMAL |
|---|---|---|
| Potassium | 4.2 mEq/L (4.2 mmol/L) | 3.5–5 mEq/L (3.5–5 mmol/L) |

**Flow Sheet**
**0700**

Blood Pressure: 128/80 mm Hg
Heart Rate: 80/min
Respiratory Rate: 16/min
Temperature: 98.6°F (37°C)

**Orders**
**0700**

Timolol ophthalmic 0.5% solution, 1 drop in each eye twice daily

The nurse returns to reassess the client at **0900** to evaluate for expected effects and side effects of the administered medication.

**For each assessment finding, click to indicate whether the nurse would assess for an increase, decrease, or expect no change at 0900.**

*Each row must have only one response option selected.*

| ASSESSMENT FINDING | INCREASE | DECREASE | NO CHANGE ANTICIPATED |
|---|---|---|---|
| Blood Pressure | | | |
| Temperature | | | |
| Heart Rate | | | |
| Pupil Size | | | |
| Eye Dryness | | | |
| Potassium | | | |

See answer on Evolve at http://evolve.elsevier.com/Visovsky/LPNpharmacology/.

# Over-the-Counter Drug Therapy

## Learning Outcomes

1. Explain what to teach patients and families about over-the-counter drugs.
2. List side effects and precautions needed for herbal preparations and those used for complementary and alternative medicine.
3. Discuss the benefits and drawbacks of medical cannabis.
4. List the actions, side effects, and precautions to take when giving the vitamins most commonly prescribed for supplementation.
5. Explain what to teach patients and families about supplemental vitamins.
6. List the actions, side effects, and precautions to take when giving the minerals most commonly prescribed for supplementation.
6. Explain what to teach patients and families about supplemental minerals.

## Key Terms

**alternative medicine**  Medical therapies such as herbalism, homeopathy, and acupuncture that are not considered mainstream.

**ascorbic acid**  Vitamin C.

**complementary medicine**  Alternative medicine therapies used in conjunction with a conventional or mainstream approach.

**herbal products**  Ground-up parts of plants made into pills, capsules, or liquids; refers to plants used in medicine as well as in cooking.

**hypervitaminosis**  Excessive intake and high storage level of one or more vitamins (notably vitamins A, D, E, and K) that can lead to toxic symptoms.

**integrative practices**  Complementary and conventional approaches to healthcare that mainly focus on health and wellness.

**minerals**  Substances found in food that are necessary for normal body function.

**niacin**  Vitamin $B_3$ or nicotinic acid, which is used to lower triglyceride levels and prevent pellagra.

**over-the-counter (OTC) drugs**  Category of drugs approved by the US Food and Drug Administration that do not require a prescription to purchase.

**riboflavin**  Vitamin $B_2$, which is used to treat riboflavin deficiency.

**thiamine**  Vitamin $B_1$, which is used to treat beriberi.

**vitamin A**  Beta-carotene, which is used to treat vitamin A deficiency.

**vitamins**  Substances found in food that are necessary for body functions and that can be broken down by heat, air, or acid.

## DOCUMENTING PATIENT HEALTHCARE PRACTICES

We often forget that many of the drugs patients use are bought in stores without a prescription or are recommended by a healthcare provider. According to the Consumer Healthcare Products Association, Americans spent about $35.2 billion on nonprescription remedies in 2018, more than double the amount spent in 2008. Over-the-counter (OTC) drugs are drugs that have been approved by the US Food and Drug Administration (FDA) that do not require a prescription to purchase because they have been judged to be safe when directions are followed and to have a low risk of abuse.

It is important for you to be familiar with the many nonprescription products available to patients. Many of these products contain chemicals that are useful in treating common health problems but carry with them safety concerns. Dangerous interactions can occur. You must become familiar with these OTC drugs to help patients choose the safest product for their current health concern, problem, or illness.

Patients do not always think to mention herbal products because they may regard them as natural and harmless or not drugs at all. Many Americans consider OTC products to be safe because they are available without prescription. Herbal products and OTC drugs may not be safe when considering the particular disease process and all other drugs, legal or otherwise, that the patient may be taking. When taking a drug history, always ask patients if they are taking OTC or herbal drugs and document the answers. Questionable products need to be brought to the attention of the healthcare provider.

Ask patients to bring in all herbs or drug remedies they are using so they may be accurately recorded.

Patients sometimes do not know the active ingredients that are in the products. Products in their original bottles or boxes give you information that may help determine whether they are safe and whether drug interactions or complications are possible.

Patients who rely on **complementary medicine, alternative medicine, or integrative practices** may take herbs, supplements, or other drugs instead of prescription drugs because of the cost, or they may use such products in addition to prescription drugs. There are several terms to describe the drugs that are taken by patients who seek complementary, alternative, or integrative healthcare, including botanical, holistic, natural, unconventional, and new age medicine. In this chapter, the term *alternative drug* is used.

There are several reasons patients use OTC, herbal, or complementary products:

- Patients seek products they hope will keep them in good health, prevent disease, or provide treatment for the health problems they have.
- They have tried traditional drugs and treatments without success.
- The traditionally prescribed drugs had undesirable side effects.
- There is no known drug therapy that can cure their problem, but alternative drugs can provide them with some relief.
- Trusted people in their family or community have told them about the product.
- They are seeking a cheaper drug to replace a prescription drug.
- Traditional drugs or treatments violate their religious or spiritual beliefs.
- They seek a more integrative medicinal approach to their healthcare.

## OVER-THE-COUNTER DRUGS

The role of OTC agents in healthcare today is growing. The FDA estimates between 100,000 and 300,000 products are available OTC. These products contain one or more of about 800 active chemicals and come in a variety of formulations, sizes, and strengths. The annual sales of OTC products are estimated at $38 billion.

Nonprescription OTC products are considered to be safe and effective for people to use without instructions from a healthcare provider about how they are to be taken. OTC products are different from prescription drugs in the following ways:

- The label information is more complete than the information on prescription drug labels. Be aware, however, the information can be difficult for some patients to read because it is printed in small type.
- OTC drugs have a wider margin of safety because of the substantial testing they have undergone before advertising. The formulations of many OTC products have been changed by the manufacturer based on information gathered after years of use by consumers.
- OTC drugs are widely available and advertised.
- The dose is often lower than the same drugs available with a prescription.
- OTC products are usually not covered by insurance.

The most common categories of OTC drugs are similar to those available by prescription. For example, laxatives, products to treat peptic acid disorders (antacids and $H_2$-receptor antagonists), analgesics, cough and cold products (antihistamines, decongestants, expectorants, and antitussives), vaginal antifungals, smoking cessation products, and topical steroids are available OTC.

Drugs that were once available only by prescription have been given OTC status, often in lower dosages than the prescription formulations. For example, ibuprofen is available as an OTC drug sold in 200-mg tablets, but it is available by prescription in 800-mg tablets.

OTC drugs are sold in pharmacies, grocery stores, gas stations, and department stores. It is important to learn the generic drug name along with the product (trade) name because there are so many different names and versions of these products. Many of these products have multiple ingredients. The cost of combination products can be more than buying all of their ingredients singly, and it is important to compare prices of commonly used products such as the OTC drug Tylenol PM, which contains acetaminophen (Tylenol) and diphenhydramine (Benadryl).

## PRODUCT LABELING

The FDA requires that OTC product labels contain important information in a manner that a typical person can read and understand (Fig. 23.1). Drug companies are required to use a standard labeling format for all OTCs sold in the United States. Key information begins with the names of the active ingredients, followed by the drug's purposes, uses, warnings, directions, and other information including the names of inactive ingredients. The labeling information is placed in the same order on all OTC packages in an easy-to-read format.

Surveys show that women are the family members most likely to buy OTC products. They are also more likely than men to read labels before taking drugs.

One of the most important things to look for on the OTC label is the presence of other chemicals in a product that may pose a risk. These "hidden" chemicals are used to help make the drug taste better, to help preserve the drug, to give color, and to help deliver the product or make it more stable. Consumers who have an allergy or intolerance to even small amounts of these hidden chemicals may not be aware of the risk unless they read the list of active and inactive ingredients on the label. Table 23.1 lists a number of common hidden chemicals in OTC products.

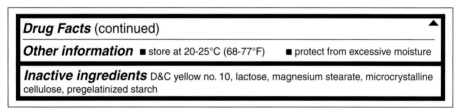

> # *Drug Facts*
>
> ## *Active ingredient (in each tablet)*               **Purpose**
> Chlorpheniramine maleate 2 mg.......................................................Antihistamine
>
> ## *Uses* temporarily relieves these symptoms due to hay fever or other upper respiratory allergies: ■ sneezing    ■ runny nose    ■ itchy, watery eyes    ■ itchy throat
>
> ## *Warnings*
> **Ask a doctor before use if you have**
> ■ glaucoma    ■ a breathing problem such as emphysema or chronic bronchitis
> ■ trouble urinating due to an enlarged prostate gland
>
> **Ask a doctor or pharmacist before use if you are** taking tranquilizers or sedatives
>
> **When using this product**
> ■ drowsiness may occur    ■ avoid alcoholic drinks
> ■ alcohol, sedatives, and tranquilizers may increase drowsiness
> ■ be careful when driving a motor vehicle or operating machinery
> ■ excitability may occur, especially in children
>
> **If pregnant or breast-feeding,** ask a health professional before use.
> **Keep out of reach of children.** In case of overdose, get medical help or contact a Poison Control Center right away.
>
> ## *Directions*
>
> | adults and children 12 years and over | take 2 tablets every 4 to 6 hours; not more than 12 tablets in 24 hours |
> |---|---|
> | children 6 years to under 12 years | take 1 tablet every 4 to 6 hours; not more than 6 tablets in 24 hours |
> | children under 6 years | ask a doctor |

> # *Drug Facts* (continued)
>
> ## *Other information*   ■ store at 20-25°C (68-77°F)    ■ protect from excessive moisture
>
> ## *Inactive ingredients* D&C yellow no. 10, lactose, magnesium stearate, microcrystalline cellulose, pregelatinized starch

**Fig. 23.1** An over-the-counter drug label. (Courtesy US Food and Drug Administration.)

## PATIENT TEACHING

Healthcare providers should tell patients some basic facts about OTC products. This important information is sometimes printed and given to the patient. Whether given verbally or in writing, the following are some of the key facts patients should learn:

- Always read the instructions on the label.
- Do not take OTC drugs in higher dosages or for a longer time than the label states.
- If you do not get well within 2 weeks, stop treating yourself, and talk with a healthcare professional.
- Side effects from OTC drugs are relatively uncommon, but read the label to know what they are.
- Responses to drugs vary from person to person.
- OTC drugs often interact with other drugs and with food or alcohol, or they might have an effect on other health problems you may have. Ask a pharmacist if you are not sure about interactions.
- If you do not understand the label, check with the pharmacist.
- Do not take the drug if the package does not have a label on it.
- Throw away drugs that have expired (are older than the date on the package).

- Do not use drugs that belong to a friend.
- Buy products that treat only the symptoms you have.
- If cost is an issue, generic OTC products may be cheaper than brand name items.
- Avoid buying these products online, outside of well-known Internet insurance company sites, because many OTC preparations sold through the Internet are counterfeit products. They may not be what you ordered, and they may be dangerous.

Parents should know the following special information about using OTC drugs for children:

- Never guess about the amount of drug to give a child. One-half an adult dose may be too much or not enough to be effective. This is true of drugs such as acetaminophen (Tylenol) or ibuprofen (Advil): Repeated overdoses may lead to poisoning of the child, liver destruction, or coma.
- If the label says to take 2 teaspoons and the dosing cup is marked with ounces only, get another measuring device. Do not try to guess about how much should be given.
- Always follow the age limits listed. If the label says the product should not be given to a child younger than 2 years, do not give it.

**Table 23.1**   **Common Active Ingredients in Over-the-Counter Products**

| HIDDEN DRUG | OTC CLASS | RISK FACTORS |
|---|---|---|
| Alcohol | Cough syrups, cold medications, mouthwash | Contraindicated for recovering alcoholics |
| Phenylephrine, pseudoephedrine | Antihistamines, analgesics, antiemetics, asthma products, cold and allergy products, menstrual products, motion sickness, sleep aids, decongestants | Difficult urination in enlarged prostate; can worsen diabetes; interact with antihypertensive and cardiac drugs; antihistamines complicate glaucoma; interact with drugs for ADHD; hyperthyroidism |
| Calcium carbonate, magnesium, sodium | Antacids | Kidney or heart disease (sodium and magnesium salts negatively affect disease process) |
| Bismuth subsalicylate | Kaopectate, Pepto-Bismol | Hard to excrete in kidney disease |
| Ibuprofen, naproxen | Ibuprofen | Kidney and liver disease, stomach ulcers, bleeding disorders |
| Acetaminophen | Analgesics; antidiarrheal; cold, allergy, and sleep products | Liver disease or alcoholism; easy to overdose with acetaminophen because it is hidden in many products |
| Caffeine | Analgesics; cold, migraine, and allergy products; diuretics; menstrual products; stimulants and weight control products | Can worsen heart disease, hypertension, sleep disorders |
| Sugar | Cough syrups and other syrup-based OTC drugs | Diabetes |
| Salicylates (e.g., aspirin, salsalate) | Anacin, Excedrin, Alka-Seltzer | Bleeding disorders, ulcers; can cause Reye's syndrome in children with flu symptoms; use with caution with renal-impaired patients as salicylates are excreted by the kidneys |
| Diphenhydramine | Antihistamines, sleep aids, cough and cold products | Confusion, falls, disorientation (especially in older adults) |

*ADHD*, attention deficit/hyperactivity disorder; *OTC*, over-the-counter.
Modified from Katzung, B. G. (2006). *Basic and clinical pharmacology* (10th ed.). McGraw-Hill Medical; Lynch, S. S. (2022). Precautions with over-the-counter drugs. In *Merck Manual Consumer Version*. http://www.merckmanuals.com/home/drugs/over-the-counter_drugs/precautions_with_over-the-counter_drugs.html

- Always use the child-resistant cap, relock the cap after use, and keep drugs in a safe place away from children.
- Throw away old, discolored, or expired drugs and any drug that has lost its label instructions.
- Do not give children a drug that contains alcohol.

## HERBAL PRODUCTS AND COMPLEMENTARY AND ALTERNATIVE MEDICINE

According to the National Institutes of Health (NIH), a survey conducted in 2012 found that 30% of adults and 12% of children use some form of alternative practices. Dietary supplements (botanicals and herbals), acupuncture, massage, mind-body medicine, and traditional Chinese medicine have been used by people in the search for health and wellness for thousands of years.

Evidence-based research for many alternative therapies is often absent, and the safety and efficacy of many are unclear. The NIH Center for Complementary and Integrative Health (NCCIH) sponsors and publishes research based on scientific evidence regarding many alternative therapies. You can better educate yourself and your patients using the evidence-based research findings available on the NIH NCCIH Web site (https://nccih.nih.gov).

 **Bookmark This!**

NIH Center for Complementary and Integrative Health: https://nccih.nih.gov.

It is important to have up-to-date, balanced, and scientific materials to help you understand herbal therapies. Such materials can help you know more about the strengths, weaknesses, clinical indications, proper dosages, toxicities, and interactions of alternative drug therapies so that you are able to accurately answer patient questions.

## PRODUCT LABELING OF DIETARY SUPPLEMENTS

The federal government has regulated dietary supplements through the FDA since 1994. A *dietary supplement* contains one or more ingredients such as vitamins, herbals, botanicals, or amino acids. However, regulations for dietary supplements are not the same as those for prescription or OTC drugs.

According to the FDA, a dietary supplement must be labeled as such and must be intended to be taken only as a dietary supplement (Fig. 23.2). Labeling information must not be deceptive. Producers of dietary supplements are responsible for ensuring that products are safe; however, they do not have to provide the

## Supplement Facts

Serving Size 1 Capsule

| Amount Per Capsule | | % Daily Value |
|---|---|---|
| Calories  20 | | |
| Calories from Fat  20 | | |
| Total Fat  2 g | | 3%* |
| Saturated Fat  0.5 g | | 3%* |
| Polyunsaturated Fat  1 g | | † |
| Monounsaturated Fat  0.5 g | | † |
| Vitamin A  4250 IU | | 85% |
| Vitamin D  425 IU | | 106% |
| Omega-3 fatty acids  0.5 g | | † |

\* Percent Daily Values are based on a 2,000 calorie diet.
† Daily Value not established.

Ingredients: Cod liver oil, gelatin, water, and glycerin.

Fig. 23.2 A dietary supplement label. (Courtesy US Food and Drug Administration.)

FDA with information that demonstrates the safety of the product before it is marketed. In contrast, prescription and OTC drugs must demonstrate to the FDA that they are safe and effective before they are marketed.

If a claim is made about the effects of a dietary supplement, the producer must have data to support the claim. Any claims about how a supplement may affect the body must have the following statement on the label: "This statement has not been evaluated by the US Food and Drug Administration (FDA). This product is not intended to diagnose, treat, cure, or prevent any disease."

The FDA has the authority to remove a product from the market, but this can happen only after the agency has proof that the product is unsafe or ineffective. Ephedra is an example. Ephedra was an ingredient in some dietary supplements used for weight loss, increased energy, and enhanced athletic performance. The FDA banned its use from all products in 2004 because of increased rates of heart problems and serious side effects when combined with caffeine.

Labeling on herbal products is generally designed to promote sales and product use and not necessarily to educate the consumer. Health professionals with a general understanding of popular herbs and supplements can talk to patients about efficacy, common side effects, risks, and interactions. The LPN/VN should ask about the patient's use of alternative herbal or Chinese medicines so that the healthcare prescriber can explore the products in detail to avoid interactions with drugs ordered in the hospital or clinic.

Patients with medical problems should not use herbs or dietary supplements without medical supervision. When patients rely on themselves for diagnosis and treatment, they may delay the essential diagnosis of a serious medical problem, and this delay may worsen their condition. Some herbal products have adverse effects, and many herbal products interact with prescribed drugs.

## PROS AND CONS OF HERBAL PRODUCTS

Safety, purity, and effectiveness are the major issues in evaluating herbal products. Many important concerns and questions must be addressed.

**Herbal products** are made by grinding up parts of plants and making them into pills, capsules, or liquids. One of the major criticisms of herbal products is that the plants vary widely in concentration or dosage. Because plants make different amounts of chemicals depending on the soil, water, and sun where they were grown, two leaves may weigh the same but contain different amounts of biologically active chemicals. Some plants may contain harmful pesticides or other chemicals. An emerging herbal drug of interest is cannabis, which includes THC and CBD (discussed later.:

Hormone replacement therapy has become a hot market for the use of "natural" products. Natural estrogens are really estrogen-like chemicals called *phytoestrogens*. Plants that contain natural estrogens or phytoestrogens include flaxseed, red clover sprouts, and soy flour. Supplements with these ingredients have not been clearly shown to improve the symptoms of menopause. Moreover, the evidence does not support claims that custom-mixed bioidentical hormones are more effective than conventional hormone therapy.

Many nonprescription products are advertised to have the same function as prescription drugs. For example, there are herbal preparations that are supposed to act like sildenafil (Viagra) to treat erectile dysfunction. Herbal products for weight loss, depression, high cholesterol levels, and asthma are also for sale. Some products may include amphetamine-like compounds that can cause high blood pressure, heart rate irregularities, stroke, and death.

St. John's wort, another example, has been shown to improve mild to moderate depression but has potentially dangerous interactions if taken with selective serotonin reuptake inhibitors, benzodiazepines, warfarin, statins, verapamil, digoxin, cyclosporine, antiviral HIV drugs, or oral contraceptives. Goldenseal has a high potential for herb–drug interactions, and ginseng may affect the blood levels of drugs with narrow therapeutic ranges because it increases liver enzyme activity.

## CANNABIS

### Endocannabinoid System

The human body contains an endocannabinoid system that maintains homeostasis and certain body processes. This system is active with or without the use of cannabis. Research has shown that the endocannabinoid system affects appetite, digestion, pain, inflammation, moods, sleep, and stress. For example, the lifting of a person's mood experienced by runners, known as a *runner's high*, results from the production of endocannabinoids in the body. Receptor sites for the endocannabinoid system are found mainly in the brain but also in peripheral tissues, glands, and organs of the body. Cannabis (marijuana) and its active compounds interact with the endocannabinoid system and have an array of effects on the human body.

More than 400 compounds occur naturally in the cannabis plant. The main active compounds are delta-9-tetrahydrocannabinol (THC) and cannabidiol (CBD). THC is a psychoactive compound that produces euphoria. CBD, while affecting receptor sites in the brain, does not produce euphoria and is not as psychoactive as THC.

Cannabis affects individuals in different ways, and little is known regarding the safety of the 400+ compounds present in cannabis. Because cannabis is listed as a Schedule I drug and is illegal at the federal level, the FDA has not approved the cannabis plant as a drug that has curative properties. However, the United States Agricultural Improvement Act of 2018 removed CBD derived from hemp from Schedule I status. Basic and clinical research on the use, safety, and efficacy of CBD is now legal, and clinical trials to determine the risks and benefits of CBD can be conducted.

The Marijuana Opportunity Reinvestment and Expungement Act (MORE Act) of 2019 passed the US House of Representatives in April 2022. The proposed legislation would decriminalize cannabis and impose taxes on imports, exports, and production facilities. The act would also remove cannabis from the Controlled Substances Act. The US Senate and the President still need to approve the act before it can become law.

As of April 2023, 38 states, the District of Columbia, and three US territories have legalized the use of cannabis for medical purposes. Each of these states has a list of diseases and disorders that are considered qualifying conditions for the use of medical cannabis. The initial dosage varies according to the route of administration and the qualifying condition.

In August of 2023, The US Department of Health and Human Services (HHS) recommended to the Drug Enforcement Agency (DEA) that cannabis be removed from a schedule I controlled substance to a schedule III controlled substance. Should this recommendation be followed, it will affect all aspects of the cannabis industry.

### Action and Uses

Cannabis can be administered through the oral, sublingual, topical, rectal, and inhalation routes. Research shows that THC decreases nausea and increases appetite. THC may also decrease pain and inflammation. Animal studies have shown that extracts from the cannabis plant can kill, reduce, and slow the growth of some cancer cells. Research is being done to treat the symptoms of illnesses such as HIV/AIDS, multiple sclerosis, disease-related pain, seizures, and mental illness and substance abuse.

According to animal studies, THC use by pregnant or nursing mothers can have negative long-term effects on the child. Pregnant women should not use medical cannabis without approval by their healthcare provider.

CBD may be useful in treating inflammatory conditions, pain, seizures, and mental health disorders such as substance abuse. An FDA-approved CBD liquid drug, Epidiolex (Cannabidiol), is used to treat Dravet syndrome and Lennox-Gastaut syndrome, which are forms of childhood epilepsy.

### Common Side Effects

Some common side effects of cannabis are dry mouth, sedation, cough, dysphoria, anxiety (with higher doses), reddened eyes, altered visual perceptions, lack of coordination, and altered sense of time.

### Adverse Effects

According to the American College of Cardiology (2023), People who used cannabis daily were found to be one-third more likely to develop coronary artery disease (CAD) when compared with people who had never used the drug . Daily cannabis use was also associated with an increased risk of psychotic and non psychotic unipolar depression and bipolar disorder (JAMA Psychiatry, 2023).

### Drug Interactions

THC and CBD are metabolized by cytochrome P-450 (CYP) enzymes. For this reason, THC, which is known to be a CYP1A2 inducer, may decrease serum concentrations of clozapine, duloxetine, cyclobenzaprine, olanzapine, haloperidol, chlorpromazine, and naproxen. CBD is an inhibitor of CYP34A and CYP2D6. CBD may increase serum concentrations of macrolide antibiotics, calcium channel blockers, benzodiazepines, cyclosporine, sildenafil, antihistamines, haloperidol, antiretrovirals, atorvastatin, and simvastatin.

The drug interaction studies that have been done on warfarin show that THC and CBD can increase warfarin levels and the international normalized ratio (INR). Cannabis has an additive CNS depressant effect when used with alcohol, barbiturates, or benzodiazepines.

### ❖ Nursing Implications and Patient Teaching

The active dose of cannabis is well below the lethal dose, and serious adverse effects of using cannabis are considered rare. An absolute contraindication of cannabis use is acute psychosis or unstable mental illness. Cannabis use among adolescents has been associated with changes in cognitive and executive functioning.

Symptoms of bronchitis are associated with smoking cannabis, and those symptoms worsen if it is used concurrently with tobacco. Although vaporization causes fewer respiratory symptoms, more than 2000 cases of lung injury associated with vaping (E-cigarettes with and without cannabis) have been reported to the

Centers for Disease Prevention and Control (CDC) as of January 2020. No single product has been identified as a cause, but most of those affected reported vaping cannabis.

Although medical cannabis is considered safer than unregulated cannabis, contamination by pesticides, fungi, and bacteria can occur and increase the risk for pneumonia or other respiratory problems.

The American Cannabis Nursing Association, established in 2015, has up-to-date resources and information for nurses and patients that can be accessed at https://www.cannabisnurses.org.

**Bookmark This!**

The American Cannabis Nursing Association: https://www.cannabisnurses.org.

**Memory Jogger**

St. John's wort, ginseng, and goldenseal are common herbal products that are most likely to cause dangerous interactions with many prescription drugs.

The Council for Responsible Nutrition is a trade association that represents dietary supplements. Companies that are members are expected to comply with federal and state regulations, additional voluntary guidelines, and the organization's code of ethics. It also provides news releases on dietary supplements and government recommendations. For more information, check out its Web site (https://www.crnusa.org).

**Bookmark This!**

Council for Responsible Nutrition: https://www.crnusa.org.

Some European countries have more extensive experience than the United States with selected herbal products. Many of the products gaining attention in the United States have been used for years in other countries as OTC products or by prescription. Much has been learned about the effects of these products and how they interact with other foods and drugs. For example, natural products that reduce the blood glucose level or blood pressure or have a sedating effect may be dangerous when taken along with prescription drugs with the same actions. Use the NIH Web site (https://www.nccih.nih.gov/health/herbsataglance) to check on specific herbal preparations.

A few nonherbal natural remedies in common use are considered safe and effective. Sometimes the products (e.g., calcium) may be of proven use. However, if the calcium came from oyster shells taken from polluted waters, the shells may contain large amounts of lead, zinc, or arsenic. A similar problem occurs with melatonin, a hormone that in its natural state is extracted from the pineal gland of a cow. If the drug maker does not ensure that the cow is

disease free, the consumer may be at risk for Creutzfeldt-Jakob disease (known as *mad cow disease*), which can be fatal. Melatonin is also manufactured synthetically.

## VITAMINS

**Vitamins** are chemical compounds that are found naturally in plant and animal tissues, but most are not made in the human body. Some are available in their active form; others come from food as a *precursor* or *provitamin* that is later converted to the active form. People take vitamins to maintain health or to correct specific nutritional deficiencies. Most people who take vitamins decide to do so on their own without the advice of a healthcare professional.

Vitamins are necessary for life and essential to normal metabolism. They can act as coenzymes to regulate the creation of compounds in the body. Vitamins are classified as two types: *Fat-soluble* vitamins are found primarily in various plant and animal oils or fats and can be stored in the body so that daily intake is not essential, and *water-soluble* vitamins are readily excreted in the urine and are not stored in the body can cause fetal. Water-soluble vitamins are found in fruits, vegetables, dairy, meat, legumes, eggs and fortified foods. Water-soluble vitamins are destroyed by heat, and deficiencies are quickly seen in patients who have a deficient diet.

Normally, if a well-balanced, nutritious diet is followed, vitamin supplements are not necessary. However, when certain conditions prevent eating solid food or when vitamins are poorly absorbed (as in ulcerative colitis), increased vitamin intake is needed. Vitamin supplements are also advised for conditions in which metabolism is increased, such as hyperthyroidism, pregnancy, and burns.

**Memory Jogger**

To remember the fat-soluble vitamins, think "The fat cat is on ADEK."

If a variety of healthy foods are eaten, the necessary vitamins can likely be obtained from diet alone. Government health agencies have determined the usual vitamin levels that are needed daily to maintain health. These are known as the *recommended dietary allowances* (RDAs). The FDA recently updated the amounts and units of dietary supplements and required new labeling. For labeling purposes, the *reference daily intake* (RDI) values are used for each vitamin; they represent population-adjusted RDAs that are sufficient to meet the needs of almost every healthy individual in every demographic category in the United States. Table 23.2 shows the updated RDI values for common vitamins. When patients are deficient in one or more vitamins, supplements are needed. For supplementation, vitamins should contain 50% to 150% of the RDA per dose.

Table 23.2    Function, Deficiency, and Reference Daily Intake Values of Vitamins

| VITAMIN | FUNCTION | DEFICIENCY | RDI* | RDI FOR PREGNANT AND LACTATING WOMEN |
|---|---|---|---|---|
| **Fat-Soluble Vitamins** | | | | |
| Vitamin A | Immune function<br>Vision<br>Red blood cell formation<br>Growth and development<br>Reproduction | Celiac disease (sprue), colitis, night blindness, impaired immunity, and hematopoiesis | Adults: 900 mcg<br>Children: 300 mcg<br>Infants: 500 mcg | 1300 mcg |
| Vitamin D | Promotes calcium and phosphorous absorption<br>Bone growth<br>Nervous system function<br>Blood pressure regulation | Rickets, osteoporosis, hypoparathyroidism, fractures, depression | Adults: 20 mcg<br>Children: 15 mcg<br>Infants: 10 mcg | 15 mcg |
| Vitamin E | Antioxidant<br>Immune function<br>Blood vessel formation | Low birth weight<br>Impaired fat metabolism | Adults: 15 mg<br>Children: 6 mg<br>Infants: 5 mg | 19 mg |
| Vitamin K | Blood clotting | Blood clotting disorders | Adults: 120 mcg<br>Children: 30 mcg<br>Infants: 2.5 mcg | 90 mcg |
| **Water-Soluble Vitamins** | | | | |
| Vitamin C (ascorbic acid) | Collagen formation<br>Healing<br>Immune function<br>Iron absorption | Scurvy | Adults: 90 mg<br>Children: 15 mg<br>Infants: 50 mg | 120 mg |
| Vitamin $B_{12}$ (cyanocobalamin) | Red blood cell production<br>Nervous system function<br>Converts food to energy | Pernicious anemia | Adults: 2.4 mcg<br>Children: 0.9 mcg<br>Infants: 0.5 mcg | 2.8 mcg |
| Vitamin $B_9$ (folic acid/folate) | Birth defect prevention<br>Red blood cell formation | Folic acid anemia | Adults: 400 mcg<br>Children: 150 mcg<br>Infants: 80 mcg | 600 mcg |
| Vitamin $B_3$ (niacin) | Cholesterol production<br>Nervous system function<br>Converts food into energy<br>Digestion | Pellagra | Adults: 16 mg<br>Children: 6 mg<br>Infants: 4 mg | 18 mg |
| Vitamin $B_6$ (pyridoxine) | Immune function<br>Nervous system function<br>Red blood cell formation<br>Protein, carbohydrate, and fat metabolism | $B_6$ anemia | Adults: 1.7 mg<br>Children: 0.5 mg<br>Infants: 0.3 mg | 2 mg |
| Vitamin $B_2$ (riboflavin) | Conversion of food into energy<br>Growth and development<br>Red blood cell formation | Discomfort eating, sore throat, stomatitis, mouth and tongue redness | Adults: 1.3 mg<br>Children: 0.5 mg<br>Infants: 0.4 mg | 1.6 mg |
| Vitamin $B_1$ (thiamine) | Converts food into energy<br>Nervous system function | Beriberi | Adults: 1.2 mg<br>Children: 0.5 mg<br>Infants: 0.3 mg | 1.4 mg |

*Adults, older than 4 years of age; children, age 1–3 years; infants, age 0–1 year.
*RDI*, Reference Daily Intake.
Modified from Office of Dietary Supplements and the National Library of Medicine National Institute of Health (2019, May). https://www.dsld.nlm.nih.gov/dsld/dailyvalue.jsp; US Food & Drug Administration. (2009, February). Nutritional educational fact sheet. https://www.accessdata.fda.gov/scripts/interactivenutritionfactslabel/assets/InteractiveNFL_Vitamins&MineralsChart_March2020.pdf; US Food & Drug Administration. (n.d.). Frequently asked questions for industry on nutrition facts labeling requirements. https://www.fda.gov/media/99069/download

There are known dangers to vitamin use, especially with high doses. When megadoses of water-soluble vitamins are taken, the excess amount is quickly excreted in the urine with no additional benefit to the patient. However, excesses of fat-soluble vitamins (i.e., vitamins A, D, E, and K) can be stored, and high levels can cause toxic side effects. Most vitamins can be toxic to children who are accidentally exposed to high levels, and iron can be deadly to small children.

Advertisers suggest that natural products are better than synthetic vitamins. However, the human body processes vitamins in the same way whether they are natural or synthetic, costly or cheap. The most important differences are that some preparations may dissolve better than others or may contain the active product in amounts that increase the absorption of other vitamins and minerals taken at the same time. Some vitamins contain fillers that may cause stomach upset if taken on an empty stomach. All vitamins should be kept in airtight dark containers out of the reach of children.

## VITAMIN A

### Action and Uses

Vitamin A is important for vision, gene expression, reproduction, embryo growth and development, and healthy immune system function. Vitamin A supplementation is used to treat disorders associated with fat malabsorption, such as celiac disease or colitis. It is also used for the treatment of specific eye diseases and night blindness. This vitamin may be given orally, intravenously (IV), or intramuscularly (IM), depending on how fast replacement is needed.

Hypervitaminosis can occur if vitamin A is given in high doses for a long time. Hypervitaminosis results from excessive intake and a high storage level of one or more vitamins, notably the fat-soluble vitamins, and can lead to toxic symptoms. Any patient who is receiving more than three times the vitamin A RDA of 900 mcg should be closely supervised. Pregnant women should not receive more than 1300 mcg daily, or they may risk fetal abnormalities.

Women who are taking oral contraceptives often show elevated plasma vitamin A levels and should be closely monitored for hypervitaminosis. Giving cod liver oil and vitamin A together is contraindicated.

### ❖ Nursing Implications and Patient Teaching

Common food sources of vitamin A include dairy products, fish, liver, spinach, broccoli, and dark orange vegetables.

Women who are using oral contraceptives should take only prescribed amounts of vitamin A to avoid hypervitaminosis. Vitamin A can cause birth defects in women who are pregnant, and excess vitamin A ingestion during pregnancy can cause fetal defects of the CNS.

Early indications of vitamin A overdose are anorexia (lack of appetite), abdominal pain, malaise, and yellowing of the skin, especially on the nose and ears.

## VITAMIN B₁ (THIAMINE)

### Action and Uses

Vitamin $B_1$, or thiamine, is water soluble and is a coenzyme needed in many physiologic pathways for carbohydrate metabolism and energy production. It also is thought to assist in nervous system function. Thiamine is excreted in the urine.

Vitamin $B_1$ is used to treat beriberi, which is a rare disorder in North America. Other conditions that lead to vitamin $B_1$ deficiency include alcoholism, gastric lesions, and hyperemesis of pregnancy. Symptoms of deficiency include anorexia (lack of appetite), vomiting, fatigability, aching muscles, ataxia (poor coordination) of gait, and emotional disturbances such as moodiness, depression, or excessive alcohol use.

Usual reactions to thiamine are mild itching, sweating, and nausea. However, adverse reactions can be severe and, when thiamine is given IV, include anaphylactic shock and death. Sensitivity tests are performed before parenteral doses are started if sensitivity is suspected. IV doses must be given very slowly. If giving thiamine to an alcoholic or thiamine-deficient patient, IV glucose should also be given to prevent precipitation or worsening of Wernicke encephalopathy.

> ### 🔺 Top Tip for Safety
>
> When giving parenteral thiamine, assess the patient continually for indications of allergic reactions: feelings of warmth, pruritus (itching), urticaria (hives), nausea, angioedema (lip and facial swelling), shortness of breath, sweating, tightness of the throat, and cyanosis (blue color of the skin). If these occur, stop the infusion, and notify the emergency team.

### ❖ Nursing Implications and Patient Teaching

Common food sources of thiamine include meats, whole grains, peas, dried beans, and peanuts. Thiamine in food is destroyed when food is boiled, fried, or cooked for a long time under pressure.

## VITAMIN B₂ (RIBOFLAVIN)

### Action and Uses

Vitamin $B_2$, or riboflavin, is water soluble and is important in the metabolism of proteins, fats, and carbohydrates. It combines with proteins to form enzymes that are important for tissue metabolism. Riboflavin is used to prevent or treat riboflavin deficiency. Symptoms of deficiency include cracks in the corners of the mouth, soreness and burning of the tongue and lips, and sore throat.

Riboflavin levels in the body can be decreased by oral contraceptives, even in low doses. The risk of deficiency is increased for women who have been taking oral contraceptives for 3 years or longer.

### ❖ Nursing Implications and Patient Teaching

Teach patients that common food sources of riboflavin include dairy products, eggs, green leafy vegetables, organ meats, and peanuts. Warn patients that riboflavin supplements can turn urine a deeper yellow color.

## NIACIN (VITAMIN B₃)

### Action and Uses

Niacin, previously called *vitamin B₃*, is water soluble and an essential part of two compounds that are important in generating cellular energy. It is used to prevent or treat deficiency states that can cause pellagra or as a nutritional supplement in cases of limited dietary intake. Niacin is also used to treat conditions of high blood fat levels such as hyperlipidemia, hypertriglyceridemia, and atherosclerosis.

Symptoms of deficiency include *glossitis* (smooth, swollen, beefy-red tongue), *stomatitis* (inflammation of the mouth), and diarrhea. Dermatitis of body parts exposed to sun or trauma may develop, as well as lesions on the skin that result from sun, fire, or heat. Mental changes that are mild early in deficiency may progress to disorientation, loss of memory, confusion, hysteria, and sometimes manic outbursts.

Expected side effects of niacin supplementation are skin warmth, flushing, and itching that can be relieved by giving aspirin with the niacin. Adverse reactions to niacin include allergies and anaphylactic reactions.

### ❖ Nursing Implications and Patient Teaching

Food sources of niacin include peanuts, yeast, cereals (especially bran and wheat germ), eggs, liver, red meats, whole grains, and enriched bread.

When taken with beta-blocking drugs and calcium channel blockers for hypertension, the side effects of niacin increase, especially skin warmth, flushing, and blood vessel dilation. This effect may lead to *postural hypotension* (low blood pressure when a person suddenly stands up). If dizziness occurs with niacin, tell the patient to sit or lie down.

Taking niacin or red yeast rice may cause rhabdomyolysis, which is muscle breakdown that can lead to kidney dysfunction.

### VITAMIN B₆ (PYRIDOXINE)

#### Action and Uses

Vitamin $B_6$, or pyridoxine hydrochloride, is water soluble and functions as a coenzyme in the metabolism of protein, carbohydrates, and fat. It is used to treat pyridoxine deficiency, vitamin $B_6$–responsive chronic anemia, neuritis, and other rare vitamin problems.

Pyridoxine deficiency is most likely to develop in the older adult population and in women of childbearing age, especially those who are pregnant or breastfeeding. Women who are taking oral contraceptives, individuals who are alcoholics, and those whose diets are poor in the quality and quantity of protein or high in refined foods are also at risk.

Symptoms of deficiency include malaise, nervousness, irritability, and difficulty in walking. There may also be personality changes in adults, such as depression and loss of a sense of responsibility. High doses of pyridoxine may produce neurotoxicity, with symptoms of ataxia (loss of control of body movements), numb feet, and clumsiness.

Oral contraceptives can induce pyridoxine deficiency. Pyridoxine may prevent chloramphenicol-induced optic neuritis. Some drugs interfere with vitamin activity enough to block action and produce symptoms of deficiency—for example, pyridoxine should never be given with levodopa.

### ❖ Nursing Implications and Patient Teaching

Good food sources of vitamin $B_6$ include bananas, avocados, potatoes, poultry, egg yolk, liver, kidney, muscle meats, fish (e.g., salmon), chickpeas, and whole grains. Limited amounts are available from milk and vegetables.

Appropriate food preparation is important in preserving vitamin $B_6$. Freezing vegetables results in a 20% loss of pyridoxine, and milling wheat results in a 90% loss.

### FOLIC ACID (VITAMIN B₉)

#### Action and Uses

Folic acid (vitamin $B_9$) is required for normal *erythropoiesis* (red blood cell formation) and DNA synthesis. It is metabolized in the liver, where it is changed to its more active form. Folic acid is used to treat anemias caused by folic acid deficiency. It is also used for alcoholism, hepatic disease, hemolytic anemia, infancy (especially for infants receiving artificial formulas), lactation, oral contraceptive use, and pregnancy. Folic acid supplements may be needed in low-birth-weight infants, infants nursed by mothers who are deficient in folic acid, or infants with infections or prolonged diarrhea.

Guidelines emphasize the importance of increased folic acid intake by all women of childbearing age, especially those who are intending to get pregnant, and during early pregnancy to help prevent spinal cord malformations in the fetus (neural tube defects). The folic acid additives in commercial bread and grain products have been increased in an attempt to provide more adequate supplies of this important vitamin.

Low levels of vitamin $B_6$, vitamin $B_{12}$, and folate are associated with high levels of homocysteine, which is a common amino acid in the blood. High levels of homocysteine are linked to the early development of heart disease.

Folic acid interacts with several drugs. It may decrease the anticancer effect of methotrexate. Antiseizure drugs reduce folic acid levels, and sulfasalazine (a sulfa drug used to treat the pain and swelling of arthritis) inhibits intestinal absorption of folate.

### ❖ Nursing Implications and Patient Teaching

Proper nutrition is essential, and dietary measures are preferable to drug therapy. Vegetables and fruits are good sources of folate. In the United States, bread, cereal, flour, pasta, rice, and cornmeal are fortified with folic acid. Beef liver, peas, beans, nuts, and eggs are also sources of folate.

### VITAMIN B₁₂ (CYANOCOBALAMIN)

#### Action and Uses

Vitamin $B_{12}$, or cyanocobalamin, is water soluble and contains cobalt. It functions in many processes for protein, fat, and carbohydrate metabolism. The coenzymes of $B_{12}$ also take part in red blood cell maturation and are needed to make DNA in new cells. Vitamin $B_{12}$ is needed to form red blood cells, and it is essential for growth, cell reproduction, and making the myelin sheath that surrounds nerve cells. Intrinsic factor must be present in the stomach and small intestine to absorb

$B_{12}$. Vitamin $B_{12}$ interacts with folate in metabolic functions, and a deficiency of vitamin $B_{12}$ makes folate useless in the body.

Vitamin $B_{12}$ is used to treat all $B_{12}$ deficiency conditions, including pernicious anemia, megaloblastic and macrocytic anemias, malabsorption syndromes, hemorrhage, intestinal bacterial overgrowth, chronic liver disease complicated by deficiency of vitamin $B_{12}$, malignancy, pregnancy, thyrotoxicosis (in which deficiency is seen because of an increased metabolic rate), and kidney disorders.

Symptoms of deficiency occur mainly in people on strict vegetarian (vegan) diets. Although vitamin $B_{12}$ is water soluble, it is found only in animal products. Symptoms of $B_{12}$ deficiency include constipation, upset stomach, tiredness, palpitations, shortness of breath, pale skin, smooth tongue, numbness, tingling, muscle weakness, and behavioral changes.

Most patients with vitamin $B_{12}$ deficiency have a malabsorption problem in the gastrointestinal (GI) tract, pernicious anemia, or alcoholism or are on a vegan diet. Vitamin replacement is injected to bypass the GI tract. Parenteral, nasal, or oral therapy may be used to maintain normal $B_{12}$ levels.

Cyanocobalamin (vitamin $B_{12}$) comes as a nasal spray or nasal gel and can be used as a maintenance drug for persons in remission after undergoing IM therapy for pernicious anemia. The dose is usually 500 mcg intranasally once weekly. If the patient develops adverse effects after taking the nasal spray—such as infection, headache, glossitis, nausea, and rhinitis—it is often necessary to start IM vitamin $B_{12}$ again. The maintenance dose of cyanocobalamin is 100 mcg IM every month. Cyanocobalamin is also packaged as a sublingual tablet.

Allergy to vitamin $B_{12}$ is rare. The patient may report pruritus, a feeling of swelling of the entire body, or a severe anaphylactic reaction. A few patients may experience mild pain, localized skin irritation, or mild transient diarrhea after an injection of cyanocobalamin.

Alcohol, colchicine, and *para*-aminosalicylic acid (an antibiotic used to treat tuberculosis) lower the absorption of vitamin $B_{12}$. Some antibiotics lower the response to vitamin $B_{12}$ therapy.

❖ **Nursing Implications and Patient Teaching**
The best food sources of vitamin $B_{12}$ include organ meats, fish and seafood (e.g., clams, lobster, sardines, flounder, tuna), eggs, nonfat dry milk, fortified non-dairy milks, and fermented cheeses (e.g., Camembert, Limburger).

## VITAMIN C (ASCORBIC ACID)
### Action and Uses
Vitamin C, or **ascorbic acid**, is necessary for formation of collagen in connective tissue, cartilage, tooth dentin, and skin as well as for bone matrix and tissue repair. It is essential for energy-producing reactions and in metabolizing some neurotransmitters, hormones, carbohydrates, and amino acids. It helps maintain the integrity of blood vessels and may promote resistance to infection. Vitamin C regulates iron distribution and plays a role in antioxidant renewal. It may be used to treat severe burns and chronic iron intoxication and to prevent recurrent urinary tract infections by acidification of urine.

The use and dosage of vitamin C in the prevention and treatment of diseases other than scurvy is uncertain. Research indicates a possible positive role for vitamin C in preventing coronary heart disease (especially in women), managing diabetes mellitus, reducing stroke, preventing osteoporosis, reducing the risk of Alzheimer's disease (in combination with high-dose vitamin E), and preventing cataracts.

With modern refrigeration and processing methods for citrus fruits, scurvy is rarely seen in the United States, but it may be found when other vitamin deficiencies are present. Symptoms include tender, painful muscles, joints, and bones; muscle cramps; anorexia; fatigue; malaise; and sore gums. Wound healing is impaired, and excessive bleeding is demonstrated by petechial hemorrhages. Bruising, faulty bone and tooth development, loosened teeth, and gingivitis also may develop.

Vitamin C may be given by oral, IM, IV, and subcutaneous routes to treat scurvy. The dosage ranges from 100 to 250 mg orally, IM, or IV twice daily in adults, but larger doses may be given.

The patient may experience mild, brief soreness at injection sites if the drug is given IM or subcutaneously. Patients may also experience brief episodes of faintness or dizziness when IV injections are given too rapidly. Excessive doses are usually rapidly excreted into the urine. Doses in excess of 1 g to 3 g daily may result in GI problems, glycosuria, and development of kidney stones, especially in patients who are prone to these problems.

Ascorbic acid may affect anticoagulants, blocking the action of some and prolonging the intensity and duration of others. Ascorbic acid increases the effect of salicylates through increased kidney reabsorption. There is also an increased chance of crystallization of sulfonamides in the urine when ascorbic acid is given at the same time as sulfa drugs. Ascorbic acid decreases the effect of tricyclic antidepressants by decreasing kidney reabsorption. Calcium ascorbate may cause *cardiac dysrhythmias* (irregular heartbeats) in patients receiving digoxin. Ascorbic acid is chemically incompatible with potassium penicillin G and should not be mixed in the same syringe.

Smoking may increase the need for vitamin C by decreasing ascorbic acid serum levels. Intermittent use of ascorbic acid by patients who are taking ethinyl estradiol (a compound in many birth control pills) may increase the risk of contraceptive failure.

❖ **Nursing Implications and Patient Teaching**
Vitamin C comes in three major forms that may be given orally or parenterally: ascorbic acid, sodium

ascorbate, and calcium ascorbate. The recommended daily intake is 90 mg for adults.

Vitamin C is easily destroyed by air, heat, and light. This drug should be kept tightly capped in its own container. Foods high in vitamin C should not be boiled for long periods or left uncovered in the refrigerator. Good food sources of vitamin C include oranges, grapefruit, strawberries, cauliflower, cantaloupe, beef liver, asparagus, green leafy vegetables, and potatoes.

## VITAMIN D

### Action and Uses

Vitamin D is a label used for a group of fat-soluble, chemically similar *sterols* (plant steroids). There are three main categories in this group:

1. *Ergocalciferol* (vitamin $D_2$), which is very limited in nature in distribution and concentration but can be artificially manufactured by ultraviolet irradiation of ergot and yeasts
2. *Cholecalciferol* (vitamin $D_3$), which occurs naturally in fish liver oils and can be formed in animals and humans by ultraviolet irradiation of the skin
3. Other lesser compounds, such as vitamins $D_4$, $D_5$, $D_6$, and $D_7$

The main action of this group of vitamins is movement of calcium and phosphorous ions into three main sites: the small intestine (to promote absorption of calcium and phosphorus from the gut), the kidneys (to cause phosphate reabsorption and, to a lesser extent, to stimulate calcium and sodium reabsorption), and bone (to help increase the mineralization of newly formed bone). Vitamin $D_3$ contributes to skin growth and repair. It is used in the treatment of some skin disorders.

Vitamin D preparations are used to treat childhood rickets and adult osteomalacia, hypoparathyroidism, and familial hypophosphatemia. In childhood, the first symptoms of rickets are excessive sweating and GI disturbances. These may appear before any obvious changes in bone have occurred. In adult cases of osteomalacia, patients may have skeletal pain and progressive muscular weakness.

Estrogen levels drop during menopause, which decreases an enzyme that is responsible for vitamin D activation. This mechanism causes vitamin D deficiency in menopausal women. Vitamin D may help mood disorders and hot flashes in menopause, so supplementation is reasonable. Menopausal women should take 600 IU of vitamin D every day.

Symptoms of vitamin D toxicity include anorexia, nausea, malaise, weight loss, vague aches and stiffness, constipation, diarrhea, convulsions, anemia, mild acidosis, and impairment of kidney function. The kidney effects are usually reversible. A variety of more serious systemic effects may be seen in adults. Dwarfism may affect infants and children. Most toxic effects persist for several months in adults at doses of 2500 mcg or more daily or in children at doses of 500 mcg or more daily. Reactions gradually disappear if treatment is discontinued at the first sign of symptoms.

Mineral oil and some of the antihyperlipidemic (blood fat–lowering) drugs may interfere with the absorption of fat-soluble vitamins. Thiazide diuretics and vitamin D together contribute to hypercalcemia. There is a possible connection between phenytoin (Dilantin) and phenobarbital (Luminal) use and the development of hypocalcemia, which can contribute to rickets or osteomalacia.

### ❖ Nursing Implications and Patient Teaching

The dosage of vitamin D must be planned for each patient and given under close supervision because the range between the therapeutic and toxic levels is narrow. Calcium intake should be enough to give a serum calcium level between 9 mg/dL and 10 mg/dL. Vitamin D levels do not need to be measured for everyone but are recommended for those who are homebound or in long-term care centers or other institutions. A normal vitamin D level is 20 ng/mL (50 nmol/L). Vitamin D levels of 12 ng/mL (30 nmol/L) are considered to be deficient. Treatment with vitamin D depends on each individual, whether she or he can absorb vitamin D, and the severity of the deficiency.

Other than sun exposure, natural sources of vitamin D are few, and most vitamin D is obtained from fortified sources. Fortified foods high in this vitamin include milk, evaporated milk, infant formula, and powdered skim milk. Cereals, margarine, and diet foods also contain vitamin D supplementation. Breast milk is usually rich in vitamin D. Oily fish (e.g., mackerel) and cod liver oil can supply adequate vitamin D. Vitamin D supplements should be protected from light in light-resistant containers.

## VITAMIN E

### Action and Uses

Vitamin E is fat soluble and consists of naturally occurring tocopherols. Vitamin E is considered an essential nutrient for humans, even though all of its specific functions are not understood. Vitamin E is an antioxidant with neuroprotective and anti-inflammatory properties. As an antioxidant, it may prevent damage to cell membranes. It stabilizes red blood cell walls and protects them from breakage or destruction. It may also increase the effect of vitamin A and stop platelet aggregation. The RDA for adults is 15 mg.

Many suggested uses of vitamin E are controversial and unproven. The only established use is to prevent or treat vitamin E deficiency, which is rare in the United States and usually the result of impaired metabolism. Vitamin E has been touted as a powerful antioxidant and may play a role in reducing heart disease and atherosclerosis.

Vitamin E appears to be the least toxic of the fat-soluble vitamins. No signs and symptoms of toxicity or hypervitaminosis have been identified in humans.

### ❖ Nursing Implications and Patient Teaching

Food sources of vitamin E are primarily plants. The highest amounts are found in vegetable oils (e.g., soybean, corn) and in nuts, wheat germ, rice germ, and green leafy vegetables. Meat and dairy products provide less vitamin E.

An accurate assessment of tocopherol levels in food is difficult to obtain. The amount in the body depends on the initial concentration of vitamin E and the processing, storage, and preparation of the food. Vitamin E products should be stored in tightly closed, light-resistant containers. Vitamin E may increase clotting times in people taking anticoagulants or antiplatelet medications. Vitamin E can reduce high-density lipoprotein (HDL) cholesterol levels and therefore may interfere with the actions of simvastatin and niacin.

## VITAMIN K

### Action and Uses
Vitamin K is a group of compounds. Vitamin $K_3$ is a synthetic, lipid-soluble form of vitamin K. Vitamin $K_2$ is most abundant in fermented foods, eggs, dark chicken meat, and goose liver. Vitamin $K_1$ is found in leafy greens and some other vegetables, and it is the main form of vitamin K supplement available in the United States.

Vitamin K helps liver formation of factors II, VII, IX, and X, which are essential for normal blood clotting, although the exact mechanism is unknown. Vitamin K is used to treat or prevent various blood clotting disorders that result in damaged formation of factors II, VII, IX, and X. The American Academy of Pediatrics recommends routine phytonadione ($K_1$) injection at birth to prevent hemorrhagic disease of the newborn. Vitamin K does not counteract the anticoagulant activity of heparin, although it is helpful in reversing the effects of warfarin (Coumadin) overdosage.

Specific adverse reactions to phytonadione ($K_1$) are transient flushing, dizziness, a strange taste in the mouth, sweating, hypotension, and pain or swelling at the injection site. Severe hypersensitivity reactions can occur. Anaphylactic shock, including cardiac arrest, respiratory arrest, and death, has occurred during and immediately after IV injection.

Use of vitamin K along with oral anticoagulants, especially warfarin, may decrease the effects of the anticoagulant. Mineral oil and cholestyramine inhibit GI absorption of oral vitamin K.

### ❖ Nursing Implications and Patient Teaching
Vitamin K is preferably administered by subcutaneous or IM routes. IV administration is not recommended because of the risk of anaphylaxis. Naturally occurring vitamin K is found in liver and green leafy vegetables.

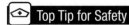
**Top Tip for Safety**

Vitamin K is the antidote for warfarin (Coumadin) overdosage.

## MINERALS

**Minerals** are inorganic substances and are found in food. Nineteen minerals are found in the body, and at least 13 are essential for normal metabolism and function. These minerals occur in body fluids as *ions* with positive and negative charges; they combine with other molecules to form salts. Minerals act as catalysts to speed up various biochemical reactions. They are obtained from a diet that includes a variety of animal and vegetable products and meets the energy and protein needs of the body.

The Food and Nutrition Board of the National Research Council has established recommended daily intakes for calcium and iron. Calcium, iron, and iodine are the three elements most frequently missing in the diet. Zinc, iron, copper, magnesium, and potassium are the five minerals most frequently involved in disturbances of metabolism. As electrolytes, these preparations are commonly infused to critically ill patients who are unable to take food orally.

## CALCIUM

### Action and Uses
Calcium is a major mineral in the body and is essential for muscular and neurologic activity, especially in the cardiac system. Calcium is important in the following actions:

- It assists in the formation and repair of skeletal tissues (bones and teeth).
- It activates several enzymes that influence cell membrane permeability and muscle contraction.
- It aids in blood clotting by stimulating the release of thromboplastin and the conversion of fibrinogen to fibrin.
- It activates pancreatic enzymes for digestion.
- It increases the intestinal absorption of cobalamin.
- It is involved in the transmission of neurotransmitters and in metabolic processes.
- It helps regulate some white blood cell functions.

Calcium is used as a supplement when dietary levels of calcium are not adequate. Calcium requirements may be increased during adolescence, pregnancy, and breast-feeding and in postmenopausal women. Calcium is also used to treat neonatal hypocalcemia and to prevent and treat postmenopausal and senile osteoporosis. It may also be used as a supplement to parenterally given vitamin D in cases of hypoparathyroidism, pseudohypoparathyroidism (an uncommon condition in which the body fails to respond to parathyroid hormone), rickets, and *osteomalacia* (a condition resulting in the formation of soft bones).

Signs of *hypocalcemia* (low blood calcium levels) are muscle spasms; numbness and tingling of the lips and fingers; weak, brittle nails; and fractures. Signs of *hypercalcemia* are polyuria (excretion of a large amount of urine), constipation, abdominal pain, mouth dryness, anorexia, nausea, and vomiting.

Vitamin D is essential for the absorption of calcium in the body. Calcium status is affected by the calcium-to-phosphorus ratio in the body and by the level of protein in the diet. Phytic acid (found in bran and whole-grain cereals) and oxalic acid (found in spinach and rhubarb) may interfere with calcium absorption by combining with calcium to form insoluble salts in the intestine.

Calcium compounds and calcium-rich substances such as milk interfere with the absorption of oral tetracycline, and their use together should be avoided. Use of corticosteroids may also decrease the absorption of calcium.

### ❖ Nursing Implications and Patient Teaching

In patients with low calcium levels, hand (carpal) spasm may be elicited by compressing the upper arm with a blood pressure cuff, causing ischemia (decreased blood supply) to the distal nerves. The patient may report a tingling sensation and may inadvertently flex the arm. This is called a *Trousseau sign*. Excessive amounts of calcium may lead to hypercalcemia and hypercalciuria, especially in patients with hyperthyroidism. Calcium should not be given to patients who already have kidney stones.

Calcium, in concentrations between 6% and 40%, is combined with other chemicals in a variety of products. Preparations come in parenteral and oral forms. OTC antacids containing calcium (e.g., TUMS) are composed of calcium carbonate, the most elemental form of calcium. It is better absorbed and is a smaller tablet than many other calcium products, making administration easier.

The recommended daily intake of calcium is 1300 mg for adults and adolescents, 700 mg for children, 260 mg for infants 1 to 3 years of age, and 1300 mg for nursing mothers. Milk, cheese, yogurt, bok choy, tofu, okra, broccoli, almonds, and fish canned with bones are the richest sources of calcium. Egg yolks and most dark green leafy vegetables are also good sources.

### IRON

### Action and Uses

Iron is a mineral that is essential for the body to produce myoglobin and hemoglobin. It stimulates the hematopoietic system and increases the production of hemoglobin to correct iron deficiency. Iron from cellular hemoglobin is recycled, and most is used again. During pregnancy, reabsorption of iron increases to 15% as the body's way of adapting to physiologic anemia.

Iron is used to treat symptomatic iron deficiency anemia only after the cause of the anemia has been identified, and it is used to prevent hypochromic anemia during infancy, childhood, pregnancy, and breast-feeding; in patients recovering from other anemias; and after some GI surgeries.

Expected reactions to iron supplements include constipation and cramping. Adverse reactions such as diarrhea and epigastric or abdominal pain may occur. Symptoms of overdosage may occur after 30

minutes to several hours and include *lethargy* (sleepiness), nausea, vomiting, abdominal pain, diarrhea, *melena* (blood in stools), and *dyspnea* (uncomfortable breathing). Coma, metabolic acidosis, and symptoms of systemic absorption may occur. Children are particularly sensitive to large amounts of iron, and if they mistake vitamins for candy, they may consume a fatal overdose.

> **⚠ Drug Alert**
>
> Fatal anaphylactic reactions can occur with iron dextran IV or IM administration. Hypersensitivity reactions include rash, itching, joint pain, muscle aches, and fever.

Large iron doses may cause a false-positive test result for occult blood using the benzidine based tests (Hematest, Occultist, Clinistix). Absorption of oral iron is inhibited by tannic acid in tea, antacids (particularly magnesium-containing antacids), milk, and eggs. Patients who are receiving chloramphenicol concurrently with iron may show a delayed response to iron therapy. Absorption of iron increases when it is given with orange juice or ascorbic acid (vitamin C) in doses of 200 mg per 30 mg of iron. Iron interferes with absorption of oral tetracycline. Vitamin E decreases the response to iron therapy. Many other drugs have interactions with iron.

### ❖ Nursing Implications and Patient Teaching

Replacement of iron in iron deficiency anemia requires 60 mg of elemental iron in one to three divided doses daily for 4 weeks. If treatment is adequate, symptoms usually go away within 2 weeks, and laboratory findings are normal within 2 months. Therapy for 4 to 6 months after the anemia has been corrected is advised to replenish iron stores.

More iron is absorbed if the iron is taken on an empty stomach with water or in an acid environment, although taking it after meals can reduce stomach irritation. Taking iron after a meal can reduce the absorption by 40% to 50%. Liquid iron preparations can discolor teeth and should be taken through a straw after dilution with liquid.

All simple oral iron preparations are available OTC. The absorption of iron taken orally or through dietary foods is typically about 10%. The body can increase iron absorption during times of physiologic stress, such as pregnancy or severe blood loss.

The recommended daily intake of elemental iron is 18 mg for adults, 11 mg for infants, 7 mg for children, and 27 mg for pregnant and lactating women. A diet high in natural iron should be encouraged to meet these needs. Fish, red meat, spinach, and dried fruits are the best sources of dietary iron.

Iron supplements can cause dark green or black stools. Tell patients to report constipation, diarrhea, nausea, or abdominal pain to the healthcare provider.

## MAGNESIUM

### Action and Uses

Magnesium is an electrolyte that is essential for several enzyme systems. It is important in maintaining osmotic pressure, ion balance, bone structure, muscular contraction, and nerve conduction. This mineral is especially important in cardiac function, and only slight deficiencies may prolong the QT interval and lead to a very dangerous form of *ventricular tachycardia* (rapid heartbeat) called *torsades de pointes*. Excessive magnesium intake may produce diarrhea. Alcohol use increases magnesium excretion by the kidneys, and body stores of magnesium can be dangerously depleted with chronic alcohol use.

### ❖ Nursing Implications and Patient Teaching

Magnesium deficiencies are seen primarily when malabsorption syndromes are present. Magnesium is typically used with other vitamins as a general dietary supplement when multiple deficiencies are suspected. Deficiency states have been associated with convulsions, slowed growth, digestive disturbances, spasticity of muscles and nerves, accelerated heartbeat, dysrhythmias, nervous conditions, and vasodilation (opening of blood vessels).

Magnesium is available in adequate quantities in meat, milk, fruits, and vegetables, and special dietary planning is unnecessary. Large amounts of magnesium are present in spinach, chard, and pumpkin seeds.

## POTASSIUM

### Action and Uses

Potassium is the principal intracellular positive ion *(cation)* of most body tissues, acting in the maintenance of normal kidney function, contraction of muscle, and transmission of nerve impulses. It is found in the body within a very narrow concentration range.

Potassium may be taken *prophylactically* (for prevention) when the patient has nephrotic syndrome, by patients with liver cirrhosis and ascites, and by patients with hyperaldosteronism who have normal kidney function. Potassium products are used prophylactically or to replace potassium lost as a result of long-term diuretic therapy, digoxin intoxication, or low dietary intake of potassium. Supplementation may be necessary for deficits resulting from vomiting and diarrhea, diabetic acidosis, metabolic alkalosis, or corticosteroid therapy or to counteract increased kidney excretion of potassium caused by acidosis, certain kidney tubular disorders, or diseases that produce increased secretion of glucocorticoids or aldosterone.

An excess or a deficit of potassium can cause symptoms. Adverse reactions to potassium supplements include nausea, vomiting, diarrhea, abdominal discomfort, and GI bleeding. Potassium intoxication or *hyperkalemia* (increased potassium in the blood) may result from overdosage of potassium or from a change in the patient's underlying condition that makes potassium buildup possible. Signs and symptoms of potassium intoxication include flaccid paralysis, *paresthesias* (numbness and tingling) of the hands and feet, mental confusion, restlessness, listlessness, malaise, and heaviness of the legs. Hypotension and cardiac dysrhythmias leading to heart block may also develop. Potentially fatal dysrhythmias may develop if potassium cannot be excreted (or if it is given too rapidly via IV). When it is detected, hyperkalemia requires immediate treatment because lethal levels of potassium may be reached in a few hours in untreated patients. Potentially fast and irregular lethal dysrhythmias may also occur with *hypokalemia* (decreased potassium in the blood).

Potassium should not be used in patients who are receiving potassium-sparing agents such as aldosterone antagonists or triamterene because overdosage may develop.

### ❖ Nursing Implications and Patient Teaching

All potassium supplements must be diluted properly or taken with plenty of liquid to avoid producing GI ulcers. The usual adult dietary intake of potassium is 40 to 60 mEq/day. The loss of 200 mEq or more potassium from the total body store is enough to produce hypokalemia. Less than 3.5 mEq/L indicates hypokalemia.

The dosage must be *titrated* (increased or decreased slowly) based on the patient's needs, and the patient must be closely watched, especially in the initial stages of therapy. For patients who are receiving diuretic therapy, 20 mEq/day is usually adequate for prevention of hypokalemia. In cases of potassium depletion, 40 to 100 mEq/day or more may be required for replacement. Blood levels must be closely monitored.

Potassium comes in various salt combinations. Potassium chloride is the form most frequently prescribed; it may be ordered by the percentage of potassium chloride or by milliequivalents of potassium chloride; 10 mEq KCl per 15 mL is equivalent to 5% KCl. Other salt combinations are potassium gluconate, potassium citrate, potassium acetate, and potassium bicarbonate.

A potassium-rich diet includes foods such as bananas, tomatoes, citrus fruits (especially oranges), apricots, and dried fruits such as raisins, prunes, and dates. Fresh cantaloupe and watermelon, nuts, dried beans, beef, and fowl also contain ample quantities of potassium.

 **Memory Jogger**

Both low blood potassium levels and high blood potassium levels can cause fatal heart dysrhythmias.

## ZINC

### Action and Uses

Zinc is a part of many enzymes and is essential for normal growth and tissue repair. Zinc functions in the mineralization of bone and in the detoxification of methanol and ethylene glycol. It plays a role in the creation of DNA and the synthesis of proteins from amino acids. It is important in wound healing and functions in moving vitamin A from liver stores.

Zinc supplements are used to prevent zinc deficiency and to treat delayed wound healing. Some evidence supports the use of zinc OTC products to reduce the severity of symptoms of the common cold.

Patients who are taking zinc may report abnormalities of taste and smell, rough skin, and anorexia with profound disinterest in food. Patients who lack zinc may demonstrate sexual immaturity, delayed wound healing, and decreased absorption of dietary folate.

Adverse reactions to zinc supplements include gastric ulceration, nausea, and vomiting. Doses in excess of 2 g produce *emesis* (vomiting). Acute zinc intoxication produces drowsiness, lethargy, lightheadedness, staggering gait, restlessness, and vomiting leading to dehydration.

Calcium competes with zinc for absorption. Phytates form insoluble complexes with zinc and interfere with its absorption. Zinc impairs the absorption of tetracycline derivatives.

### ❖ Nursing Implications and Patient Teaching
Seafood and meats are rich sources of natural zinc. Cereals and legumes also have significant amounts of this mineral.

## Get Ready for the Next-Generation NCLEX® Examination!

### Key Points

- Patients think that herbal and OTC products are safe. Ask patients to bring all herbal products and OTC drugs with them to every appointment.
- Some OTC, herbal, and complementary therapy drugs can interact and interfere with a patient's prescribed therapy.
- St. John's wort, goldenseal, and ginseng are the top three herbal products that people take, and they have dangerous interactions with many prescribed drugs.
- Cannabis is metabolized by P-450 enzymes and can interact with many medications
- Almost all vitamins can be destroyed by air, light, and heat. Keep vitamins in a tightly capped bottle away from light and heat.
- Fat-soluble vitamins (ADEK), if not taken as prescribed or recommended, can have toxic effects called *hypervitaminosis*.
- If giving vitamin $B_1$ (thiamine) to alcoholics or thiamine-deficient persons, IV glucose must also be given to prevent Wernicke encephalopathy.
- Vitamin $B_{12}$ requires intrinsic factor to be absorbed. In pernicious anemia, give vitamin $B_{12}$ by nasal, sublingual, or IM routes.
- Use of vitamin K may decrease the effectiveness of oral anticoagulants.
- Vitamin D is essential for calcium absorption.
- A deficit or excess of potassium can lead to fatal cardiac dysrhythmias.

### Clinical Judgment and Next-Generation NCLEX® Examination-Style Questions

#### Case Study
John Clarke is a 66-year-old recently retired steelworker who is being seen with a lack of appetite, constipation, weakness, and fatigue. He is COVID-19 negative and, as far as he knows, has never had the virus. He is vaccinated with boosters. His daughter is very concerned about his mental state as he lives alone and does not eat well. She says he has been somewhat confused and agitated lately. His vital signs are stable, he has no known allergies, and he takes lisinopril 20 mg every day for hypertension. He says he drinks three beers at night and smokes weed occasionally. **Instructions: Highlight the findings that indicate Mr. Clarke may have a vitamin or mineral deficiency.**

1. **Which nursing actions are most helpful when determining nutritional status of a patient? Select all or any that apply.**

   1. Ask the patient to complete a diary of what he eats in a week.
   2. Calculate the patient's body mass index.
   3. Ask the patient about his hobbies.
   4. Ask the patient about any OTC medications he takes.
   5. Ask the patient about any ethnic/cultural/religious needs.
   6. Ask the patient about any changes in the taste of food.
   7. Ask the patient about his pain level.
   8. Inspect the patient's general appearance.
   9. Inspect the patient's lab work for abnormal findings.

2. **The dietician has seen the patient and reveals that his diet consists mostly of white bread and processed foods. He also admits to drinking half a liter of vodka with the three beers to which he originally admitted. Which conditions will the nurse be concerned about? Select all or any that apply.**

   1. Beriberi
   2. Scurvy
   3. Alcoholism
   4. Wernicke-Korsakoff syndrome
   5. Osteopenia
   6. Pernicious anemia
   7. Night blindness
   8. Stomatitis
   9. Hemolytic anemia

3. **Mr. Clarke's labs came back, and his thiamine level is very low. The healthcare provider has requested thiamine to be given intravenously. Which precautions will the nurse take before and during thiamine therapy?**

   1. Administer diphenhydramine before the thiamine to decrease allergic reaction.
   2. Administer glucose after thiamine to prevent worsening of Wernicke encephalopathy.
   3. Administer thiamine IV push rapidly.
   4. Administer glucose before thiamine to prevent worsening of Wernicke encephalopathy.

4. A 56-year-old patient is taking CBD every day for hip pain. Which prescription medications taken by the patient should the nurse be most concerned about?

   1. Warfarin
   2. Diphenhydramine
   3. Atorvastatin
   4. Naprosyn

5. A patient has been diagnosed with megaloblastic anemia. Which diet change by the patient may have precipitated the diagnosis?

   1. A keto diet
   2. A DASH diet
   3. A Mediterranean diet
   4. A vegetarian diet

6. The nurse is preparing to give medications. Which drug combinations will not interact with each other?

   1. Vitamin B12 and ibuprofen
   2. Niacin and aspirin
   3. Folate and methotrexate
   4. Vitamin C and magnesium

7. Instructions: Highlight the findings that indicate the child may have an iron deficiency.

   A 6-year-old child looks very pale, and his mother states he is tired all the time and doesn't want to play. Vital signs are stable. The family does not eat red meat, only white meat, vegetables, and fruit.

8. The nurse is preparing to give medications. Which drug combinations will interact with each other? **Select all or any that apply.**

   1. St. John's wort and fluoxetine
   2. Digoxin and goldenseal
   3. Gingko biloba and coumadin
   4. Valerian root and zolpidem
   5. Cannabis and alprazolam
   6. Oral contraceptives and vitamin A

9. A 66-year-old woman asks why she needs to take extra supplements of vitamin D during menopause. Which is the best response given by the nurse?

   1. Vitamin D prevents rickets.
   2. Vitamin D may help to reduce menopausal symptoms.
   3. Vitamin D will help increase osteopenia.
   4. Vitamin D may help depressive episodes.

## Next-Generation NCLEX® (NGN) Examination–Style Question

**History and Physical**
**2 Months Ago, 1000**

CC: "I would like to try a medication to boost my mood."
HPI: A 43-year-old female client presents to the primary care office and wishes to discuss medication to help with depression. Client reports "feeling down, sad, and fatigued over the last few months." The client denies suicidal ideations. The client states, "Ever since my divorce 6 months ago, I just haven't felt like myself."
Past Medical History: diabetes, gout
Current Medications: metformin 500 mg orally twice daily

**Today, 0800**

"I'm feeling much better. My mood is better, and my sleeping is better. I started taking a few over-the-counter medications to help with my medical problems also."
Past Medical History: depression, diabetes, hypertension, gout
Current Medications: metformin 1000 mg orally twice daily, lisinopril 20 mg orally daily, sertraline 50 mg orally daily, St. John's wort 375 mg orally daily, vitamin D 5,000 IU orally daily, niacin 500 mg orally daily, folic acid 5 mg orally daily, vitamin C 500 mg orally daily

**Laboratory Results**
**2 Months Ago, 1000**

| TEST/PANEL | RESULT | NORMAL |
|---|---|---|
| Hemoglobin A1c | 8.6% | 4%–5.9% |

**Flow Sheet**
**2 Months Ago, 1000**

Blood Pressure: 158/90 mm Hg

Heart Rate: 70/min
Respiratory Rate: 18/min
Temperature: 98.6°F (37°C)

**Today, 0800**

Blood Pressure: 138/80 mm Hg
Heart Rate: 68/min
Respiratory Rate: 18/min
Temperature: 98.6°F (37°C)

**Orders**
**2 Months Ago, 1000**

Start sertraline 50 mg orally daily
Start lisinopril 20 mg orally daily
Increase metformin to 1000 mg orally twice daily
   A nurse is caring for a client in the outpatient primary care provider's office.

**Choose the most likely options for the information missing from the statement(s) by selecting from the lists of options provided.**

The nurse should educate the client that the over-the-counter medication ____1____ may ____2____.

| OPTIONS FOR 1 | OPTIONS FOR 2 |
|---|---|
| vitamin D | interact with sertraline |
| niacin | cause glossitis |
| folic Acid | cause fetal abnormalities if the client becomes pregnant |
| St. John's Wort | interact with lisinopril |
| vitamin C | contribute to hypoglycemia |

See answer on Evolve at http://evolve.elsevier.com/Visovsky/LPNpharmacology/.

# Answers to Clinical Judgment Questions

## CHAPTER 1

| | |
|---|---|
| 1. **Answer:** 2 | 6. **Answer:** 1 |
| 2. **Answer:** 2, 3, 6, 7 | 7. **Answer:** 3 |
| 3. **Answer:** 1, 2, 4, 5, 6 | 8. **Answer:** 1 |
| 4. **Answer:** 2 | 9. **Answer:** 4 |
| 5. **Answer:** 2 | 10. **Answer:** |

| NURSING ACTIONS FOR DRUG ADMINISTRATION | ESSENTIAL | NON-ESSENTIAL | CONTRA-INDICATED |
|---|---|---|---|
| Assess the patient's mental status. | X | | |
| Use two patient identifiers before giving the drug. | X | | |
| Check the patient's blood sugar. | | X | |
| Lay the patient flat in bed. | | | X |
| Check the patient's blood pressure before administration of the drug. | X | | |
| Document that the drug has been given following administration. | X | | |
| Teach the patient that drugs for blood pressure may cause dizziness. | X | | |
| Get the patient up in the chair before giving her the medication. | | X | |

## CHAPTER 2

1. **Answer:** Option 1, In a double-locked cabinet; Option 2, Overseeing the use and recording of all opioids given; Option 3, Sign out all controlled drugs given during the shift.

2. **Answer:** 4, 5. Drug diversion is defined as the illegal transfer of regulated drugs (like narcotics) from the patient for whom it was prescribed, to another person, such as a nurse, for their own (or others') use. Drug diversion should also be suspected if patients continually report pain despite appropriate drug treatment, and if inaccurate narcotic counts are noted. While it is not acceptable for patients to bring or use home-based drugs in the hospital, it is not a sign of drug diversion by a staff member.

3. **Answer:** 2. A standing order indicates that the drug is to be given until discontinued or for a certain number of doses. Hospital or institutional policy usually dictates that most standing orders expire after a certain number of days. Number 1 is a single dose or one-time order; number 3 is an emergency order (stat); and number 4 is a prn order.

4. **Answer:** 2

5. **Answer:** 4

6. **Answer:** 1, 2, 3, 4, 6, 8, 9

7. **Answer:** 2

## CHAPTER 3

Ms. Dayan is a member of the Women's Professional Golf Association (PGA). She is being seen in the clinic today for a urinary tract infection (UTI). She has an allergy to penicillin. Her medications include a birth control pill every morning and an antidepressant (amitriptyline) every evening. The healthcare provider has prescribed the antibiotic cephalexin 250 mg every 6 hours for 7 days. Ms. Dayan tells the nurse she is worried she will forget to take the medication as her schedule is very busy and asks why she must take this drug every 6 hours instead of once a day.

1. **Answer:** 3. Drugs with a short half-life are dosed more frequently so therapeutic drug levels remain constant. Cephalexin is often prescribed for patients allergic to penicillin, and cephalexin can also be prescribed as 500 mg taken twice a day, but that does not answer the patient's question.

2. **Answer:** 4. Bone receives 5% to 10% of cardiac output, and the urinary system receives about 25% of cardiac output. Less blood to an area makes antibiotic penetration more difficult. For this reason, many antibiotics for bone infections are given for a longer period. Cephalexin has a low percentage of protein binding, but that does not increase the amount getting to the tissue. Antibiotics used for bone tissue do work differently, but that is not the patient's concern. Resistance to antibiotics is a problem for all infections, not just bones.

3. **Answer:** 1. The patient is allergic to penicillin, and the rash is the result of a hypersensitivity caused by an antibody response to the allergy. An allergy is not unusual when prescribing antibiotics from different classes when one class causes an allergic response. An idiosyncratic reaction is an unexpected response to a drug. A drug rash is not considered a simple side effect but rather an adverse side effect that implies a problem is developing. Generic drugs are manufactured identical to brand name drugs and are considered bioequivalent apart from some cardiac and antiseizure drugs.

4. **Answer:**

| OPTION 1 | OPTION 2 | OPTION 3 |
|---|---|---|
| Administered | Distributed | Elimination |
| Absorbed | Diffused | First Pass |
| Distributed | Metabolized | Biotransformation |

Once a drug is absorbed and distributed in the body, the body transforms the drug. This process is called *biotransformation.*

5. **Answer:** 2, 4, 5, 7, 8. Double vision, rash, wheezing, throat tightness, and heart palpitations are all serious effects that can occur after administration of a drug. Nausea, diarrhea, and headache are all side effects that occur after administration of any drug and are not considered serious or life threatening.

6. **Answer:** 3. Osmosis is the movement of water across a semipermeable membrane to maintain balanced sodium levels. Water filters across the cell membranes dilute the excess salt and excrete it with urine. Diffusion is the movement of molecules across a semipermeable membrane. Filtration is passage of a substance through a filter, and active transport requires energy to move solutes from an area of lesser to an area of greater concentration. A key point to remember about osmosis is that water goes to salt.

7. **Answer:** 2. Codeine is a prodrug and as such must be transformed and activated by enzymes in the liver before the drug can be used in the body. Liver cancer or cirrhosis diminishes the enzymes and makes prodrugs ineffective. Asian ethnicity, a past history of alcoholism, and a normal creatinine clearance level are not related to the use of prodrugs.

8. **Answer:** 1, 2, 4, 6, 7. Drugs are excreted mostly by the renal system, but drugs are also excreted to a lesser degree in the bile, gastrointestinal tract via feces, tears, lungs, saliva, and breast milk. Drug metabolites can be found in the skin, hair, and semen, but these are not areas of elimination.

9. **Answer:** 4. The rich blood vessels under the tongue rapidly absorb drugs that do not need to go through the first pass because they are directly absorbed into the bloodstream instead of going through the gastrointestinal tract first. The rate of absorption is rapid for drugs of all potencies. Side effects of sublingual drugs can still occur because the drugs are still absorbed into the body.

10. **Answer:** 1, 2, 3, 4, 7, 8. Before administration, the nurse should always review all medications patients are on in

case there is a contraindication to administering any of them together. Because this drug is being given for high blood pressure, it is important to make sure the blood pressure is within normal limits or there is a danger of lowering the blood pressure too much. A diuretic removes water from the body through urination, and after administration the patient will need to urinate often. Self-ambulation is important so the patient can walk to the bathroom without falling and without being incontinent. Because the diuretic causes water loss, it is important for the patient to have a normal fluid intake, or they can become dehydrated. Electrolytes are lost with the water and can cause heart dysrhythmias or seizures if not within normal limits, and therefore levels should be checked. Creatinine clearance rate should be checked to make sure that the renal system can excrete the metabolized drug. Arthritis and dementia are concerns for the patient at home, but this patient is being cared for in the nursing home and not giving her own meds.

## CHAPTER 4

1A. **Answer:** 2.5 mL according to the label directions

1B. **Answer:** 1.5 mL

2. **Answer:** 1

3. **Answer:** 1

4. **Answer:** 3

5. **Answer:** 4

6. **Answer:** 2

7. **Answer:** 1

8. **Answer:** 1, 3, 4

9. **Answer:** 2

10. **Answer:**

| NURSING ACTION | INDICATED | CONTRA-INDICATED | NON-ESSENTIAL |
|---|---|---|---|
| Change the IV tubing. | | | X |
| Lower the IV pole height. | | X | |
| Check the IV tubing for kinks. | X | | |
| Check the position of the needle. | X | | |
| Examine the IV site for infiltration. | X | | |
| Check the IV solution type. | | | X |
| Reposition the patient's wrist and elbow. | X | | |

Failure of an IV to infuse properly warrants the following nursing actions: Check for bent or kinked tubing, reposition the patient's wrist and elbow, check the needle position (it should be against a vein wall), the IV pole may be too low, or the needle may be out of the vein and infiltrated.

## CHAPTER 5

1. **Answer**: 4, The action of protein synthesis inhibitors like tetracycline is bacteriostatic. They do not kill the bacteria but rather interfere with the bacterial processes necessary to make proteins. If the bacteria cannot make proteins, the bacterial reproduction is reduced. Answers 1, 2, and 3, although true, do not clearly answer a 16-year-old patient's question on how tetracycline works.

2. **Answer**: Option 1, GI system; Option 2, Sunburn; Option 3, Skin

3. **Answer**: 1, 2, 3, 5, 6, 7, 9. Tetracycline is contraindicated in women who are pregnant and breast-feeding, and Jane should be on birth control while taking the drug. Yeast infections can occur, but only the healthcare provider can advise the patient about additional drug use. Tetracycline can cause a severe sunburn, so sunscreen should be used. Isotretinoin and acitretin are drugs used for acne that can raise intracranial pressure if taken with tetracycline. Antacids and dairy products can interfere with the absorption of tetracycline. Tetracycline should be taken on an empty stomach 1 hour before or 2 hours after eating. Topical retinol can be used but will increase the chances of sunburn if sunscreen is not used when outdoors.

4. **Answer 1**: 80 kg; **Answer 2**: 240 mg; **Answer 3**: 6 mL

5. **Answer**: 2. If more than 3 mL of a solution is required, the nurse must divide the total dose by 2 and give 2 injections in different sites. The dorsogluteal area is no longer used due to tissue damage to the nerves and blood vessels in that area.

6. **Answer**: 1, 2, 3, 4, 6, 9. Renal function and ototoxicity can occur with administration of aminoglycosides. Peak and trough levels of gentamicin must be monitored so the patient is not given a toxic dose of gentamicin. Ototoxicity is increased with the use aspirin, furosemide, and ethacrynic acid among other drugs, so the pharmacist or healthcare provider should be alerted. Chest pain and palpitations do occur after administration of macrolides. Fluids should be increased, if not contraindicated, to ensure a urine output of at least 1500 mL a day or 1–1.5 mL/kg. Gentamicin is irritating to the tissue and should always be given through the Z-track method.

7. **Answer**: 2, 3, 4, 5, 6, 7. Fluoroquinolones should be administered with food. Joint pain and disease can occur, so the drug should be stopped and the healthcare provider notified. Urine output should be at least 1500 mL a day to dilute the urine. Hyperglycemia or hypoglycemia can occur in diabetics while taking these drugs, so blood sugar levels should be checked more frequently. Lethal rhythms can occur if given to patients on antidysrhythmics, such as quinidine or amiodarone. These drugs should not be given with dairy products or enteral tube feedings. Stomatitis is a side effect of sulfonamides and not fluoroquinolones. Fluoroquinolones should not be given to children under 18 because they interfere with bone, muscle, and tendon growth.

8. **Answer**: 4. Fluconazole will rid the patient of a yeast infection, but she is asking how to prevent it. Over-the-counter Monistat cream will not prevent a yeast infection, and it is not within the LPN's scope of practice to recommend any medications. *Lactobacillus acidophilus* capsules will also prevent a yeast infection, but they are considered a medication. Greek yogurt contains *Lactobacillus acidophilus*, and it is within the LPN's scope of practice to recommend nutritional products.

9. **Answer**: 2, 3. Aminoglycosides are used for serious gram-negative bacteria. *Klebsiella* and *E. coli* are gram-negative bacteria. All the other bacteria mentioned are gram-positive bacteria.

10. **Answer**: 2, 4, 7, 9. Cephalosporins should never be given to a patient who has had an anaphylactic reaction to penicillin. Gentamicin is unrelated to penicillin and can be used for gram-negative bacteria. Erythromycin and clarithromycin are macrolides that are safe to use, and of the two, clarithromycin has a longer duration, less side effects, and is effective against bacteria that are sensitive to penicillin. Vancomycin is a narrow-spectrum antibiotic that is frequently used in place of penicillin. Penicillin, Augmentin, and amoxicillin are all penicillins.

## CHAPTER 6

1. **Answer**: 2
2. **Answer**: 2, 4, 5
3. **Answer**: 1
4. **Answer**: 3
5. **Answer**: 3
6. **Answer**: 1, 2, 5, 6
7. **Answer**: 3
8. **Answer**: 2
9. **Answer**: 3
10. **Answer**: 3

### Case Study
**Answer**:

| OPTIONS FOR 1 | OPTIONS FOR 2 | OPTIONS FOR 3 |
|---|---|---|
| Antibiotic treatment for pyelonephritis Moderate obesity Birth control pills Diabetes type 2 Wiping genital area from back to front when defecating | *E. coli* Candida Trichomoniasis Plasmodium | fluconazole 150 mg griseofulvin 300 mg metronidazole 500 mg iodoquinol 650 mg |

### Drug Calculation Review
1. **Answer**: 8 tablets
2. **Answer**: a. 637.5 mg, b. 1.8 mL

## CHAPTER 7

1. **Answer**: 3. The child should be placed on oxygen immediately before desaturation occurs. Acetaminophen can be given and a history can be taken after oxygenation has been stabilized.

2. **Answer**: 1. The albuterol should be initiated as soon as possible to assist with breathing. Lung infections in children cause inflammation in the airways. The airways in children are much smaller than those of an adult and can close off very quickly. An IV to rehydrate the child is most important, but airway and breathing remain the priority. Based on wheezing and nasal flaring, he is still facing issues with airway and breathing.

3. **Answer:** 1, 6. Ribavirin can cause anemia and worsening of infection because red blood cells and white blood cells are suppressed with this medication. The door to the room should be closed at all times so as not to contaminate the hallway. Patients with RSV should be placed on contact precautions with gloves and gown. A mask should always be worn during administration of the ribavirin. The mother should not be in the room while the ribavirin is being administered because she is pregnant and ribavirin is a highly teratogenic drug. Male nurses are also at risk for male-mediated teratogenicity, so if a male nurse is actively trying to get his partner pregnant, he should not be assigned to care for Nick. Ribavirin is excreted by the kidneys. Ribavirin is a prodrug that is minimally metabolized by the liver, so monitoring for liver dysfunction is not necessary.

4. **Answer:** 1, 2, 3, 4, 5, 7. BUN/Creatinine, WBC, RBC, and platelet count baseline must be taken before administration and for several days after administration of ganciclovir because it can cause severe anemia, nephrotoxicity, and bone marrow suppression. Higher-than-normal liver enzyme levels are common in a liver transplant and need to be followed, but ganciclovir does not affect liver function. The infusion nurse should be told that the patient is on TPN as it will interfere with the administration of ganciclovir. An allergy to acyclovir is a contraindication to the administration of ganciclovir. Ganciclovir has a black box warning for teratogenicity and mutagenicity. The patient should be counseled before administration that she should protect against pregnancy for at least 90 days after administration. Birth control pills will not interfere with administration.

5. **Answer:** 2, 3. Baloxavir must be given to children 12 and over; rimantadine and amantadine are no longer widely used for influenza because of increased resistance to influenza. Peramivir can be given intravenously to children age 6 years and older, but only for those who are unable to take oral oseltamivir.

6. **Answer:** 1-A, 2-C, 3-A, 4-F, 5-G, 6-D, 7-I, 8-J.

7A. **Answer:** 20 lb = 9.07 kg
15 mg × 9.07 kg = 136.5 mg to be given
100 mg/1mL = 136.5 mg/XmL
X = 1.356 mL
X = 1.4 mL to be administered IM

7B. **Answer:** 2. One mL of solution is the maximum amount to be injected into either the vastus lateralis or the ventrogluteal muscle of a child older than 7 months.

8. **Answer:** John H is an overweight 67-year-old Hispanic male who presents to the clinic with a fever of 101°F (38.3°C) and an oxygen saturation of 90% on room air. He has a cough productive of yellowish-green sputum. He is visibly short of breath and states he has body aches and fatigue. His medical history is positive for diabetes type 2 and rheumatoid arthritis.

   COVID-19 patients have a dry cough that is sometimes productive of clear sputum. Yellow-green sputum suggests a bacterial pneumonia.

9. **Answer:** 4. Emtricitabine/tenofovir alafenamide (Descovy) is a pre-exposure prophylactic drug (PrEP) taken once a day for as long as the patient is at risk for infection.

10. **Answer:** 4. Peginterferon alfa-2b can cause life-threatening neuropsychiatric events, so it is no longer used to treat hepatitis C.

11. **Answer:**

| OPTION 1 | OPTION 2 |
| --- | --- |
| Skin-to-skin contact | Remdesivir |
| Contaminated surface transmission | Nirmatrelvir, ritonavir |
| Droplet transmission | Emtricitabine, tenofovir, and efavirenz |
| Sexual transmission | Tipranavir |

| OPTION 3 | OPTION 4 |
| --- | --- |
| Phenytoin | Rheumatoid arthritis |
| Voriconazole | Asthma |
| Ritonavir | Stage 4 renal disease |
| Indinavir | Elevated liver enzymes |

## CHAPTER 8

1. **Answer:** 3. The nurse should first don PPE and then apply oxygen. The patient has symptoms of COVID-19, and until the antigen test is confirmed negative, the staff must wear full PPE and an N95 or higher mask. The patient has chest discomfort, so placing the patient on a cardiac monitor is warranted but not after safety and oxygenation needs are met. The patient is not unstable, so the rapid rescue team should not be called.

2. **Answer:** 1, 2, 3, 4, 6, 7, 8. CBC will reveal the patient's white blood count and differential (neutrophils, lymphocytes, monocytes, basophils, and eosinophils), which can indicate an infection. The patient has COVID-19–type symptoms, so an antigen test is warranted. The patient is on 28% oxygen now, so increasing the oxygen to 30% is warranted, and a venturi mask is indicated because of the patient's history of COPD. A nicotine patch will help ease the symptoms of nicotine withdrawal. Diphenhydramine should not be used in elderly patients. Formoterol nebulizer is a long-acting beta agonist (LABA) and will open the airways. A peak flow will determine how much air is flowing out of the lungs (expiration). A chest x-ray will reveal abnormalities in the lungs such as an infection. Azithromycin should not be ordered until a sputum specimen for culture and sensitivity is performed first.

3. **Answer:** 1, 3, 4, 5, 6. Pets, mold, cigarettes, and weight can all contribute to his asthma. Although his right-sided weakness from his stroke history cannot be changed, it can be assessed and adjusted. Occupational therapy can be consulted to improve the weakness and recommend arm splinting, which might make help Mr. Clarke better able to use the inhalers he needs to prevent asthma and COPD exacerbations.

4. **Answer:** 3. Tiotropium is a cholinergic antagonist that blocks the opposing action of acetylcholine of adrenaline in the body allowing for maximum bronchial dilation.

Pseudoephedrine is a decongestant; fexofenadine is an antihistamine and montelukast is a leukotriene inhibitor that will assist with exacerbations but do not cause direct bronchial dilation.

5. **Answer:** 2, 3, 4, 5, 6,7, 9 are all true. The patient should wait only 1 minute between puffs. A side effect of SABA is shaking, which is a side effect beta$_2$ stimulation. This side effect usually stops after continued use.

6. **Answer:** 6, 9, 1, 7, 4, 2, 5, 3, 8

7. **Answer:** 3. Grapefruit will minimize the amount of drug that is released into the bloodstream, decreasing its effectiveness. A nasal antihistamine should only be used for 3 to 5 days, and diphenhydramine should not be used for elderly patients. If fexofenadine no longer works, the patient should discontinue its use and try a different antihistamine. Grapefruit will minimize the amount of drug that is released into the bloodstream, decreasing its effectiveness.

8. **Answer:** 3. When using all three inhalers, the SABA should be used first because it will immediately open the airway to allow the LABA and the IC to penetrate the airway more effectively.

9. **Answer:** 3. Epinephrine should be administered first as it will open the airways. Oxygen can be administered second. Oxygen will not be able to reach the airways when bronchoconstriction occurs, so the constriction of the bronchus must be relieved first before oxygen. It will take 911 responders too long to get to the office. Diphenhydramine is usually administered after epinephrine but will be given intravenously for the fastest action.

10. **Answer:** 1,3,4,5,6. All are true, except clothes and bedding should be washed in hot water to get rid of dust mites.

## CHAPTER 9

1. **Answer:** 1, 5
2. **Answer:** 4
3. **Answer:** 1, 2, 3, 4
4. **Answer:** 3
5. **Answer:** 1
6. **Answer:** 1, 2, 3
7. **Answer:** 1
8. **Answer:** 1-C, 2-A, 3-D, 4-B, 5-A, 6-B
9. **Answer:** 4
10. **Answer:** 1-e, 2-c, 3-b, 4-a, 5-d

### Case Study

1. **Answer:** 2
2. **Answer:** Gout is an adverse effect associated with thiazide diuretics. The nurse would notify the healthcare provider to report the adverse effect.

### Drug Calculation Review

1. **Answer:** A, B, C, G
2. **Answer:** The nurse recognizes that amlodipine, a drug from the calcium channel blocker category, is the most likely cause of the increase in peripheral edema. Evaluation of Mr. Johnson's lab work reveals a decreased potassium level that is commonly associated with thiazide-like diuretics. Besides his high blood pressure, Mr. Johnson is showing symptoms associated with heart failure.

## CHAPTER 10

1. **Answer:**

| POTENTIAL PRESCRIPTION | ANTICIPATED | NON-ESSENTIAL | CONTRA-INDICATED |
|---|---|---|---|
| Carbidopa/levodopa | X | | |
| Tolcapone | X | | |
| Pimavanserin | | | X |
| Pramipexole | X | | |
| Tramadol | | | X |
| Selegiline | X | | |
| Phenylephrine | | | X |
| Amantadine | | X | |

Carbidopa/levodopa is essential for dopamine replacement. Tolcapone is a COMT inhibitor that suppresses the breakdown of dopamine and dopamine agonists to allow the blood levels of dopamine to remain high. Pramipexole is a dopamine agonist used in conjunction with carbidopa/levodopa. Selegiline is an MAO-B inhibitor that prevents the breakdown of neurotransmitters, including dopamine. Pimavanserin is contraindicated in elderly patients with dementia as it carries a risk of death. Tramadol has opiate activity, and therefore it is contraindicated with use of MAO-B inhibitors as it might initiate a hypertensive crisis. Phenylephrine is contraindicated because it is a sympathetic nervous system stimulant and can cause a hypertensive crisis. Amantadine is nonessential because it is used for worsening tremors which the patient is not experiencing.

2. **Answer:** 3. Tyramine-rich foods should be avoided when taking any MAO inhibitor because they can cause a severe hypertensive crisis. Raisins are a tyramine-rich food, as are cured or smoked meats (e.g., salami), fish (e.g., anchovies), cheeses, avocados, bananas, figs, beer, red wine, sauerkraut, sour cream, soy sauce and soy-containing foods (e.g., miso soup), and yeast extract found in some breads, canned foods, and snacks.

3. **Answer:** 4. Difficulty chewing can increase the risk of food getting stuck in the upper airway and causing choking and aspiration. Airway patency is always the first safety issue and takes precedence over fall or suicide risks.

4. **Answer:** 2. The wearing-off effect occurs when levodopa loses effectiveness. Levodopa's action peaks in 1 hour after administration and wears off in 4 to 5 hours.

5. **Answer:** 3. Phenytoin can cause gum hyperplasia. It is important for patients to practice good oral care. A rash can occur with phenytoin, but it could be a serious manifestation of Stevens-Johnson syndrome. Phenytoin is the one antiepileptic that does not cause drowsiness or dizziness.

**6. Answer:**

| OPTION 1 | OPTION 2 | OPTION 3 |
|---|---|---|
| Utilize an Alzheimer's Disease Assessment scale | Be placed on the back every day | Urinary retention |
| Obtain a 12-lead EKG | Be covered with plastic wrap when showering | Headaches |
| Obtain a chest x-ray | Be changed at the same time every 48 hours | Cough |
| Assess for swallowing problems | Be rotated to different sites on the arms and legs | BUN/creatinine levels |

An Alzheimer's Disease Assessment scale is evaluated before medication so that an objective evaluation can be made regarding any condition in improvement. The patch must be placed on the patient's back every 24 hours so it cannot be taken off easily. It can be used when showering without the need for a plastic covering. Cholinesterase inhibitors mimic the parasympathetic nervous system, which can cause increased secretions and a bronchospasm, so the nurse will monitor for shortness of breath, which is **most** important because the patient has a history of asthma. Coughing is an early sign of a bronchospasm. Urinary incontinence and headaches can occur, and abnormalities in the BUN/creatinine levels can affect drug levels.

**7. Answer:** 2. 1 hour before meals so the muscles will be strongest to assist swallowing and prevent aspiration.

**8. Answer:** 1, 2, 3, 4, 8 are all signs of infection. Monoclonal antibody uses in patients with MS inactivate and destroy lymphocytes (immune cells) that destroy the myelin. They increase the risk of infection by reducing immunity, and they can also trigger allergic reactions.

**9. Answer:** 4, 5, 6. Lennox-Gastaut syndrome is a severe form of epilepsy with many different types of seizures that begin in childhood. Treatment with multiple epileptics is warranted, but cannabidiol, rufinamide, and felbamate are the only adjuvant therapies that have shown the best efficacy in controlling the seizures.

**10. Answer:** 5, 7. Phenobarbital can cause both physical and psychological dependence. Lacosamide can cause psychological dependence due to the side effect of euphoria. Cannabidiol does not contain THC and, like the other antiepileptics, listed does not affect either physical or psychological dependence.

## CHAPTER 11

**1. Answer:** 3

**2. Answer:** 4

**3. Answer:** 4

**4. Answer:** 3

**5. Answer:** 1, 2, 6

**6. Answer:** 4

**7. Answer:** 4

**8. Answer:** The nurse teaches the patient to take the zolpidem immediately before bedtime and to take the paroxetine first thing in the morning.

### Unfolding Case Study for Discussion

**1. Answer:** Maintenance of safety within the environment is critical. Patients who experience symptoms of acute mania may engage in destructive behaviors to themselves and to others. Speaking in a non-threatening yet firm voice will be important in decreasing the chance of escalation. It will be important to administer medications as directed recognizing that onset of action varies according to the medication given.

**2. Answer:** The most common side effect associated with initial treatment with haloperidol is drowsiness. One adverse effect that may occur with higher doses of haloperidol is acute dystonia. Acute dystonia can occur within 24-96 hours after initiating therapy. Side effects associated with early lithium use include mild nausea, vomiting and diarrhea as well as mild dizziness and fatigue may occur early in therapy but typically subside over time. In addition, patients may experience mild hand tremor. If severe, report to the healthcare provider.

**3. Answer:** Symptoms of acute dystonia include spasm of neck muscles, difficulty swallowing or breathing, spasm of the eye muscles, and protrusion of the tongue. These are more likely in patients receiving higher doses and of younger age (especially younger males). If the patient experiences any of these symptoms, make sure to notify the healthcare provider immediately.

**4. Answer:** 1, 2, 4, 6, 7, 8, 9

### Drug Calculation Review

**1. Answer:** Four capsules

**2. Answer:** 0.5 mL

## CHAPTER 12

**1. Answer:** B, D, E. Morphine is a strong opioid agonist against which all other analgesics are compared. Fentanyl and hydromorphone are more powerful than morphine. Codeine, hydrocodone, and oxycodone are weaker opioid agonists.

**2. Answer:**

| ASSESSMENT FINDING | ADVERSE REACTIONS REQUIRING IMMEDIATE ATTENTION |
|---|---|
| Constipation | |
| Drowsiness | |
| Respiratory rate of 8 breaths/min | X |
| Blood pressure of 80/60 mm Hg | X |
| Decreased pupil size | X |
| Cool, clammy skin | |
| Temperature of 98.24°F (36.8°C) | |

Hypotension, decreased respirations with shallow breathing and cool, clammy skin are signs of opiate adverse effects or overdose. The remaining choices are expected side effects and not urgent.

3. **Answer:** 1

4. **Answer:** 3

5. **Answer:** 3

6. **Answer:** 3

7. **Answer:**

| NURSING ACTION | EFFECTIVE | INEFFECTIVE | UNRELATED |
|---|---|---|---|
| Assess the patient's extremities for fluid retention. | | | X |
| Assess the patient for seizures. | X | | |
| Assess skeletal muscle reactivity. | X | | |
| Assess the patient for visual changes. | | | X |
| Assess for understanding of patient teaching. | | X | |
| Assess the radial pulse. | X | | |
| Assess sense of touch. | | | X |

8. **Answer:** 1, 3, 6. A side effect of aspirin and many other NSAIDs is increased risk of bleeding that can present as bloody stools. If the bleeding continues, the patient may show signs of anemia such as fatigue and rapid heart rate.

9. **Answer:** 3

10. **Answer:** 3

**Drug Calculation Review**

1A. **Answer:** 0.8 mL

1B. **Answer:** 3.3 mL

2. **Answer:** 1.5 mL

**Case Study**

1. **Answer:** Acute pain

2. **Answer:** You can assess the patient's pain level by using a visual analog scale to determine the level of pain.

3. **Answer:** Vicodin (hydrocodone plus acetaminophen) is a Schedule II drug classified as an opioid narcotic medication.

4. **Answer:** The drug schedule can be altered (with approval by the healthcare provider) to provide the maximum dose of 2 tables administered 30 minutes prior to physical therapy so that he would have the effect of the drug during his exercise session and upon returning.

5. **Answer:** 1800 mg/day (300 mg × 6 (6 times per day) = 1800)

# CHAPTER 13

1. **Answer:**

| | |
|---|---|
| Skip all missed drug doses | |
| If it is close to the next time the drug is due, skip the missed dose. | X |
| All missed doses of the drug should be returned to the pharmacy. | |
| Never take a double dose of this drug. | X |
| If possible, take the missed dose within an hour of the scheduled time. | X |
| Once you miss a dose, you should double up on the drug dose at the next time it is due. | |

Never take a double dose of this drug. If a drug dose is missed, it may be taken within an hour of when it was scheduled. If the patient remembers the missed dose close to the time when the next dose is to be taken, he should take the regular dose and miss the skipped dose.

2. **Answer:** 3

3. **Answer:** 2

4. **Answer:** 1, 3, 4. Corticosteroids are very useful in managing chronic inflammation. They are very powerful in decreasing the production of all known mediators that trigger inflammation. Corticosteroids inhibit enzymes and proteins that start and continue the arachidonic acid production of inflammatory mediators. They also slow the production of white blood cells (WBCs) in the bone marrow. The actions of corticosteroids occur in all cells, not just those involved in inflammation. As a result, their therapeutic effects, side effects, and adverse effects are widespread.

5. **Answer:** 1

6. **Answer:**

| | |
|---|---|
| Ask whether the patient has received an immunization within the past month. | X |
| Instruct the patient to take the first dose at home right before bedtime. | |
| Instruct the patient to report the signs and symptoms of infection to the healthcare provider immediately. | X |
| Instruct the patient to avoid drinking cold or cool liquids. | |
| Instruct the patient to prevent sun exposure with hats, long sleeves, and sunscreen. | |
| Teach the patient the principles of self-injection. | X |
| Ask the patient if she has had shingles or hepatitis in the past. | X |
| Instruct the patient to eat a high purine diet. | |
| Instruct the patient to get tested for TB before starting a DMARD. | X |

DMARDs reduce immunity, and therefore immunizations containing live viruses are contraindicated, and signs and symptoms of infection should be reported immediately. Due to the risk for anaphylaxis, the first injected does is give by a physician or RN with appropriate emergency equipment on standby. There is no reason to avoid cool or cold liquids. Photosensitivity is not a side effect of DMARDs. DMARDs are given parenterally, and patients who are injecting themselves will need to be taught how to do so with a return demonstration.

Past viral infections (shingles, hepatitis) and TB infections can be reactivated by DMARDs, so the nurse must ask about these before the patient receives the first dose. The patient taking DMARDs is not prescribed a high purine diet.

7. **Answer:** 1
8. **Answer:** 2
9. **Answer:** 1
10. **Answer:** 3
11. **Answer:** 1.5 mL

## CHAPTER 14

1. **Answer:** 1
2. **Answer:** 3
3. **Answer:** 2
4. **Answer:** 1, 2, 3, 7
5. **Answer:** 1, 3, 4
6. **Answer:** 1, 2, 4, 5
7. **Answer:** 2
8. **Answer:** 2
9. **Answer:** 3
10. **Answer:** 1

### Drug Calculation Review

1. **Answer:** 2 tablets
2. **Answer:** 10 mL
3. **Answer:** 40 mL
4. **Answer:** 22.5 mL

### Case Study 1

Answer:
- Temperature = 98.6°F (37°C)
- Heart rate = 106 beats/min and regular
- Respirations = 22 breaths/min
- Blood pressure = 96/52 mm Hg
- Skin cool and moist to touch
- Reports feeling unusually tired today
- Oriented to person, place, and time
- States that her abdominal pain is currently a 7 (on a 0-to-10 pain intensity scale)

### Case Study 2

**Answer:** A, B, C, F

## CHAPTER 15

1. **Answer:** 3, 4, 7, 8, 11. The child has measles, which is a highly contagious disease that has recently resurged in the United States. According to the CDC, measles is spread through airborne contact, so the child must be isolated immediately and for 4 days after the appearance of the rash. Healthcare personnel who encounter the child should wear an N95 respirator. Vitamin A is administered to children with the measles because vitamin A deficiency is a risk factor for developing severe measles infections. Fluids should be increased to minimize fluid loss from fever. Aspirin should never be given to children with viral diseases. They could develop Reye's syndrome (swelling of the liver and brain). The infection control nurse should be contacted so postexposure prophylaxis can begin with the child's family and others who may have met the child. Most healthcare professionals have been vaccinated, but if they have not, they should have an MMR vaccination within 72 hours and intramuscular immune globulin as postexposure prophylaxis within 6 days.

2. **Answer:** 3, 4. Using the hospital's over-the-phone interpreting service is useful, but if the nurse needs to leave the room while she is taking care of an acutely ill child, it would not be feasible. However, newer hospital phone interpreters can use cell phones when a special number is reached, and that would be acceptable in this situation. iTranslate Medical is a translation app specifically designed to meet HIPAA standards on an iPhone and covers 42 languages. Other HIPAA-compliant apps are also available. Using a coworker on the other unit is not the best action as it would take the coworker off their unit and leave the unit short staffed and leave patients unattended. The brother might not translate the information correctly, and the nurse would not know. Removing the family from the scene is inappropriate and would create further harm, and a handout would not relay information that is happening in real time.

3. **Answer:** 3. Before notifying the healthcare provider, the nurse should observe the patient and perform a focused assessment on the lungs because the patient has developed a cough. Pneumonia is a common occurrence after measles and a common cause of death in children. The patient is not in acute distress, so the healthcare provider does not need to be notified immediately, and the nurse will be able to relay more pertinent information to the healthcare provider about the patient if the patient is observed and assessed before calling.

4. **Answer:** 1-(a,b); 2-(f); 3-(e); 4-(g); 5-(c,d); 6-(d)

5. **Answer:** 1, 2, 4, 5. It might be difficult for a 34-year-old to get copies of his vaccination from his primary care provider because of his age. Medical records are only kept for 7 years after the patient's last visit. The department of public health might have the records, but there isn't a national organization that keeps records. However, it is worth a call. Antibody titer levels can be drawn to see whether the patient's immunity is high for those diseases so that revaccination would not be necessary. It is acceptable for all vaccinations to be given at once. According to the CDC, there is no upper limit for the number of vaccines that can be administered during one visit. Vaccinations should not be deferred because multiple vaccines are needed. The patient does not need to take a leave of absence until all vaccines are given but should be advised that it takes a few weeks for immunity to develop.

6. **Answer:** 1. Ibuprofen and acetaminophen should not be taken with either calcineurin inhibitor because calcineurin inhibitor can cause significant kidney and liver toxicity. Ibuprofen is kidney toxic, and acetaminophen is liver toxic. The other drugs do not cause significant side effects when given together; however, all other drugs given in tandem with calcineurin inhibitors can cause inconsistent drug levels that can negatively affect transplanted tissues.

7. **Answer:** 4. The incident of an allergic reaction from the flu vaccine for people with egg allergies is very rare. However, for the 2022 flu season, an egg-free vaccine was available. It is called Flublok Quadrivalent. Advising the patient to wear a mask and wash hands frequently and asking the patient what kind of symptoms he gets from eating eggs are important as well but do not protect the patient from the flu. Documenting the patient's allergy to eggs should be done, but it is unclear whether he is allergic to the vaccine or just allergic to eggs. Follow-up on the symptoms of a vaccine reaction, if there was one, needs to be clear.

8. **Answer:** 5. Anyone allergic to a drug or cosmetic that contains PEG should NOT receive the mRNA COVID-19 vaccine.

9. **Answer:** 3. The patient might have an infection. If the patient is rejecting the kidney, the temperature will be over 100°F (32°C), and the patient would have flulike symptoms, such as chills, headache, nausea, vomiting. Tenderness or painful kidneys and swelling might also be present. If the kidneys are failing, the symptoms can include decreased urine, confusion, fatigue, and weakness. Tremor, restlessness, and diarrhea are side effects of cyclosporine.

10. **Answer:** 1, 2, 3, 4, 5, 6. Immunosuppressed people need to stay away from sickness and wash hands frequently because their immune defenses have been blunted. Immunocompromised conditions can lead to increased risk of skin and other tumors. Live virus vaccines should never be given to immunocompromised people. Fruits and vegetables can carry disease from people handling them and should be washed before eating. Yellowing of the eyes and skin is indicative of liver failure, an adverse effect of immunosuppressants.

## CHAPTER 16

1. **Answer:**

| | |
|---|---|
| Report signs of abnormal bleeding. | X |
| Increase your intake of green, leafy vegetables. | |
| You may continue all herbal supplements that you are currently taking. | |
| Avoid drinking alcohol. | X |
| Keep all laboratory testing appointments. | X |
| Continue warfarin when you have dental or surgical procedures to prevent clots. | |
| Use a soft toothbrush. | X |
| Avoid using electric razors. | |

2. **Answer:** 3

3. **Answer:** 4

4. **Answer:** 3

5. **Answer:**

| | |
|---|---|
| Acetylsalicylic acid | |
| Apixaban | X |
| Clopidogrel | |
| Dabigatran | X |
| Heparin | |
| Protamine sulfate | |
| Rivaroxaban | X |
| Warfarin | |

Apixaban, dabigatran, and rivaroxaban are agents considered to be direct thrombin inhibitors.

6. **Answer:** 1

7. **Answer:** 0.4

8. **Answer:** 3

## CHAPTER 17

1. **Answer:** 2, 4, 5, 6. Chemotherapy affects both normal cells and cancer cells, which explains why fast-growing cells, such as hair, and cells of the GI tract are affected. Since chemotherapy is toxic to the patient and nurse, the chemotherapy-certified RN must wear PPE when administering the chemotherapy, as must anyone coming in contact with the IV fluids containing chemotherapy. The severe toxicities that can occur with chemotherapy make these drugs high-alert drugs. Combination chemotherapy is used to kill more cancer cells throughout the cell cycle.

2. **Answer:** 1. The time period of 5 to 10 days following chemotherapy is known as the *nadir*—when the lowest blood cell counts, especially white blood cells, can be expected, making the patient vulnerable to infection.

3. **Answer:**

| NURSING ACTION | INDICATED | CONTRA-INDICATED | NON-ESSENTIAL |
|---|---|---|---|
| Check the patient for signs of hypersensitivity reaction. | X | | |
| Explain to the patient that a fluid restriction is needed for patients taking this drug. | | X | |
| Provide small snacks throughout the infusion period. | | | X |
| Check the patient's vital signs before, during, and after the infusion. | X | | |
| Assess the patient's IV site. | X | | |
| Instruct the patient to take antiemetics as soon as nausea begins. | | X | |
| Teach the patient that the urine color will be dark pink or red after the infusion. | | X | |

Cyclophosphamide can cause hypersensitivity reactions. This drug can also result in kidney damage, so fluids are encouraged, and the urine should NOT be pink or red, which can indicate hematuria. While small frequent snacks are not prohibited, they are not essential.

Patients should take antiemetics around the clock and not wait for nausea to begin, as then nausea and vomiting are much harder to control. Cyclophosphamide can cause hypotension, so vital signs should be monitored. This drug can cause irritation, so the IV site should be monitored for redness, swelling, or infiltration.

4. **Answer:** 2, 5, 6. Antimitotics can result in cardiovascular complications such as bradycardia, neutropenia, and peripheral neuropathy.

5. **Answer:** 3. While documentation of this side effect is needed, the best action is to reassure the patient that menopausal symptoms such as sweating and hot flashes are expected side effects of this therapy.

# CHAPTER 18

1. **Answer:** 2
2. **Answer:** 1
3. **Answer:**

- You may increase the dose of testosterone after 2 weeks if no effect is seen.
- You should report signs of fluid retention to your healthcare provider.
- You should avoid crowds because this drug decreases your immunity.
- You may experience enlargement of the breasts with this drug.
- Testosterone can increase the effects of the drugs you take for your diabetes.
- To enhance absorption, drink a warm fluid when taking the buccal form of this drug.
- The expected response to testosterone may not be seen for several months.
- Notify your healthcare provider if you experience a painful or prolonged erection.
- This drug can only be given by injection.
- You should report the presence of jaundice to your healthcare provider.

The dose of testosterone should not be increased without the specific instructions of the healthcare provider, as effects may not be seen until after 1 to 2 months. Fluid retention; painful, prolonged erections; jaundice; and male breast enlargement are adverse effects of testosterone, but a decrease in immunity is not expected.

Testosterone can increase the effects of antidiabetic agents and anticoagulants.

Before taking the buccal or sublingual form of the drug, refrain from eating or drinking until the drug is dissolved.

4. **Answer:** 1
5. **Answer:**

| OPTIONS FOR 1 | OPTIONS FOR 2 |
|---|---|
| Placing the gel only on the penis and scrotum | Allowing the gel to dry for 5 minutes before dressing |
| Applying the gel to the covered skin of the abdomen, shoulders, or upper arms | Using a sterile tongue blade to apply the gel |
| Applying the gel only before sexual intercourse | Covering the gel once applied with a sterile bandage |

# CHAPTER 19

1. **Answer:** 3
2. **Answer:** 1
3. **Answer:** 4
4. **Answer:** 1
5. **Answer:** 2
6. **Answer:** 3
7. **Answer:**

| | |
|---|---|
| "Adrenal hormones differ by age and gender." | |
| "Aldosterone controls sodium and water balance." | X |
| "Glucocorticoid hormones are necessary for life." | X |
| "The most common cause of adrenal gland hyperfunction is an adrenal gland tumor." | X |
| "Low levels of adrenal hormones can lead to stroke." | |
| "The adrenal cortex secretes aldosterone and cortisol." | X |
| "When adrenal hormones are overproduced, cancer can result." | |

The adrenal cortex secretes aldosterone and cortisol. Aldosterone controls sodium and water balance. Cortisol, of which there are many types, has many more functions that are essential for life. Cortisol helps maintain critical blood glucose levels, the stress response, excitability of cardiac muscle, immunity, and blood sodium levels. Since cortisol was first discovered to affect blood glucose levels, it is also known as a *glucocorticoid.*

8. **Answer:** A, D, F, G. Alendronate, ibandronate, risedronate, and zoledronic acid all belong to the bisphosphonate class of drug. Denosumab is a monoclonal antibody. Estrogen/bazedoxifene and raloxifene are from the estrogen agonist/antagonist class of drugs.

# CHAPTER 20

1. **Answer:**

| OPTIONS FOR 1 | OPTIONS FOR 2 |
|---|---|
| notify the pharmacy | shaking the insulin vial vigorously before drawing the drug up into the syringe |
| shake the vial to disperse the drug | assessing and rotating the injection sites |
| administer the insulin as scheduled | giving the insulin at a 45-degree angle |
| administer a rapid-acting insulin instead as they are interchangeable | giving the insulin at a cold temperature, directly from the refrigerator |
| **OPTIONS FOR 3** | **OPTIONS FOR 4** |
| massage the injection site to prevent bleeding | hyperglycemia |
| eat a meal within 15 minutes of receiving the injection to prevent hypoglycemia | hypoglycemia |
| recap the syringe before disposing of it in a sharps container | hypertension |
| check their blood sugar 1 hour after the injection | respiratory distress |

2. **Answer:** 3

3. **Answer:** 3

4. **Answer:**

| | |
|---|---|
| Take this drug daily with food. | |
| Weight loss and fatigue can occur when taking pramlintide. | X |
| If a dose is missed, double the next dose to be taken. | |
| Warm this drug to room temperature before injecting it. | |
| Check your blood glucose level regularly. | X |
| Avoid alcohol when taking this drug. | X |
| Pramlintide can result in excessive blood clotting. | |
| You can add your insulin to the same syringe with pramlintide. | |
| Dizziness can occur with pramlintide. | X |

5. **Answer:** 4. Oral contraceptives and antibiotics can interact with drugs for diabetes, reducing their effectiveness.

6. **Answer:** 2. Metformin should be stopped for 24 hours before and for 48 hours after a test that uses a radioactive dye to prevent kidney damage.

# CHAPTER 21

1. **Answer:** 1, 5, 6, 7. Smoking increases the risk for osteoporosis. Sedentary lifestyle increases risk, whereas a lifestyle with weight-bearing exercise, such as running, can reduce risk. Typically, lower weight and lower BMI are higher risks for osteoporosis. Estrogen replacement does not increase risk of osteoporosis, but high doses can be avoided in older women due to cardiovascular effects.

2. **Answer:** 1. Oral bisphosphonates must be taken on an empty stomach with only plain water (no juice or milk). It is important that all dentists are aware of the risk of osteonecrosis of the jaw. Patients must sit or stand at least 30 minutes after taking the drug to decrease the risk of esophageal erosion. It must be taken a minimum of 30 minutes before eating or drinking.

3. **Answer:** 2. Raloxifene is a selective estrogen receptor modulator. This drug has an increased risk of clotting and is contraindicated in patients with a history of blood clots.

4. **Answer:** 1, 2, 3, 5. Calcitonin can be irritating to the nostrils, so it is important to rotate every day. It is important to maintain adequate calcium and vitamin D. The nasal spray should be discarded after 30 days, if not empty. Oral bisphosphonates but not calcitonin require the patient to sit or stand after taking the drug.

5. **Answer:** 4. Each egg has about 27 mg of calcium; white toast (6 mg/slice) and coffee with cream have 21 mg. All other menu items provide more calcium.

6. **Answer:**

| OPTIONS FOR 1 | OPTIONS FOR 2 |
|---|---|
| Osteonecrosis of the jaw | Low blood calcium |
| Hypercalcemia | History of hip fracture |
| Esophageal necrosis | Intake of high calcium foods |
| Nausea and vomiting | History of dental problems |

Sclerostin inhibitors are associated with a risk of osteonecrosis of the jaw. This is more often associated with someone with dental problems or who has undergone dental surgery. Make sure patients taking these drugs are evaluated by their dentist.

7. **Answer:**

| OPTIONS FOR 1 | OPTIONS FOR 2 |
|---|---|
| Alendronate 10 mg orally once daily | Takes a 600 mg calcium vitamin D supplement daily |
| Raloxifene 60 mg once daily | Has a history of occasional constipation |
| Calcitonin 100 IU subcutaneously daily | Complains of difficulty swallowing |
| Romosozumab 210 mg subcutaneously once a month | Recently had a fractured forearm from a fall |

Patients taking oral bisphosphonates for osteoporosis must be able to sit or stand anywhere from 30 minutes to 2 hours (depending on the specific drug) and must be able to swallow the drug and at least a full glass of plain water.

8. **Answer:**

> - You will be able to give this drug at home every 6 months.
> - Make sure to let your dentist knows you are on this drug.
> - Schedule a dental exam at least every 2 years.
> - This drug helps to build bone.
> - This drug may increase your risk for infection.
> - Make sure to eat plenty of fruits and vegetables as this drug can cause constipation.
> - Some patients experience a flulike syndrome about 3 days after administration of denosumab. Notify your healthcare provider if you have fever, chills, or muscle and joint ache.
> - This drug can be given intranasally as a spray.
> - Make sure you include enough calcium and vitamin D in your diet.
> - Notify your provider if you have signs of low blood calcium such as fast heartbeat, muscle pain, or tingling or numbness in the hands or feet.

Denosumab needs to be given in a healthcare rather than home setting. Patients should notify their dentist and schedule a dental evaluation every 6 months because of the risk of osteonecrosis of the jaw. Denosumab decreases the breakdown of bone and increases the risk for infection, so patients should avoid conditions that increase risk. It can cause constipation, so patients should maintain a healthy diet, including plenty of fruits and vegetables. Patients can experience an acute-phase reaction about 3 days after administration, so they should notify their healthcare provider. Denosumab is available for subcutaneous use. Hypocalcemia is an adverse effect that can occur with denosumab.

9. **Answer:** Two tablets with each dose.

## Case Study

1. **Answer:**

   1. Does the patient have a normal swallowing reflex?
   2. Is the patient able to sit or stand (walking is fine) for at least 30 minutes to 1 hour after taking the bisphosphonate?
   3. Does the patient have any history of GI bleeding or esophageal reflux? This should be reported to the provider?
   4. Does the patient currently use aspirin or NSAIDs? These can increase the risk of esophageal adverse effects.

2. **Answer:** The Dietary Guidelines for Americans provides a number of excellent sources for calcium. Examples include low-fat or skim milk, yogurt, cheese, spinach, collard greens, sardines, and orange juice.

3. **Answer:** The Dietary Guidelines for Americans provides a number of excellent sources for vitamin D. Examples include salmon, tilapia, canned sardines, milk fortified with vitamin D, yogurt, cheese, fortified orange juice, and almond milk.

4. **Answer:** Include the following recommendations.

   1. Take your ibandronate with a full glass of plain water first thing in the morning before any food or any other medications. Do not eat or drink for at least 30 minutes after taking it. You should remain sitting or standing for at least 1 hour after taking ibandronate. Do not lie down.
   2. Avoid smoking.
   3. Eat a balanced diet with plenty of fruits and vegetables.
   4. Limit alcoholic beverages.
   5. Get at least 1200 mg calcium and 600 IU vitamin D daily.
   6. Include weight-bearing exercise in your weekly activity such as walking, running, low-impact aerobics, or gardening. Include balance and strengthening activities. Avoid high-impact exercises.

## CHAPTER 22

1. **Answer:** 1
2. **Answer:** 3, 4, 5
3. **Answer:** 1
4. **Answer:** 1, 2, 4
5. **Answer:** 1, 2, 4
6. **Answer:** 1
7. **Answer:** 4
8. **Answer:** 1, 3, 4
9. **Answer:** The drug will last 175 days.
10. **Answer:** 300 mg
11. **Answer:** 4
12. **Answer:** 4, 1, 5, 2, 3, 6

## Case Study 1

1. **Answer:** Risks include African Americans > 40 years, older age > 60 years, especially Mexican Americans with a family history of glaucoma and childhood eye trauma.

2. **Answer:** Prostaglandin agonists

3. **Answer:** The most common side effects are eye itching and redness, change in color of the iris over time, as well as thickening and lengthening of eye lashes.

4. **Answer:** Wash your hands before instilling eye drops. Tilt your head back, looking up at the ceiling. Using your nondominant hand, pull the lower eye lid towards your cheek, and using your dominant hand, place the appropriate amount of drops into the eye pocket. Close the eye gently (hold closed for 2 min) and gently wipe with a tissue.

5. **Answer:** Wash hands carefully every time you use eye makeup. Avoid using eye makeup after using it for 3 months as it can be a source of infection. Never share eye makeup with anyone, including friends and family. Contact an ophthalmologist before applying any eyelash extensions or false eyelashes.

6. **Answer:** Explain risk factors for glaucoma and that early and consistent treatment reduces risk of vision loss. Emphasize the importance of reaching out to her healthcare provider if she has any side effects that are bothersome.

7. **Answer:** National Eye Institute (https://nei.nih.gov); American Academy of Ophthalmology (https://www.aao.org/eye-health).

## Case Study 2

**Answer:** The nurse is working with a patient who was recently diagnosed with glaucoma. She has been prescribed latanoprost (Xalatan) 0.005% solution one drop in the right eye daily. When administering the latanoprost the nurse will check for any scratches or signs of trauma prior to administering, then will double-check that they have selected the correct solution concentration and administer one drop to the right eye. The nurse will teach the patient that eyelashes on the affected eye may become longer and thicker and that the eyelid may become darker.

Always check that there is no evidence of trauma to the eye prior to giving any prostaglandin agonist. Ensure that you are giving the correct solution concentration of all eye medications. The nurse will confirm the correct eye (the right eye in this case). Prostaglandin agonists can cause an increase in eyelash length in the affected eye and can make the iris and the eyelid darker. This change can be permanent.

## CHAPTER 23

1. **Answer:** John Clarke is a 66-year-old recently retired steelworker who is being seen with a lack of appetite, constipation, weakness, and fatigue. He is COVID-19 negative and, as far as he knows, has never had the virus. He is vaccinated with boosters. His daughter is very concerned about his mental state as he lives alone and does not eat well. She says he has been somewhat confused and agitated lately. His vital signs are stable, he has no known allergies, and he takes lisinopril 20 mg every day for hypertension. He says he drinks three beers at night and smokes weed occasionally.

2. **Answer:** 2, 5, 6, 7, 8, 9. A food diary is very cumbersome for a patient to complete, especially if he is weak, tired, and confused. A better way to find out the patient's food intake is to have him fill out a food frequency questionnaire or have a dietician evaluate his intake. A BMI must be completed because it is objective data regarding body fat. Hobbies the patient has and OTC drugs he takes are not likely to provide any information about nutritional status. Ethnic, cultural, and religious needs can affect nutritional status and should be asked about. Changes in the taste of food can affect appetite, as can any changes in dentition, which should also be asked about. Pain from indigestion, heartburn, and bloating affects nutritional status. General appearance of the skin, hair, and nails and abnormal findings on lab work all give clues about nutritional deficits.

3. **Answer:** 1, 3, 4. Beriberi affects the cardiovascular and central nervous system and is associated with thiamine ($B_1$) deficiency from the white bread and processed food diet. Meats and whole grains, beans, and peanuts are high in thiamine. Scurvy is associated with a deficiency of vitamin C. Alcoholism also leads to thiamine deficiency. Wernicke-Korsakoff syndrome is a brain disorder that occurs from a severe lack of thiamine. Osteopenia is associated with lack of vitamin D and calcium. Pernicious anemia occurs when vitamin $B_{12}$ is malabsorbed in the GI tract. Night blindness is associated with a vitamin A deficiency. Stomatitis occurs with a lack of niacin. Hemolytic anemia can occur if there is a deficiency of folic acid.

   Thiamine is administered before glucose to prevent worsening of Wernicke encephalopathy. Thiamine is necessary to metabolize glucose, and glucose prevents cell damage in the brain.

4. **Answer:** 1. CBD is an inhibitor of CYP34A and CYP2D6 and can increase levels of all those drugs except for naproxen (Naprosyn). CBD can increase warfarin levels, and as bleeding is a priority, the nurse should be most concerned about the effect of CBD on the patient's INR levels.

5. **Answer:** 4. The most common causes of megaloblastic, macrocytic anemia are deficiencies of vitamin $B_{12}$ or folate ($B_9$), which are obtained from red meat and vegetables.

6. **Answer:** 3. If folate is given with methotrexate, it can decrease the effectiveness of methotrexate, which is a chemotherapy drug used for cancer and some autoimmune diseases, such as rheumatoid arthritis. Niacin and aspirin are given together to decrease the flushing and itching that niacin supplementation can cause.

7. **Answer:** A 6-year-old child looks very pale, and his mother states that he is tired all the time and does not want to play. Vital signs are stable. The family does not eat red meat—only white meat, vegetables, and fruit.

   The diet should include red meat, dark green vegetables, and iron-fortified cereal.

8. **Answer:** All the listed herbs interact by either lowering or increasing the prescription drug.

9. **Answer:** 2. Vitamin D maintains bone health by absorbing calcium in menopause. It plays a role in reducing inflammation and might also help lower symptoms of mood irregularities and hot flashes in patients with menopause.

# Index

Page numbers followed by "*f*" indicate figures, "*t*" indicate tables, and "*b*" indicate boxes.